SINCE 1820

Founded in 1820, the **U.S.P. Convention** is responsible for establishing legally recognized drug quality standards in the United States—and for disseminating authoritative information for the use of medicines and related articles by health care professionals, patients and consumers. Over 1000 experts serve on USP Subcommittees and Advisory Panels and as *ad hoc* reviewers to ensure the accuracy and current relevance of USP standards and information.

THE

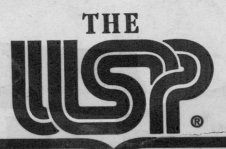

GUIDE TO
MEDICINES

FIRST EDITION

By authority of U. S. PHARMACOPEIA

AVON BOOKS ◆ NEW YORK

The information on page v constitutes an extension of this copyright page.

AVON BOOKS
A division of
The Hearst Corporation
1350 Avenue of the Americas
New York, New York 10019

Copyright © 1996 by The United States Pharmacopeial Convention, Inc.
Medicine chart insert copyright © 1996 by The United States Pharmacopeial Convention, Inc.
Published by arrangement with The United States Pharmacopeial Convention, Inc.
Visit our website at http://AvonBooks.com
Library of Congress Catalog Card Number: 95-94723
ISBN: 0-380-78092-5

First Avon Books Printing: February 1996

AVON TRADEMARK REG. U.S. PAT. OFF. AND IN OTHER COUNTRIES, MARCA REGISTRADA, HECHO EN U.S.A.

Printed in the U.S.A.

WCD   10   9   8   7   6   5   4   3

Contents

To the Reader   ix
  How to Use This Book   ix
  Notice   xi
  About USP   xii
  About *USP DI*   xiii

General Information About Use of Medicines   xv
  Before Using Your Medicine   xv
  Storage of Your Medicine   xvi
  Proper Use of Your Medicine   xvii
  Precautions While Using Your Medicine   xxiii
  Side Effects of Your Medicine   xxiv
  Additional Information   xxiv

Avoiding Medicine Mishaps   xxvi
  Tips Against Tampering   xxvi
  Unintentional Poisoning   xxix

Getting the Most Out of Your Medicines   xxxiv
  Communicating with Your Health Care
    Provider   xxxiv
  Your Health Care Team   xl
  Managing Your Medicines   xlix
  Taking Your Medicine   liii
  The "Expiration Date" on Medicine Labels   lvi

About the Medicines You Are Taking   lviii
  New Drugs—From Idea to Marketplace   lviii
  Drug Names   lxii
  Drug Quality   lxii
  Differences in Drug Products   lxiii

Drug Monographs   1

Medicine chart follows page 638

Glossary   1251

USP Division of Information
    Development Advisory Panels   1296

Index   1309

To the Reader

When purchasing a medicine, whether over-the-counter (non-prescription) or with a doctor's prescription, you may have questions about its usefulness to you, the best way to take it, possible side effects, and precautions to take to avoid complications. For instance, some medicines should be taken with meals, others between meals. Some may make you drowsy while others may tend to keep you awake. Alcoholic or other beverages, other medicines, certain foods, or smoking may affect the way your medicine works. As for side effects, some are merely bothersome and may go away while others may require medical attention.

The USP Guide to Medicines contains information which may provide general answers to some of your questions as well as suggestions for the correct use of your medicine. *It is important to remember, however, that the human body is very complex and medicines may act differently on different people—and even in the same person at different times. If you want additional information about your medicine or its possible side effects, ask your doctor, nurse, or pharmacist. They are there to help you.*

How to Use This Book

The USP Guide to Medicines contains a section of general information about the correct use of any medicine, as well as individual discussions of a wide variety of commonly and not so commonly used medicines. *You should read both the general information and the information specific to the medicine you are taking.*

Each medicine has a generic name that all manufacturers who make that medicine must use. Some manufacturers also create a brand name to put on the label and to use in advertising. *Look in the index* for the generic name or the brand name of the medicine about which you have questions. We have put the generic names and common brand names in the same index, so you do not have to know whether the name you have is a generic name or a brand name. However, it is a good idea for you to learn both the generic and the brand names of the medicines you are using and to write them down and keep them for future use.

Although the informational monographs generally appear in alphabetical order by generic name, there are numerous occasions when closely related medicines are grouped under a family name. Therefore, the surest way to quickly find the page number of the information about each medicine is to *look in the index first*.

The information for each medicine is presented according to the area of the body which is affected. As a general rule, information for one type of use will not be the same as for other types of use. For example, if you take tetracycline capsules by mouth for their systemic effect in treating an infection, the information will not be the same as for tetracycline ointment, which is applied directly to the skin for its topical effects. And both of these will be different from the information for tetracyclines used in the eye. The common divisions used in this publication are:

- *BUCCAL*—For general effects throughout the body when a medicine is placed in the cheek pocket and slowly absorbed.
- *DENTAL*—For local effects when applied to the teeth or gums.
- *INHALATION*—For local, and in some cases systemic, effects when inhaled into the lungs.
- *INTRA-AMNIOTIC*—For local effects when a medicine is injected into the sac that contains the fetus and amniotic fluid.
- *INTRACAVERNOSAL*—For local effects in the penis when a medicine is given by injection.
- *LINGUAL*—For general effects throughout the body when a medicine is absorbed through the lining of the mouth.
- *MUCOSAL*—For local effects when applied directly to mucous membranes (for example, the inside of the mouth).
- *NASAL*—For local effects when used in the nose.
- *OPHTHALMIC*—For local effects when applied directly to the eyes.

- *ORAL-LOCAL*—For local effects in the gastrointestinal tract when taken by mouth (i.e., not absorbed into the body).
- *OTIC*—For local effects when used in the ear.
- *PARENTERAL-LOCAL*—For local effects in a specific area of the body when given by injection.
- *RECTAL*—For local, and in some cases systemic, effects when used in the rectum.
- *SUBLINGUAL*—For general effects throughout the body when a medicine is placed under the tongue and slowly absorbed.
- *SYSTEMIC*—For general effects throughout the body; applies to most medicines when taken by mouth or given by injection.
- *TOPICAL*—For local effects when applied directly to the skin.
- *VAGINAL*—For local, and in some cases systemic, effects when used in the vagina.

Notice

The information about the drugs contained herein is general in nature and is intended to be used in consultation with your health care providers. It is not intended to replace specific instructions or directions or warnings given to you by your physician or other prescriber or accompanying a particular product. The information is selective and it is not claimed that it includes all known precautions, contraindications, effects, or interactions possibly related to the use of a drug. The information may differ from that contained in the product labeling which is required by law. The information is not sufficient to make an evaluation as to the risks and benefits of taking a particular drug in a particular case and is not medical advice for individual problems and should not alone be relied upon for these purposes. Since the inclusion or exclusion of particular information about a drug is judgmental in nature and since opinion as to drug usage may differ, you may wish to consult additional sources. Should you desire additional information or if you have any questions as to how this information may relate to you in particular, ask your doctor, nurse, pharmacist, or other health care professional.

Monographs for only the more commonly used medicines have been included in this volume.

Since new drugs are constantly being marketed and since previously unreported side effects, newly recognized precautions, or other new information for any given drug may come to light at any time, continuously updated drug information sources should be consulted as necessary.

There are many brands of drugs on the market. The listing of selected brand names is intended only for ease of reference. The inclusion of a brand name does not mean the USP has any particular knowledge that the brand listed has properties different from other brands of the same drug, nor should it be interpreted as an endorsement by the USP. Similarly, the fact that a brand name has not been included does not indicate that that particular brand has been judged to be unsatisfactory or unacceptable.

If any of the information in this book causes you special concern, do not decide against taking any medicine prescribed for you without first checking with your doctor.

About USP

The information in this volume is prepared by the United States Pharmacopeia (USP), the organization that sets the official standards of strength, quality, purity, packaging, and labeling for medical products used in the United States.

The United States Pharmacopeia is an independent, not-for-profit corporation composed of delegates from the accredited colleges of medicine and pharmacy in the U.S.; state medical and pharmaceutical associations; many national associations concerned with medicines, such as the American Medical Association, the American Nurses Association, the American Dental Association, the National Association of Retail Druggists, and the American Pharmaceutical Association; and various departments of the federal government, including the Food and Drug Administration. In addition, four members have been appointed by the Board of Trustees specifically to represent the public. USP was established 175 years ago, and is the only national body that represents the professions of both pharmacy and medicine.

The first convention came into being on January 1, 1820, and within the year published the first national drug formulary of the United States. The *U.S. Pharmacopeia* of 1820 contained 217 drug names, divided into two groups according to the level of general acceptance and usage.

When Congress passed the first major drug safety law in 1906, the standards recognized by that statute were those set forth in the *United States Pharmacopeia* and in the *National Formulary*. Today, the *USP* and *NF* continue to be the official U.S. compendia for standards for drugs and for the inactive ingredients in drug dosage forms. The *United States Pharmacopeia* is the world's oldest regularly revised national pharmacopeia and is generally accepted as being the most influential.

The work of the USP is carried out by the Committee of Revision. This committee of experts is elected by the members and currently consists of 114 outstanding physicians, pharmacists, dentists, nurses, chemists, microbiologists, and other individuals particularly qualified to judge the merits of drugs and the standards and information that should apply to them. Committee members serve without pay and are assisted by numerous advisory panels, other outside reviewers, and USP staff.

About *USP DI*

The USP Guide to Medicines contains information extracted from *Advice for the Patient* (Volume II of *USP DI*). Volume I contains drug use information in technical language for the physician, dentist, pharmacist, nurse, or other health care professional, and Volume II is its lay language counterpart for use by consumers. Volume III provides information on approved drug products and legal requirements. The monthly *USP DI Update* keeps all volumes up-to-date with selected new drug entries and related information. Together, the volumes form the foundation of a coordinated approach to drug-use education. Many health care professionals, institutions, and associations in the United States and Canada provide individual drug leaflets based on *Advice for the Patient*. Spanish translations for many medicines are also available.

USP DI was first published in 1980. It is continuously reviewed and revised and is intended for use by prescribers, dispensers, and consumers of medications. The information is developed by the consensus of the USP Committee of Revision and its Advisory Panels and anyone, including users of medicines, may contribute through review and comment on drafts of the monographs when they are published for comment in *USP DI Review*, a part of the monthly *USP DI Update*.

For further information about *USP DI* or to comment on how the information published in this volume might better meet your information needs, please contact:

USP Division of Information Development
12601 Twinbrook Parkway
Rockville, Maryland 20852
(301) 816-8351

GENERAL INFORMATION ABOUT USE OF MEDICINES

Information about the proper use of medicines is of two types. One type is drug specific and applies to a certain medicine or group of medicines only. The other type is general in nature and applies to the use of any medicine.

The information that follows is general in nature. For your own safety, health, and well-being, however, it is important that you learn about the proper use of your specific medicines as well. You can get this information from your health care professional, or find it in the individual listings of this book.

Before Using Your Medicine

Before you use any medicine, your health care professional should be told:

—if you have ever had an allergic or unusual reaction to any medicine, food, or other substance, such as yellow dye or sulfites.

—if you are on a low-salt, low-sugar, or any other special diet. Most medicines contain more than their active ingredient, and many liquid medicines contain alcohol.

—*if you are pregnant or if you plan to become pregnant.* Certain medicines may cause birth defects or other problems in the unborn child. For other medicines, safe use during pregnancy has not been established. *The use of any medicine during pregnancy must be carefully considered* and should be discussed with a health care professional.

—*if you are breast-feeding.* Some medicines may pass into the breast milk and cause unwanted effects in the baby.

—*if you are now taking or have taken any medicines or dietary supplements in the recent past.* Do not forget over-the-counter (nonprescription) medicines such as pain relievers, laxatives, and antacids or dietary supplements.

—*if you have any medical problems* other than the one(s) for which your medicine was prescribed.

—*if you have difficulty remembering things or reading labels.*

Storage of Your Medicine

It is important to store your medicines properly. Guidelines for proper storage include:

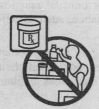

- *Keep out of the reach of children.*
- Keep medicines in their original containers.
- Store away from heat and direct light.

- Do not store capsules or tablets in the bathroom, near the kitchen sink, or in other damp places. Heat or moisture may cause the medicine to break down. Also, do not leave the cotton plug in a medicine container that has been opened, since it may draw moisture into the container.
- Keep liquid medicines from freezing.

- Do not store medicines in the refrigerator unless directed to do so.
- Do not leave your medicines in an automobile for long periods of time.
- Do not keep outdated medicine or medicine that is no longer needed. Be sure that any discarded medicine is out of the reach of children.

Proper Use of Your Medicine

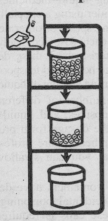

Take medicine only as directed, at the right time, and for the full length of your prescribed treatment. If you are using an over-the-counter (nonprescription) medicine, follow the directions on the label unless otherwise directed by your health care professional. If you feel that your medicine is not working for you, check with your health care professional.

Unless your pharmacist has packaged different medicines together in a "bubble-pack," different medicines should never be mixed in one container. It is best to keep your medicines tightly capped in their original containers when not in use. Do not remove the label, since directions for use and other important information may appear on it.

To avoid mistakes, do not take medicine in the dark. Always read the label before taking, especially noting the expiration date and any directions for use.

For oral (by mouth) medicines:

- In general, it is best to take oral medicines with a full glass of water. However, follow your health care

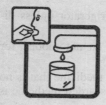

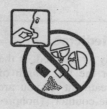

professional's directions. Some medicines should be taken with food, while others should be taken on an empty stomach.

- When taking most long-acting forms of a medicine, each dose should be swallowed whole. Do not break, crush, or chew before swallowing unless you have been specifically told that it is all right to do so.

- If you are taking liquid medicines, you should consider using a specially marked measuring spoon or other device to measure each dose accurately. Ask your pharmacist about these devices. The average household teaspoon may not hold the right amount of liquid.

- Oral medicine may come in a number of different dosage forms, such as tablets, capsules, and liquids. If you have trouble swallowing the dosage form prescribed for you, check with your health care professional. Another dosage form that you can swallow more easily may be available.

- Child-resistant caps on medicine containers have decreased greatly the number of accidental poisonings that occur each year. Use of these caps is required by law. However, if you find it hard to open such caps, you may ask your pharmacist for a regular, easier-to-open cap. He or she can provide you with a regular cap if you request it. However, you must make this request each time you get a prescription filled.

For skin patches:
- Apply the patch to a clean, dry skin area with little or no hair and free of scars, cuts, or irritation. Remove the previous patch before applying a new one.

- Apply a new patch if the first one becomes loose or falls off.

- Apply each patch to a different area of skin to prevent skin irritation or other problems.
- Do not try to trim or cut the adhesive patch to adjust the dosage. Check with your health care professional if you think the medicine is not working as it should.

For inhalers:

- Medicines that come in inhalers usually come with patient directions. *Read the directions carefully before using the medicine.* If you do not understand the directions, or if you are not sure how to use the inhaler, check with your health care professional.
- Since different types of inhalers may be used in different ways, it is very important to follow carefully the directions given to you.

For ophthalmic (eye) drops:

- To prevent contamination, do not let the tip of the eye drop applicator touch any surface (including the eye) and keep the container tightly closed.

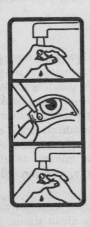

- The bottle may not be full; this is to provide proper drop control.
- How to apply: First, wash your hands. Tilt your head back and, with the index finger, pull the lower eyelid away from the eye to form a pouch. Drop the medicine into the pouch and gently close your eyes. Do not blink. Keep your eyes closed for one to two minutes.
- If your medicine is for glaucoma or inflammation of the eye: Follow the directions for application that are listed above. However, immediately after placing the drops in your eye, apply pressure to the in-

side corner of the eye with your middle finger. Continue to apply pressure for 1 to 2 minutes after the medicine has been placed in the eye. This will help prevent the medicine from being absorbed into the body and causing side effects.

- After applying the eye drops, wash your hands to remove any medicine.

For ophthalmic (eye) ointments:

- To prevent contamination of the eye ointment, do not let the tip of the applicator touch any surface (including the eye). After using, wipe the tip of the ointment tube with a clean tissue and keep the tube tightly closed.

- How to apply: First, wash your hands. Pull the lower eyelid away from the eye to form a pouch. Squeeze a thin strip of ointment into the pouch. A 1-cm (approximately ⅓-inch) strip of ointment is usually enough unless otherwise directed. Gently close your eyes and keep them closed for 1 to 2 minutes.

- After applying the eye ointment, wash your hands to remove any medicine.

For nasal (nose) drops:

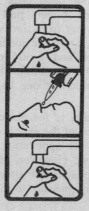

- How to use: Blow your nose gently, without squeezing. Tilt your head back while standing or sitting up, or lie down on your back on a bed and hang your head over the side. Place the drops into each nostril and keep your head tilted back for a few minutes to allow the medicine to spread throughout the nose.

- Rinse the dropper with hot water and dry with a clean tissue. Replace the cap right after use. To avoid the spread of infection, do not use the container for more than one person.

For nasal (nose) spray:

- How to use: Blow your nose gently, without squeezing. With your head upright, spray the medicine into each nostril. Sniff briskly while squeezing the bottle quickly and firmly.

- Rinse the tip of the spray bottle with hot water, taking care not to suck water into the bottle, and dry with a clean tissue. Replace the cap right after cleaning. To avoid the spread of infection, do not use the container for more than one person.

For otic (ear) drops:

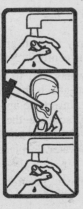

- To prevent contamination of the ear drops, do not touch the applicator tip to any surface (including the ear).

- The bottle may not be full; this is to provide proper drop control.

- How to apply: Lie down or tilt the head so that the ear that needs treatment faces up. For adults, gently pull the earlobe up and back to straighten the ear canal. (For children, gently pull the earlobe down and back.) Drop the medicine into the ear canal. Keep the ear facing up for about 5 minutes to allow the medicine to run to the bottom of the ear canal. (For young children and other patients who cannot stay still for 5 minutes, try to keep the ear facing up for at least 1 or 2 minutes.)

- Do not rinse the dropper after use. Wipe the tip of the dropper with a clean tissue and keep the container tightly closed.

For rectal suppositories:

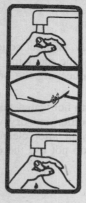

- How to insert suppository: First, wash your hands. Remove the foil wrapper and moisten the suppository with water. Lie down on your side. Push the suppository well up into the rectum with your finger. If the suppository is too soft to insert, chill it in the refrigerator for 30 minutes or run cold water over it before removing the foil wrapper.

- Wash your hands after you have inserted the suppository.

For rectal cream or ointment:

- Bathe and dry the rectal area. Apply a small amount of cream or ointment and rub it in gently.

- If your health care professional wants you to insert the medicine into the rectum: First, attach the plastic applicator tip onto the opened tube. Insert the applicator tip into the rectum and gently squeeze the tube to deliver the cream. Remove the applicator tip from the tube and wash with hot, soapy water. Replace the cap of the tube after use.

- Wash your hands after you have inserted the medicine.

For vaginal medicines:

- How to insert the medicine: First, wash your hands. Use the special applicator. Follow any special directions that are provided by the manufacturer. However, if you are pregnant, check with your health care professional before using the applicator to insert the medicine.

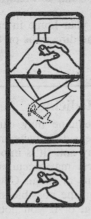

- Lie on your back, with your knees drawn up. Using the applicator, insert the medicine into the vagina as far as you can without using force or causing discomfort. Release the medicine by pushing on the plunger. Wait several minutes before getting up.
- Wash the applicator and your hands with soap and warm water.

Precautions While Using Your Medicine

Never give your medicine to anyone else. It has been prescribed for your personal medical problem and may not be the correct treatment for or may even be harmful to another person.

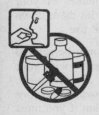

Many medicines should not be taken with other medicines or with alcoholic beverages. Follow your health care professional's directions to help avoid problems.

Before having any kind of surgery (including dental surgery) or emergency treatment, tell the physician or dentist about any medicine you are taking.

If you think you have taken an overdose of any medicine or if a child has taken a medicine by accident: Call your poison control center or your health care professional at once. Keep those telephone numbers handy. Also, keep a bottle of Ipecac Syrup safely stored in your home in case you are told to cause vomiting. Read the directions on the label of Ipecac Syrup before using.

Side Effects of Your Medicine

Along with its intended effects, a medicine may cause some unwanted effects. Some of these side effects may need medical attention, while others may not. It is important for you to know what side effects may occur and what you should do if you notice signs of them. Check with your health care professional about the possible side effects of the medicines you are taking, or if you notice any unusual reactions or side effects.

Additional Information

It is a good idea for you to learn both the generic and brand names of your medicine and even to write them down and keep them for future use.

Many prescriptions may not be refilled until your pharmacist checks with your health care professional. *To save time, do not wait until you have run out of medicine before requesting a refill.* This is especially important if you must take your medicine every day.

When traveling:

- Carry your medicine with you rather than putting it in your checked luggage. Checked luggage may get lost or misplaced or may be stored in very cold or very hot areas.
- Make sure a source of medicine is available where you are traveling, or take a large enough supply to

last during your visit. It is also a good idea to take a copy of your written prescription with you.

If you want more information about your medicines, ask your health care professional. *Do not be embarrassed to ask questions* about any medicine you are taking. To help you remember, it may be helpful to write down any questions and bring them with you on your next visit to your health care professional.

AVOIDING MEDICINE MISHAPS

Tips Against Tampering

Over-the-counter (OTC) or nonprescription medicines are now packaged so that it will be easier to notice signs of tampering. A tamper-evident package is required either to be unique so that it cannot be copied easily, or to have a barrier or indicator (that has an identifying characteristic, such as a pattern, picture, or logo) that will be easily noticed if it is broken. For two-piece, unsealed, hard gelatin capsules, two tamper-evident features are required. Improved packaging also includes the use of special wrappers, seals, or caps on the outer and/or inner containers, or sealing each dose in its own pouch.

Even with such packaging, however, no system is completely safe. It is important that you do your part by checking for signs of tampering whenever you buy or use a medicine.

The following information may help you detect possible signs of tampering.

Protecting yourself

General common sense suggestions include the following:

• When buying a drug product, *consider* the dosage form (for example, capsules, tablets, syrup), the type of packaging, and the tamper-evident features. Ask yourself: Would it be easy for someone to tamper with this product? Will I be able to determine whether or not this product has been tampered with?

• *Look very carefully* at the outer packaging of the drug product before you buy it. After you buy it, also check the inner packaging as soon as possible.

• If the medicine has a protective packaging feature, it should be described in the labeling. This description is required to be placed so that it will not be affected if the feature is broken or missing. If the feature is broken or missing, *do not buy or use* the product. If you have already purchased the product, return it to the store. Always be sure to tell someone in charge about any problems.

• *Do not take* medicines that show even the slightest signs of tampering or don't seem quite right.

• Never take medicines in the dark or in poor lighting. *Read* the label and check each dose of medicine before you take it.

What to look for

Packaging

• Are there breaks, cracks, or holes in the outer or inner wrapping or protective cover or seal?

• Does the outer or inner covering appear to have been disturbed, unwrapped, or replaced?

• Does a plastic or other shrink band (tight-fitting wrap) around the top of the bottle appear distorted or stretched, as though it had been rolled down and then put back into place? Is the band missing? Has the band been slit and retaped?

• Is the bottom of the container intact?

• Does the container appear to be too full or not full enough?

• Is the cap on tight?

• Are there bits of paper or glue stuck on the rim of the container that make it seem the container once had a bottle seal?

• Is the cotton plug or filler in the bottle torn, sticky, or stained, or does it appear to have been taken out and put back?

• Do eye drops have a protective seal? All eye drops must be sealed when they are made, in order to keep them germ-free. Do not use if there is any sign of a broken or removed seal.

• Check the bottom as well as the top of a tube. Is the tube properly sealed? Metal tubes crimped up from the bottom like a tube of toothpaste should be firmly sealed.

• Are the expiration date, lot number, and other information the same on both the container and its outer wrapping or box?

Liquids

• Is the medicine the usual color? Thickness?

• Is a normally clear liquid cloudy or colored?

• Are there particles (small pieces) in the bottom of the bottle or floating in the solution? For some liquids, called suspensions, floating particles are normal.

• Does the medicine have a strange or different taste or odor (for example, bleach, acid, gasoline-like, or other pungent or sharp odor)? Do not taste the medicine if it has a strange odor.

Tablets

• Do the tablets look different than they usually do? Do they have unusual spots or markings? If they normally are shiny and smooth, are some dull or rough? Is there anything unusual about the color?

• Are the tablets all the same size and thickness?

• If there is printing on the tablets, do they all have the same imprint? Is the imprint missing from any?

• Do the tablets have a strange or different odor or taste?

• Are any of the tablets broken?

Capsules

• Do the capsules look different than they usually do? Are any cracked or dented? Are they all the same size and color?

• Do they have their normal shiny appearance or are

some dull or have fingerprints on them as though they have been handled?

• Are the capsules all the same length?

• If there is printing on the capsules, do they all have the same imprint? Is the imprint missing from any? Do the imprints all line up the same way?

• Do the capsules have an unexpected or unusual odor or taste?

Tubes and jars (ointments, creams, pastes, etc.)

• Does the product or container look different than usual?

• Are ointments and creams smooth and non-gritty? Have they separated?

Be a wise consumer. Look for signs of tampering before you buy a medicine and again each time you take a dose. Also, pay attention to the daily news in order to learn about any reported tampering.

It is important to understand that a change in the appearance or condition of a product may not mean that the package has been tampered with. The manufacturer may have changed the color of a medicine or its packaging. Also, the product may be breaking down with age or it may have had rough or unusual handling in shipping. In addition, some minor product variations may be normal.

Whenever you suspect that something is unusual about a medicine or its packaging, take it to your pharmacist. He or she is familiar with most products and their packaging. If there are serious concerns or problems, your pharmacist should report it to the USP Practitioners' Reporting Network^{SM} (USP PRN) at 1-800-487-7776, or other appropriate authorities.

Unintentional Poisoning

According to information provided by the American Association of Poison Control Centers, nearly one million children 6 years of age and under were unintentionally poisoned in 1993; 27 children 6 years of age and younger died as a result of poisoning.

Adults also may be unintentionally poisoned. This happens most often through carelessness or lack of information. For example, the sleepy adult who takes a medicine in the dark and winds up getting the wrong one, or the adult who decides to take the medicine prescribed for a friend to treat "the same symptoms."

Drug poisoning from an unintentional overdose is one type of accidental poisoning that contributes to these figures. Other causes include household chemical poisoning from unintentional ingestion or contact, and inhaled poisoning— for example, carbon monoxide, usually from a car.

Children are ready victims

The natural curiosity of children makes them ready victims of poisoning. Children explore everywhere and investigate their environment. What they find frequently goes into their mouths. They do not understand danger and possibly cannot read warning labels.

Accidental poisoning from medicine is especially dangerous in small children because the strength of most medicines that may be ingested is often based on their use in adults. Even a small quantity of an adult dose can sometimes poison a child.

Preventing poisoning from medicines

• Store medicines out of the sight and reach of children, preferably in a locked cabinet—not in the bathroom medicine cabinet or in a food cabinet.

• If you have children living with you or only as occasional guests, you should have child-resistant caps on your medicine containers. These will help to ensure that an accidental poisoning does not occur in your home. Always store your medicines in a secure place.

- Adults who have difficulty opening child-resistant closures may request traditional, easy-to-open packaging for their medicines.

- Always replace lids and return medicines to their storage place after use, even if you will be using them again soon.

- If you are called to the telephone or to answer the door while you are taking medicine, take the container with you or put the medicine out of the reach of small children. Children act quickly—usually when no one is watching.

- Date medicines when purchased and clean out your medicines periodically. Discard prescription medicines that are past their expiration or "beyond use" date. As medicines grow old, the chemicals in them may change. In general, medicines that do not have an expiration date should not be kept for more than one year. Carefully discard any medicines so that children cannot get them. Rinse containers well before discarding in the trash.

- Take only those medicines prescribed for you and give medicines only to those for whom prescribed. A medicine that worked well for one person may harm another.

- It is best to keep all medicines in their original containers with their labels intact. The label contains valuable information for taking the medicine properly. Also, in case of accidental poisoning, it is important to know the ingredients in a drug product and any emergency instructions from the manufacturer. While prescription medicines usually do not list ingredients, information on the label makes it possible for your pharmacist to identify the contents.

- Ask your pharmacist to include on the label the number of tablets or capsules that he or she put in the container. In case of poisoning, it may be important to know roughly how many tablets or capsules were taken.

• Do not trust your memory—read the label before using the medicine, and take it as directed.

• If a medicine container has no label or the label has been defaced so that you are not absolutely sure what it says, do not use it.

• Turn on a light when taking or giving medicines at night or in a dark room.

• Label medicine containers with poison symbols, especially if you have children, individuals with poor vision, or other persons in your home who cannot read well.

• Teach children that medicine is not candy by calling each medicine by its proper name.

• Do not take medicines in front of children. They may wish to imitate you.

• Communicate these safety rules to any babysitters you have and remember them if you babysit or are visiting a house with children. Children are naturally curious and can get into a pocketbook, briefcase, or overnight bag that contains medicines.

What to do if a poisoning happens

Remember:

• There may be no immediate, significant symptoms or warning signs, particularly in a child.

• Nothing you can give will work equally well in all cases of poisoning. In fact, one "antidote" may counteract the effects of another.

• Many poisons act quickly, leaving little time for treatment.

Therefore:

• If you think someone has swallowed medicine or a household product, and the person is unconscious, having seizures (convulsions), or is not breathing, immediately call for an ambulance. Otherwise, do not wait to see what effect the poison will have or if symptoms of overdose develop; immediately call a Poison Control Center (listed in the white pages of your telephone book under ''Poison Control'' or inside the front cover with other emergency numbers). These numbers should be posted beside every telephone in the house, as should those of your pharmacist, the police, the fire department, and ambulance services. (Some poison control centers have TTY capability for the deaf. Check with your local center if you or someone in your family requires this service.)

• Have the container with you when you call so you can read the label on the product for ingredients.

• Describe what, when, and how much was taken and the age and condition of the person poisoned—for example, if the person is vomiting, choking, drowsy, shows a change in color or temperature of skin, is conscious or unconscious, or is convulsing.

• *Do not induce vomiting* unless instructed by medical personnel. *Do not induce vomiting or force liquids* into a person who is convulsing, unconscious, or very drowsy.

• Stay calm and in control of the situation.

Keep a bottle of Ipecac Syrup stored in a secure place in your home for emergency use. It is available at pharmacies in 1 ounce bottles without prescription. Ipecac Syrup is often recommended to induce vomiting in cases of poisoning.

Activated Charcoal is also sometimes recommended in certain types of poisoning and you may wish to add a supply to your emergency medicines. It is available without a prescription. Before using this medicine for poisoning, however, call a poison control center for advice.

GETTING THE MOST OUT OF YOUR MEDICINES

To get the most out of your medicines, there are certain things that you must do. Although your health care professionals will be working with you, you also have a responsibility for your own health.

Communicating with Your Health Care Provider

Communication between you and your health care professional is central to good medical care. Your health care professional needs to know about you, your medical history, and your current problems. In turn, you need to understand the recommendations he or she is making and what you will need to do to follow the treatment. You will have to ask questions—and answer some too. Communication is a two-way street.

Giving information

To provide effective care, your health care professional needs to know some details about your past and present medical history. In discussing these details, you should always be completely open and honest. Your health professional's diagnosis and treatment will be based in part on the information that you provide. A complete list of the details that should be included in a full medical history is provided below.

"Medical history" checklist

A "medical history" checklist covers the following information:

- All the serious illnesses you have ever had and the approximate dates.
- Your current symptoms, if any.

• **All** the medicines and dietary supplements you are taking or have taken in the recent past. This includes prescription and nonprescription medicines (such as pain relievers, antacids, laxatives, cold medicines, etc.) and home remedies. This is especially important if you are seeing more than one health care professional; if you are having surgery, including dental or emergency treatment; or if you get your medicines from more than one source.

• **Any** allergies or sensitivities to medicines, foods, or other substances.

• Your smoking, drinking, and exercise habits.

• Any recent changes in your lifestyle or personal habits. New job? Retired? Change of residence? Death in family? Married? Divorced? Other?

• Any special diet you are on—low-sugar, low-sodium, low-fat, or a diet to lose or gain weight.

• If you are pregnant, plan to become pregnant, or if you are breast-feeding.

• All the vaccinations and vaccination boosters you have had, with dates if possible.

• Any operations you have had, including dental and those performed on an outpatient basis, and any accidents that have required hospitalization.

• Illnesses or conditions that run in your family.

• Cause of death of closest relatives.

Remember, be sure to tell your health care professional at each visit if there have been any changes since your last visit.

Many health care professionals have a standard "medical history" form they will ask you to fill out when they see you for the first time. Some may ask the questions and write down the answers for you. If you will be visiting a health care professional for the first time, prepare yourself before you go by thinking about the questions that might be asked and jotting down the answers—including dates—so that you will not forget an important detail. Once your "medical history" is in the files, subsequent visits will take less time.

You will have to supply each health care provider you see—every time you see one—with complete information about what happened since your last visit. It is important that your records are updated so he or she can make sound recommendations for your continued treatment, or treatment of any new problems.

It will simplify things if you develop a "medical history" file at home for yourself and each family member for whom you are responsible. Setting up the file will take time. However, once it is established, you need only to keep it up-to-date and remember to take it with you when you see a health care professional. This will be easier than having to repeat the information each time and running the risk of confusing or forgetting details.

It is also a good idea to carry in your wallet a card that summarizes your chronic medical conditions, the medicines you are taking, and your allergies and drug sensitivities. You should keep this card as up-to-date as possible. Many pharmacists provide these cards as a service.

Getting information

For your health care professional to be able to serve you well, you must communicate all that you know about your present health condition at every visit. In order to benefit from the advice for which you have paid, your health care professional must communicate full instructions for your care. More importantly, you must understand completely everything that he or she tells you. Do not be embarrassed to ask questions, or to ask him or her to explain again any instruction or detail that you do not understand. Then it is up to you to carry out those instructions precisely. If there is a failure in any part of this system, you will pay an even higher price—physically and financially—for your health care.

Your health care professional may provide instructions to you in written form. If he or she does not, you may want to write them down or ask the health care professional to write them down for you. If you do not have time to jot down everything while you are still with your health care professional, sit down in the waiting room before you leave and write down the information while it is still fresh in your mind and you can still ask questions. If you have been given a prescription, ask for written information about the drug and how to take it. Your pharmacist can also answer questions when you have your prescription filled.

What you need to know about your medicines

There are a number of things that you should know about each medicine you are taking. These include:

- The medicine's generic and brand name.
- How it will help you and the expected results. How it makes you feel. How long it takes to begin working.
- How much to take at one time.
- How often to take the medicine.
- How long it will be necessary to take the medicine.
- When to take it. Before, during, after meals? At bedtime? At any other special times?
- How to take it. With water? With fruit juice? How much?
- What to do if you forget to take it (miss a dose).
- Foods, drinks, or other medicines that you should not take while taking the medicine.

xxxviii The USP Guide to Medicines

• Restrictions on activities while taking the medicine. May I drive a car or operate other motor vehicles?

• Possible side effects. What to do if they appear. How to minimize the side effects. How soon they will go away.

• When to seek help if there are problems.

• How long to wait before reporting no change in symptoms.

• How to store the medicine.

• The expiration date.

• The cost of the medicine.

• How to have your prescription refilled, if necessary.

Other information

Following are some other issues and information that you may want to consider:

• Ask your health care professional about the ingredients in the medicines (both prescription and over-the-counter [OTC]) you are taking and whether there may be a conflict with other medicines. Your health care professional can help you avoid dangerous combinations or drug products that contain ingredients to which you are allergic or sensitive.

• Ask your health care professional for help in developing a system for taking your medicines properly, particularly if you are taking a number of them on a daily basis. (When you are a patient in a hospital, ask for instructions before you are discharged.) Do not hesitate or be embarrassed to ask questions or ask for help.

• If you are over 60 years of age, ask your health care professional if the dose of the medicine prescribed is right for you. Some medicines should be given in lower doses to certain older individuals.

• If you are taking several different medicines, ask your health care professional if all of them are necessary for you. You should take only those medicines that you need.

• Medicines should be kept in the container they came in. If this is not possible when you are at work or away from home, ask your pharmacist to provide or recommend a container to transport your medicines safely. The use of "pill boxes" can also cause some problems, such as broken or chipped tablets, mistaking one medicine for another, and even interactions between the medicine and the metal of these boxes.

• Some people have trouble taking tablets or capsules. Your health care professional will know if another dosage form is available, and if tablets or capsule contents can be taken in a liquid. If this is an ongoing problem, ask your prescriber to write the prescription for the dosage form you can take most comfortably.

• Child-resistant caps are required by law on most prescription medicines for oral use to protect children from accidental poisoning. These containers are designed so that children will have difficulty opening them. Since many adults also find these containers hard to open, the law allows consumers to request traditional, easy-to-open packaging for their drugs. If you do not use child-resistant packaging, make sure that your medicines are stored where small children cannot see or reach them. If you use child-resistant containers, ask your pharmacist to show you how to open them.

Consumer education is one of the most important responsibilities of your health care professional. To supplement what you learn during your visit, ask if there is any written information about your medicines that you can take home with you. Your health care professional may also have available various reference books or

computerized drug information that you can consult for
details about precautions, side effects, and proper use
of your medicines.

Your Health Care Team

Your health care team will be made up of several
different health care professionals. Each of these individuals will play an important part in the overall provision
of your health care. It is important that you understand
the roles of each of these providers and what you
should be able to expect from each of them.

Your dentist

In addition to providing care and maintenance of your
mouth, teeth, and gums, your dentist is also an essential
member of your overall health care team since your
oral health and general health often affect one another.

In providing dental treatment, your dentist should base
his or her decisions upon an extensive knowledge of
your current condition and past medical and dental
history. Because the dentist is a prescriber of medications, it is very important that he or she is aware of
your full medical and dental history. A complete medical and dental history should include the information
that is listed in the ''Medical history checklist'' section
above. Even if you do not consider this information
important, you should inform your dentist as fully as
possible.

In the treatment of any dental/oral problem your dentist
should make every effort to inform you as fully as
possible about the nature of the problem. He or she
should explain why this problem has occurred, the ad-
vantages and disadvantages of available treatments (including no treatment), and what types of preventive

measures can be employed to avoid future problems. These measures may include periodic visits to the dentist, and a general awareness of the manner in which dental and overall health may affect one another. In any type of treatment, your dentist should always allow you to ask questions, and should be willing to answer them to your satisfaction.

In selecting a dentist, it is important to keep in mind the role of the dentist as a member of the health care team, and the extent of the information that he or she should be asking for and providing. There are also several practical issues that you should consider, such as:

- Is the dentist a specialist or general practitioner?
- What are the office hours?
- Is the dentist or his/her associates available after office hours by phone? In emergencies, will you be able to contact a dentist?
- What is the office policy on cancellations?
- What types of payment are accepted at the office?
- What is the office policy on x-ray procedures?
- Is the dentist willing to work with other medical and/or dental specialists that you may be seeing?

Your dentist should be an integral part of your health care team. In treating problems and providing general maintenance of your oral health, your dentist should base decisions upon a full dental and medical history. He or she should also be willing to answer any questions that you have regarding your oral health, any medications prescribed, and preventive measures to avoid future problems.

Your nurse

Depending upon the setting, type of therapy being administered, and state regulations, the role of the nurse in your health care team may vary. Registered nurses practice in diverse health care settings, such as hospitals, out-patient clinics or physicians' offices, schools, work-places, homes, and long-term care facilities like nursing homes and retirement centers. Some nurses, including certified nurse practitioners and midwives, hold a master's degree in nursing and may assume the role of primary health care professional, either in practice by themselves or in joint practices with physicians. In most states, nurse practitioners may prescribe selected medications. Clinical nurse specialists also have a master's degree in nursing and specialize in a particular area of health care. In some hospitals, long-term care facilities, and out-patient care settings, licensed practical nurses (LPNs) have certain responsibilities in administering medication to patients. LPNs usually work under the supervision of a RN or physician. Nursing aides assist RNs and LPNs with different kinds of patient care activities. In most places where people receive health care, RNs may be the primary source of information for drug therapies and other medical treatments. It is important that you be aware of the roles and responsibilities of the nurses participating in your health care.

Professional nurses participate with other health professionals, such as physicians and pharmacists, to ensure that your medication therapy is safe and effective and to monitor any effects (both desired and negative) from the medication. You may be admitted to the hospital so that nurses can administer medications and monitor your response to therapy. In hospitals or long-term care facilities, nurses are responsible for administering your medications in their proper dosage form and dose, and at correct time intervals, as well as monitoring your response to these medications. At home or in outpatient settings, nurses should ensure that you have the proper information and support of others, if needed, to get the medication and take it as prescribed. When nurses administer medication, they should explain why you are receiving this medication, how it works, any possible side effects, special precautions or actions that you must take while using the medication, and any potential interactions with other medications.

If you experience any side effects or symptoms from a medication, you should always tell your health care provider. It is important that these reactions be detected before they become serious or permanent. You can seek advice about possible ways to minimize these side effects from your nurse. Your health care professional should also be made aware of any additional medical problems or conditions (such as pregnancy) that you may have, since these can also affect the safety and effectiveness of a medication.

The professional nurse is someone who can help to clarify drug information. In most health care settings, nurses are accessible and can answer your questions or direct you to others who can assist you. Professional nurses are skilled in the process of patient teaching. To make sure that patients learn important information about their health problem and its treatment, RNs often use a combination of teaching methods, such as verbal instruction, written materials, demonstration, and audiovisual instructions. Above all, professional nurses should teach at a pace and level that are appropriate for you. RNs can also help you design a medication schedule that fits your lifestyle and may be less likely to cause unwanted side effects.

Your pharmacist

Your pharmacist is an important member of your health care team. In addition to performing traditional services, such as dispensing medications, your pharmacist can help you understand your medications and how to take them safely and effectively. By keeping accurate and up-to-date records and monitoring your use of medications, your pharmacist can help to protect you from improper medication therapy, unwanted side effects, and dangerous drug interactions. Because your pharmacist can play a vital role in protecting and improving your health, you should seek a pharmacist who will provide these services.

To provide you with the best possible care, your pharmacist should be informed about your current condition and medication history. Your personal medication history should include the information that is listed in the "Medical history checklist" section above. Your pharmacist should also be aware of any special packaging needs that you may have (such as child-resistant or easy-to-open containers). Your pharmacist should keep accurate and up-to-date records that contain this information. If you visit a new pharmacy that does not have access to your medication records, it is important that you inform that pharmacist as fully as possible about your medical history or provide him or her with a copy of your medication records from your previous pharmacy. In general, in order to get the most out of your pharmacy services, it is best to get all of your medications (including OTCs) from the same pharmacy.

Your pharmacist should be a knowledgeable and approachable source of information about your medications. Some of the information that your pharmacist should explain to you about your medications is listed in the "What you need to know about your medicines" section above. Ideally, this information should also be provided in written form, so that you may refer to it later if you have any questions or problems. The pharmacist should always be willing to answer any questions that you have regarding your medications, and should also be willing to contact your physician or other health care professionals (dentist, nurses, etc.) on your behalf if necessary.

Your pharmacist can also help you with information on the costs of your medicines. Many medicines are available from more than one company. They may have equal effects, but may have different costs. Your insurance company, HMO, or other third-party payment group may reimburse you for only some of these medications or only for part of their costs. Your pharmacist will be able to tell you which of these medications are covered by your payment plan or which cost less.

In selecting a pharmacist, it is important that you understand the role of the pharmacist as a member of your health care team and the extent of information that he or she should be asking for and providing. Because pharmacies can offer different types of services and have different policies regarding patient information, some of the issues that you should consider in selecting a pharmacist also relate to the pharmacy where that person practices. There are several issues regarding the pharmacist and pharmacy that you should consider, such as:

• Does the pharmacy offer written information that you can take home? Home delivery?

• Are you able to talk to your pharmacist without other people hearing you?

• Can the pharmacist be reached easily by phone? In an emergency, is a pharmacist available twenty-four hours (including weekends and holidays) by phone?

• What types of payment are accepted in the pharmacy?

• Does the pharmacy accept your HMO or third-party payment plan?

• Does the pharmacy offer any specialized services, such as diabetes education?

You should select your pharmacist and pharmacy as carefully as you select your physician, and stay with the same pharmacy so that all of your medication records are in the same place. This will help to ensure that your records are accurate and up-to-date and will allow you to develop a beneficial relationship with your pharmacist.

Your physician

One of the most important health care decisions that you will make is your choice of a personal physician. The physician is central to your health care team, and is responsible for helping you maintain your overall health. In addition to detecting and treating ailments or adverse conditions, your physician and his or her co-workers should also serve as primary sources of health care information. Because the physician plays such an important role in your overall health care, it is important that you understand the full range of the physician's role as health care and information provider.

In providing any type of treatment or counseling, your physician should base his or her decisions upon an extensive knowledge of your current condition and past medical history. A complete medical history should include the information that is listed in the "Medical history checklist" section above. Your physician should keep accurate and comprehensive medical records containing this information. Because your treatment (and your health) is dependent upon a full disclosure of your medical history, as well as any factors that may currently be affecting your health (i.e., stress, smoking, drug use, etc.), it is important that you inform your physician as fully as possible, even if you might not consider this information important.

It is important that you inform your personal physician of any other physicians (such as specialists or subspecialists), dentists, or other health care professionals that you are seeing. You should also inform your physician of the pharmacy that you use or intend to use, so that he or she can contact the pharmacist if necessary.

In treating any health problem, your physician should make every effort to help you understand completely the nature of the problem and its treatment. He or she should take the time to explain the problem, why it may have occurred, and what preventive measures (if any) can be taken to avoid it in the future. Your physician should explain fully the reasons for any prescribed treatment. He or she should also be willing to discuss alternative therapies, especially if you are uncomfortable with the one that has been prescribed. Your physician should always be willing to answer all of your questions to your satisfaction.

In selecting a physician, you should look for one who will provide a full range of services. Asking for a full medical history and providing complete information about your treatment and medications are some of these services. There are several other issues that you may want to consider. Does your physician:

- Consult peers with specialty training for difficult problems?
- Inquire about your general health as well as specific problems?
- Have a good working relationship with your pharmacist? With the nurses and staff at his/her office?
- Periodically have you bring in bottles or labels from all of the medications (prescription and nonprescription) that you are taking or have at home?
- Periodically check the status of your vaccinations?

You may also want to consider your physician's medical credentials. Your local medical society should be able to provide specific facts about your physician's training, experience, and membership in professional societies.

One of the most important issues in contemporary health care is that of cost and payment. Your physician should be sensitive to the costs of your treatment and the manner in which you intend to pay for this and related medications. If you belong to an HMO or third-party payment plan, be sure that your physician is aware of your involvement in the plan. You should also be aware of the different types of payment that are accepted at the physician's office.

In prescribing medications, your physician should take into account the manner in which you intend to pay for your drugs, and should be aware of any specific concerns regarding the costs of your treatment and medication. He or she should also explain why brand or generic medication may be preferable in certain situations.

In selecting a physician, there are also several practical issues and matters of convenience that you should consider, such as:

- Is the office convenient to your home or work?
- What are the office hours?
- Is your physician or his/her associates or partners available (twenty-four hours) by phone? In emergencies, will you be able to contact a physician?
- Are you able to arrange appointments to fit your schedule? What is the office policy on cancellations?
- Is the physician well regarded in the community? Does he or she have a reputation for listening to patients and answering questions?
- Does the physician have admitting privileges at a hospital of your preference?
- Does he/she participate in your health plan?

In addition to the considerations already mentioned, your physician should be sensitive to the special concerns of treating the elderly. Older patients can present disease processes differently from younger adults, can react differently to certain drugs and dosages, and may have preexisting conditions that require special treatments to be prescribed.

There are also several special issues to consider in your selection of a pediatrician or family physician. If your child is not old enough to understand all instructions and information, it is important that your child's physician explain to you any information pertaining to the nature of a problem and all instructions for medications. When your child is of school age, the physician should speak directly to the child as well, asking and answering questions, and providing information about cause and prevention of medical problems and the use of medications. He or she should choose a dosage form and dose that is appropriate for your child's age and explain what to do if your child has certain symptoms, such as fever, vomiting, etc. (including the amount and type of medicine to give, if any, and when to call him or her for advice).

Your physician should be a primary source of information about your health and any medications that you are taking. In providing treatment for medical problems or conditions, the physician should base decisions upon a full medical history and be willing to answer any questions that you have regarding your health, treatment, and medications.

Managing Your Medicines

To get the full benefit and reduce risks in taking your prescribed medicines, it is important to take the right medicine and dose at correct time intervals for the length of time prescribed. Bad effects can result from taking too much or too little of a medicine, or taking it too often or not often enough.

Establishing a system

Whether you are taking one or several medicines, you should develop a system for taking them. It can be just as difficult to remember whether you took your once-a-day medicine as it can be to keep track of a number of medicines that need to be taken several times a day. Many medicines also have special instructions that can further complicate proper use.

Establish a way of knowing whether you took your medicines properly, then make that a part of your daily routine. If you take one or two medicines a day, you may only need to take them at the same time that you perform some other regular task, such as brushing your teeth or getting dressed.

For most people, a check-off record can also be a handy way of managing multiple medicines. Keep your medicine record in a handy, visible place next to where you take your medicines. Check off each dose as you take it. If you miss a dose, make a note about what happened and what you did on the back of the record or the bottom of the sheet.

Be sure to note any unwanted effects or anything unusual that you think may be connected with your medicines. Also note if a medicine does not do what you expect. Remember that some medicines take a while before they start having a noticeable effect.

If you keep a check-off record faithfully, you will know for sure whether or not you took your medicine. You will also have a complete record for your health care professionals to review when you visit them again. This information can help them determine if the medicine is working properly or causing unwanted side effects, or whether adjustments should be made in your medicines and/or doses.

If your medicines or the instructions for taking them are changed, correct your record or make a new one. Keep the old record until you are sure you or your health care professionals no longer need that information.

You might want to color code your medicine containers to help tell them apart. If you are having trouble reading labels or if you are color-blind, codes that can be recognized by touch (rubber bands, a cotton ball, or a piece of emery board, for instance) can be attached to the container. If you code your medicines, be sure these identifications are included on any medicine record you use. If necessary, ask your pharmacist to type medicine labels in large letters for easier reading.

A check-off list is not the only method to record medicine use. If this system does not work for you, ask your health care professional to help you develop an alternative. Be sure he or she knows all the medicines prescribed for you and any nonprescription medicines you take regularly, the hours you usually eat your meals, and any special diet you are following.

Informed management

Your medicines have been prescribed for you and your condition. Ask your health care professional what benefits to expect, what side effects may occur, and when to report any side effects. If your symptoms go away, do not decide you are well and stop taking your medicine. If you stop too soon, the symptoms may come back. Finish all of the medicine if you have been told to do so. However, if you develop diarrhea or other unpleasant side effects, do not continue with the medicine just because you were told to finish it. Call your health care professional and report these effects. A change in dose or in the kind of medicine you are taking may be necessary.

When you are given a prescription for a medicine, ask the person who wrote it to explain it to you. For example, does "four times a day" mean one in the morning, one at noon, one in the evening, and one at bedtime; or does it mean every six hours around the clock? When a prescription says "take as needed," ask how close together the doses can be taken and what the maximum number of doses you can take in one day should be. Does "take with liquids" mean with water, milk, or something else? Are there some liquids that should avoided? What does "take with food" mean? At every meal time (some people must eat six meals a day), or with a snack? Do not trust your memory—have the instructions written down. To follow the instructions for taking your medicines, you must understand exactly what the prescriber wants you to do in order to "take as directed."

When the pharmacist dispenses your medicine, you have another opportunity to clarify information or to ask other questions. Before you leave, check the label on your medicine to be sure it matches the prescription and your understanding of what you are to do. If it does not, ask more questions.

The key to getting the most from your prescribed treatments is following instructions accurately and intelligently. If you have questions or doubts about the prescribed treatment, do not decide not to take the medicine or fail to follow the prescribed regimen. Discuss your questions and doubts with your health care professional.

The time and effort put into setting up a system to manage your medicines and establish a routine for taking them will pay off by relieving anxiety and helping you get the most from your prescribed treatment.

Taking Your Medicine

To take medicines safely and get the greatest benefit from them, it is important to establish regular habits so that you are less likely to make mistakes.

Before taking any medicine, read the label and any accompanying information. You can also consult books to learn more about the medicine. If you have unanswered questions, check with your health care professional.

The label on the container of a prescription medicine should bear your first and last name; the name of the prescriber; the pharmacy address and telephone number; the prescription number; the date of dispensing; and directions for use. Some states or provinces may have additional requirements. If the name of the drug product is not on the label, ask the pharmacist to include the brand (if any) and generic names. An expiration date may also appear. All of this information is important in identifying your medicines and using them properly. The labels on containers should never be removed and all medicines should be kept in their original containers.

Some tips for taking medicines safely and accurately include the following:

- Read the label of each medicine container three times:
  —before you remove it from its storage place,
  —before you take the lid off the container to remove the dose, and
  —before you replace the container in its storage place.

• Never take medicines in the dark, even if you think you know exactly where to find them.

• Use standard measuring devices to take your medicines (the household teaspoon, cup, or glass vary widely in the amount they hold). Ask your pharmacist for help with measuring.

• Set bottles and boxes of medicines on a clear area, well back from the edge of the surface to prevent containers and/or caps from being knocked to the floor.

• When pouring liquid medicines, pick up the container with the label against the palm of your hand to protect it from being stained by dripping medicine.

• Wipe off the top and neck of bottles of liquid medicines to keep labels from being obscured, and to make it less likely that the lid will stick.

• Shake all liquid suspensions of drug products before pouring so that ingredients are mixed thoroughly.

• If you are to take medicine with water, take a full, 8 ounce glassful, not just enough to get it down. Too little liquid with some medicines can prevent the medicine from working properly, and can cause throat irritation if the medicine does not get completely to the stomach.

• To avoid accidental confusion of lids, labels, and medicines, replace the lid on one container before opening another.

• When you are interrupted while taking your medicine, take the container with you or put the medicine up out of the reach of small children. It only takes a second for them to take an overdose. When you return, check the label of the medicine to be sure you have the right one before taking it.

• Only crush tablets or open capsules to take with food or beverages if your health care professional has told you that this will not affect the way the medicine works. If you have difficulty swallowing a tablet or capsule, check with your health care professional about the availability of a different dosage form.

• Follow any diet instructions or other treatment measures prescribed by your health care professional.

• If at any point you realize you have taken the wrong medicine or the wrong amount, call your health care professional immediately. In an emergency, call your local emergency number.

When you have finished taking your medicines, mark it down immediately on your medication calendar to avoid "double dosing." Also, make notes of any unusual changes in your body: change in weight, color or amount of urine, perspiration, or sputum; your pulse, temperature, or any other items you may have been instructed to observe for your condition or your medicine.

Try to take your medicines on time, but a half hour early or late will usually not upset your schedule. If you are more than several hours late and are getting close to your next scheduled dose, check any instructions that were given to you by your health care professional. If you did not receive instructions for what to do about a missed dose, check with your health care professional. You may also find missed dose information in the entries included in this book.

When your medicines are being managed by someone else (for example, when you are a patient in a hospital or nursing home), question what is happening to you and communicate what you know about your previous drug therapy or any other treatments. If you know you always take one, not two, of a certain tablet, say so and ask that your record be checked before you take the medicine. If you think you are receiving the wrong treatment or medication, do not hesitate to say so. You should always remain involved in your own therapy.

Many hospitals and nursing homes now offer counseling in medicine management as part of their discharge planning for patients. If you or a family member are getting ready to come home, ask your health care professional if you can be part of such instruction.

The "Expiration Date" on Medicine Labels

To assure that a drug product meets applicable standards of identity, strength, quality, and purity at the time of use, an "expiration date" is added by the manufacturer to the label of most prescription and nonprescription drug products.

The expiration date on a drug product is valid only as long as the product is stored in the original, unopened container under the storage conditions specified by the manufacturer. Among other things, drugs can be affected by humidity, temperature, light, and even air. A medicine taken after the expiration date may have changed in potency or may have formed harmful material as it deteriorates. In other instances, contamination with germs may have occurred. The safest rule is not to use any medicine beyond the expiration date.

Preventing deterioration

A drug begins to deteriorate the minute it is made. This rate of deterioration is factored in by the manufacturer in calculating the expiration date. Keeping the drug product in the container supplied by the pharmacist helps slow down deterioration. Storing the drug in the prescribed manner—for example, in a light-resistant container or in a cool, dry place (not the bathroom medicine cabinet)—also helps. The need for medicines to be kept in their containers and stored properly cannot be overstressed.

Patients sometimes ask their health care professionals to prescribe a large quantity of a particular medicine in order to "economize." Although this may be all right in some cases, this practice may backfire. If you have a large supply of your medicine and it deteriorates before you can use it all, or if your doctor changes your medicine, you may lose out.

Sometimes deterioration can be recognized by physical changes in the drug, such as a change in odor or appearance. For example, aspirin tablets develop a vinegar odor when they break down. These changes are not true of all drugs, however, and the absence of physical changes should not be assumed to mean that no deterioration has occurred.

Some liquid medicines mixed at the pharmacy will have a "beyond use" date on the label. This is an expiration date that is calculated from the date of preparation in the pharmacy. This is a definite date, after which you should discard any of the medicine that remains.

If your prescription medicines do not bear an "expiration" or "beyond use" date, your dispensing pharmacist is the best person to advise you about how long they can be safely utilized.

ABOUT THE MEDICINES
YOU ARE TAKING

New Drugs—From Idea to Marketplace

To be sold legitimately in the United States, new drugs must pass through a rigorous system of approval specified in the Food, Drug, and Cosmetic Act and supervised by the Food and Drug Administration (FDA). Except for certain drugs subject to other regulatory provisions, no new drug for human use may be marketed in this country unless FDA has approved a "New Drug Application" (NDA) for it.

The idea

The creation of a new drug usually starts with an idea. Most likely that idea results from the study of a disease or group of symptoms. Ideas can also come from observations of clinical research. This may involve many years of study, or the idea may occur from an accidental discovery in a research laboratory. Some may be coincidental discoveries, as in the case of penicillin.

Idea development takes place most often in the laboratory of a pharmaceutical company, but may also happen in laboratories at research institutions like the National Institutes of Health, at medical centers and universities, or in the laboratory of a chemical company.

Animal testing

The idea for a new drug is first tested on animals to help determine how toxic the substance may be. Most drugs interfere in some way with normal body functions. These animal studies are designed to discover the degree of that interference and the extent of the toxic effects.

After successful animal testing, perhaps over several years, the sponsors of the new drug apply to the FDA for an Investigational New Drug (IND) application. This status allows the drug to be tested in humans. As part of their request, the sponsoring manufacturer must submit the results of the animal studies, plus a detailed outline of the proposed human testing and information about the researchers that will be involved.

Human testing

Drug testing in humans usually consists of three consecutive phases. "Informed consent" must be secured from all volunteers participating in this testing.

Phase I testing is most often done on young, healthy adults. This testing is done on a relatively small number of subjects, generally between 20 and 80. Its purpose is to learn more about the biochemistry of the drug: how it acts on the body, and how the body reacts to it. The procedure differs for some drugs, however. For example, Phase I testing of drugs used to treat cancer involves actual patients with the disease from the beginning of testing.

During Phase II, small controlled clinical studies are designed to test the effectiveness and relative safety of the drug. These are done on closely monitored patients who have the disease for which the drug is being tested. Their numbers seldom go beyond 100 to 200 patients. Some volunteers for Phase II testing who have severely complicating conditions may be excluded.

A "control" group of people of comparable physical and disease types is used to do double-blind, controlled experiments for most drugs. These are conducted by medical investigators thoroughly familiar with the disease and this type of research. In a double-blind experiment, the patient, the health care provider, and other personnel do not know whether the patient is receiving the drug being tested, another active drug, or no medicine at all (a placebo or "sugar pill"). This helps eliminate bias and assures the accuracy of results. The findings of these tests are statistically analyzed to determine whether they are "significant" or due to chance alone.

Phase III consists of larger studies. This testing is performed after effectiveness of the drug has been established and is intended to gather additional evidence of effectiveness for specific uses of the drug. These studies also help discover adverse drug reactions that may occur with the drug. Phase III studies involve a few hundred to several thousand patients who have the disease the drug is intended to treat.

Patients with additional diseases or those receiving other therapy may be included in later Phase II and Phase III studies. They would be expected to be representative of certain segments of the population who would receive the drug following approval for marketing.

Final approval

When a sponsor believes the investigational studies on a drug have shown it to be safe and effective in treating specific conditions, a New Drug Application (NDA) is submitted to FDA. This application is accompanied by all the documentation from the company's research, including complete records of all the animal and human testing. This documentation can run to many thousands of pages.

The NDA application and its documentation must then be reviewed by FDA physicians, pharmacologists, chemists, statisticians, and other professionals experienced in evaluating new drugs. Proposed labeling information for the physician and pharmacist is also screened for accuracy, completeness, and conformity to FDA-approved wording.

Regulations call for the FDA to review an NDA within 180 days. This period may be extended and actually takes an average of 2 to 3 years. When all research phases are considered, the actual time it takes from idea to marketplace may be 8 to 10 years or even longer. However, for drugs representing major therapeutic advances, FDA may "fast-track" the approval process to try to get those drugs to patients who need them as soon as possible.

After approval

After a drug is marketed, the manufacturer must inform the FDA of any unexpected side effects or toxicity that comes to its attention. Consumers and health care professionals have an important role in helping to identify any previously unreported effects. If new evidence indicates that the drug may present an "imminent hazard," the FDA can withdraw approval for marketing or add new information to the drug's labeling at any time.

Generic drugs

After a new drug is approved for marketing, a patent will generally protect the financial interests of the drug's developer for a number of years. The traditional protection period is for 17 years. In reality, however, the period is much less due to the extended period of time needed to gain approval before marketing can begin. Recognizing that a considerable part of a drug's patent life may be tied up in the approval process, in 1984 Congress passed a law providing patent extension for drugs whose commercial sale may have been unduly delayed by the approval process.

Any manufacturer can apply for permission to produce and market a drug after the patent for the drug has expired. Following a procedure called an Abbreviated New Drug Application (ANDA), the applicant must show that its product is bioequivalent to the originator's product. Although the extensive clinical testing the originator had to complete during the drug's development does not have to be repeated, comparative testing between the products must be done to ensure that they will be therapeutically equivalent.

Drug Names

Every drug must have a nonproprietary name; a name that is available for each manufacturer to use. These names are commonly called generic names.

The FDA requires that the generic name of a drug product be placed on its labeling. However, manufacturers often coin brand (trade) names to use in promoting their products. In general, brand names are shorter, catchier, and easier to use than the corresponding generic name. The brand name manufacturer will then emphasize its brand name (which cannot be used by anyone else) in its advertising and other promotions. In many instances, the consumer may not recognize that a drug being sold under one particular brand name is indeed available under other brand names or by generic name. Ask your pharmacist if you have any questions about the names of your medicines.

Drug Quality

After an NDA or an ANDA has been approved for a product, the manufacturer must then meet all requirements relating to production. These include current Good Manufacturing Practice regulations of the Food and Drug Administration (FDA) and any applicable standards relating to strength, quality, purity, packaging, and labeling that are established by the *United States Pharmacopeia* (USP).

Simply placing a brand name on a label does not assure the quality of the product inside the container. Rather, the quality of a product depends on the manufacturer's ability to create a value product consistently from batch to batch.

Routine product testing by the manufacturer is required by the Good Manufacturing Practice regulations of the FDA (the FDA itself does not routinely test all products, except in cases where there is a suspicion that something might be wrong). In addition to governmental requirements, drug products must meet public standards of strength, quality, and purity that are published in the USP. In order to market their products, all manufacturers in the United States must meet USP-established standards unless they specifically choose not to meet the standards for a particular product. In this case, that product's label must state that it is ''not USP'' and how it differs from USP standards (this occurs very rarely).

Differences in Drug Products

Although standards to ensure strength, quality, purity, and bioequivalence exist for drug products, the standards allow for variations in certain factors that may produce other differences from product to product. These product variations may be important to some patients, since not all patients are ''equivalent.'' For example, the size, shape, and coating may vary and, therefore, be harder or easier for some patients to swallow; an oral liquid will taste good to some patients and awful to others; one manufacturer may use lactose as an inactive ingredient in its product while a therapeutically equivalent product may use some other inactive ingredient; one product may contain sugar or alcohol while another product may not.

In deciding to use one therapeutically equivalent product over another, consumers should keep the following in mind:

• Consider convenience factors of drug products (for example, ease of taking a particular dosage form).

• Don't overlook the convenience of the package. The package must protect the drug in accordance with USP requirements, but packages can be quite different in their ease of carrying, storing, opening, and measuring.

• If you have a known allergy or any type of dietary restriction, you need to be aware of the pharmaceutic or "inactive" ingredients that may be present in medicines you have to take. These inactive ingredients may vary from product to product.

• Price is always a consideration. The price difference between products (e.g., different brands, or brands versus generics) may be a major factor in the overall price of a prescription. Talk to your pharmacist about price considerations. Some states require that the pharmacist dispense exactly what is prescribed. However, other states allow the pharmacist to dispense less expensive medicines when appropriate.

Aside from differences in the drug product, there are many other factors that may influence the effectiveness of a medicine. For example, your diet, body chemistry, medical conditions, or other drugs you are taking may affect how much of a dose of a particular medicine gets into the body.

For the majority of drugs, slight differences in the amount of drug made available to the body will not make any therapeutic difference. For other drugs, the precise amount that gets into the body is more critical. For example, some heart or epilepsy medicines may create problems for the patient if the dose delivered to the body varies for some reason.

For those drugs that fall in the critical category, it is a good idea to stay on the specific product you started on. Changes should only be made after consultation with the health care professional who prescribed the medicine for you. If you feel that a certain batch of your medicine is more potent or does not work as well as other batches, or if you have other questions, check with your health care professional.

Drug
Monographs

Entries appear alphabetically by generic or "family" names (groupings of closely related medicines). To find the location of brand name entries, refer to the Index at the back of the book.

ACYCLOVIR Systemic

Some commonly used brand names are:

In the U.S.—
  Zovirax

In Canada—
  Avirax   Zovirax

Other commonly used names are aciclovir.

Description

Acyclovir (ay-SYE-kloe-veer) belongs to the family of medicines called antivirals, which are used to treat infections caused by viruses. Usually these medicines work for only one kind or group of virus infections.

Acyclovir is used to treat the symptoms of herpes virus infections of the genitals (sex organs), the skin, the brain, and mucous membranes (lips and mouth). Acyclovir is also used to treat chickenpox and shingles. Although acyclovir will not cure herpes, it does help relieve the pain and discomfort and helps the sores (if any) heal faster.

Acyclovir may also be used for other virus infections as determined by your doctor. However, it does not work in treating certain viruses, such as the common cold.

Acyclovir is available only with your doctor's prescription, in the following dosage forms:

Oral
  • Capsules (U.S. and Canada)
  • Oral suspension (U.S. and Canada)
  • Tablets (U.S. and Canada)

Parenteral
  • Injection (U.S. and Canada)

Before Using This Medicine

In deciding to use a medicine, the risks of taking the medicine must be weighed against the good it will do.

This is a decision you and your doctor will make. For acyclovir, the following should be considered:

Allergies—Tell your doctor if you have ever had any unusual or allergic reaction to acyclovir or ganciclovir. Also tell your health care professional if you are allergic to any other substances, such as foods, sulfites or other preservatives, or dyes.

Pregnancy—Acyclovir has been used in pregnant women and has not been reported to cause birth defects or other problems. However, studies have not been done in humans. Studies in rabbits have shown that acyclovir given by injection may keep the fetus from becoming attached to the lining of the uterus (womb). However, acyclovir has not been shown to cause birth defects or other problems in mice given many times the usual human dose, or in rats or rabbits given several times the usual human dose.

Breast-feeding—Acyclovir passes into the breast milk. However, it has not been reported to cause problems in nursing babies.

Children—A limited number of studies have been done using oral acyclovir in children, and it has not caused different effects or problems in children than it does in adults.

Older adults—Acyclovir has been used in the elderly and has not been shown to cause different side effects or problems in older people than it does in younger adults.

Other medicines—Although certain medicines should not be used together at all, in many cases two different medicines may be used together even if an interaction might occur. In these cases, changes in dose or other precautions may be necessary. If you are receiving acyclovir by injection it is especially important that your health care professional know if you are taking any of the following:

- Carmustine (e.g., BiCNU) or
- Cisplatin (e.g., Platinol) or
- Combination pain medicine containing acetaminophen and aspirin (e.g., Excedrin) or other salicylates or
- Cyclosporine (e.g., Sandimmune) or
- Deferoxamine (e.g., Desferal) (with long-term use) or
- Gold salts (medicine for arthritis) or
- Inflammation or pain medicine, except narcotics, or
- Lithium (e.g., Lithane) or
- Methotrexate (Mexate) or
- Other medicine for infection or
- Penicillamine (e.g., Cuprimine) or
- Plicamycin (e.g., Mithracin) or
- Streptozocin (e.g., Zanosar) or
- Tiopronin (Thiola)—Concurrent use of these medicines with acyclovir by injection may increase the chance for side effects, especially when kidney disease is present

Other medical problems—The presence of other medical problems may affect the use of acyclovir. Make sure you tell your doctor if you have any other medical problems, especially:

- Kidney disease—Kidney disease may increase blood levels of acyclovir, increasing the chance of side effects
- Nerve disease—Acyclovir by injection may increase the chance for nervous system side effects

---

Proper Use of This Medicine

Patient information about the treatment of herpes is available with this medicine. Read it carefully before using this medicine.

Acyclovir is best used as soon as possible after the symptoms of herpes infection (for example, pain, burning, blisters) begin to appear.

Acyclovir capsules, tablets, and oral suspension may be taken with meals.

If you are taking acyclovir for the *treatment of chickenpox*, it is best to start taking acyclovir as soon as possible after the first sign of the chickenpox rash, usually within one day.

If you are using *acyclovir oral suspension*, use a specially marked measuring spoon or other device to measure each dose accurately. The average household teaspoon may not hold the right amount of liquid.

Acyclovir is best taken with a full glass (8 ounces) of water.

To help clear up your herpes infection, *keep taking acyclovir for the full time of treatment,* even if your symptoms begin to clear up after a few days. *Do not miss any doses.* However, *do not use this medicine more often or for a longer time than your doctor ordered.*

Dosing—The dose of acyclovir will be different for different patients. *Follow your doctor's orders or the directions on the label.* The following information includes only the average doses of acyclovir. Your dose may be different if you have kidney disease. *If your dose is different, do not change it* unless your doctor tells you to do so.

The number of capsules or tablets or teaspoonfuls of suspension that you take depends on the strength of the medicine. Also, *the number of doses you take each day, the time allowed between doses, and the length of time you take the medicine depend on the medical problem for which you are taking acyclovir.*

- For *oral* dosage forms (capsules, oral suspension, or tablets):

  —For treatment of herpes of the genitals or mucous membranes, or for shingles:

    • Adults and children 12 years of age and older—200 to 800 milligrams (mg) two to five times a day for up to ten days.

- Children younger than 12 years of age—Use and dose must be determined by the doctor.

—For treatment of chickenpox:

- Adults and children 2 years of age and older—Dose is based on body weight. The usual dose is 20 mg per kilogram (kg) of body weight, up to 800 mg, four times a day for five days.

- Children younger than 2 years of age—Use and dose must be determined by the doctor.

- For *injection* dosage form:

—For treatment of herpes of the genitals or mucous membranes, or for shingles:

- Adults and children 12 years of age and older—Dose is based on body weight. The usual dose is 5 to 10 mg of acyclovir per kg (2.3 to 4.6 mg per pound) of body weight, injected slowly into a vein over at least a one-hour period, and repeated every eight hours for five to ten days.

- Children younger than 12 years of age—Dose is based on body weight or body size. The medicine is injected slowly into a vein over at least a one-hour period and repeated every eight hours for five to ten days.

Missed dose—If you do miss a dose of this medicine, take it as soon as possible. However, if it is almost time for your next dose, skip the missed dose and go back to your regular dosing schedule. Do not double doses.

Storage—To store this medicine:

- Keep out of the reach of children.
- Store away from heat and direct light.
- Do not store the capsule or tablet form of this medicine in the bathroom, near the kitchen sink, or in other damp places. Heat or moisture may cause the medicine to break down.

• Do not keep outdated medicine or medicine no longer needed. Be sure that any discarded medicine is out of the reach of children.

Precautions While Using This Medicine

Women with genital herpes may be more likely to get cancer of the cervix (entrance to the womb). Therefore, it is very important that a Pap test be taken at least once a year to check for cancer. Cervical cancer can be cured if found and treated early.

If your symptoms do not improve within a few days, or if they become worse, check with your doctor.

The areas affected by herpes should be kept as clean and dry as possible. Also, wear loose-fitting clothing to avoid irritating the sores (blisters).

It is important to remember that acyclovir will not keep you from spreading herpes to others.

Herpes infection of the genitals can be caught from or spread to your partner during any sexual activity. Even though you may get herpes if your partner has no symptoms, the infection is more likely to be spread if sores are present. This is true until the sores are completely healed and the scabs have fallen off. *Therefore, it is best to avoid any sexual activity if either you or your sexual partner has any symptoms of herpes.* The use of a latex condom ("rubber") may help prevent the spread of herpes. However, spermicidal (sperm-killing) jelly or a diaphragm will probably not help.

Side Effects of This Medicine

Along with its needed effects, a medicine may cause some unwanted effects. Although not all of these side effects

may occur, if they do occur they may need medical attention.

Check with your doctor immediately if any of the following side effects occur:

> *For acyclovir injection only*
>> *More common*
>>> Pain, swelling, or redness at place of injection
>>
>> *Less common (more common with rapid injection)*
>>> Abdominal or stomach pain; decreased frequency of urination or amount of urine; increased thirst; loss of appetite; nausea or vomiting; unusual tiredness or weakness
>>
>> *Rare*
>>> Confusion; convulsions (seizures); hallucinations (seeing, hearing, or feeling things that are not there); trembling

Other side effects may occur that usually do not need medical attention. These side effects may go away during treatment as your body adjusts to the medicine. However, check with your doctor if any of the following side effects continue or are bothersome:

> *For oral acyclovir only*
>> *Less common (especially seen with long-term use or high doses)*
>>> Diarrhea; headache; lightheadedness; nausea or vomiting

Other side effects not listed above may also occur in some patients. If you notice any other effects, check with your doctor.

Additional Information

Once a medicine has been approved for marketing for a certain use, experience may show that it is also useful for other medical problems. Although not specifically included in product labeling, acyclovir by injection is used in certain patients with the following medical conditions:

- Disseminated neonatal herpes simplex (widespread infection in the newborn)
- Herpes simplex (prevention of repeated infections)

Other than the above information, there is no additional information relating to proper use, precautions, or side effects for these uses.

ALLOPURINOL   Systemic

Some commonly used brand names are:

In the U.S.—
    Lopurin   Zyloprim
    Generic name product may also be available.

In Canada—
    Apo-Allopurinol   Zyloprim
    Purinol

Description

Allopurinol (al-oh-PURE-i-nole) is used to treat chronic gout (gouty arthritis). This condition is caused by too much uric acid in the blood.

This medicine works by causing less uric acid to be produced by the body. Allopurinol will not relieve a gout attack that has already started. Also, it does not cure gout, but it will help prevent gout attacks. However, it works only after you have been taking it regularly for a few months. Allopurinol will help prevent gout attacks only as long as you continue to take it.

Allopurinol is also used to prevent or treat other medical problems that may occur if too much uric acid is present in the body. These include certain kinds of kidney stones or other kidney problems.

Certain medicines or medical treatments can greatly increase the amount of uric acid in the body. This can cause gout or kidney problems in some people. Allopurinol is also used to prevent these problems.

Allopurinol is available only with your doctor's prescription in the following dosage form:

Oral
- Tablets (U.S. and Canada)

Before Using This Medicine

In deciding to use a medicine, the risks of taking the medicine must be weighed against the good it will do. This is a decision you and your doctor will make. For allopurinol, the following should be considered:

Allergies—Tell your doctor if you have ever had any unusual or allergic reaction to allopurinol. Also tell your health care professional if you are allergic to any other substances, such as foods, preservatives, or dyes.

Pregnancy—Although studies on birth defects have not been done in pregnant women, allopurinol has not been reported to cause problems in humans. In one study in mice, large amounts of allopurinol caused birth defects and other unwanted effects. However, allopurinol did not cause birth defects or other problems in rats or rabbits given doses up to 20 times the amount usually given to humans.

Breast-feeding—Allopurinol passes into the breast milk. Mothers who are taking this medicine and who wish to breast-feed should discuss this with their doctor.

Children—This medicine has been tested in children and, in effective doses, has not been shown to cause different side effects or problems than it does in adults.

Older adults—Many medicines have not been studied specifically in older people. Therefore, it may not be known whether they work exactly the same way they do in younger adults or if they cause different side effects or problems in older people. There is no specific information comparing use of allopurinol in the elderly with use in other age groups.

Other medicines—Although certain medicines should not be used together at all, in other cases two different medicines may be used together even if an interaction might occur. In these cases, your doctor may want to change the dose, or other precautions may be necessary. When you are taking allopurinol, it is especially important that your doctor and pharmacist know if you are taking any of the following:

- Anticoagulants (blood thinners)—Allopurinol may increase the chance of bleeding; changes in the dose of the anticoagulant may be needed, depending on blood test results
- Azathioprine (e.g., Imuran) or
- Mercaptopurine (e.g., Purinethol)—Allopurinol may cause higher blood levels of azathioprine or mercaptopurine, leading to an increased chance of serious side effects

Other medical problems—The presence of other medical problems may affect the use of allopurinol. Make sure you tell your doctor if you have any other medical problems, especially:

- Congestive heart disease or
- Diabetes mellitus (sugar diabetes) or
- High blood pressure or
- Kidney disease—There is an increased risk of severe allergic reactions or other serious effects; a change in the dose of allopurinol may be needed

Proper Use of This Medicine

If this medicine upsets your stomach, it may be taken after meals. If stomach upset (indigestion, nausea, vomiting, diarrhea, or stomach pain) continues, check with your doctor.

In order for this medicine to help you, it must be taken regularly as ordered by your doctor.

To help prevent kidney stones while taking allopurinol, adults should drink at least 10 to 12 full glasses (8 ounces each) of fluids each day unless otherwise directed by their doctor. Check with the doctor about the amount of fluids that children should drink each day while receiving this medicine. Also, your doctor may want you to take another medicine to make your urine less acid. It is important that you follow your doctor's instructions very carefully.

For patients taking allopurinol for *chronic gout:*

- After you begin to take allopurinol, gout attacks may continue to occur for a while. However, if you take this medicine regularly as directed by your doctor, the attacks will gradually become less frequent and less painful. After you have been taking allopurinol regularly for several months, the attacks may stop completely.

- Allopurinol is used to help prevent gout attacks. It will not relieve an attack that has already started. *Even if you take another medicine for gout attacks, continue to take this medicine also.*

Dosing—The dose of allopurinol will be different for different patients. *Follow your doctor's orders or the directions on the label.* The following information includes only the average doses of allopurinol. *If your dose is different, do not change it* unless your doctor tells you to do so.

The number of tablets that you take each day and the number of times that you take the medicine every day depend on the strength of the medicine, on the dose that you need, and on the reason you are taking allopurinol. Up to 300 milligrams (mg) of allopurinol can be taken at one time. Doses larger than 300 mg a day should be divided into smaller amounts that are taken two, three, or even four times a day.

- For the *oral* dosage form (tablets):
  —For gout:
  - Adults—At first, most people will take 100 mg a day. After about a week, your doctor will probably increase the dose gradually until the amount of uric acid in your blood has been lowered to normal levels. The total amount of allopurinol is usually not more than 800 mg a day. After the uric acid has remained at normal levels for a while, your doctor may lower your dose gradually until you are taking the smallest amount of medicine that will keep the uric acid from increasing again.
  - Children and teenagers—Use and dose must be determined by the doctor.
  —For kidney stones:
  - Adults—100 to 800 mg a day, depending on the kind of kidney stones.
  - Children and teenagers—Use and dose must be determined by the doctor.
  —For preventing or treating medical problems that may occur if certain treatments increase the amount of uric acid in the blood:
  - Adults—600 to 800 mg a day, starting one to three days before the treatment.
  - Children—The dose depends on the child's age.
    —Children up to 6 years of age: 50 mg (one-half of a 100-mg tablet) three times a day.
    —Children 6 to 10 years of age: One 100-mg

tablet three times a day or one 300-mg tablet a day.

—Children 11 years of age and older: The dose may be the same as for adults.

Missed dose—If you miss a dose of this medicine, take it as soon as possible. However, if it is almost time for your next dose, skip the missed dose and go back to your regular dosing schedule. Do not double doses.

Storage—To store this medicine:

- Keep out of the reach of children.
- Store away from heat and direct light.
- Do not store this medicine in the bathroom, near the kitchen sink, or in other damp places. Heat or moisture may cause the medicine to break down.
- Do not keep outdated medicine or medicine no longer needed. Be sure that any discarded medicine is out of the reach of children.

Precautions While Using This Medicine

Your doctor should check your progress at regular visits. Blood tests may be needed to make sure that this medicine is working properly and is not causing unwanted effects.

Drinking too much alcohol may increase the amount of uric acid in the blood and lessen the effects of allopurinol. Therefore, people with gout and other people with too much uric acid in the body should be careful to limit the amount of alcohol they drink.

Taking too much vitamin C may make the urine more acidic and increase the possibility of kidney stones forming while you are taking allopurinol. Therefore, check with your doctor before you take vitamin C while taking this medicine.

Check with your doctor immediately:
- *If you notice a skin rash, hives, or itching while you are taking allopurinol.*
- *If chills, fever, joint pain, muscle aches or pains, sore throat, or nausea or vomiting occur, especially if they occur together with or shortly after a skin rash.*

Very rarely, these effects may be the first signs of a serious reaction to the medicine.

Allopurinol may cause some people to become drowsy or less alert than they are normally. *Make sure you know how you react to this medicine before you drive, use machines, or do anything else that could be dangerous if you are not alert.*

Side Effects of This Medicine

Along with its needed effects, a medicine may cause some unwanted effects. Although not all of these side effects may occur, if they do occur they may need medical attention.

Stop taking this medicine and check with your doctor immediately if any of the following side effects occur:

More common

Skin rash or sores, hives, or itching

Rare

Black, tarry stools; bleeding sores on lips; blood in urine or stools; chills, fever, muscle aches or pains, nausea, or vomiting—especially if occurring with or shortly after a skin rash; difficult or painful urination; pinpoint red spots on skin; redness, tenderness, burning, or peeling of skin; red and/or irritated eyes; red, thickened, or scaly skin; shortness of breath, troubled breathing, tightness in chest, or wheezing; sores, ulcers, or white spots in mouth or on lips; sore throat and fever; sudden decrease in amount of urine; swelling in upper abdominal (stomach) area; swelling of face, fingers, feet, or lower legs; swollen and/or painful glands; unusual bleeding or bruising; unusual tiredness or weakness; weight gain (rapid); yellow eyes or skin

Also, check with your doctor as soon as possible if any of the following side effects occur:

Rare

Loosening of fingernails; numbness, tingling, pain, or weakness in hands or feet; pain in lower back or side; unexplained nosebleeds

Other side effects may occur that usually do not need medical attention. These side effects may go away during treatment as your body adjusts to the medicine. However, check with your doctor if any of the following side effects continue or are bothersome:

Less common or rare

Diarrhea; drowsiness; headache; indigestion; nausea or vomiting occurring without a skin rash or other side effects; stomach pain occurring without other side effects; unusual hair loss

Other side effects not listed above may also occur in some patients. If you notice any other effects, check with your doctor.

AMANTADINE   Systemic

Some commonly used brand names are:

In the U.S.—
Symadine
Symmetrel
Generic name product may also be available.

In Canada—
Symmetrel

Description

Amantadine (a-MAN-ta-deen) is an antiviral. It is used to prevent or treat certain influenza (flu) infections (type A).

It may be given alone or along with flu shots. Amantadine will not work for colds, other types of flu, or other virus infections.

Amantadine also is an antidyskinetic. It is used to treat Parkinson's disease, sometimes called paralysis agitans or shaking palsy. It may be given alone or with other medicines for Parkinson's disease. By improving muscle control and reducing stiffness, this medicine allows more normal movements of the body as the disease symptoms are reduced. Amantadine is also used to treat stiffness and shaking caused by certain medicines used to treat nervous, mental, and emotional conditions.

Amantadine may be used for other conditions as determined by your doctor.

Amantadine is available only with your doctor's prescription, in the following dosage forms:

Oral

- Capsules (U.S. and Canada)
- Syrup (U.S. and Canada)

Before Using This Medicine

In deciding to use a medicine, the risks of taking the medicine must be weighed against the good it will do. This is a decision you and your doctor will make. For amantadine, the following should be considered:

Allergies—Tell your doctor if you have ever had any unusual or allergic reaction to amantadine. Also tell your health care professional if you are allergic to any other substances, such as foods, preservatives, or dyes.

Pregnancy—Studies have not been done in humans. However, studies in some animals have shown that amantadine is harmful to the fetus and causes birth defects.

Breast-feeding—Amantadine passes into breast milk. However, the effects of amantadine in newborn babies and infants are not known.

Children—This medicine has been tested in children over one year of age and has not been shown to cause different side effects or problems in these children than it does in adults. There is no specific information comparing the use of amantadine in children under one year of age with use in other age groups.

Older adults—Elderly people are especially sensitive to the effects of amantadine. Confusion, difficult urination, blurred vision, constipation, and dry mouth, nose, and throat may be especially likely to occur.

Other medicines—Although certain medicines should not be used together at all, in other cases two different medicines may be used together even if an interaction might occur. In these cases, your doctor may want to change the dose, or other precautions may be necessary. When you are taking amantadine, it is especially important that your health care professional know if you are taking any of the following:

- Amphetamines or
- Appetite suppressants (diet pills), except fenfluramine (e.g., Pondimin), or
- Caffeine (e.g., NoDoz) or
- Chlophedianol (e.g., Ulone) or
- Cocaine or
- Medicine for asthma or other breathing problems or
- Medicine for colds, sinus problems, or hay fever or other allergies (including nose drops or sprays) or
- Methylphenidate (e.g., Ritalin) or
- Nabilone (e.g., Cesamet) or
- Pemoline (e.g., Cylert)—The use of amantadine with these medicines may increase the chance of unwanted effects such as nervousness, irritability, trouble in sleeping, and possibly seizures or irregular heartbeat

- Anticholinergics (medicine for abdominal or stomach spasms or cramps)—The use of amantadine with these medicines may increase the chance of unwanted effects such as blurred vision, dryness of the mouth, confusion, hallucinations, and nightmares

Other medical problems—The presence of other medical problems may affect the use of amantadine. Make sure you tell your doctor if you have any other medical problems, especially:

- Eczema (recurring)—Amantadine may cause or worsen eczema
- Epilepsy or other seizures (history of)—Amantadine may increase the frequency of convulsions (seizures) in patients with a seizure disorder
- Heart disease or other circulation problems or
- Swelling of feet and ankles—Amantadine may increase the chance of swelling of the feet and ankles, and may worsen heart disease or circulation problems
- Kidney disease—Amantadine is removed from the body by the kidneys; patients with kidney disease will need to receive a lower dose of amantadine
- Mental or emotional illness—Higher doses of amantadine may cause confusion, hallucinations, and nightmares

---

Proper Use of This Medicine

For patients *taking amantadine to prevent or treat flu infections:*

- Talk to your doctor about the possibility of getting a flu shot if you have not had one yet.
- This medicine is *best taken before exposure, or as soon as possible after exposure,* to people who have the flu.
- To help keep yourself from getting the flu, *keep taking this medicine for the full time of treatment.* Or if you already have the flu, continue taking this medi-

cine for the full time of treatment even if you begin to feel better after a few days. This will help to clear up your infection completely. If you stop taking this medicine too soon, your symptoms may return. This medicine should be taken for at least 2 days after all your flu symptoms have disappeared.

- This medicine works best when there is a constant amount in the blood. *To help keep the amount constant, do not miss any doses. Also, it is best to take the doses at evenly spaced times day and night.* For example, if you are to take 2 doses a day, the doses should be spaced about 12 hours apart. If this interferes with your sleep or other daily activities, or if you need help in planning the best times to take your medicine, check with your health care professional.

- If you are using the oral liquid form of amantadine, use a specially marked measuring spoon or other device to measure each dose accurately. The average household teaspoon may not hold the right amount of liquid.

For patients *taking amantadine for Parkinson's disease or movement problems* caused by certain medicines used to treat nervous, mental, and emotional conditions:

- *Take this medicine exactly as directed by your doctor.* Do not miss any doses and do not take more medicine than your doctor ordered.

- Improvement in the symptoms of Parkinson's disease usually occurs in about 2 days. However, in some patients this medicine must be taken for up to 2 weeks before full benefit is seen.

Dosing—The dose of amantadine will be different for different patients. *Follow your doctor's orders or the directions on the label.* The following information includes only the average doses of amantadine. Your dose may be different if you have kidney disease. *If your dose is different, do not change it* unless your doctor tells you to do so.

- The number of capsules or teaspoonfuls of suspension that you take depends on the strength of the medicine. Also, *the number of doses you take each day, the time allowed between doses, and the length of time you take the medicine depend on the medical problem for which you are taking amantadine.*

- For the *treatment or prevention of flu:*

  —Older adults: 100 milligrams once a day.

  —Adults and children 12 years of age and older: 200 milligrams once a day, or 100 milligrams two times a day.

  —Children 9 to 12 years of age: 100 milligrams two times a day.

  —Children 1 to 9 years of age: Dose is based on body weight and must be determined by the doctor.

- For the *treatment of Parkinson's disease or movement problems:*

  —Older adults: 100 milligrams once a day to start. The dose may be increased slowly over time, if needed.

  —Adults: 100 milligrams one or two times a day.

  —Children: Dose has not been determined.

Missed dose—If you miss a dose of this medicine, take it as soon as possible. This will help to keep a constant amount of medicine in the blood. However, if it is almost time for your next dose, skip the missed dose and go back to your regular dosing schedule. Do not double doses.

Storage—To store this medicine:

- Keep out of the reach of children.
- Store away from heat and direct light.
- Do not store the capsule form of this medicine in the bathroom, near the kitchen sink, or in other damp places. Heat or moisture may cause the medicine to break down.

- Keep the oral liquid form of this medicine from freezing.
- Do not keep outdated medicine or medicine no longer needed. Be sure that any discarded medicine is out of the reach of children.

Precautions While Using This Medicine

Drinking alcoholic beverages while taking this medicine may cause increased side effects such as circulation problems, dizziness, lightheadedness, fainting, or confusion. Therefore, *do not drink alcoholic beverages while you are taking this medicine.*

This medicine may cause some people to become dizzy, confused, or lightheaded, or to have blurred vision or trouble concentrating. *Make sure you know how you react to this medicine before you drive, use machines, or do anything else that could be dangerous if you are dizzy or are not alert or able to see well.* If these reactions are especially bothersome, check with your doctor.

Getting up suddenly from a lying or sitting position may also be a problem because of the dizziness, lightheadedness, or fainting that may be caused by this medicine. Getting up slowly may help. If this problem continues or gets worse, check with your doctor.

Amantadine may cause dryness of the mouth, nose, and throat. For temporary relief of mouth dryness, use sugarless candy or gum, melt bits of ice in your mouth, or use a saliva substitute. However, if your mouth continues to feel dry for more than 2 weeks, check with your doctor or dentist. Continuing dryness of the mouth may increase the chance of dental disease, including tooth decay, gum disease, and fungus infections.

This medicine may cause purplish red, net-like, blotchy spots on the skin. This problem occurs more often in females and usually occurs on the legs and/or feet after this medicine has been taken regularly for a month or more. Although the blotchy spots may remain as long as you are taking this medicine, they usually go away gradually within 2 to 12 weeks after you stop taking the medicine. If you have any questions about this, check with your doctor.

For patients *taking amantadine to prevent or treat flu infections:*

- If your symptoms do not improve within a few days, or if they become worse, check with your doctor.

For patients *taking amantadine for Parkinson's disease or movement problems* caused by certain medicines used to treat nervous, mental, and emotional conditions:

- *Patients with Parkinson's disease must be careful not to overdo physical activities as their condition improves and body movements become easier* since injuries resulting from falls may occur. Such activities must be gradually increased to give your body time to adjust to changing balance, circulation, and coordination.

- Some patients may notice that this medicine gradually loses its effect while they are taking it regularly for a few months. If you notice this, check with your doctor. Your doctor may want to adjust the dose or stop the medicine for a while and then restart it to restore its effect.

- *Do not suddenly stop taking this medicine without first checking with your doctor* since your Parkinson's disease may get worse very quickly. Your doctor may want you to reduce your dose gradually before stopping the medicine completely.

Side Effects of This Medicine

Along with its needed effects, a medicine may cause some unwanted effects. Although not all of these side effects

may occur, if they do occur they may need medical attention.

Check with your doctor immediately if any of the following side effects occur:

Less common

Blurred vision; confusion (especially in elderly patients); difficult urination (especially in elderly patients); fainting; hallucinations (seeing, hearing, or feeling things that are not there)

Rare

Convulsions (seizures); decreased vision or any change in vision; difficulty in coordination; irritation and swelling of the eye; mental depression; skin rash; swelling of feet or lower legs; unexplained shortness of breath

Other side effects may occur that usually do not need medical attention. These side effects may go away during treatment as your body adjusts to the medicine. However, check with your doctor if any of the following side effects continue or are bothersome:

More common

Difficulty concentrating; dizziness or lightheadedness; headache; irritability; loss of appetite; nausea; nervousness; purplish red, net-like, blotchy spots on skin; trouble in sleeping or nightmares

Less common or rare

Constipation; dryness of the mouth, nose, and throat; vomiting

Other side effects not listed above may also occur in some patients. If you notice any other effects, check with your doctor.

Additional Information

Once a medicine has been approved for marketing for a certain use, experience may show that it is also useful for

other medical problems. Although this use is not included in product labeling, amantadine is used in certain patients with the following medical condition:

- Unusual tiredness or weakness associated with multiple sclerosis

Other than the above information, there is no additional information relating to proper use, precautions, or side effects for this use.

AMLODIPINE   Systemic†

A commonly used brand name in the U.S. is Norvasc.

†Not commercially available in Canada.

Description

Amlodipine (am-LOE-di-peen) is a calcium channel blocker used to treat angina (chest pain) and high blood pressure. Amlodipine affects the movement of calcium into the cells of the heart and blood vessels. As a result, amlodipine relaxes blood vessels and increases the supply of blood and oxygen to the heart while reducing its workload.

High blood pressure adds to the workload of the heart and arteries. If it continues for a long time, the heart and arteries may not function properly. This can damage the blood vessels of the brain, heart, and kidneys, resulting in a stroke, heart failure, or kidney failure. High blood pressure may also increase the risk of heart attacks. These problems may be less likely to occur if blood pressure is controlled.

This medicine is available only with your doctor's prescription, in the following dosage form:

Oral

- Tablets (U.S.)

Before Using This Medicine

In deciding to use a medicine, the risks of taking the medicine must be weighed against the good it will do. This is a decision you and your doctor will make. For amlodipine, the following should be considered:

Allergies—Tell your doctor if you have ever had any unusual or allergic reaction to amlodipine. Also tell your health care professional if you are allergic to any other substances, such as foods, preservatives, or dyes.

Pregnancy—Amlodipine has not been studied in pregnant women. However, studies in animals have shown that, at very high doses, amlodipine may cause fetal death. Before taking this medicine, make sure your doctor knows if you are pregnant or if you may become pregnant.

Breast-feeding—It is not known whether amlodipine passes into breast milk. Although most medicines pass into breast milk in small amounts, many of them may be used safely while breast-feeding. Mothers who are taking this medicine and who wish to breast-feed should discuss this with their doctor.

Children—Studies on this medicine have been done only in adult patients, and there is no specific information comparing use of amlodipine in children with use in other age groups.

Older adults—Elderly people may be especially sensitive to the effects of amlodipine. This may increase the chance of side effects during treatment.

Other medicines—Although certain medicines should not be used together at all, in other cases two different medicines may be used together even if an interaction might occur. In these cases, your doctor may want to change the dose, or other precautions may be necessary. Tell your health care professional if you are using any other pre-

scription or nonprescription (over-the-counter [OTC])
medicine.

Other medical problems—The presence of other medical
problems may affect the use of amlodipine. Make sure
you tell your doctor if you have any other medical problems, especially:

- Congestive heart failure—There is a small chance that amlodipine may make this condition worse
- Liver disease—Higher blood levels of amlodipine may result and a smaller dose may be needed
- Very low blood pressure—Amlodipine may make this condition worse

---

Proper Use of This Medicine

Take this medicine exactly as directed even if you feel
well and do not notice any chest pain. Do not take more
of this medicine and do not take it more often than your
doctor ordered. Do not miss any doses.

For patients taking this medicine *for high blood pressure:*

- In addition to the use of the medicine your doctor
  has prescribed, treatment for your high blood pressure
  may include weight control and care in the types of
  food you eat, especially foods high in sodium (salt).
  Your doctor will tell you which of these are most
  important for you. You should check with your doctor
  before changing your diet.

- Many patients who have high blood pressure will not
  notice any signs of the problem. In fact, many may
  feel normal. It is very important that you *take your
  medicine exactly as directed* and that you keep your
  appointments with your doctor even if you feel well.

- Remember that this medicine will not cure your high
  blood pressure but it does help control it. Therefore,
  you must continue to take it as directed if you expect

to lower your blood pressure and keep it down. *You may have to take high blood pressure medicine for the rest of your life.* If high blood pressure is not treated, it can cause serious problems such as heart failure, blood vessel disease, stroke, or kidney disease.

Dosing—The dose of amlodipine will be different for different patients. *Follow your doctor's orders or the directions on the label.* The following information includes only the average doses of amlodipine. *If your dose is different, do not change it* unless your doctor tells you to do so.

The number of tablets that you take depends on the strength of the medicine.

- For *oral* dosage form (tablets):
  - —For angina (chest pain):
    - Adults—5 to 10 milligrams (mg) once a day.
    - Children—Use must be determined by your doctor.
  - —For high blood pressure:
    - Adults—2.5 to 10 mg once a day.
    - Children—Use must be determined by your doctor.

Missed dose—If you miss a dose of this medicine, take it as soon as possible. However, if it is almost time for your next dose, skip the missed dose and go back to your regular dosing schedule. Do not double doses.

Storage—To store this medicine:

- Keep out of the reach of children.
- Store away from heat and direct light.
- Do not store in the bathroom, near the kitchen sink, or in other damp places. Heat or moisture may cause the medicine to break down.
- Keep the medicine from freezing. Do not refrigerate.

- Do not keep outdated medicine or medicine no longer needed. Be sure that any discarded medicine is out of the reach of children.

Precautions While Using This Medicine

It is important that your doctor check your progress at regular visits. This will allow your doctor to make sure the medicine is working properly and to change the dosage if needed.

If you have been using this medicine regularly for several weeks, do not suddenly stop using it. Stopping suddenly may cause your chest pain or high blood pressure to come back or get worse. Check with your doctor for the best way to reduce gradually the amount you are taking before stopping completely.

Chest pain resulting from exercise or physical exertion usually is reduced or prevented by this medicine. This may tempt you to be too active. *Make sure you discuss with your doctor a safe amount of exercise for your medical problem.*

After taking a dose of this medicine you may get a headache that lasts for a short time. This should become less noticeable after you have taken this medicine for a while. If this effect continues, or if the headaches are severe, check with your doctor.

In some patients, tenderness, swelling, or bleeding of the gums may appear soon after treatment with this medicine is started. Brushing and flossing your teeth carefully and regularly and massaging your gums may help prevent this. *See your dentist regularly* to have your teeth cleaned. Check with your medical doctor or dentist if you have any questions about how to take care of your teeth and gums, or if you notice any tenderness, swelling, or bleeding of your gums.

For patients taking this medicine *for high blood pressure:*

- *Do not take other medicines unless they have been discussed with your doctor.* This especially includes over-the-counter (nonprescription) medicines for appetite control, asthma, colds, cough, hay fever, or sinus problems, since they may tend to increase your blood pressure.

Side Effects of This Medicine

Along with its needed effects, a medicine may cause some unwanted effects. Although not all of these side effects may occur, if they do occur they may need medical attention.

Check with your doctor as soon as possible if any of the following side effects occur:

More common
     Swelling of ankles or feet

Less common
     Dizziness; pounding heartbeat

Rare
     Chest pain; dizziness or lightheadedness when getting up from a lying or sitting position; slow heartbeat

Other side effects may occur that usually do not need medical attention. These side effects may go away during treatment as your body adjusts to the medicine. However, check with your doctor if any of the following side effects continue or are bothersome:

More common
     Flushing; headache

Less common
     Nausea; unusual tiredness or weakness

Other side effects not listed above may also occur in some patients. If you notice any other effects, check with your doctor.

ANGIOTENSIN-CONVERTING ENZYME (ACE) INHIBITORS
Systemic

Some commonly used brand names are:

In the U.S.—

Accupril[7]	Monopril[5]
Altace[8]	Prinivil[6]
Capoten[2]	Vasotec[3,4]
Lotensin[1]	Zestril[6]

In Canada—

Capoten[2]	Vasotec[3,4]
Prinivil[6]	Zestril[6]

Note: For quick reference, the following angiotensin-converting enzyme (ACE) inhibitors are numbered to match the corresponding brand names.

This information applies to the following medicines:

1. Benazepril (ben-AY-ze-pril)†
2. Captopril (KAP-toe-pril)
3. Enalapril (e-NAL-a-pril)
4. Enalaprilat (e-NAL-a-pril-at)
5. Fosinopril (foe-SIN-oh-pril)†
6. Lisinopril (lyse-IN-oh-pril)
7. Quinapril (KWIN-a-pril)†
8. Ramipril (ra-MI-pril)†

†Not commercially available in Canada.

Description

ACE inhibitors belong to the class of medicines called high blood pressure medicines (antihypertensives). They are used to treat high blood pressure (hypertension).

High blood pressure adds to the work load of the heart

and arteries. If it continues for a long time, the heart and arteries may not function properly. This can damage the blood vessels of the brain, heart, and kidneys, resulting in a stroke, heart failure, or kidney failure. High blood pressure may also increase the risk of heart attacks. These problems may be less likely to occur if blood pressure is controlled.

Captopril is used in some patients after a heart attack. After a heart attack, some of the heart muscle is damaged and weakened. The heart muscle may continue to weaken as time goes by. This makes it more difficult for the heart to pump blood. Captopril helps slow down the further weakening of the heart.

Captopril is also used to treat kidney problems in some diabetic patients who use insulin to control their diabetes. Over time, these kidney problems may get worse. Captopril may help slow down the further worsening of kidney problems.

In addition, some ACE inhibitors are used to treat congestive heart failure, or may be used for other conditions as determined by your doctor.

The exact way that these medicines work is not known. They block an enzyme in the body that is necessary to produce a substance that causes blood vessels to tighten. As a result, they relax blood vessels. This lowers blood pressure and increases the supply of blood and oxygen to the heart.

These medicines are available only with your doctor's prescription, in the following dosage forms:

Oral

Benazepril
- Tablets (U.S.)

Captopril
- Tablets (U.S. and Canada)

Enalapril
  • Tablets (U.S. and Canada)
Fosinopril
  • Tablets (U.S.)
Lisinopril
  • Tablets (U.S. and Canada)
Quinapril
  • Tablets (U.S.)
Ramipril
  • Capsules (U.S.)

Parenteral

Enalaprilat
  • Injection (U.S. and Canada)

Before Using This Medicine

In deciding to use a medicine, the risks of taking the medicine must be weighed against the good it will do. This is a decision you and your doctor will make. For the angiotensin-converting enzyme (ACE) inhibitors, the following should be considered:

Allergies—Tell your doctor if you have ever had any unusual or allergic reaction to benazepril, captopril, enalapril, fosinopril, lisinopril, quinapril, or ramipril. Also tell your health care professional if you are allergic to any other substances, such as foods, preservatives, or dyes.

Pregnancy—Use of angiotensin-converting enzyme (ACE) inhibitors during pregnancy, especially in the second and third trimesters (after the first three months) can cause low blood pressure, severe kidney failure, too much potassium, or even death in the newborn. *Therefore, it is important that you check with your doctor immediately if you think that you may be pregnant.* Be sure that you have discussed this with your doctor before taking this medicine. In addition, if you are taking:

  • *Benazepril*—Benazepril has not been shown to cause

birth defects in animals when given in doses more than 3 times the highest recommended human dose.

- *Captopril*—Studies in rabbits and rats at doses up to 400 times the recommended human dose have shown that captopril causes an increase in deaths of the fetus and newborn. Also, captopril has caused deformed skulls in the offspring of rabbits given doses 2 to 70 times the recommended human dose.

- *Enalapril*—Studies in rats at doses many times the recommended human dose have shown that use of enalapril causes the fetus to be smaller than normal. Studies in rabbits have shown that enalapril causes an increase in fetal death. Enalapril has not been shown to cause birth defects in rats or rabbits.

- *Fosinopril*—Studies in rats have shown that fosinopril causes the fetus to be smaller than normal. Studies in rabbits have shown that fosinopril causes fetal death, probably due to extremely low blood pressure. In rats, birth defects such as skeletal and facial deformities were seen. However, it is not clear that the deformities were related to fosinopril. Birth defects were not seen in rabbits.

- *Lisinopril*—Studies in mice and rats at doses many times the recommended human dose have shown that use of lisinopril causes a decrease in successful pregnancies, a decrease in the weight of infants, and an increase in infant deaths. It has also caused a decrease in successful pregnancies and abnormal bone growth in rabbits. Lisinopril has not been shown to cause birth defects in mice, rats, or rabbits.

- *Quinapril*—Studies in rats have shown that quinapril causes lower birth weights and changes in kidney structure of the fetus. However, birth defects were not seen in rabbits given quinapril.

- *Ramipril*—Studies in animals have shown that ramipril causes lower birth weights.

Breast-feeding—

- *Benazepril, captopril, and fosinopril*—These medicines pass into breast milk.
- *Enalapril, lisinopril, quinapril, or ramipril*—It is not known whether these medicines pass into breast milk. However, these medicines have not been reported to cause problems in nursing babies.

Children—Children may be especially sensitive to the blood pressure–lowering effect of ACE inhibitors. This may increase the chance of side effects or other problems during treatment. Therefore, it is especially important that you discuss with the child's doctor the good that this medicine may do as well as the risks of using it.

Older adults—This medicine has been tested in a limited number of patients 65 years of age or older and has not been shown to cause different side effects or problems in older people than it does in younger adults.

Other medicines—Although certain medicines should not be used together at all, in other cases two different medicines may be used together even if an interaction might occur. In these cases, your doctor may want to change the dose, or other precautions may be necessary. When you are taking or receiving ACE inhibitors it is especially important that your health care professional know if you are taking any of the following:

- Diuretics (water pills)—Effects on blood pressure may be increased. In addition, some diuretics make the increase in potassium in the blood caused by ACE inhibitors even greater
- Potassium-containing medicines or supplements or
- Salt substitutes or
- Low-salt milk—Use of these substances with ACE inhibitors may result in an unusually high potassium level in the blood, which can lead to heart rhythm and other problems

Other medical problems—The presence of other medical problems may affect the use of the ACE inhibitors. Make sure you tell your doctor if you have any other medical problems, especially:

- Diabetes mellitus (sugar diabetes)—Increased risk of potassium levels in the body becoming too high
- Heart or blood vessel disease or
- Heart attack or stroke (recent)—Lowering blood pressure may make problems resulting from these conditions worse
- Kidney disease or
- Liver disease—Effects may be increased because of slower removal of medicine from the body
- Kidney transplant—Increased risk of kidney disease caused by ACE inhibitors
- Systemic lupus erythematosus (SLE)—Increased risk of blood problems caused by ACE inhibitors
- Previous reaction to any ACE inhibitor involving hoarseness; swelling of face, mouth, hands, or feet; or sudden trouble in breathing—Reaction is more likely to occur again

---

Proper Use of This Medicine

To help you remember to take your medicine, try to get into the habit of taking it at the same time each day.

For patients taking *captopril:*

- This medicine is best taken on an empty stomach 1 hour before meals, unless you are otherwise directed by your doctor.

For patients taking this medicine *for high blood pressure:*

- In addition to the use of the medicine your doctor has prescribed, treatment for your high blood pressure may include weight control and care in the types of foods you eat, especially foods high in sodium. Your doctor will tell you which of these are most important for you. You should check with your doctor before changing your diet.

- Many patients who have high blood pressure will not notice any signs of the problem. In fact, many may feel normal. It is very important that you *take your medicine exactly as directed* and that you keep your appointments with your doctor even if you feel well.

- Remember that this medicine will not cure your high blood pressure but it does help control it. Therefore, you must continue to take it as directed if you expect to lower your blood pressure and keep it down. *You may have to take high blood pressure medicine for the rest of your life*. If high blood pressure is not treated, it can cause serious problems such as heart failure, blood vessel disease, stroke, or kidney disease.

Dosing—The dose of the ACE inhibitor will be different for different patients. *Follow your doctor's orders or the directions on the label*. The following information includes only the average doses. *If your dose is different, do not change it* unless your doctor tells you to do so.

The number of capsules or tablets that you take depends on the strength of the medicine. Also, *the number of doses you take each day, the time allowed between doses, and the length of time you take the medicine depend on the medical problem for which you are taking the ACE inhibitor*.

For benazepril

- For *oral* dosage form (tablets):

    —For high blood pressure:

    - Adults—10 milligrams (mg) once a day at first. Then, your doctor may increase your dose to 20 to 40 mg a day taken as a single dose or divided into two doses.

    - Children—Use and dose must be determined by your doctor.

For captopril
- For *oral* dosage form (tablets):
  —For congestive heart failure:
  - Adults—12.5 to 100 mg two or three times a day.
  - Children—Dose must be determined by your doctor.

  —For high blood pressure:
  - Adults—12.5 to 25 mg two or three times a day.
  - Children—Dose must be determined by your doctor.

  —For kidney problems related to diabetes:
  - Adults—25 mg three times a day.

  —For treatment after a heart attack:
  - Adults—12.5 to 50 mg three times a day.

For enalapril
- For *oral* dosage form (tablets):
  —For congestive heart failure:
  - Adults—2.5 mg once a day or two times a day at first. Your doctor may increase your dose to 5 to 20 mg a day taken as a single dose or divided into two doses.
  - Children—Use and dose must be determined by your doctor.

  —For high blood pressure:
  - Adults—5 mg once a day at first. Then, your doctor may increase your dose to 10 to 40 mg a day taken as a single dose or divided into two doses.
  - Children—Use and dose must be determined by your doctor.

  —For treating weakened heart muscle:
  - Adults—2.5 mg two times a day at first. Then,

your doctor may increase your dose up to 20 mg a day taken in divided doses.

- For *injection* dosage form:

—For high blood pressure:

- Adults—1.25 mg every six hours injected into a vein.

- Children—Use and dose must be determined by your doctor.

For fosinopril

- For *oral* dosage form (tablets):

—For high blood pressure:

- Adults—10 to 40 mg once a day.

- Children—Use and dose must be determined by your doctor.

For lisinopril

- For *oral* dosage form (tablets):

—For congestive heart failure:

- Adults—2.5 to 20 mg once a day.

- Children—Use and dose must be determined by your doctor.

—For high blood pressure:

- Adults—10 to 40 mg once a day.

- Children—Use and dose must be determined by your doctor.

For quinapril

- For *oral* dosage form (tablets):

—For high blood pressure:

- Adults—10 mg once a day at first. Then, your doctor may increase your dose to 20 to 80 mg a day taken as a single dose or divided into two doses.

- Children—Use and dose must be determined by your doctor.

For ramipril

- For *oral* dosage form (capsules):

  —For high blood pressure:

    • Adults—2.5 mg once a day at first. Then, your doctor may increase your dose up to 20 mg a day taken as a single dose or divided into two doses.

    • Children—Use and dose must be determined by your doctor.

Missed dose—If you miss a dose of this medicine, take it as soon as possible. However, if it is almost time for your next dose, skip the missed dose and go back to your regular dosing schedule. Do not double doses.

Storage—To store this medicine:

- Keep out of the reach of children.

- Store away from heat and direct light.

- Do not store in the bathroom, near the kitchen sink, or in other damp places. Heat or moisture may cause the medicine to break down.

- Do not keep outdated medicine or medicine no longer needed. Be sure that any discarded medicine is out of the reach of children.

Precautions While Using This Medicine

It is important that your doctor check your progress at regular visits to make sure that this medicine is working properly and to check for unwanted effects.

For patients taking this medicine *for high blood pressure:*

- *Do not take other medicines unless they have been discussed with your doctor.* This especially includes over-the-counter (nonprescription) medicines for appetite control, asthma, colds, cough, hay fever, or sinus problems, since they may tend to increase your blood pressure.

Dizziness or lightheadedness may occur after the first dose of this medicine, especially if you have been taking a diuretic (water pill). Make sure you know how you react to this medicine before you drive, use machines, or do anything else that could be dangerous if you are dizzy.

Check with your doctor right away if you become sick while taking this medicine, especially with severe or continuing nausea and vomiting or diarrhea. These conditions may cause you to lose too much water and lead to low blood pressure.

Dizziness, lightheadedness, or fainting may also occur if you exercise or if the weather is hot. Heavy sweating can cause loss of too much water and low blood pressure. Use extra care during exercise or hot weather.

Avoid alcoholic beverages until you have discussed their use with your doctor. Alcohol may make the low blood pressure effect worse and/or increase the possibility of dizziness or fainting.

Before having any kind of surgery (including dental surgery) or emergency treatment, tell the medical doctor or dentist in charge that you are taking this medicine.

For patients taking *captopril or fosinopril:*

• Before you have any medical tests, tell the doctor in charge that you are taking this medicine. The results of some tests may be affected by this medicine.

Side Effects of This Medicine

Along with its needed effects, a medicine may cause some unwanted effects. Although not all of these side effects

may occur, if they do occur they may need medical attention.

Check with your doctor immediately if any of the following side effects occur:

Rare

Fever and chills; hoarseness; swelling of face, mouth, hands, or feet; trouble in swallowing or breathing (sudden); stomach pain, itching of skin, or yellow eyes or skin

Check with your doctor as soon as possible if any of the following side effects occur:

Less common

Dizziness, lightheadedness, or fainting; skin rash, with or without itching, fever, or joint pain

Rare

Abdominal pain, abdominal distention, fever, nausea, or vomiting; chest pain

Signs and symptoms of too much potassium in the body

Confusion; irregular heartbeat; nervousness; numbness or tingling in hands, feet, or lips; shortness of breath or difficulty breathing; weakness or heaviness of legs

Other side effects may occur that usually do not need medical attention. These side effects may go away during treatment as your body adjusts to the medicine. However, check with your doctor if any of the following side effects continue or are bothersome:

More common

Cough (dry, continuing)

Less common

Diarrhea; headache; loss of taste; nausea; unusual tiredness

Other side effects not listed above may also occur in some patients. If you notice any other effects, check with your doctor.

Additional Information

Once a medicine has been approved for marketing for a certain use, experience may show that it is also useful for other medical problems. Although these uses are not included in product labeling, ACE inhibitors are used in certain patients with the following medical conditions:

- Hypertension in scleroderma (high blood pressure in patients with hardening and thickening of the skin)
- Renal crisis in scleroderma (kidney problems in patients with hardening and thickening of the skin)

Other than the above information, there is no additional information relating to proper use, precautions, or side effects for these uses.

ANTICHOLINERGICS/ ANTISPASMODICS   Systemic

Some commonly used brand names are:

In the U.S.—

Anaspas[8]	Levsinex Timecaps[8]
Antispas[5]	Levsin S/L[8]
A-Spas[5]	Neoquess[5,8]
Banthine[11]	Norpanth[15]
Bentyl[5]	Or-Tyl[5]
Cantil[10]	Pamine[12]
Cystospaz[8]	Pathilon[17]
Cystospaz-M[8]	Pro-Banthine[15]
Darbid[9]	Quarzan[4]
Daricon[13]	Robinul[6]
Di-Spaz[5]	Robinul Forte[6]
Gastrosed[8]	Spasmoject[5]
Homapin[7]	Transderm-Scōp[16]
Levsin[8]	Valpin 50[1]

In Canada—

Bentylol[5]	Gastrozepin[14]
Buscopan[16]	Levsin[8]
Formulex[5]	Lomine[5]

In Canada (cont'd)—

Pro-Banthine[15]   Robinul Forte[6]

Propanthel[15]   Spasmoban[5]

Robinul[6]   Transderm-V[16]

Other commonly used names are:

dicycloverine[5]   hyoscine methobromide[12]

glycopyrronium bromide[6]   methanthelinium[11]

hyoscine hydrobromide[16]   octatropine[1]

Note: For quick reference, the following anticholinergics/antispasmodics are numbered to match the corresponding brand names.

This information applies to the following medicines:

1. Anisotropine (an-iss-oh-TROE-peen)†‡
2. Atropine (A-troe-peen)‡§
3. Belladonna (bell-a-DON-a)†‡
4. Clidinium (kli-DI-nee-um)†
5. Dicyclomine (dye-SYE-kloe-meen)‡
6. Glycopyrrolate (glye-koe-PYE-roe-late)‡
7. Homatropine (hoe-MA-troe-peen)†
8. Hyoscyamine (hye-oh-SYE-a-meen)
9. Isopropamide (eye-soe-PROE-pa-mide)†
10. Mepenzolate (me-PEN-zoe-late)†
11. Methantheline (meth-AN-tha-leen)†
12. Methscopolamine (meth-skoe-POL-a-meen)†
13. Oxyphencyclimine (ox-i-fen-SYE-kli-meen)†
14. Pirenzepine (peer-EN-ze-peen)*
15. Propantheline (proe-PAN-the-leen)‡
16. Scopolamine (scoe-POL-a-meen)‡
17. Tridihexethyl (trye-dye-hex-ETH-il)†

---

*Not commercially available in the U.S.
†Not commercially available in Canada.
‡Generic name product may also be available in the U.S.
§Generic name product may also be available in Canada.

Description

The anticholinergics/antispasmodics are a group of medicines that include the natural belladonna alkaloids (atropine, belladonna, hyoscyamine, and scopolamine) and related products.

The anticholinergics/antispasmodics are used to relieve cramps or spasms of the stomach, intestines, and bladder. Some are used together with antacids or other medicine in the treatment of peptic ulcer. Others are used to prevent nausea, vomiting, and motion sickness.

Anticholinergics/antispasmodics are also used in certain surgical and emergency procedures. In surgery, some are given by injection before anesthesia to help relax you and to decrease secretions, such as saliva. During anesthesia and surgery, atropine, glycopyrrolate, hyoscyamine, and scopolamine are used to help keep the heartbeat normal. Atropine is also given by injection to help relax the stomach and intestines for certain types of examinations. Some anticholinergics are also used to treat poisoning caused by medicines such as neostigmine and physostigmine, certain types of mushrooms, and poisoning by "nerve" gases or organic phosphorous pesticides (for example, demeton [Systox], diazinon, malathion, parathion, and ronnel [Trolene]). Also, anticholinergics can be used for painful menstruation, runny nose, and to prevent urination during sleep.

These medicines may also be used for other conditions as determined by your doctor.

The anticholinergics/antispasmodics are available only with your doctor's prescription in the following dosage forms:

Oral

Anisotropine
- Tablets (U.S.)

Atropine
- Tablets (U.S.)
- Soluble tablets (U.S.)

Belladonna
- Tincture (U.S.)

Clidinium
- Capsules (U.S.)

Dicyclomine
- Capsules (U.S. and Canada)
- Syrup (U.S. and Canada)
- Tablets (U.S. and Canada)

- Extended-release Tablets (Canada)

Glycopyrrolate
- Tablets (U.S. and Canada)

Homatropine
- Tablets (U.S.)

Hyoscyamine
- Extended-release capsules (U.S.)
- Elixir (U.S.)
- Oral solution (U.S. and Canada)
- Tablets (U.S.)

Isopropamide
- Tablets (U.S.)

Mepenzolate
- Tablets (U.S.)

Methantheline
- Tablets (U.S.)

Methscopolamine
- Tablets (U.S.)

Oxyphencyclimine
- Tablets (U.S.)

Pirenzepine
- Tablets (Canada)

Propantheline
- Tablets (U.S. and Canada)

Scopolamine
- Tablets (Canada)

Tridihexethyl
- Tablets (U.S.)

Parenteral

Atropine
- Injection (U.S. and Canada)

Dicyclomine
- Injection (U.S. and Canada)

Glycopyrrolate
- Injection (U.S. and Canada)

Hyoscyamine
- Injection (U.S. and Canada)

Scopolamine
- Injection (U.S. and Canada)

Rectal

Scopolamine
- Suppositories (Canada)

Transdermal
Scopolamine
  • Transdermal disk (U.S. and Canada)

Before Using This Medicine

In deciding to use a medicine, the risks of taking the medicine must be weighed against the good it will do. This is a decision you and your doctor will make. For anticholinergics/antispasmodics the following should be considered:

Allergies—Tell your doctor if you have ever had any unusual or allergic reaction to any of the natural belladonna alkaloids (atropine, belladonna, hyoscyamine, and scopolamine), iodine or iodides, or any related products. Also, tell your health care professional if you are allergic to any other substances, such as foods, preservatives, or dyes.

Pregnancy—If you are pregnant or if you may become pregnant, make sure your doctor knows if your medicine contains any of the following:

  • *Atropine*—Atropine has not been shown to cause birth defects or other problems in animals. However, when injected into humans during pregnancy, atropine has been reported to increase the heartbeat of the fetus.

  • *Belladonna*—Studies on effects in pregnancy have not been done in either humans or animals.

  • *Clidinium*—Clidinium has not been studied in pregnant women. However, clidinium has not been shown to cause birth defects or other problems in animal studies.

  • *Dicyclomine*—Dicyclomine has been associated with a few cases of human birth defects but dicyclomine has not been confirmed as the cause.

- *Glycopyrrolate*—Glycopyrrolate has not been studied in pregnant women. However, glycopyrrolate did not cause birth defects in animal studies, but did decrease the chance of becoming pregnant and in the newborn's chance of surviving after weaning.

- *Hyoscyamine*—Studies on effects in pregnancy have not been done in either humans or animals. However, when injected into humans during pregnancy, hyoscyamine has been reported to increase the heartbeat of the fetus.

- *Isopropamide*—Studies on effects in pregnancy have not been done in either humans or animals.

- *Mepenzolate*—Mepenzolate has not been studied in pregnant women. However, studies in animals have not shown that mepenzolate causes birth defects or other problems.

- *Propantheline*—Studies on effects in pregnancy have not been done in either humans or animals.

- *Scopolamine*—Studies on effects in pregnancy have not been done in either humans or animals.

Breast-feeding—Although these medicines may pass into the breast milk, they have not been reported to cause problems in nursing babies. However, the flow of breast milk may be reduced in some patients. The use of dicyclomine in nursing mothers has been reported to cause breathing problems in infants.

Children—Unusual excitement, nervousness, restlessness, or irritability and unusual warmth, dryness, and flushing of skin are more likely to occur in children, who are usually more sensitive to the effects of anticholinergics. Also, when anticholinergics are given to children during hot weather, a rapid increase in body temperature may occur. In infants and children, especially those with spastic paralysis or brain damage, this medicine may be more likely to cause severe side effects. Shortness of breath or difficulty in breathing has occurred in children taking dicyclomine.

Older adults—Confusion or memory loss; constipation; difficult urination; drowsiness; dryness of mouth, nose, throat, or skin; and unusual excitement, nervousness, restlessness, or irritability may be more likely to occur in the elderly, who are usually more sensitive than younger adults to the effects of anticholinergics. Also, eye pain may occur, which may be a sign of glaucoma.

Other medicines—Although certain medicines should not be used together at all, in other cases two different medicines may be used together even if an interaction might occur. In these cases, your doctor may want to change the dose, or other precautions may be necessary. When you are taking anticholinergics/antispasmodics, it is especially important that your health care professional know if you are taking any of the following:

- Antacids or
- Diarrhea medicine containing kaolin or attapulgite or
- Ketoconazole (e.g., Nizoral)—Using these medicines with an anticholinergic may lessen the effects of the anticholinergic
- Central nervous system (CNS) depressants (medicines that cause drowsiness)—Taking scopolamine with CNS depressants may increase the effects of either medicine
- Other anticholinergics (medicine for abdominal or stomach spasms or cramps) or
- Tricyclic antidepressants (amitriptyline [e.g., Elavil], amoxapine [e.g., Asendin], clomipramine [e.g., Anafranil], desipramine [e.g., Pertofrane], doxepin [e.g., Sinequan], imipramine [e.g., Tofranil], nortriptyline [e.g., Aventyl], protriptyline [e.g., Vivactil], trimipramine [e.g., Surmontil])—Taking anticholinergics with tricyclic antidepressants or other anticholinergics may cause an increase in the effects of the anticholinergic
- Potassium chloride (e.g., Kay Ciel)—Using this medicine with an anticholinergic may make gastrointestinal problems caused by potassium worse

Other medical problems—The presence of other medical problems may affect the use of anticholinergics/antispasmodics. Make sure you tell your doctor if you have any other medical problems, especially:

- Bleeding problems (severe)—These medicines may increase heart rate, which would make bleeding problems worse
- Brain damage (in children)—May increase the CNS effects of this medicine
- Colitis (severe) or
- Dryness of mouth (severe and continuing) or
- Enlarged prostate or
- Fever or
- Glaucoma or
- Heart disease or
- Hernia (hiatal) or
- High blood pressure (hypertension) or
- Intestinal blockage or other intestinal problems or
- Lung disease (chronic) or
- Myasthenia gravis or
- Toxemia of pregnancy or
- Urinary tract blockage or difficult urination—These medicines may make these conditions worse
- Down's syndrome (mongolism)—These medicines may cause an increase in pupil dilation and heart rate
- Kidney disease or
- Liver disease—Higher blood levels may occur and cause an increase in side effects
- Overactive thyroid—These medicines may further increase heart rate
- Spastic paralysis (in children)—This condition may increase the effects of the anticholinergic

Proper Use of This Medicine

Take this medicine only as directed. Do not take more of it, do not take it more often, and do not take it for a longer time than your doctor ordered. To do so may increase the chance of side effects.

Missed dose—If you miss a dose of this medicine, take it as soon as possible. However, if it is almost time for your next dose, skip the missed dose and go back to your regular dosing schedule. Do not double doses.

For patients *taking any of these medicines by mouth:*

• Take this medicine 30 minutes to 1 hour before meals unless otherwise directed by your doctor.

To use the *rectal suppository* form of *scopolamine:*

• If the suppository is too soft to insert, chill it in the refrigerator for 30 minutes or run cold water over it before removing the foil wrapper.

• To insert the suppository: First remove the foil wrapper and moisten the suppository with cold water. Lie down on your side and use your finger to push the suppository well up into the rectum.

To use the *transdermal disk* form of *scopolamine:*

• This medicine usually comes with patient directions. Read them carefully before using this medicine.

• Wash and dry your hands thoroughly before and after handling.

• Apply the disk to the hairless area of skin behind the ear. Do not place over any cuts or irritations.

Storage—To store this medicine:

• Keep out of the reach of children. Overdose is especially dangerous in young children.

• Store away from heat and direct light.

• Do not store the capsule or tablet form of this medicine in the bathroom, near the kitchen sink, or in other damp places. Heat or moisture may cause the medicine to break down.

• Keep the liquid form of this medicine tightly closed and keep it from freezing. Do not refrigerate the syrup form of this medicine.

- Do not keep outdated medicine or medicine no longer needed. Be sure that any discarded medicine is out of the reach of children.

Precautions While Using This Medicine

If you think you or someone else may have taken an overdose, get emergency help at once. Taking an overdose of any of the belladonna alkaloids or taking scopolamine with alcohol or other CNS depressants may lead to unconsciousness and possibly death. Some signs of overdose are clumsiness or unsteadiness; dizziness; severe drowsiness; fever; hallucinations (seeing, hearing, or feeling things that are not there); confusion; shortness of breath or troubled breathing; slurred speech; unusual excitement, nervousness, restlessness, or irritability; fast heartbeat; and unusual warmth, dryness, and flushing of skin.

These medicines may make you sweat less, causing your body temperature to increase. *Use extra care not to become overheated during exercise or hot weather while you are taking this medicine,* since overheating may result in heat stroke. Also, hot baths or saunas may make you dizzy or faint while you are taking this medicine.

Check with your doctor before you stop using this medicine. Your doctor may want you to reduce gradually the amount you are using before stopping completely. Stopping this medicine may cause withdrawal side effects such as vomiting, sweating, and dizziness.

Anticholinergics may cause some people to have blurred vision. *Make sure your vision is clear before you drive or do anything else that could be dangerous if you are not able to see well.* These medicines may also cause your eyes to become more sensitive to light than they are normally. Wearing sunglasses may help lessen the discomfort from bright light.

These medicines, especially in high doses, may cause some people to become dizzy or drowsy. *Make sure you know how you react to this medicine before you drive, use machines, or do anything else that could be dangerous if you are dizzy or are not alert.*

Dizziness, lightheadedness, or fainting may occur, especially when you get up from a lying or sitting position. Getting up slowly may help lessen this problem.

These medicines may cause dryness of the mouth, nose, and throat. For temporary relief of mouth dryness, use sugarless candy or gum, melt bits of ice in your mouth, or use a saliva substitute. However, if your mouth continues to feel dry for more than 2 weeks, check with your medical doctor or dentist. Continuing dryness of the mouth may increase the chance of dental disease, including tooth decay, gum disease, and fungus infections.

For patients taking *isopropamide:*

- Make sure your doctor knows if you are planning to have any future thyroid tests. The results of the thyroid test may be affected by the iodine in this medicine.

For patients taking *scopolamine:*

- This medicine will add to the effects of alcohol and other CNS depressants (medicines that slow down the nervous system, possibly causing drowsiness). Some examples of CNS depressants are antihistamines or medicine for hay fever, other allergies, or colds; sedatives, tranquilizers, or sleeping medicine; prescription pain medicine or narcotics; barbiturates; medicine for seizures; muscle relaxants; or anesthetics, including some dental anesthetics. *Check with your doctor before taking any of the above while you are using this medicine.*

For patients *taking any of these medicines by mouth:*

- Do not take this medicine within 2 or 3 hours of

taking antacids or medicine for diarrhea. Taking antacids or antidiarrhea medicines and this medicine too close together may prevent this medicine from working properly.

Side Effects of This Medicine

Along with its needed effects, a medicine may cause some unwanted effects. Although not all of these side effects may occur, if they do occur they may need medical attention.

Check with your doctor as soon as possible if any of the following side effects occur:

Rare

Confusion (especially in the elderly); dizziness, lightheadedness (continuing), or fainting; eye pain; skin rash or hives

Symptoms of overdose

Blurred vision (continuing) or changes in near vision; clumsiness or unsteadiness; confusion; convulsions (seizures); difficulty in breathing, muscle weakness (severe), or tiredness (severe); dizziness; drowsiness (severe); dryness of mouth, nose, or throat (severe); fast heartbeat; fever; hallucinations (seeing, hearing, or feeling things that are not there); slurred speech; unusual excitement, nervousness, restlessness, or irritability; unusual warmth, dryness, and flushing of skin

Other side effects may occur that usually do not need medical attention. These side effects may go away during treatment as your body adjusts to the medicine. However, check with your doctor if any of the following side effects continue or are bothersome:

More common

Constipation (less common with hyoscyamine); decreased sweating; dryness of mouth, nose, throat, or skin

Less common or rare

> Bloated feeling; blurred vision; decreased flow of breast milk; difficult urination; difficulty in swallowing; drowsiness (more common with high doses of any of these medicines and with usual doses of scopolamine when given by mouth or by injection); false sense of well-being (for scopolamine only); headache; increased sensitivity of eyes to light; lightheadedness (with injection); loss of memory; nausea or vomiting; redness or other signs of irritation at place of injection; trouble in sleeping (for scopolamine only); unusual tiredness or weakness

For patients using *scopolamine:*

- After you stop using scopolamine, your body may need time to adjust. The length of time this takes depends on the amount of scopolamine you were using and how long you used it. During this period of time check with your doctor if you notice any of the following side effects:

> Anxiety; irritability; nightmares; trouble in sleeping

For patients using the *transdermal disk* of *scopolamine:*

- While using the disk or even after removing it, your eyes may become more sensitive to light than usual. You may also notice the pupil in one eye is larger than the other. Check with your doctor if this side effect continues or is bothersome.

Other side effects not listed above may also occur in some patients. If you notice any other effects, check with your doctor.

Additional Information

Once a medicine has been approved for marketing for a certain use, experience may show that it is also useful for other medical problems. Although these uses are not in-

cluded in product labeling, anticholinergics/antispasmodics are used in certain patients with the following medical conditions:

- Diarrhea
- Excessive watering of mouth

Other than the above information, there is no additional information relating to proper use, precautions, or side effects for these uses.

ANTICOAGULANTS Systemic

Some commonly used brand names are:

In the U.S.—

Coumadin[3]	Panwarfin[3]
Miradon[1]	Sofarin[3]

In Canada—

Coumadin[3]	Warfilone[3]

Note: For quick reference, the following anticoagulants are numbered to match the corresponding brand names.

This information applies to the following medicines:

1. Anisindione (an-iss-in-DYE-one)†
2. Dicumarol (dye-KOO-ma-role)†‡
3. Warfarin (WAR-far-in)‡

This information does *not* apply to heparin.

†Not commercially available in Canada.
‡Generic name product may also be available in the U.S.

Description

Anticoagulants decrease the clotting ability of the blood and therefore help to prevent harmful clots from forming in the blood vessels. These medicines are sometimes called blood thinners, although they do not actually thin the blood. They also will not dissolve clots that already have formed, but they may prevent the clots from becoming larger and causing more serious problems. They are often used as treatment for certain blood vessel, heart, and lung conditions.

In order for an anticoagulant to help you without causing serious bleeding, it must be used properly and all of the precautions concerning its use must be followed exactly. Be sure that you have discussed the use of this medicine with your doctor. It is very important that you understand all of your doctor's orders and that you are willing and able to follow them exactly.

Anticoagulants are available only with your doctor's prescription, in the following dosage forms:

Oral

Anisindione
   • Tablets (U.S.)
Dicumarol
   • Tablets (U.S.)
Warfarin
   • Tablets (U.S. and Canada)

Parenteral

Warfarin
   • Injection (U.S.)

Before Using This Medicine

In deciding to use a medicine, the risks of taking the medicine must be weighed against the good it will do. This is a decision you and your doctor will make. For anticoagulants, the following should be considered:

Allergies—Tell your doctor if you have ever had any unusual or allergic reaction to an anticoagulant. Also tell your health care professional if you are allergic to any other substances, such as foods, preservatives, or dyes.

Pregnancy—Anticoagulants may cause birth defects. They may also cause other problems affecting the physical or mental growth of the fetus or newborn baby. In addition, use of this medicine during the last 6 months of pregnancy may increase the chance of severe, possibly fatal, bleeding in the fetus. If taken during the last few weeks of pregnancy, anticoagulants may cause severe bleeding in both the fetus and the mother before or during delivery and in the newborn infant.

Do not begin taking this medicine during pregnancy, and do not become pregnant while taking it, unless you have first discussed the possible effects of this medicine with your doctor. Also, if you suspect that you may be pregnant and you are already taking an anticoagulant, check with your doctor at once. Your doctor may suggest that you take a different anticoagulant that is less likely to harm the fetus or the newborn infant during all or part of your pregnancy. Anticoagulants may also cause severe bleeding in the mother if taken soon after the baby is born.

Breast-feeding—Warfarin is not likely to cause problems in nursing babies. Other anticoagulants may pass into the breast milk. A blood test can be done to see if unwanted effects are occurring in the nursing baby. If necessary, another medicine that will overcome any unwanted effects of the anticoagulant can be given to the baby.

Children—Very young babies may be especially sensitive to the effects of anticoagulants. This may increase the chance of bleeding during treatment.

Older adults—Elderly people are especially sensitive to the effects of anticoagulants. This may increase the chance of bleeding during treatment.

Other medicines—Although certain medicines should not be used together at all, in other cases two different medicines may be used together even if an interaction might occur. In these cases, your doctor may want to change the dose, or other precautions may be necessary. *Many different medicines can affect the way anticoagulants work in* *your body.* Therefore, it is very important that your health care professional knows if you are taking *any* other prescription or nonprescription (over-the-counter [OTC]) medicine, even aspirin, laxatives, vitamins, or antacids.

Other medical problems—The presence of other medical problems may affect the use of anticoagulants. Make sure you tell your doctor if you have *any* other medical problems, or if you are now being treated by any other medical doctor or dentist. Many medical problems and treatments will affect the way your body responds to this medicine.

Also, it is important that you tell your doctor if you have recently had any of the following conditions or medical procedures:

- Childbirth or
- Falls or blows to the body or head or
- Fever lasting more than a couple of days or
- Heavy or unusual menstrual bleeding or
- Insertion of intrauterine device (IUD) or
- Medical or dental surgery or
- Severe or continuing diarrhea or
- Spinal anesthesia or
- X-ray (radiation) treatment—The risk of serious bleeding may be increased

---

Proper Use of This Medicine

Take this medicine only as directed by your doctor. Do not take more or less of it, do not take it more often, and do not take it for a longer time than your doctor ordered. This is especially important for elderly patients, who are especially sensitive to the effects of anticoagulants.

Your doctor should check your progress at regular visits. A blood test must be taken regularly to see how fast your blood is clotting. This will help your doctor decide on the proper amount of anticoagulant you should be taking each day.

Dosing—The dose of these medicines will be different for different patients. *Follow your doctor's orders or the directions on the label.* The following information includes only the average doses of these medicines. *If your dose is different, do not change it* unless your doctor tells you to do so.

For anisindione

- For *oral* dosage form (tablets):

  —For preventing harmful blood clots:

  - Adults and teenagers—The usual dose is 25 to 250 milligrams (mg) per day.
  - Children—Dose must be determined by your doctor.

For dicumarol

- For *oral* dosage form (tablets):

  —For preventing harmful blood clots:

  - Adults and teenagers—The usual dose is 25 to 200 milligrams (mg) per day.
  - Children—Dose must be determined by your doctor.

For warfarin

- For *oral* dosage form (tablets):

  —For preventing harmful blood clots:

  - Adults and teenagers—The starting dose is usually 10 to 15 milligrams (mg) per day for two to four days. Then, your doctor may decrease the dose to 2 to 10 mg per day, depending on your condition.
  - Children—Dose must be determined by your doctor.

- For *injection* dosage form:

  —For preventing harmful blood clots:

  - Adults and teenagers—The starting dose is usually 10 to 15 mg, injected into a muscle or a vein, once a day for two to four days. Then, your doctor may decrease the dose to 2 to 10 mg per day, depending on your condition.

• Children—Dose must be determined by your doctor.

Missed dose—If you miss a dose of this medicine, take it as soon as possible. Then go back to your regular dosing schedule. If you do not remember until the next day, do not take the missed dose at all and do not double the next one. *Doubling the dose may cause bleeding.* Instead, go back to your regular dosing schedule. It is recommended that you keep a record of each dose as you take it to avoid mistakes. Also, be sure to give your doctor a record of any doses you miss. If you have any questions about this, check with your doctor.

Storage—To store this medicine:

• Keep out of the reach of children.

• Store away from heat and direct light.

• Do not store this medicine in the bathroom, near the kitchen sink, or in other damp places. Heat or moisture may cause the medicine to break down.

• Do not keep outdated medicine or medicine no longer needed. Be sure that any discarded medicine is out of the reach of children.

Precautions While Using This Medicine

Tell all medical doctors, dentists, and pharmacists you go to that you are taking this medicine.

Check with your health care professional before you start or stop taking any other medicine. This includes any nonprescription (over-the-counter [OTC]) medicine, even aspirin or acetaminophen. Many medicines change the way this medicine affects your body. You may not be able to take the other medicine, or the dose of your anticoagulant may need to be changed.

It is important that you carry identification stating that you are using this medicine. If you have any questions about what kind of identification to carry, check with your health care professional.

While you are taking this medicine, it is very important that you avoid sports and activities that may cause you to be injured. Report to your doctor any falls, blows to the body or head, or other injuries, since serious internal bleeding may occur without your knowing about it.

Be careful to avoid cutting yourself. This includes taking special care in brushing your teeth and in shaving. Use a soft toothbrush and floss gently. Also, it is best to use an electric shaver rather than a blade.

Drinking too much alcohol may change the way this anticoagulant affects your body. You should not drink regularly on a daily basis or take more than one or two drinks at any time. If you have any questions about this, check with your doctor.

The foods that you eat may also affect the way this medicine affects your body. Eat a normal, balanced diet while you are taking this medicine. Do not go on a reducing diet, make other changes in your eating habits, start taking vitamins, or begin using other nutrition supplements unless you have first checked with your health care professional. Also, check with your doctor if you are unable to eat for several days or if you have continuing stomach upset, diarrhea, or fever. These precautions are important because the effects of the anticoagulant depend on the amount of vitamin K in your body. Therefore, it is best to have the same amount of vitamin K in your body every day. Some multiple vitamins and some nutrition supplements contain vitamin K. Vitamin K is also present in meats, dairy products (such as milk, cheese, and yogurt), and green, leafy vegetables (such as broccoli, cabbage, collard greens, kale, lettuce, and spinach). It is especially important that you do not make large changes in the amounts of these foods that you eat every day while you are taking an anticoagulant.

After you stop taking this medicine, your body will need time to recover before your blood clotting ability returns to normal. Your health care professional can tell you how long this will take depending on which anticoagulant you were taking. Use the same caution during this period of time as you did while you were taking the anticoagulant.

Side Effects of This Medicine

Along with its needed effects, a medicine may cause some unwanted effects. Although not all of these side effects may occur, if they do occur they may need medical attention.

Check with your doctor immediately if any of the following side effects occur:

  Less common or rare
    Blue or purple color of toes and pain in toes; cloudy or
    dark urine; difficult or painful urination; sores, ulcers,
    or white spots in mouth or throat; sore throat and fever
    or chills; sudden decrease in amount of urine; swelling
    of face, feet, or lower legs; unusual tiredness or weak-
    ness; unusual weight gain; yellow eyes or skin

Since many things can affect the way your body reacts to this medicine, you should always watch for signs of unusual bleeding. Unusual bleeding may mean that your body is getting more medicine than it needs. *Check with your doctor immediately if any of the following signs of overdose occur:*

  Bleeding from gums when brushing teeth; unexplained bruis-
    ing or purplish areas on skin; unexplained nosebleeds; un-

> usually heavy bleeding or oozing from cuts or wounds; unusually heavy or unexpected menstrual bleeding

Signs and symptoms of bleeding inside the body

> Abdominal or stomach pain or swelling; back pain or backaches; blood in urine; bloody or black tarry stools; constipation; coughing up blood; dizziness; headache (severe or continuing); joint pain, stiffness, or swelling; vomiting blood or material that looks like coffee grounds

Also, check with your doctor as soon as possible if any of the following side effects occur:

Less common or rare

> Diarrhea (more common with dicumarol); nausea or vomiting; skin rash, hives, or itching; stomach cramps or pain

For patients taking *anisindione* (e.g., Miradon):

- Depending on your diet, this medicine may cause your urine to turn orange. Since it may be hard to tell the difference between blood in the urine and this normal color change, check with your doctor if you notice any color change in your urine.

Other side effects may occur that usually do not need medical attention. These side effects may go away during treatment as your body adjusts to the medicine. However, check with your doctor if any of the following side effects continue or are bothersome:

More common

> Bloated feeling or gas (with dicumarol)

Less common

> Blurred vision or other vision problems (with anisindione); loss of appetite; unusual hair loss

Other side effects not listed above may also occur in some patients. If you notice any other effects, check with your doctor.

ANTICONVULSANTS, HYDANTOIN Systemic

Some commonly used brand names are:

In the U.S.—

Dilantin[3]

Dilantin-125[3]

Dilantin Infatabs[3]

Dilantin Kapseals[3]

Diphenylan[3]

Mesantoin[2]

Peganone[1]

Phenytex[3]

In Canada—

Dilantin[3]

Dilantin-30[3]

Dilantin-125[3]

Dilantin Infatabs[3]

Mesantoin[2]

Another commonly used name for phenytoin is diphenylhydantoin.

Note: For quick reference, the following hydantoin anticonvulsants are numbered to match the corresponding brand names.

This information applies to the following medicines:

1. Ethotoin (ETH-oh-toyn)†
2. Mephenytoin (me-FEN-i-toyn)
3. Phenytoin (FEN-i-toyn)‡

---

†Not commercially available in Canada.

‡Generic name product may also be available in the U.S.

Description

Hydantoin anticonvulsants (hye-DAN-toyn an-tye-kon-VUL-sants) are used most often to control certain convulsions or seizures in the treatment of epilepsy. Phenytoin may also be used for other conditions as determined by your doctor.

In seizure disorders, these medicines act on the central nervous system (CNS) to reduce the number and severity of seizures. Hydantoin anticonvulsants may also produce some unwanted effects. These depend on the patient's individual condition, the amount of medicine taken, and how long it has been taken. It is important that you know what the side effects are and when to call your doctor if they occur.

Hydantoin anticonvulsants are available only with your doctor's prescription, in the following dosage forms:

Oral

  Ethotoin
    • Tablets (U.S.)

  Mephenytoin
    • Tablets (U.S. and Canada)

  Phenytoin
    • Extended capsules (U.S. and Canada)
    • Prompt capsules (U.S.)
    • Oral suspension (U.S. and Canada)
    • Chewable tablets (U.S. and Canada)

Parenteral

  Phenytoin
    • Injection (U.S. and Canada)

Before Using This Medicine

In deciding to use a medicine, the risks of taking the medicine must be weighed against the good it will do. This is a decision you and your doctor will make. For hydantoin anticonvulsants, the following should be considered:

Allergies—Tell your doctor if you have ever had any unusual or allergic reaction to any hydantoin anticonvulsant medicine. Also tell your health care professional if you are allergic to any other substance, such as foods, preservatives, or dyes.

Pregnancy—Although most mothers who take medicine for seizure control deliver normal babies, there have been reports of increased birth defects when these medicines were used during pregnancy. It is not definitely known if any of these medicines are the cause of such problems.

Also, pregnancy may cause a change in the way hydantoin anticonvulsants are absorbed in your body. You may have more seizures, even though you are taking your medicine regularly. Your doctor may need to increase the anticonvulsant dose during your pregnancy.

In addition, when taken during pregnancy, this medicine may cause a bleeding problem in the mother during delivery and in the newborn. This may be prevented by giving vitamin K to the mother during delivery, and to the baby immediately after birth.

Breast-feeding—Ethotoin and phenytoin pass into the breast milk in small amounts. It is not known whether mephenytoin passes into breast milk. Be sure you have discussed the risks and benefits of the medicine with your doctor.

Children—Some side effects, especially bleeding, tender, or enlarged gums and enlarged facial features, are more likely to occur in children and young adults. Also, unusual and excessive hair growth may occur, which is more noticeable in young girls. In addition, some children may not do as well in school after using high doses of this medicine for a long time.

Older adults—Some medicines may affect older patients differently than they do younger patients. Overdose is more likely to occur in elderly patients and in patients with liver disease.

Other medicines—Although certain medicines should not be used together at all, in other cases two different medicines may be used together even if an interaction might occur. In these cases, your doctor may want to change the dose, or other precautions may be necessary. When you are taking or receiving hydantoin anticonvulsants, it is especially important that your health care professional know if you are taking any of the following:

- Alcohol or
- Central nervous system (CNS) depressants (medicine that causes drowsiness)—Long-term use of alcohol may decrease the blood levels of hydantoin anticonvulsants, resulting in decreased effects; use of hydantoin anticonvulsants in cases where a large amount of alcohol is consumed may increase the blood levels of the hydantoin, resulting in an increased risk of side effects

- Aminophylline (e.g., Somophyllin) or
- Caffeine (e.g., NoDoz) or
- Oxtriphylline (e.g., Choledyl) or
- Theophylline (e.g., Somophyllin-T)—Hydantoin anticonvulsants may make these medicines less effective

- Amiodarone (e.g., Cordarone)—Use with phenytoin and possibly with other hydantoin anticonvulsants may increase blood levels of the hydantoin, resulting in an increase in serious side effects

- Antacids or
- Medicine containing calcium—Use of antacids or calcium supplements may decrease the absorption of phenytoin; doses of antacids and phenytoin or calcium supplements and phenytoin should be taken 2 to 3 hours apart

- Anticoagulants (blood thinners) or
- Chloramphenicol (e.g., Chloromycetin) or
- Cimetidine (e.g., Tagamet) or
- Disulfiram (e.g., Antabuse) (medicine for alcoholism) or
- Isoniazid (INH) (e.g., Nydrazid) or
- Fluconazole (e.g., Diflucan) or
- Fluoxetine (e.g., Prozac) or
- Phenylbutazone (e.g., Butazolidin) or
- Sulfonamides (sulfa drugs)—Blood levels of hydantoin anticonvulsants may be increased, increasing the risk of serious side effects; hydantoin anticonvulsants may increase the effects of the anticoagulants at first, but with continued use may decrease the effects of these medicines

- Corticosteroids (cortisone-like medicines) or
- Estrogens (female hormones) or
- Oral contraceptives (birth-control pills) containing estrogens—Hydantoin anticonvulsants may decrease the effects of these medicines; use of hydantoin anticonvulsants with

oral, estrogen-containing contraceptives may result in breakthrough bleeding and contraceptive failure; the amount of estrogen in the oral contraceptive may need to be increased to stop the bleeding and decrease the risk of pregnancy

- Diazoxide (e.g., Proglycem)—Use with hydantoin anticonvulsants may decrease the effects of both medicines; therefore, these medicines should not be taken together

- Lidocaine—Risk of slow heartbeat may be increased. Other effects of lidocaine may be decreased because hydantoin anticonvulsants may cause it to be removed from the body more quickly

- Methadone (e.g., Dolophine, Methadose)—Long-term use of phenytoin may bring on withdrawal symptoms in patients being treated for drug dependence

- Phenacemide (e.g., Phenurone)—Use with hydantoin anticonvulsants may increase the risk of serious side effects

- Rifampin (e.g., Rifadin)—Use with phenytoin may decrease the effects of phenytoin; your doctor may need to adjust your dosage

- Streptozocin (e.g., Zanosar)—Phenytoin may decrease the effects of streptozocin; therefore, these medicines should not be used together

- Sucralfate (e.g., Carafate)—Use of sucralfate may decrease the absorption of hydantoin anticonvulsants

- Valproic acid (e.g., Depakene, Depakote)—Use with phenytoin, and possibly other hydantoin anticonvulsants, may increase seizure frequency and increase the risk of serious liver side effects, especially in infants

Other medical problems—The presence of other medical problems may affect the use of hydantoin anticonvulsants. Make sure you tell your doctor if you have any other medical problems, especially:

- Alcohol abuse—Blood levels of phenytoin may be decreased, decreasing its effects

- Blood disease—Risk of serious infections rarely may be increased by hydantoin anticonvulsants

- Diabetes mellitus (sugar diabetes) or

- Porphyria or
- Systemic lupus erythematosus—Hydantoin anticonvulsants may make the condition worse
- Fever above 101°F for longer than 24 hours—Blood levels of hydantoin anticonvulsants may be decreased, decreasing the medicine's effects
- Heart disease—Administration of phenytoin by injection may change the rhythm of the heart
- Kidney disease or
- Liver disease—Blood levels of hydantoin anticonvulsants may be increased, leading to an increase in serious side effects
- Thyroid disease—Blood levels of thyroid hormones may be decreased

---

Proper Use of This Medicine

For patients taking the *liquid form* of this medicine:

- Shake the bottle well before using.
- Use a specially marked measuring spoon, a plastic syringe, or a small measuring cup to measure each dose accurately. The average household teaspoon may not hold the right amount of liquid.

For patients taking the *chewable tablet form* of this medicine:

- Tablets may be chewed or crushed before they are swallowed, or may be swallowed whole.

For patients taking the *capsule form* of this medicine:

- Swallow the capsule whole.

If this medicine upsets your stomach, take it with food, unless otherwise directed by your doctor. The medicine should always be taken at the same time in relation to meals to make sure that it is absorbed in the same way.

To control your medical problem, *take this medicine every day* exactly as ordered by your doctor. Do not take more or less of it than your doctor ordered. To help you remember to take the medicine at the correct times, try to get into the habit of taking it at the same time each day.

Dosing—The dose of hydantoin anticonvulsants will be different for different patients. *Follow your doctor's orders or the directions on the label.* The following information includes only the average doses of ethotoin, mephenytoin, and phenytoin. *If your dose is different, do not change it* unless your doctor tells you to do so.

The number of capsules or tablets or teaspoonfuls of suspension that you take depends on the strength of the medicine. Also, *the number of doses you take each day, the time allowed between doses, and the length of time you take the medicine depend on the medical problem for which you are using an hydantoin anticonvulsant.*

For ethotoin

- For *oral* dosage form (tablets):
  —As an anticonvulsant:
    - Adults and teenagers—To start, 125 to 250 milligrams (mg) four to six times a day. Your doctor may increase your dose gradually over several days if needed. However, the dose is usually not more than 3000 mg a day.
    - Children—To start, up to 750 mg a day, based on the age and weight of the child. The doctor may increase the dose gradually if needed.

For mephenytoin

- For *oral* dosage form (tablets):
  —As an anticonvulsant:
    - Adults and teenagers—To start, 50 to 100 milligrams (mg) once a day. Your doctor may increase your dose by 50 to 100 mg a day at weekly intervals if needed. However, the dose is usually not more than 1200 mg a day.
    - Children—To start, 25 to 50 mg once a day.

The doctor may increase the dose by 25 to 50 mg a day at weekly intervals if needed. However, the dose is usually not more than 400 mg a day.

For phenytoin

- For *oral* dosage forms (capsules, chewable tablets, or suspension):

  —As an anticonvulsant:

  - Adults and teenagers—To start, 100 to 125 milligrams (mg) three times a day. Your doctor may adjust your dose at intervals of seven to ten days if needed.

  - Children—Dose is based on body weight or body surface area. The usual dose is 5 mg of phenytoin per kilogram (kg) (2.3 mg per pound) of body weight to start. The doctor may adjust the dose if needed.

  - Older adults—Dose is based on body weight. The usual dose is 3 mg per kg (1.4 mg per pound) of body weight. The doctor may need to adjust the dose based on your response to the medicine.

- For *injection* dosage form:

  —As an anticonvulsant:

  - Adults and children—Dose is based on illness being treated, and body weight or body surface area of the patient. The medicine is usually injected into a vein.

Missed dose—*If you miss a dose of this medicine* and your dosing schedule is:

- One dose a day—Take the missed dose as soon as possible. However, if you do not remember the missed dose until the next day, skip it and go back to your regular dosing schedule. Do not double doses.

- More than one dose a day—Take the missed dose as soon as possible. However, if it is within 4 hours of

your next dose, skip the missed dose and go back to your regular dosing schedule. Do not double doses.

If you miss doses for 2 or more days in a row, check with your doctor.

Storage—To store this medicine:

- Keep out of the reach of children.
- Store away from heat and direct light.
- Do not store in the bathroom, near the kitchen sink, or in other damp places. Heat or moisture may cause the medicine to break down.
- Keep the liquid form of this medicine from freezing. Do not refrigerate.
- Do not keep outdated medicine or medicine no longer needed. Be sure any discarded medicine is out of the reach of children.

Precautions While Using This Medicine

Your doctor should check your progress at regular visits, especially during the first few months of treatment with this medicine. During this time the amount of medicine you are taking may have to be changed often to meet your individual needs.

Do not start or stop taking any other medicine without your doctor's advice. Other medicines may affect the way this medicine works.

This medicine will add to the effects of alcohol and other CNS depressants (medicines that slow down the nervous system, possibly causing drowsiness). Some examples of CNS depressants are antihistamines or medicine for hay fever, other allergies, or colds; sedatives, tranquilizers, or sleeping medicine; prescription pain medicine or narcotics; barbiturates; other medicine for seizures; muscle relaxants; or anesthetics, including some dental anesthetics. *Check with your doctor before taking any of the above while you are using this medicine.*

Do not take this medicine within 2 to 3 hours of taking antacids or medicine for diarrhea. Taking these medicines and hydantoin anticonvulsants too close together may make the hydantoins less effective.

Do not change brands or dosage forms of phenytoin without first checking with your doctor. Different products may not work the same way. If you refill your medicine and it looks different, check with your pharmacist.

If you have been taking this medicine regularly for several weeks or more, do not suddenly stop taking it. Your doctor may want you to reduce gradually the amount you are taking before stopping completely.

Your doctor may want you to carry a medical identification card or bracelet stating that you are taking this medicine.

For diabetic patients:
• This medicine may affect blood sugar levels. If you notice a change in the results of your blood or urine sugar tests or if you have any questions, check with your doctor

Before you have any medical tests, tell the doctor in charge that you are taking this medicine. The results of some tests (including the dexamethasone, metyrapone, or Schilling tests, and certain thyroid function tests) may be affected by this medicine.

Before having any kind of surgery, dental treatment, or emergency treatment, tell the medical doctor or dentist in charge that you are taking this medicine. Taking hydantoin anticonvulsants together with medicines that are used during surgery or dental or emergency treatments may cause increased side effects.

This medicine may cause some people to become dizzy, lightheaded, drowsy, or less alert than they are normally. After you have taken this medicine for a while, this effect may not be so bothersome. However, *make sure you know how you react to this medicine before you drive, use machines, or do anything else that could be dangerous if you are dizzy or are not alert.*

Oral contraceptives (birth control pills) containing estrogen may not work properly if you take them while you are taking hydantoin anticonvulsants. Unplanned pregnancies may occur. You should use a different or additional means of birth control while you are taking hydantoin anticonvulsants. If you have any questions about this, check with your health care professional.

For patients taking *phenytoin* or *mephenytoin*:

- In some patients (usually younger patients), tenderness, swelling, or bleeding of the gums (gingival hyperplasia) may appear soon after phenytoin or mephenytoin treatment is started. To help prevent this, brush and floss your teeth carefully and regularly and massage your gums. Also, *see your dentist every 3 months to have your teeth cleaned. If you have any questions about how to take care of your teeth and gums, or if you notice any tenderness, swelling, or bleeding of your gums, check with your doctor or dentist.*

Side Effects of This Medicine

Along with its needed effects, a medicine may cause some unwanted effects. Although not all of these side effects may occur, if they do occur they may need medical attention.

Check with your doctor as soon as possible if any of the following side effects or signs of overdose occur:

More common

Bleeding, tender, or enlarged gums (rare with ethotoin); clumsiness or unsteadiness; confusion; continuous, uncontrolled back-and-forth and/or rolling eye movements—may be sign of overdose; enlarged glands in neck or underarms; fever; increase in seizures; mood or mental changes; muscle weakness or pain; skin rash or itching; slurred speech or stuttering—may be sign of overdose; sore throat; trembling—may be sign of overdose; unusual excitement, nervousness, or irritability

Rare

Bone malformations; burning pain at place of injection; chest discomfort; chills and fever; dark urine; dizziness; frequent breaking of bones; headache; joint pain; learning difficulties—in children taking high doses for a long time; light gray–colored stools; loss of appetite; nausea or vomiting; pain of penis on erection; restlessness or agitation; slowed growth; stomach pain (severe); troubled or quick, shallow breathing; uncontrolled jerking or twisting movements of hands, arms, or legs; uncontrolled movements of lips, tongue, or cheeks; unusual bleeding (such as nosebleeds) or bruising; unusual tiredness or weakness; weight loss (unusual); yellow eyes or skin

Rare (with long-term use of phenytoin)

Numbness, tingling, or pain in hands or feet

Symptoms of overdose

Blurred or double vision; clumsiness or unsteadiness (severe); confusion (severe); dizziness or drowsiness (severe); staggering walk

Other side effects may occur that usually do not need medical attention. These side effects may go away during treatment as your body adjusts to the medicine. However, check with your doctor if any of the following side effects continue or are bothersome:

More common

Constipation; dizziness (mild); drowsiness (mild)

Less common

> Diarrhea (with ethotoin); enlargement of jaw; muscle twitching; swelling of breasts—in males; thickening of lips; trouble in sleeping; unusual and excessive hair growth on body and face (more common with phenytoin); widening of nose tip

Other side effects not listed above may also occur in some patients. If you notice any other effects, check with your doctor.

Additional Information

Once a medicine has been approved for marketing for a certain use, experience may show that it is also useful for other medical problems. Although these uses are not included in product labeling, phenytoin is used in certain patients with the following medical conditions:

- Cardiac arrhythmias (changes in your heart rhythm) caused by digitalis medicine
- Episodic dyscontrol (certain behavior disorders)
- Myotonia congenita or
- Myotonic muscular dystrophy or
- Neuromyotonia
  (certain muscle disorders)
- Paroxysmal choreoathetosis (certain movement disorders)
- Tricyclic antidepressant poisoning
- Trigeminal neuralgia (tic douloureux)

Other than the above information, there is no additional information relating to proper use, precautions, or side effects for these uses.

ANTIDEPRESSANTS, MONOAMINE OXIDASE (MAO) INHIBITOR   Systemic

Some commonly used brand names are:

In the U.S.—

Marplan[1]   Parnate[3]

Nardil[2]

In Canada—

Marplan[1]   Parnate[3]

Nardil[2]

Note: For quick reference, the following antidepressants are numbered to match the corresponding brand names.

This information applies to the following medicines:

1. Isocarboxazid (eye-soe-kar-BOX-a-zid)
2. Phenelzine (FEN-el-zeen)
3. Tranylcypromine (tran-ill-SIP-roe-meen)

Note: This information does *not* apply to furazolidone, procarbazine, or selegiline.

Description

Monoamine oxidase (MAO) inhibitors are used to relieve certain types of mental depression. They work by blocking the action of a chemical substance known as monoamine oxidase (MAO) in the nervous system.

Although these medicines are very effective for certain patients, they may also cause some unwanted reactions if not taken in the right way. It is very important to avoid certain foods, beverages, and medicines while you are being treated with an MAO inhibitor. Your health care professional will help you obtain a list to carry in your wallet or purse as a reminder of which products you should avoid.

MAO inhibitors are available only with your doctor's prescription, in the following dosage forms:

Oral

Isocarboxazid
  • Tablets (U.S. and Canada)
Phenelzine
  • Tablets (U.S. and Canada)
Tranylcypromine
  • Tablets (U.S. and Canada)

Before Using This Medicine

In deciding to use a medicine, the risks of taking the medicine must be weighed against the good it will do. This is a decision you and your doctor will make. For monoamine oxidase (MAO) inhibitors, the following should be considered:

Allergies—Tell your doctor if you have ever had any unusual or allergic reaction to any MAO inhibitor. Also tell your health care professional if you are allergic to any other substances, such as foods, preservatives, or dyes.

Diet—Dangerous reactions such as sudden high blood pressure may result when MAO inhibitors are taken with certain foods or drinks. The following foods should be avoided:

  • Foods that have a high tyramine content (most common in foods that are aged or fermented to increase their flavor), such as cheeses; fava or broad bean pods; yeast or meat extracts; smoked or pickled meat, poultry, or fish; fermented sausage (bologna, pepperoni, salami, summer sausage) or other fermented meat; sauerkraut; or any overripe fruit. If a list of these foods and beverages is not given to you, ask your health care professional to provide one.

  • Alcoholic beverages or alcohol-free or reduced-alcohol beer and wine.

- Large amounts of caffeine-containing food or beverages such as coffee, tea, cola, or chocolate.

Pregnancy—A limited study in pregnant women showed an increased risk of birth defects when these medicines were taken during the first 3 months of pregnancy. In animal studies, MAO inhibitors caused a slowing of growth and increased excitability in the newborn when very large doses were given to the mother during pregnancy.

Breast-feeding—Tranylcypromine passes into the breast milk; it is not known whether isocarboxazid or phenelzine passes into breast milk. Problems in nursing babies have not been reported.

Children—Studies on these medicines have been done only in adult patients, and there is no specific information comparing use of MAO inhibitors in children with use in other age groups. However, animal studies have shown that these medicines may slow growth in the young. Therefore, be sure to discuss with your doctor the use of these medicines in children.

Older adults—Dizziness or lightheadedness may be especially likely to occur in elderly patients, who are usually more sensitive than younger adults to these effects of MAO inhibitors.

Other medicines—Although certain medicines should not be used together at all, in other cases two different medicines may be used together even if an interaction might occur. In these cases, your doctor may want to change the dose, or other precautions may be necessary. When you are taking MAO inhibitors, it is especially important that your health care professional know if you are taking any of the following:

- Amphetamines or
- Antihypertensives (high blood pressure medicine) or
- Appetite suppressants (diet pills) or

- Cyclobenzaprine (e.g., Flexeril) or
- Fluoxetine (e.g., Prozac) or
- Levodopa (e.g., Dopar, Larodopa) or
- Maprotiline (e.g., Ludiomil) or
- Medicine for asthma or other breathing problems or
- Medicines for colds, sinus problems, or hay fever or other allergies (including nose drops or sprays) or
- Meperidine (e.g., Demerol) or
- Methylphenidate (e.g., Ritalin) or
- Monoamine oxidase (MAO) inhibitors, other, including furazolidone (e.g., Furoxone), procarbazine (e.g., Matulane), or selegiline (e.g., Eldepryl), or
- Paroxetine (e.g., Paxil), or
- Sertraline (e.g., Zoloft), or
- Tricyclic antidepressants (amitriptyline [e.g., Elavil], amoxapine [e.g., Asendin], clomipramine [e.g., Anafranil], desipramine [e.g., Pertofrane], doxepin [e.g., Sinequan], imipramine [e.g., Tofranil], nortriptyline [e.g., Aventyl], protriptyline [e.g., Vivactil], trimipramine [e.g., Surmontil])—Using these medicines while you are taking or within 2 weeks of taking MAO inhibitors may cause serious side effects such as sudden rise in body temperature, extremely high blood pressure, severe convulsions, and death; however, sometimes certain of these medicines may be used with MAO inhibitors under close supervision by your doctor
- Antidiabetics, oral (diabetes medicine you take by mouth) or
- Insulin—MAO inhibitors may change the amount of antidiabetic medicine you need to take
- Bupropion (e.g., Wellbutrin)—Using bupropion while you are taking or within 2 weeks of taking MAO inhibitors may cause serious side effects such as seizures
- Buspirone (e.g., BuSpar)—Use with MAO inhibitors may cause high blood pressure
- Carbamazepine (e.g., Tegretol)—Use with MAO inhibitors may increase seizures
- Central nervous system (CNS) depressants (medicines that cause drowsiness)—Using these medicines with MAO inhibitors may increase the CNS and other depressant effects

- Cocaine—Cocaine use by persons taking MAO inhibitors, including furazolidone and procarbazine, may cause a severe increase in blood pressure
- Dextromethorphan—Use with MAO inhibitors may cause excitement, high blood pressure, and fever
- Trazodone or
- Tryptophan used as a food supplement or a sleep aid— Use of these medicines by persons taking MAO inhibitors, including furazolidone and procarbazine, may cause mental confusion, excitement, shivering, trouble in breathing, or fever

Other medical problems—The presence of other medical problems may affect the use of MAO inhibitors. Make sure you tell your doctor if you have any other medical problems, especially:

- Alcohol abuse—Drinking alcohol while you are taking an MAO inhibitor may cause serious side effects
- Angina (chest pain) or
- Headaches (severe or frequent)—These conditions may interfere with warning signs of serious side effects of MAO inhibitors
- Asthma or bronchitis—Some medicines used to treat these conditions may cause serious side effects when used while you are taking an MAO inhibitor
- Diabetes mellitus (sugar diabetes)—These medicines may change the amount of insulin or oral antidiabetic medication that you need
- Epilepsy—Seizures may occur more often
- Heart or blood vessel disease or
- Liver disease or
- Mental illness (or history of) or
- Parkinson's disease or
- Recent heart attack or stroke—MAO inhibitors may make the condition worse
- High blood pressure—Condition may be affected by these medicines
- Kidney disease—Higher blood levels of MAO inhibitors may occur, which increases the chance of side effects

- Overactive thyroid or
- Pheochromocytoma (PCC)—Serious side effects may occur

Proper Use of This Medicine

Sometimes this medicine must be taken for several weeks before you begin to feel better. Your doctor should check your progress at regular visits, especially during the first few months of treatment, to make sure that this medicine is working properly and to check for unwanted effects.

Take this medicine only as directed by your doctor. Do not take more of it, do not take it more often, and do not take it for a longer time than your doctor ordered.

MAO inhibitors may be taken with or without food or on a full or empty stomach. However, if your doctor tells you to take the medicine a certain way, take it exactly as directed.

Dosing—The dose of MAO inhibitors will be different for different patients. *Follow your doctor's orders or the directions on the label.* The following information includes only the average doses of isocarboxazid, phenelzine, and tranylcypromine. *If your dose is different, do not change it* unless your doctor tells you to do so.

The number of tablets that you take depends on the strength of the medicine. Also, *the number of doses you take each day, the time allowed between doses, and the length of time you take the medicine depend on the medical problem for which you are using an MAO inhibitor.*

For isocarboxazid

- For *oral* dosage form (tablets):
  —For treatment of depression:
    - Adults—To start, 30 milligrams (mg) a day. Your doctor may decrease or increase your dose

as needed. However, the dose is usually not more than 60 mg a day.

• Children up to 16 years of age—Use and dose must be determined by the doctor.

For phenelzine

• For *oral* dosage form (tablets):

—For treatment of depression:

• Adults—Dose is based on your body weight. To start, the usual dose is 1 milligram (mg) per kilogram (kg) of body weight (0.45 mg per pound) a day. Your doctor may decrease or increase your dose as needed. However, the dose is usually not more than 90 mg a day.

• Children up to 16 years of age—Use and dose must be determined by the doctor.

• Older adults—To start, 15 mg in the morning. Your doctor may increase your dose gradually as needed. However, the dose is usually not more than 60 mg a day.

For tranylcypromine

• For *oral* dosage form (tablets):

—For treatment of depression:

• Adults—To start, 30 milligrams (mg) a day. Your doctor may increase your dose gradually as needed. However, the dose is usually not more than 60 mg a day.

• Children up to 16 years of age—Use and dose must be determined by the doctor.

• Older adults—To start, 2.5 to 5 mg a day. The doctor may increase your dose as needed. However, the dose is usually not more than 45 mg a day.

Missed dose—If you miss a dose of this medicine, take it as soon as possible. However, if it is within 2 hours of

your next dose, skip the missed dose and go back to your regular dosing schedule. Do not double doses.

Storage—To store this medicine:

- Keep out of the reach of children.
- Store away from heat and direct light.
- Do not store in the bathroom, near the kitchen sink, or in other damp places. Heat or moisture may cause the medicine to break down.
- Do not keep outdated medicine or medicine no longer needed. Be sure that any discarded medicine is out of the reach of children.

Precautions While Using This Medicine

When taken with certain foods, drinks, or other medicines, MAO inhibitors can cause very dangerous reactions such as sudden high blood pressure (also called hypertensive crisis). To avoid such reactions, *obey the following rules of caution:*

- Do not eat foods that have a high tyramine content (most common in foods that are aged or fermented to increase their flavor), such as cheeses; fava or broad bean pods; yeast or meat extracts; smoked or pickled meat, poultry, or fish; fermented sausage (bologna, pepperoni, salami, and summer sausage) or other fermented meat; sauerkraut; or any overripe fruit. If a list of these foods is not given to you, ask your health care professional to provide one.
- Do not drink alcoholic beverages or alcohol-free or reduced-alcohol beer and wine.
- Do not eat or drink large amounts of caffeine-containing food or beverages such as coffee, tea, cola, or chocolate.
- Do not take any other medicine unless approved or

prescribed by your doctor. This especially includes nonprescription (over-the-counter [OTC]) medicine, such as that for colds (including nose drops or sprays), cough, asthma, hay fever, and appetite control; "keep awake" products; or products that make you sleepy.

This medicine will add to the effects of alcohol and other CNS depressants (medicines that slow down the nervous system, possibly causing drowsiness). Some examples of CNS depressants are antihistamines or medicine for hay fever, other allergies, or colds; sedatives, tranquilizers, or sleeping medicine; prescription pain medicine or narcotics; barbiturates; medicine for seizures; muscle relaxants; or anesthetics, including some dental anesthetics. *Check with your doctor before taking any of the above while you are using this medicine.*

Check with your doctor or hospital emergency room immediately if severe headache, stiff neck, chest pains, fast heartbeat, or nausea and vomiting occur while you are taking this medicine. These may be symptoms of a serious side effect that should have a doctor's attention.

Do not stop taking this medicine without first checking with your doctor. Your doctor may want you to reduce gradually the amount you are using before stopping completely.

Dizziness, lightheadedness, or fainting may occur, especially when you get up from a lying or sitting position. *Getting up slowly may help.* When you get up from lying down, sit on the edge of the bed with your feet dangling for 1 or 2 minutes. Then stand up slowly. If the problem continues or gets worse, check with your doctor.

This medicine may cause blurred vision or make some people drowsy or less alert than they are normally. *Make sure you know how you react to this medicine before you* drive, use machines, or do anything else that could be dangerous if you are unable to see well or are not alert.

Before having any kind of surgery, dental treatment, or emergency treatment, tell the medical doctor or dentist in charge that you are using this medicine or have used it within the past 2 weeks. Taking MAO inhibitors together with medicines that are used during surgery or dental or emergency treatments may increase the risk of serious side effects.

Your doctor may want you to carry an identification card stating that you are using this medicine.

For patients with *angina* (chest pain):
- This medicine may cause you to have an unusual feeling of good health and energy. However, *do not suddenly increase the amount of exercise you get without discussing it with your doctor.* Too much activity could bring on an attack of angina.

For *diabetic* patients:
- This medicine may affect blood sugar levels. While you are using this medicine, be especially careful in testing for sugar in your blood or urine. If you have any questions about this, check with your doctor.

After you stop using this medicine, you must continue to obey the rules of caution for at least 2 weeks concerning food, drink, and other medicine, since these things may continue to react with MAO inhibitors.

Side Effects of This Medicine

Along with its needed effects, a medicine may cause some unwanted effects. Although not all of these side effects may occur, if they do occur they may need medical attention.

Stop taking this medicine and get emergency help immediately if any of the following side effects occur:

Symptoms of unusually high blood pressure (hypertensive crisis)

Chest pain (severe); enlarged pupils; fast or slow heartbeat; headache (severe); increased sensitivity of eyes to light; increased sweating (possibly with fever or cold, clammy skin); nausea and vomiting; stiff or sore neck

Check with your doctor as soon as possible if any of the following side effects occur:

More common

Dizziness or lightheadedness (severe), especially when getting up from a lying or sitting position

Less common

Diarrhea; fast or pounding heartbeat; swelling of feet or lower legs; unusual excitement or nervousness

Rare

Dark urine; fever; skin rash; slurred speech; sore throat; staggering walk; yellow eyes or skin

Symptoms of overdose

Anxiety (severe); confusion; convulsions (seizures); cool, clammy skin; dizziness (severe); drowsiness (severe); fast and irregular pulse; fever; hallucinations (seeing, hearing, or feeling things that are not there); headache (severe); high or low blood pressure; muscle stiffness; sweating; troubled breathing; trouble in sleeping (severe); unusual irritability

Other side effects may occur that usually do not need medical attention. These side effects may go away during treatment as your body adjusts to the medicine. However, check with your doctor if any of the following side effects continue or are bothersome:

More common

Blurred vision; decreased amount of urine; decreased sexual ability; dizziness or lightheadedness (mild), especially when getting up from a lying or sitting position;

drowsiness; headache (mild); increased appetite (especially for sweets) or weight gain; increased sweating; muscle twitching during sleep; restlessness; shakiness or trembling; tiredness and weakness; trouble in sleeping

Less common or rare

Chills; constipation; decreased appetite; dryness of mouth

Other side effects not listed above may also occur in some patients. If you notice any other effects, check with your doctor.

Additional Information

Once a medicine has been approved for marketing for a certain use, experience may show that it is also useful for other medical problems. Although these uses are not included in product labeling, phenelzine and tranylcypromine are used in certain patients with the following medical conditions:

- Headache
- Panic disorder

Other than the above information, there is no additional information relating to proper use, precautions, or side effects for these uses.

ANTIDEPRESSANTS, TRICYCLIC Systemic

Some commonly used brand names are:

In the U.S.—

Anafranil[3]	Enovil[1]
Asendin[2]	Norfranil[6]
Aventyl[7]	Norpramin[4]
Elavil[1]	Pamelor[7]
Endep[1]	Sinequan[5]

In the U.S. (cont'd)—
  Surmontil[9]
  Tipramine[6]
  Tofranil[6]
  Tofranil-PM[6]
  Vivactil[8]

In Canada—
  Anafranil[3]
  Apo-Amitriptyline[1]
  Apo-Imipramine[6]
  Apo-Trimip[9]
  Asendin[2]
  Aventyl[7]
  Elavil[1]
  Impril[6]
  Levate[1]
  Norpramin[4]
  Novo-Doxepin[5]
  Novopramine[6]
  Novo-Tripramine[9]
  Novotriptyn[1]
  Pertofrane[4]
  Rhotrimine[9]
  Sinequan[5]
  Surmontil[9]
  Tofranil[6]
  Triadapin[5]
  Triptil[8]

Note: For quick reference, the following tricyclic antidepressants are numbered to match the corresponding brand names.

This information applies to the following medicines:
1. Amitriptyline (a-mee-TRIP-ti-leen)‡§
2. Amoxapine (a-MOX-a-peen)‡
3. Clomipramine (cloe-MIP-ra-meen)
4. Desipramine (dess-IP-ra-meen)‡§
5. Doxepin (DOX-e-pin)‡
6. Imipramine (im-IP-ra-meen)‡§
7. Nortriptyline (nor-TRIP-ti-leen)‡
8. Protriptyline (proe-TRIP-ti-leen)
9. Trimipramine (trye-MIP-ra-meen)‡

‡Generic name product may also be available in the U.S.
§Generic name product may also be available in Canada.

Description

Tricyclic antidepressants are used to relieve mental depression.

One form of this medicine (imipramine) is also used to treat enuresis (bedwetting) in children. Another form (clomipramine) is used to treat obsessive-compulsive disorders. Tricyclic antidepressants may be used for other conditions as determined by your doctor.

These medicines are available only with your doctor's prescription, in the following dosage forms:

Oral

Amitriptyline
- Syrup (Canada)
- Tablets (U.S. and Canada)

Amoxapine
- Tablets (U.S. and Canada)

Clomipramine
- Capsules (U.S.)
- Tablets (Canada)

Desipramine
- Tablets (U.S. and Canada)

Doxepin
- Capsules (U.S. and Canada)
- Oral solution (U.S.)

Imipramine
- Capsules (U.S.)
- Tablets (U.S. and Canada)

Nortriptyline
- Capsules (U.S. and Canada)
- Oral solution (U.S.)

Protriptyline
- Tablets (U.S. and Canada)

Trimipramine
- Capsules (U.S. and Canada)
- Tablets (Canada)

Parenteral

Amitriptyline
- Injection (U.S.)

Imipramine
- Injection (U.S.)

Before Using This Medicine

In deciding to use a medicine, the risks of taking the medicine must be weighed against the good it will do. This is a decision you and your doctor will make. For tricyclic antidepressants, the following should be considered:

Allergies—Tell your doctor if you have ever had any unusual or allergic reaction to any tricyclic antidepressant or to carbamazepine, maprotiline, or trazodone. Also tell your health care professional if you are allergic to any other substances, such as foods, preservatives, or dyes.

Pregnancy—Studies have not been done in pregnant women. However, there have been reports of newborns suffering from muscle spasms and heart, breathing, and urinary problems when their mothers had taken tricyclic antidepressants immediately before delivery. Also, studies in animals have shown that some tricyclic antidepressants may cause unwanted effects in the fetus.

Breast-feeding—Tricyclic antidepressants pass into the breast milk. Doxepin has been reported to cause drowsiness in the nursing baby.

Children—Children are especially sensitive to the effects of this medicine. This may increase the chance of side effects during treatment. However, side effects in children taking this medicine for bedwetting usually disappear upon continued use. The most common of these are nervousness, sleeping problems, tiredness, and mild stomach upset. If these side effects continue or are bothersome, check with your doctor.

Older adults—Drowsiness, dizziness, confusion, vision problems, dryness of mouth, constipation, and problems in urinating are more likely to occur in elderly patients, who are usually more sensitive than younger adults to the effects of tricyclic antidepressants.

Other medicines—Although certain medicines should not be used together at all, in other cases 2 different medicines may be used together even if an interaction might occur. In these cases, your doctor may want to change the dose, or other precautions may be necessary. When you are taking a tricyclic antidepressant, it is especially important that your health care professional know if you are taking any of the following:

- Amphetamines or
- Appetite suppressants (diet pills) or
- Ephedrine or
- Epinephrine (e.g., Adrenalin) or
- Isoproterenol (e.g., Isuprel) or
- Medicine for asthma or other breathing problems or
- Medicine for colds, sinus problems, or hay fever or other allergies or
- Phenylephrine (e.g., Neo-Synephrine)—Using these medicines with tricyclic antidepressants may increase the risk of serious effects on the heart
- Antipsychotics (medicine for mental illness) or
- Clonidine (e.g., Catapres)—Using these medicines with tricyclic antidepressants may increase the CNS depressant effects and increase the chance of serious side effects
- Antithyroid agents (medicine for overactive thyroid) or
- Cimetidine (e.g., Tagamet)—Using these medicines with tricyclic antidepressants may increase the chance of serious side effects
- Central nervous system (CNS) depressants (medicine that causes drowsiness)—Using these medicines with tricyclic antidepressants may increase the CNS depressant effects
- Guanadrel (e.g., Hylorel) or
- Guanethidine (e.g., Ismelin)—Tricyclic antidepressants may keep these medicines from working as well
- Methyldopa (e.g., Aldomet) or
- Metoclopramide (e.g., Reglan) or
- Metyrosine (e.g., Demser) or
- Pemoline (e.g., Cylert) or
- Pimozide (e.g., Orap) or
- Promethazine (e.g., Phenergan) or
- Rauwolfia alkaloids (alseroxylon [e.g., Rauwiloid], deserpidine [e.g., Harmonyl], rauwolfia serpentina [e.g., Raudixin], reserpine [e.g., Serpasil]) or
- Trimeprazine (e.g., Temaril)—Tricyclic antidepressants may cause certain side effects to be more severe and occur more often
- Metrizamide—The risk of seizures may be increased

- Monoamine oxidase (MAO) inhibitors (furazolidone [e.g., Furoxone], isocarboxazid [e.g., Marplan], phenelzine [e.g., Nardil], procarbazine [e.g., Matulane], selegiline [e.g., Eldepryl], tranylcypromine [e.g., Parnate])—Taking tricyclic antidepressants while you are taking or within 2 weeks of taking MAO inhibitors may cause sudden high body temperature, extremely high blood pressure, severe convulsions, and death; however, sometimes certain of these medicines may be used together under close supervision by your doctor

Other medical problems—The presence of other medical problems may affect the use of tricyclic antidepressants. Make sure you tell your doctor if you have any other medical problems, especially:

- Alcohol abuse (or history of)—Drinking alcohol may cause increased CNS depressant effects
- Asthma or
- Bipolar disorder (manic-depressive illness) or
- Blood disorders or
- Convulsions (seizures) or
- Difficult urination or
- Enlarged prostate or
- Glaucoma or increased eye pressure or
- Heart disease or
- High blood pressure (hypertension) or
- Schizophrenia—Tricyclic antidepressants may make the condition worse
- Kidney disease or
- Liver disease—Higher blood levels of tricyclic antidepressants may result, increasing the chance of side effects
- Overactive thyroid or
- Stomach or intestinal problems—Tricyclic antidepressants may cause an increased chance of serious side effects

---

Proper Use of This Medicine

To lessen stomach upset, take this medicine with food, even for a daily bedtime dose, unless your doctor has told you to take it on an empty stomach.

Take this medicine only as directed by your doctor, to benefit your condition as much as possible. Do not take more of it, do not take it more often, and do not take it for a longer time than your doctor ordered.

Sometimes this medicine must be taken for several weeks before you begin to feel better. Your doctor should check your progress at regular visits.

To use *doxepin oral solution:*
- This medicine is to be taken by mouth even though it comes in a dropper bottle. The amount you should take should be measured with the dropper provided with your prescription and diluted just before you take each dose. Dilute each dose with about one-half glass (4 ounces) of water, milk, citrus fruit juice, tomato juice, or prune juice. Do not mix this medicine with grape juice or carbonated beverages since these may decrease the medicine's effectiveness.
- Doxepin oral solution must be mixed immediately before you take it. Do not prepare it ahead of time.

Dosing—The dose of tricyclic antidepressants will be different for different patients. *Follow your doctor's orders or the directions on the label.* The following information includes only the average doses of tricyclic antidepressants. *If your dose is different, do not change it* unless your doctor tells you to do so.

The number of capsules or tablets, or the amount of solution or syrup that you take depends on the strength of the medicine. Also, *the number of doses you take each day, the time allowed between doses, and the length of time you take the medicine depend on the medical problem for which you are taking tricyclic antidepressants.*

For amitriptyline
- For *tablet* dosage form:
    —For depression:

• Adults—At first, 25 milligrams (mg) two to four times a day. Your doctor may increase your dose gradually as needed. However, the dose is usually not more than 150 mg a day, unless you are in the hospital. Some hospitalized patients may need higher doses.

• Teenagers—At first, 10 mg three times a day, and 20 mg at bedtime. Your doctor may increase your dose gradually as needed. However, the dose is usually not more than 100 mg a day.

• Children 6 to 12 years of age—10 to 30 mg a day.

• Children up to 6 years of age—Use and dose must be determined by your doctor.

• Older adults— At first, 25 mg at bedtime. Your doctor may increase your dose gradually as needed. However, the dose is usually not more than 100 mg a day.

• For *syrup* dosage form:

—For depression:

• Adults—At first, 25 mg two to four times a day. Your doctor may increase your dose gradually as needed.

• Teenagers—At first, 10 mg three times a day, and 20 mg at bedtime. Your doctor may increase your dose gradually as needed. However, the dose is usually not more than 100 mg a day.

• Children 6 to 12 years of age—10 to 30 mg a day.

• Children up to 6 years of age—Use and dose must be determined by your doctor.

• Older adults—At first, 10 mg three times a day, and 20 mg at bedtime. Your doctor may increase your dose gradually as needed. However, the dose is usually not more than 100 mg a day.

- For *injection* dosage form:
  - —For depression:
    - Adults—20 to 30 mg four times a day, injected into a muscle.
    - Children up to 12 years of age—Use and dose must be determined by your doctor.

For amoxapine

- For *tablet* dosage form:
  - —For depression:
    - Adults—At first, 50 milligrams (mg) two to three times a day. Your doctor may increase your dose gradually as needed.
    - Children up to 16 years of age—Use and dose must be determined by your doctor.
    - Older adults—At first, 25 mg two to three times a day. Your doctor may increase your dose gradually as needed.

For clomipramine

- For *capsule or tablet* dosage forms:
  - —For obsessive-compulsive disorders:
    - Adults—At first, 25 milligrams (mg) once a day. Your doctor may increase your dose gradually as needed. However, the dose is usually not more than 250 mg a day, unless you are in the hospital. Some hospitalized patients may need higher doses.
    - Teenagers and children 10 years of age and over—At first, 25 mg once a day. Your doctor may increase your dose gradually as needed. However, the dose is usually not more than 200 mg a day.
    - Children up to 10 years of age—Use and dose must be determined by your doctor.
    - Older adults—At first, 20 to 30 mg a day. Your doctor may increase your dose gradually as needed.

For desipramine

- For *tablet* dosage form:

  —For depression:

    • Adults—100 to 200 milligrams (mg) a day. Your doctor may increase your dose gradually as needed. However, the dose is usually not more than 300 mg a day.

    • Teenagers—25 to 50 mg a day. Your doctor may increase your dose gradually as needed. However, the dose is usually not more than 100 mg a day.

    • Children 6 to 12 years of age—10 to 30 mg a day.

    • Older adults—25 to 50 mg a day. Your doctor may increase your dose gradually as needed. However, the dose is usually not more than 150 mg a day.

For doxepin

- For *capsule or solution* dosage forms:

  —For depression:

    • Adults—At first, 25 milligrams (mg) three times a day. Your doctor may increase your dose gradually as needed. However, the dose is usually not more than 150 mg a day, unless you are in the hospital. Some hospitalized patients may need higher doses.

    • Children up to 12 years of age—Use and dose must be determined by your doctor.

    • Older adults—At first, 25 to 50 mg a day. Your doctor may increase your dose gradually as needed.

For imipramine

- For *tablet* dosage form:

  —For depression:

    • Adults—25 to 50 milligrams (mg) three to four times a day. Your doctor may increase your dose gradually as needed. However, the dose is usually not more than 200 mg a day, unless you are in the hospital. Some hospitalized patients may need higher doses.

• Adolescents—25 to 50 mg a day. Your doctor may increase your dose gradually as needed. However, the dose is usually not more than 100 mg a day.

• Children 6 to 12 years of age—10 to 30 mg a day.

• Children up to 6 years of age—Use and dose must be determined by your doctor.

• Older adults—At first, 25 mg at bedtime. Your doctor may increase your dose gradually as needed. However, the dose is usually not more than 100 mg a day.

—For bedwetting:

• Children—25 mg once a day, taken one hour before bedtime. Your doctor may increase the dose as needed, based on the child's age.

• For *capsule* dosage form:

—For depression:

• Adults—At first, 75 mg a day taken at bedtime. Your doctor may increase your dose gradually as needed. However, the dose is usually not more than 200 mg a day, unless you are in the hospital. Some hospitalized patients may need higher doses.

• Children up to 12 years of age—Use and dose must be determined by your doctor.

• For *injection* dosage form:

—For depression:

• Adults—Dose must be determined by your doctor. It is injected into a muscle. The dose is usually not more than 300 mg a day.

- Children up to 12 years of age—Use and dose must be determined by your doctor.

For nortriptyline

- For *capsule or solution* dosage forms:
  —For depression:
  - Adults—25 milligrams (mg) three to four times a day. Your doctor may increase your dose gradually as needed. However, the dose is usually not more than 150 mg a day.
  - Teenagers—25 to 50 mg a day. Your doctor may increase your dose gradually as needed.
  - Children 6 to 12 years of age—10 to 20 mg a day.
  - Older adults—30 to 50 mg a day. Your doctor may increase your dose gradually as needed.

For protriptyline

- For *tablet* dosage form:
  —For depression:
  - Adults—At first, 5 to 10 milligrams (mg) three to four times a day. Your doctor may increase your dose gradually as needed. However, the dose is usually not more than 60 mg a day.
  - Teenagers—At first, 5 mg three times a day. Your doctor may increase your dose gradually as needed.
  - Children up to 12 years of age—Use and dose must be determined by your doctor.
  - Older adults—At first, 5 mg three times a day. Your doctor may increase your dose gradually as needed.

For trimipramine

- For *capsule or tablet* dosage forms:
  —For depression:
  - Adults—At first, 75 milligrams (mg) a day.

Your doctor may increase your dose as needed. However, the dose is usually not more than 200 mg a day, unless you are hospitalized. Some hospitalized patients may need higher doses.

- Teenagers—At first, 50 mg a day. Your doctor may increase your dose gradually as needed. However, the dose is usually not more than 100 mg a day.

- Children up to 12 years of age—Use and dose must be determined by your doctor.

- Older adults—At first, 50 mg a day. Your doctor may increase your dose gradually as needed. However, the dose is usually not more than 100 mg a day.

Missed dose—If you miss a dose of this medicine and your dosing schedule is:

- One dose a day at bedtime—Do not take the missed dose in the morning since it may cause disturbing side effects during waking hours. Instead, check with your doctor.

- More than one dose a day—Take the missed dose as soon as possible. However, if it is almost time for your next dose, skip the missed dose, and go back to your regular dosing schedule. Do not double doses.

If you have any questions about this, check with your doctor.

Storage—To store this medicine:

- Keep out of the reach of children. Overdose of this medicine is very dangerous in young children.

- Store away from heat and direct light.

- Do not store the tablet or capsule form of this medicine in the bathroom, near the kitchen sink, or in other damp places. Heat or moisture may cause the medicine to break down.

- Keep the liquid form of this medicine from freezing.

- Do not keep outdated medicine or medicine no longer needed. Be sure that any discarded medicine is out of the reach of children.

Precautions While Using This Medicine

It is very important that your doctor check your progress at regular visits to allow dosage adjustments and to help reduce side effects.

This medicine will add to the effects of alcohol and other CNS depressants (medicines that make you drowsy or less alert). Some examples of CNS depressants are antihistamines or medicine for hay fever, other allergies, or colds; sedatives, tranquilizers, or sleeping medicine; prescription pain medicine or narcotics; barbiturates; medicine for seizures; muscle relaxants; or anesthetics, including some dental anesthetics. *Check with your medical doctor or dentist before taking any of the above while you are taking this medicine.*

This medicine may cause some people to become drowsy. *If this occurs, do not drive, use machines, or do anything else that could be dangerous if you are not alert.*

Dizziness, lightheadedness, or fainting may occur, especially when you get up from a lying or sitting position. Getting up slowly may help. If this problem continues or gets worse, check with your doctor.

This medicine may cause dryness of the mouth. For temporary relief, use sugarless gum or candy, melt bits of ice in your mouth, or use a saliva substitute. However, if your mouth continues to feel dry for more than 2 weeks, check with your medical doctor or dentist. Continuing dryness of the mouth may increase the chance of dental disease, including tooth decay, gum disease, and fungus infections.

Tricyclic antidepressants may cause your skin to be more sensitive to sunlight than it is normally. Exposure to sunlight, even for brief periods of time, may cause a skin rash, itching, redness or other discoloration of the skin, or a severe sunburn. When you begin taking this medicine:

- Stay out of direct sunlight, especially between the hours of 10:00 a.m. and 3:00 p.m., if possible.

- Wear protective clothing, including a hat. Also, wear sunglasses.

- Apply a sun block product that has a skin protection factor (SPF) of at least 15. Some patients may require a product with a higher SPF number, especially if they have a fair complexion. If you have any questions about this, check with your health care professional.

- Apply a sun block lipstick that has an SPF of at least 15 to protect your lips.

- Do not use a sunlamp or tanning bed or booth.

If you have a severe reaction from the sun, check with your doctor.

Before you have any medical tests, tell the medical doctor in charge that you are taking this medicine. The results of the metyrapone test may be affected by this medicine.

Before having any kind of surgery, dental treatment, or emergency treatment, tell the medical doctor or dentist in charge that you are using this medicine. Taking tricyclic antidepressants together with medicines used during surgery or dental or emergency treatments may increase the risk of side effects.

For diabetic patients:

- This medicine may affect blood sugar levels. If you notice a change in the results of your blood or urine sugar tests or if you have any questions, check with your doctor.

Do not stop taking this medicine without first checking with your doctor. Your doctor may want you to reduce gradually the amount you are using before stopping completely. This may help prevent a possible worsening of your condition and reduce the possibility of withdrawal symptoms such as headache, nausea, and/or an overall feeling of discomfort.

The effects of this medicine may last for 3 to 7 days after you have stopped taking it. Therefore, all the precautions stated here must be observed during this time.

For patients taking protriptyline:

- If taken late in the day, protriptyline may interfere with nighttime sleep.

Side Effects of This Medicine

Along with its needed effects, a medicine may cause some unwanted effects. Although not all of these side effects may occur, if they do occur they may need medical attention.

Stop taking this medicine and get emergency help immediately if any of the following side effects occur:

> *Reported for amoxapine only—rare*
>
> Convulsions (seizures); difficult or fast breathing; fever with increased sweating; high or low (irregular) blood pressure; loss of bladder control; muscle stiffness (severe); pale skin; unusual tiredness or weakness

Check with your doctor as soon as possible if any of the following side effects occur:

> *Less common*
>
> Blurred vision; confusion or delirium; constipation (especially in the elderly); decreased sexual ability (more common with amoxapine and clomipramine); difficulty in speaking or swallowing; eye pain; fainting; fast or

irregular heartbeat (pounding, racing, skipping); hallucinations; loss of balance control; mask-like face; nervousness or restlessness; problems in urinating; shakiness or trembling; shuffling walk; slowed movements; stiffness of arms and legs

Reported for amoxapine only (in addition to the above)—less common

Lip smacking or puckering; puffing of cheeks; rapid or worm-like movements of tongue; uncontrolled chewing movements; uncontrolled movements of hands, arms, or legs

Rare

Anxiety; breast enlargement in both males and females; hair loss; inappropriate secretion of milk—in females; increased sensitivity to sunlight; irritability; muscle twitching; red or brownish spots on skin; ringing, buzzing, or other unexplained sounds in the ears; seizures (more common with clomipramine); skin rash and itching; sore throat and fever; swelling of face and tongue; swelling of testicles (more common with amoxapine); trouble with teeth or gums (more common with clomipramine); weakness; yellow eyes or skin

Symptoms of acute overdose

Confusion; convulsions (seizures); disturbed concentration; drowsiness (severe); enlarged pupils; fast, slow, or irregular heartbeat; fever; hallucinations (seeing, hearing, or feeling things that are not there); restlessness and agitation; shortness of breath or troubled breathing; unusual tiredness or weakness (severe); vomiting

Other side effects may occur that usually do not need medical attention. These side effects may go away during treatment as your body adjusts to the medicine. However, check with your doctor if any of the following side effects continue or are bothersome:

More common

Dizziness; drowsiness; dryness of mouth; headache; increased appetite (may include craving for sweets); nausea; tiredness or weakness (mild); unpleasant taste; weight gain

Less common

Diarrhea; heartburn; increased sweating; trouble in sleeping (more common with protriptyline, especially when taken late in the day); vomiting

Certain side effects of this medicine may occur after you have stopped taking it. Check with your doctor if you notice any of the following effects:

Headache; irritability; nausea, vomiting, or diarrhea; restlessness; trouble in sleeping, with vivid dreams; unusual excitement

Reported for amoxapine only (in addition to the above)

Lip smacking or puckering; puffing of cheeks; rapid or worm-like movements of the tongue; uncontrolled chewing movements; uncontrolled movements of arms or legs

Other side effects not listed above also may occur in some patients. If you notice any other effects, check with your doctor.

Additional Information

Once a medicine has been approved for marketing for a certain use, experience may show that it is also useful for other medical problems. Although these uses are not included in product labeling, tricyclic antidepressants are used in certain patients with the following medical conditions:

- Attention deficit hyperactivity disorder (hyperactivity in children) (desipramine, imipramine, and protriptyline)
- Bulimia (uncontrolled eating, followed by vomiting) (amitriptyline, clomipramine, desipramine, and imipramine)
- Cocaine withdrawal (desipramine and imipramine)
- Headache prevention (for certain types of frequent or continuing headaches) (most tricyclic antidepressants)

- Itching with hives due to cold temperature exposure (doxepin)
- Narcolepsy (extreme tendency to fall asleep suddenly) (clomipramine, desipramine, imipramine, and protriptyline)
- Neurogenic pain (a type of continuing pain) (amitriptyline, clomipramine, desipramine, doxepin, imipramine, nortriptyline, and trimipramine)
- Panic disorder (clomipramine, desipramine, doxepin, nortriptyline, and trimipramine)
- Stomach ulcer (amitriptyline, doxepin, and trimipramine)
- Urinary incontinence (imipramine)

Other than the above information, there is no additional information relating to proper use, precautions, or side effects for these uses.

ANTIDIABETICS, ORAL   Systemic

Some commonly used brand names are:

In the U.S.—

DiaBeta[4]	Micronase[4]
Diabinese[2]	Orinase[6]
Dymelor[1]	Tolamide[5]
Glucotrol[3]	Tolinase[5]
Glynase PresTab[4]	Tol-Tab[6]

In Canada—

Albert Glyburide[4]	Euglucon[4]
Apo-Chlorpropamide[2]	Gen-Glybe[4]
Apo-Glyburide[4]	Mobenol[6]
Apo-Tolbutamide[6]	Novo-Butamide[6]
DiaBeta[4]	Novo-Glyburide[4]
Diabinese[2]	Novo-Propamide[2]
Dimelor[1]	Orinase[6]

Another commonly used name for glyburide is glibenclamide.

Note: For quick reference, the following oral antidiabetics are numbered to match the corresponding brand names.

This information applies to the following medicines:

1. Acetohexamide (a-set-oh-HEX-a-mide)‡
2. Chlorpropamide (klor-PROE-pa-mide)‡§

3. Glipizide (GLIP-i-zide)†
4. Glyburide (GLYE-byoo-ride)
5. Tolazamide (tole-AZ-a-mide)†‡
6. Tolbutamide (tole-BYOO-ta-mide)‡§

---

†Not commercially available in Canada.
‡Generic name product may also be available in the U.S.
§Generic name product may also be available in Canada.

Description

Oral antidiabetics (diabetes medicine you take by mouth) may help reduce the amount of sugar in the blood by causing your pancreas gland to make more insulin. They are used to treat certain types of diabetes mellitus (sugar diabetes).

Oral antidiabetics can usually be used only by adults who develop diabetes after 30 years of age and who do not require insulin shots (or who usually do not require more than 20 Units of insulin a day) to control their condition. This type of diabetic patient is said to have non–insulin-dependent diabetes mellitus (or NIDDM), sometimes known as maturity-onset or Type II diabetes. Oral antidiabetics do not help diabetic patients who have insulin-dependent diabetes mellitus (or IDDM), sometimes known as juvenile-onset or Type I diabetes.

Chlorpropamide may also be used for other conditions as determined by your doctor.

Oral antidiabetic medicines do not help diabetic patients who are insulin-dependent (type I). However, non–insulin-dependent (type II) diabetic patients who are taking oral antidiabetics may have to temporarily switch to insulin if they:

- develop diabetic coma or ketoacidosis.
- have a severe injury or burn.
- develop a severe infection.
- are to have major surgery.
- are pregnant.

Before you begin treatment with this medicine, you and your doctor should talk about the good the medicine will do as well as the risks of using it. You should also find out about other possible ways to treat your diabetes such as by diet alone or by diet plus insulin.

Oral antidiabetics are available only with your doctor's prescription, in the following dosage forms:

Oral

Acetohexamide
* Tablets (U.S. and Canada)

Chlorpropamide
* Tablets (U.S. and Canada)

Glipizide
* Tablets (U.S.)

Glyburide
* Tablets (U.S. and Canada)

Tolazamide
* Tablets (U.S.)

Tolbutamide
* Tablets (U.S. and Canada)

Before Using This Medicine

In deciding to use a medicine, the risks of taking the medicine must be weighed against the good it will do. This is a decision you and your doctor will make. For oral antidiabetic medicines, the following should be considered:

Allergies—Tell your doctor if you have ever had any unusual or allergic reaction to oral antidiabetic medicines, or to sulfonamide-type (sulfa) medications, including thiazide diuretics (a certain type of water pill). Also tell your health care professional if you are allergic to any other substances, such as foods, preservatives, or dyes.

Diet—If you have non–insulin-dependent (type II) diabetes, your doctor may try to control your condition by prescribing a personal meal plan for you before prescribing medicine. Such a diet is low in refined carbohydrates (foods such as sugar and candy used for quick energy) and fat. The daily number of calories in this meal plan should be adjusted by a dietitian to help you reach and maintain a proper body weight. Oral antidiabetics are less effective if you are greatly overweight. It may be very important for you to follow a planned weight reduction diet. In addition, meals and snacks are arranged to meet the energy needs of your body at different times of the day.

Many people with type II diabetes are able to control their diabetes by carefully following their prescribed meal and exercise plan. Oral antidiabetics are prescribed only when additional help is needed.

Pregnancy—Oral antidiabetics should not be used during pregnancy. Insulin may be needed to keep blood sugar levels as close to normal as possible. Poor control of blood sugar levels may cause birth defects or death of the fetus. In addition, use of oral antidiabetics during pregnancy may cause the newborn baby to have low blood sugar levels. This may last for several days following birth.

Breast-feeding—Chlorpropamide passes into the breast milk and its use is not recommended because it could cause low blood sugar in the baby. Although it is not known if the other oral antidiabetics pass into breast milk and these medicines have not been shown to cause problems in humans, the chance always exists.

Children—There is little information about the use of oral antidiabetic agents in children. Type II diabetes is unusual in this age group.

Older adults—The elderly may be more sensitive than younger adults to the effects of oral antidiabetics. Also, elderly patients who take chlorpropamide are more likely to retain (keep) too much body water.

Other medicines—Although certain medicines should not be used together at all, in other cases two different medicines may be used together even if an interaction might occur. In these cases, your doctor may want to change the dose, or other precautions may be necessary. *Do not take any other medicine, unless prescribed or approved by your doctor.* When you are taking oral antidiabetic drugs, it is especially important that your health care professional know if you are taking any of the following:

- Anticoagulants (blood thinners)—The effect of either the blood thinner or the antidiabetic medicine may be increased or decreased if the two medicines are used together

- Appetite control medicines or
- Asthma medicines or
- Cough or cold medicines or
- Hay fever or allergy medicines—Many medicines (including nonprescription [over-the-counter]) products can affect the control of your blood glucose (sugar)

- Aspirin or other salicylates or
- Chloramphenicol (e.g., Chloromycetin) or
- Guanethidine (e.g., Ismelin) or
- Sulfonamides (sulfa medicine)—These medicines may increase the chances of low blood sugar

- Beta-blockers (acebutolol [e.g., Sectral], atenolol [e.g., Tenormin], carteolol [e.g., Cartrol], labetalol [e.g., Normodyne], metoprolol [e.g., Lopressor], nadolol [e.g., Corgard], oxprenolol [e.g., Trasicor], penbutolol [e.g., Levatol], pindolol [e.g., Visken], propranolol [e.g., Inderal], sotalol [e.g., Sotacor], timolol [e.g., Blocadren])—Beta-blockers may increase the risk of high or low blood sugar occurring. They can also block symptoms of low blood sugar (such as fast heartbeat or high blood pressure). Because of this, a diabetic patient might not know that he or she had low blood sugar and might not immediately take the proper steps to raise the blood sugar level. Beta-blockers can also cause low blood sugar to last longer

- Monoamine oxidase (MAO) inhibitors (furazolidone [e.g., Furoxone], isocarboxazid [e.g., Marplan], pargyline [e.g., Eutonyl], phenelzine [e.g., Nardil], procarbazine [e.g., Matulane], or tranylcypromine [e.g., Parnate])—Taking oral antidiabetic medicines while you are taking (or within 2 weeks of taking) monoamine oxidase (MAO) inhibitors may increase the chances of low blood sugar occurring

Other medical problems—The presence of other medical problems may affect the use of the oral antidiabetic medicines. Make sure you tell your doctor if you have any other medical problems, especially:

- Heart disease—Chlorpropamide causes some patients to retain (keep) more body water than usual. Heart disease may be worsened by this extra body water
- Infection (severe)—Insulin may be needed temporarily to control diabetes in patients with severe infection because changes in blood sugar may occur rapidly and without much warning
- Kidney disease or
- Liver disease—Low blood sugar may be more likely to occur because the kidney or liver is not able to get the medicine out of the blood stream as it normally would. Also, people with kidney disease who take chlorpropamide are more likely to retain (keep) too much body water
- Thyroid disease
- Underactive adrenal glands (untreated) or
- Underactive pituitary gland (untreated)—Patients with these conditions may be more likely to develop low blood sugar (hypoglycemia) while taking oral antidiabetic medicines

---

Proper Use of This Medicine

Follow carefully your special meal plan, since this is the most important part of controlling your diabetes and is necessary if the medicine is to work properly.

Take your oral antidiabetic medicine only as directed by your doctor. Do not take more or less of it than your doctor ordered, and take it at the same time each day. This will help to control your blood sugar levels.

Dosing—The dose of these medicines will be different for different patients. *Follow your doctor's orders or the directions on the label.* The following information includes only the average doses of these medicines. *If your dose is different, do not change it* unless your doctor tells you to do so.

The number of tablets that you take depends on the strength of the medicine. Also, *the number of doses you take each day, the time allowed between doses, and the length of time you take the medicine depend on the amount of sugar in your blood or urine.*

For acetohexamide

- For *oral* dosage form (tablets):

    —For treating sugar diabetes (diabetes mellitus):

    - Adults—At first, 250 milligrams (mg) once a day. Some elderly people may need a lower dose of 125 to 250 mg a day at first. Then, your doctor may change your dose at little at a time if needed. The dose is usually not more than 1.5 grams a day. If your dose is 1 gram or more, the dose is usually divided into two doses. These doses are taken before the morning and evening meals.

    - Children—The type of diabetes treated with this medicine is rare in children. However, if a child needs this medicine, the dose would have to be determined by the doctor.

For chlorpropamide

- For *oral* dosage form (tablets):

    —For treating sugar diabetes (diabetes mellitus):

    - Adults—At first, 250 milligrams (mg) once a day. Some elderly people may need a lower dose of 100 to 125 mg a day at first. Then, your doctor may change your dose a little at a time if needed. The dose is usually not more than 750 mg a day.

    - Children—The type of diabetes treated with this

medicine is rare in children. However, if a child needs this medicine, the dose would have to be determined by the doctor.

For glipizide

- For *oral* dosage form (tablets):

  —For treating sugar diabetes (diabetes mellitus):

  - Adults—At first, 5 milligrams (mg) once a day. Some elderly people may need a lower dose of 2.5 mg a day at first. Then, your doctor may change your dose a little at a time if needed. The dose is usually not more than 40 mg a day. If your dose is 15 mg or more, the dose is usually divided into two doses. These doses are taken before the morning and evening meals.

  - Children—The type of diabetes treated with this medicine is rare in children. However, if a child needs this medicine, the dose would have to be determined by the doctor.

For glyburide

- For *oral* dosage form (tablets):

  —For treating sugar diabetes (diabetes mellitus):

  - Adults—At first, 2.5 to 5 milligrams (mg) once a day. Some elderly people may need a lower dose of 1.25 to 2.5 mg a day at first. Then, your doctor may change your dose a little at a time if needed. The dose is usually not more than 20 mg a day. If your dose is 10 mg or more, the dose is usually divided into two doses. These doses are taken before the morning and evening meals.

  - Children—The type of diabetes treated with this medicine is rare in children. However, if a child needs this medicine, the dose would have to be determined by the doctor.

For tolazamide

- For *oral* dosage form (tablets):

—For treating sugar diabetes (diabetes mellitus):

• Adults—At first, 100 to 250 milligrams (mg) once a day in the morning. Then, your doctor may change your dose a little at a time if needed. The dose is usually not more than 1 gram a day. If your dose is 500 mg or more, the dose is usually divided into two doses. These doses are taken before the morning and evening meals.

• Children—The type of diabetes treated with this medicine is rare in children. However, if a child needs this medicine, the dose would have to be determined by the doctor.

For tolbutamide

• For *oral* dosage form (tablets):

—For treating sugar diabetes (diabetes mellitus):

• Adults—At first, 500 milligrams (mg) to 2 grams a day. Some elderly people may need lower doses to start. The dose is usually divided into two doses. These doses are taken before the morning and evening meals. Your doctor may change your dose a little at a time if needed. The dose is usually not more than 3 grams a day.

• Children—The type of diabetes treated with this medicine is rare in children. However, if a child needs this medicine, the dose would have to be determined by the doctor.

Missed dose—If you miss a dose of this medicine, take it as soon as possible. However, if it is almost time for your next dose, skip the missed dose and go back to your regular dosing schedule. Do not double doses.

Storage—To store this medicine:

• Keep out of the reach of children.

• Store away from heat and direct light.

• Do not store in the bathroom, near the kitchen sink,

or in other damp places. Heat or moisture may cause the medicine to break down.

• Do not keep outdated medicine or medicine no longer needed. Be sure that any discarded medicine is out of the reach of children.

Precautions While Using This Medicine

Your doctor will want to check your progress at regular visits, especially during the first few weeks that you take this medicine.

Test for sugar in your blood or urine as directed by your doctor. This is important in making sure your diabetes is being controlled and provides an early warning when it is not.

Do not take any other medicines, unless prescribed or approved by your doctor. This especially includes nonprescription (over-the-counter [OTC]) medicines such as those for colds, cough, asthma, hay fever, or appetite control.

Avoid drinking alcoholic beverages until you have discussed their use with your doctor. Some patients who drink alcohol while taking this medicine may suffer stomach pain, nausea, vomiting, dizziness, pounding headache, sweating, or flushing (redness of face and skin). In addition, alcohol may produce hypoglycemia (low blood sugar).

Oral antidiabetic medicines may cause your skin to be more sensitive to sunlight than it is normally. Exposure to sunlight, even for brief periods of time, may cause a skin rash, itching, redness or other discoloration of the skin, or a severe sunburn.

When you begin taking this medicine:

- Stay out of direct sunlight, especially between the hours of 10:00 a.m. and 3:00 p.m., if possible.
- Wear protective clothing, including a hat. Also, wear sunglasses.
- Apply a sun block product that has a skin protection factor (SPF) of at least 15. Some patients may require a product with a higher SPF number, especially if they have a fair complexion. If you have any questions about this, check with your health care professional.
- Apply a sun block lipstick that has an SPF of at least 15 to protect your lips.
- Do not use a sunlamp or tanning bed or booth.

If you have a severe reaction from the sun, check with your doctor.

Eat or drink something containing sugar and check with your doctor right away if mild symptoms of low blood sugar (hypoglycemia) appear. Good sources of sugar are glucose tablets or gel or fruit juice, corn syrup, honey, non-diet soft drinks, or sugar cubes or table sugar (dissolved in water). It is a good idea also to check your blood sugar to confirm that it is low.

- *If severe symptoms such as convulsions (seizures) or unconsciousness occur, diabetics should not eat or drink anything.* There is a chance that they could choke from not swallowing correctly. Emergency medical help should be obtained immediately.

- *Symptoms of low blood sugar (hypoglycemia) are:*
  Abdominal or stomach pain (mild)
  Anxious feeling
  Chills (continuing)
  Cold sweats
  Confusion
  Convulsions (seizures)
  Cool pale skin
  Difficulty in concentration

Drowsiness
Excessive hunger
Fast heartbeat
Headache (continuing)
Nausea or vomiting (continuing)
Nervousness
Shakiness
Unconsciousness
Unsteady walk
Unusual tiredness or weakness
Vision changes

- Different people may have different symptoms of hypoglycemia. It is important that you learn your own signs of low blood sugar so that you can treat it quickly.

- *These symptoms may occur if you:*

  —delay or miss a scheduled meal or snack.

  —exercise much more than usual.

  —cannot eat because of nausea and vomiting.

  —drink a significant amount of alcohol.

- *Tell someone to take you to your doctor or to a hospital right away if the symptoms do not improve after eating or drinking a sweet food.*

- Even if you correct these symptoms by eating sugar, it is very important to call your doctor or hospital emergency service right away, since the blood sugar–lowering effects of this medicine may last for days and the symptoms may return often during this time.

Before having any kind of surgery, dental treatment, or emergency treatment, tell the medical doctor or dentist in charge that you are taking this medicine.

You should wear a medical I.D. bracelet or chain at all times. In addition, you should carry an identification card that says you have diabetes and that lists your medications.

Side Effects of This Medicine

The use of oral antidiabetics has been reported to increase the risk of death from heart and blood vessel disease. A report based on a study by the University Group Diabetes Program (UGDP) compared the use of one of the oral medicines (tolbutamide) to the use of diet alone or diet plus insulin. Although only tolbutamide was studied, other oral antidiabetics may cause a similar effect since all these medicines are related chemically and in the way they work.

Along with their needed effects, oral antidiabetics may cause some unwanted effects. Although not all of these side effects may occur, if they do occur they may need medical attention.

Check with your doctor as soon as possible if any of the following side effects occur:

Rare

> Chest pain; chills; coughing up blood; dark urine; fever; general feeling of illness; increased amounts of sputum (phlegm); increased sweating; itching of the skin; light-colored stools; shortness of breath; sore throat; unusual bleeding or bruising; unusual tiredness or weakness (continuing and unexplained); yellow eyes or skin

Symptoms of overdose (hypoglycemia)

> Abdominal or stomach pain (mild); anxious feeling; chills (continuing); cold sweats; confusion; convulsions (seizures); cool, pale skin; difficulty in concentration; drowsiness; excessive hunger; fast heartbeat; headache (continuing); nausea or vomiting (continuing); nervousness; shakiness; unconsciousness; unsteady walk; unusual tiredness or weakness; vision changes

Other side effects may occur that usually do not need medical attention. These side effects may go away during treatment as your body adjusts to the medicine. However,

check with your doctor if any of the following side effects continue or are bothersome:

More common

Changes in taste (for tolbutamide); constipation; diarrhea; dizziness; drowsiness (mild); headache; heartburn; increased or decreased appetite; nausea; vomiting; stomach pain, fullness, or discomfort

Less common or rare

Hives; increased sensitivity of skin to sun; skin redness, itching, or rash

For patients taking chlorpropamide:

• Some patients who take chlorpropamide may retain (keep) more body water than usual. Check with your doctor as soon as possible if any of the following signs occur:

Breathing difficulty; shortness of breath

Other side effects not listed above may also occur in some patients. If you notice any other effects, check with your doctor.

Additional Information

Once a medicine has been approved for marketing for a certain use, experience may show that it is also useful for other medical problems. Although this use is not included in product labeling, chlorpropamide is used in certain patients with the following medical condition:

• Diabetes insipidus (water diabetes)

If you are taking this medicine for water diabetes, the advice listed above that relates to diet and urine testing for patients with *sugar* diabetes *does not apply to you*. However, the advice about hypoglycemia (low blood sugar) does apply to you. Call your doctor right away if you feel any of the symptoms described.

ANTIDYSKINETICS   Systemic

Some commonly used brand names are:

In the U.S.—

Akineton[2]   Kemadrin[4]
Artane[5]   Parsidol[3]
Artane Sequels[5]   Trihexane[5]
Cogentin[1]   Trihexy[5]

In Canada—

Akineton[2]   Kemadrin[4]
Apo-Benztropine[1]   Parsitan[3]
Apo-Trihex[5]   PMS Benztropine[1]
Artane[5]   PMS Procyclidine[4]
Artane Sequels[5]   PMS Trihexyphenidyl[5]
Cogentin[1]   Procyclid[4]

Other commonly used names are:

Benzatropine[1]   Profenamine[3]

Note: For quick reference, the following antidyskinetics are numbered to
      match the corresponding brand names.

This information applies to the following medicines:

1. Benztropine (BENZ-troe-peen)‡§
2. Biperiden (bye-PER-i-den)
3. Ethopropazine (eth-oh-PROE-pa-zeen)
4. Procyclidine (proe-SYE-kli-deen)
5. Trihexyphenidyl (trye-hex-ee-FEN-i-dill)‡

Note: This information does *not* apply to Amantadine, Carbidopa and
      Levodopa, Diphenhydramine, Haloperidol, and Levodopa.

‡Generic name product may also be available in the U.S.
§Generic name product may also be available in Canada.

Description

Antidyskinetics are used to treat Parkinson's disease,
sometimes referred to as "shaking palsy." By improving
muscle control and reducing stiffness, this medicine allows
more normal movements of the body as the disease symptoms are reduced. It is also used to control severe reactions
to certain medicines such as reserpine (e.g., Serpasil)

(medicine to control high blood pressure) or phenothiazines, chlorprothixene (e.g., Taractan), thiothixene (e.g., Navane), loxapine (e.g., Loxitane), and haloperidol (e.g., Haldol) (medicines for nervous, mental, and emotional conditions).

Antidyskinetics may also be used for other conditions as determined by your doctor.

These medicines are available only with your doctor's prescription in the following dosage forms:

Oral

Benztropine
- Tablets (U.S. and Canada)

Biperiden
- Tablets (U.S. and Canada)

Ethopropazine
- Tablets (U.S. and Canada)

Procyclidine
- Elixir (Canada)
- Tablets (U.S. and Canada)

Trihexyphenidyl
- Extended-release capsules (U.S. and Canada)
- Elixir (U.S. and Canada)
- Tablets (U.S. and Canada)

Parenteral

Benztropine
- Injection (U.S. and Canada)

Biperiden
- Injection (U.S.)

Before Using This Medicine

In deciding to use a medicine, the risks of taking the medicine must be weighed against the good it will do. This is a decision you and your doctor will make. For antidyskinetics, the following should be considered:

Allergies—Tell your doctor if you have ever had any unusual or allergic reaction to antidyskinetics. Also tell your health care professional if you are allergic to any other substances, such as foods, preservatives, or dyes.

Pregnancy—Studies on effects in pregnancy have not been done in either humans or animals. However, antidyskinetics have not been shown to cause problems in humans.

Breast-feeding—It is not known if antidyskinetics pass into breast milk. Although most medicines pass into breast milk in small amounts, many of them may be used safely while breast-feeding. Mothers who are taking these medicines and who wish to breast-feed should discuss this with their doctor.

Since antidyskinetics tend to decrease the secretions of the body, it is possible that the flow of breast milk may be reduced in some patients.

Children—Children may be especially sensitive to the effects of antidyskinetics. This may increase the chance of side effects during treatment.

Older adults—Agitation, confusion, disorientation, hallucinations, memory loss, and mental changes are more likely to occur in elderly patients, who are usually more sensitive to the effects of antidyskinetics.

Other medicines—Although certain medicines should not be used together at all, in other cases two different medicines may be used together even if an interaction might occur. In these cases, your doctor may want to change the dose, or other precautions may be necessary. When you are taking an antidyskinetic, it is especially important that your health care professional know if you are taking any of the following:

- Anticholinergics (medicine for abdominal or stomach spasms or cramps) or

- Central nervous system (CNS) depressants (medicine that causes drowsiness) or
- Tricyclic antidepressants (medicine for depression)—Using these medicines together with antidyskinetics may result in additive effects, increasing the chance of unwanted effects

Other medical problems—The presence of other medical problems may affect the use of antidyskinetics. Make sure you tell your doctor if you have any other medical problems, especially:

- Difficult urination or
- Enlarged prostate or
- Glaucoma or
- Heart or blood vessel disease or
- High blood pressure or
- Intestinal blockage or
- Myasthenia gravis or
- Uncontrolled movements of hands, mouth, or tongue—Antidyskinetics may make the condition worse
- Kidney disease or
- Liver disease—Higher blood levels of the antidyskinetics may result, increasing the chance of side effects

---

Proper Use of This Medicine

Take this medicine only as directed by your doctor. Do not take more of it, do not take it more often, and do not take it for a longer period of time than your doctor ordered. To do so may increase the chance of side effects.

To lessen stomach upset, take this medicine with meals or immediately after meals, unless otherwise directed by your doctor.

Dosing—The dose of antidyskinetics will be different for different patients. *Follow your doctor's orders or the directions on the label.* The following information includes only the average doses of benztropine, biperiden, ethopropazine, procyclidine, and trihexyphenidyl. *If your dose is* *different, do not change it* unless your doctor tells you to do so.

The number of capsules, tablets, or teaspoonfuls of elixir that you take depends on the strength of the medicine. Also, *the number of doses you take each day, the time allowed between doses, and the length of time you take the medicine depend on the medical problem for which you are taking antidyskinetics.*

For benztropine

- For *oral* dosage forms (tablets):

  —For Parkinson's disease or certain severe side effects caused by some other medicines:

  - Adults—To start, 0.5 to 4 milligrams (mg) a day, depending on your condition. Your doctor will adjust your dose as needed; however, the dose is usually not more than 6 mg a day.

  - Children—Use and dose must be determined by your doctor.

- For *injection* dosage form:

  —For Parkinson's disease or certain severe side effects caused by some other medicines:

  - Adults—1 to 4 mg a day, depending on your condition. Your doctor will adjust your dose as needed; however, the dose is usually not more than 6 mg a day.

  - Children—Use and dose must be determined by your doctor.

For biperiden

- For *oral* dosage forms (tablets):

  —For Parkinson's disease or certain severe side effects caused by some other medicines:

  - Adults—2 mg up to four times a day. Your doctor will adjust your dose, depending on your condition; however, the dose is usually not more than 16 mg a day.

• Children—Use and dose must be determined by your doctor.

• For *injection* dosage form:

—For Parkinson's disease or certain severe side effects caused by some other medicines:

• Adults—2 mg, injected into a muscle or vein. The dose may be repeated if needed; however, the dose is usually not given more than four times a day.

• Children—Use and dose is based on body weight and must be determined by your doctor.

For ethopropazine

• For *oral* dosage forms (tablets):

—For Parkinson's disease or certain severe side effects caused by some other medicines:

• Adults—50 mg one or two times a day. Your doctor will adjust your dose as needed; however, the dose is usually not more than 600 mg a day.

• Children—Use and dose must be determined by your doctor.

For procyclidine

• For *oral* dosage forms (elixir or tablets):

—For Parkinson's disease or certain severe side effects caused by some other medicines:

• Adults—To start, 2.5 mg three times a day after meals. Your doctor may need to adjust your dose, depending on your condition.

• Children—Use and dose must be determined by your doctor.

For trihexyphenidyl

• For *extended-release oral* dosage forms (extended-release capsules):

—For Parkinson's disease or certain severe side effects caused by some other medicines:

- Adults—5 mg after breakfast. Your doctor may add another 5 mg dose to be taken twelve hours later, depending on your condition.
- Children: Use and dose must be determined by your doctor.

- For other *oral* dosage forms (elixir or tablets):

  —For Parkinson's disease or certain severe side effects caused by some other medicines:

  - Adults—To start, 1 to 2 mg a day. Your doctor may adjust your dose as needed; however, the dose is usually not more than 15 mg a day.
  - Children—Use and dose must be determined by your doctor.

Missed dose—If you miss a dose of this medicine, take it as soon as possible. However, if it is within 2 hours of your next dose, skip the missed dose and go back to your regular dosing schedule. Do not double doses.

Storage—To store this medicine:

- Keep out of the reach of children.
- Store away from heat and direct light.
- Do not store the capsule or tablet form of this medicine in the bathroom, near the kitchen sink, or in other damp places. Heat or moisture may cause the medicine to break down.
- Keep the liquid form of this medicine from freezing.
- Do not keep outdated medicine or medicine no longer needed. Be sure that any discarded medicine is out of the reach of children.

Precautions While Using This Medicine

Your doctor should check your progress at regular visits, especially for the first few months you take this medicine.

This will allow your dosage to be changed as necessary to meet your needs.

Your doctor may want you to have your eyes examined by an ophthalmologist (eye doctor) before and also sometime later during treatment.

Do not stop taking this medicine without first checking with your doctor. Your doctor may want you to reduce gradually the amount you are taking before stopping completely, to prevent side effects or the worsening of your condition.

This medicine will add to the effects of alcohol and other CNS depressants (medicines that slow down the nervous system, possibly causing drowsiness). Some examples of CNS depressants are antihistamines or medicine for hay fever, other allergies, or colds; sedatives, tranquilizers, or sleeping medicine; prescription pain medicine or narcotics; barbiturates; medicine for seizures; muscle relaxants; or anesthetics, including some dental anesthetics. *Check with your doctor before taking any of the above while you are using this medicine.*

Do not take this medicine within 1 hour of taking medicine for diarrhea. Taking these medicines too close together will make this medicine less effective.

If you think you or anyone else has taken an overdose of this medicine, get emergency help at once. Taking an overdose of this medicine may lead to unconsciousness. Some signs of an overdose are clumsiness or unsteadiness; seizures; severe drowsiness; severe dryness of mouth, nose and throat; fast heartbeat; hallucinations (seeing, hearing, or feeling things that are not there); mood or mental changes; shortness of breath or troubled breathing; trouble in sleeping; and unusual warmth, dryness, and flushing of skin.

This medicine may cause your eyes to become more sensitive to light than they are normally. Wearing sunglasses and avoiding too much exposure to bright light may help lessen the discomfort.

This medicine may cause some people to have blurred vision or to become drowsy, dizzy, or less alert than they are normally. *Make sure you know how you react to this medicine before you drive, use machines, or do anything else that could be dangerous if you are dizzy or are not alert or able to see well.*

Dizziness, lightheadedness, or fainting may occur, especially when you get up from lying or sitting. Getting up slowly may help. If the problem continues or gets worse, check with your doctor.

This medicine may make you sweat less, causing your body temperature to increase. *Use extra care to avoid becoming overheated during exercise or hot weather while you are taking this medicine, since overheating may result in heat stroke.* Also, hot baths or saunas may make you feel dizzy or faint while you are taking this medicine.

This medicine may cause dryness of the mouth. For temporary relief, use sugarless candy or gum, melt bits of ice in your mouth, or use a saliva substitute. However, if your mouth continues to feel dry for more than 2 weeks, check with your medical doctor or dentist. Continuing dryness of the mouth may increase the chance of dental disease, including tooth decay, gum disease, and fungus infections.

Side Effects of This Medicine

Along with its needed effects, a medicine may cause some unwanted effects. Although not all of these side effects may occur, if they do occur they may need medical attention.

Check with your doctor as soon as possible if any of the following side effects occur:

Rare

Confusion (more common in the elderly or with high doses); eye pain; skin rash

Symptoms of overdose

Clumsiness or unsteadiness; drowsiness (severe); dryness of mouth, nose, or throat (severe); fast heartbeat; hallucinations (seeing, hearing, or feeling things that are not there); mood or mental changes; seizures; shortness of breath or troubled breathing; trouble in sleeping; warmth, dryness, and flushing of skin

Other side effects may occur that usually do not need medical attention. These side effects may go away during treatment as your body adjusts to the medicine. However, check with your doctor if any of the following side effects continue or are bothersome:

More common

Blurred vision; constipation; decreased sweating; difficult or painful urination (especially in older men); drowsiness; dryness of mouth, nose, or throat; increased sensitivity of eyes to light; nausea or vomiting

Less common or rare

Dizziness or lightheadedness when getting up from a lying or sitting position; false sense of well-being (especially in the elderly or with high doses); headache; loss of memory (especially in the elderly); muscle cramps; nervousness; numbness or weakness in hands or feet; soreness of mouth and tongue; stomach upset or pain; unusual excitement (more common with large doses of trihexyphenidyl)

After you stop using this medicine, your body may need time to adjust. The length of time this takes depends on the amount of medicine you were using and how long you used it. During this period of time check with your doctor if you notice any of the following side effects:

Anxiety; difficulty in speaking or swallowing; dizziness or lightheadedness when getting up from a lying or sitting position; fast heartbeat; loss of balance control; mask-like face; muscle spasms, especially of face, neck, and back; restlessness or desire to keep moving; shuffling walk; stiffness of arms or legs; trembling and shaking of hands and fingers; trouble in sleeping; twisting movements of body

Other side effects not listed above may also occur in some patients. If you notice any other effects, check with your doctor.

ANTIFUNGALS, AZOLE Systemic

Some commonly used brand names are:

In the U.S.—
Diflucan[1]   Nizoral[3]
Monistat i.v.[4]   Sporanox[2]

In Canada—
Diflucan[1]   Sporanox[2]
Nizoral[3]

Note: For quick reference, the following antifungals are numbered to match the corresponding brand names.

This information applies to the following medicines:

1. Fluconazole (floo-KOE-na-zole)
2. Itraconazole (i-tra-KOE-na-zole)
3. Ketoconazole (kee-toe-KON-a-zole)
4. Miconazole (mi-KON-a-zole)†

†Not commercially available in Canada.

Description

Azole antifungals are used to treat serious fungus infections that may occur in different parts of the body. These medicines may also be used for other problems as determined by your doctor.

Azole antifungals are available only with your doctor's prescription, in the following dosage forms:

Oral

Fluconazole
  • Oral suspension (U.S.)
  • Tablets (U.S. and Canada)
Itraconazole
  • Capsules (U.S. and Canada)
Ketoconazole
  • Oral suspension (Canada)
  • Tablets (U.S. and Canada)

Parenteral

Fluconazole
  • Injection (U.S. and Canada)
Miconazole
  • Injection (U.S.)

Before Using This Medicine

In deciding to use a medicine, the risks of taking the medicine must be weighed against the good it will do. This is a decision you and your doctor will make. For the azole antifungals, the following should be considered:

Allergies—Tell your doctor if you have ever had any un-usual or allergic reaction to any of the azole antifungals. Also tell your health care professional if you are allergic to any other substances, such as foods, preservatives, or dyes.

Pregnancy—Studies have not been done in pregnant women. However, studies in some animals have shown that azole antifungals, taken in high doses, may cause harm to the mother and the fetus. They have caused birth defects in animals. Before taking these medicines, make sure your doctor knows if you are pregnant or if you may become pregnant.

Breast-feeding—Azole antifungals pass into breast milk. Mothers who are taking these medicines and who wish to breast-feed should discuss this with their doctors.

Children—A small number of children have been safely treated with azole antifungals. Be sure to discuss with your child's doctor the use of these medicines in children.

Older adults—Many medicines have not been studied specifically in older people. Therefore, it may not be known whether they work exactly the same way they do in younger adults or if they cause different side effects or problems in older people. There is no specific information comparing use of azole antifungals in the elderly with use in other age groups.

Other medicines—Although certain medicines should not be used together at all, in other cases two different medicines may be used together even if an interaction might occur. In these cases, your doctor may want to change the dose, or other precautions may be necessary. When you are taking azole antifungals, it is especially important that your health care professional know if you are taking any of the following:

- Acetaminophen (e.g., Tylenol) (with long-term, high-dose use) or
- Amiodarone (e.g., Cordarone) or
- Anabolic steroids (nandrolone [e.g., Anabolin], oxandrolone [e.g., Anavar], oxymetholone [e.g., Anadrol], stanozolol [e.g., Winstrol]) or
- Androgens (male hormones) or
- Antithyroid agents (medicine for overactive thyroid) or
- Carmustine (e.g., BiCNU) or
- Chloroquine (e.g., Aralen) or
- Dantrolene (e.g., Dantrium) or
- Daunorubicin (e.g., Cerubidine) or
- Disulfiram (e.g., Antabuse) or
- Divalproex (e.g., Depakote) or
- Estrogens (female hormones) or
- Etretinate (e.g., Tegison) or
- Gold salts (medicine for arthritis) or
- Hydroxychloroquine (e.g., Plaquenil) or
- Mercaptopurine (e.g., Purinethol) or
- Methotrexate (e.g., Mexate) or
- Methyldopa (e.g., Aldomet) or

- Naltrexone (e.g., Trexan) (with long-term, high-dose use) or
- Oral contraceptives (birth control pills) containing estrogen or
- Other anti-infectives by mouth or by injection (medicine for infection) or
- Phenothiazines (acetophenazine [e.g., Tindal], chlorpromazine [e.g., Thorazine], fluphenazine [e.g., Prolixin], mesoridazine [e.g., Serentil], perphenazine [e.g., Trilafon], prochlorperazine [e.g., Compazine], promazine [e.g., Sparine], promethazine [e.g., Phenergan], thioridazine [e.g., Mellaril], trifluoperazine [e.g., Stelazine], triflupromazine [e.g., Vesprin], trimeprazine [e.g., Temaril]) or
- Plicamycin (e.g., Mithracin) or
- Valproic acid (e.g., Depakene)—Use of these medicines with azole antifungals may increase the chance of side effects affecting the liver

- Amantadine (e.g., Symmetrel) or
- Antacids or
- Anticholinergics (medicine for abdominal or stomach spasms or cramps) or
- Antidepressants (medicine for depression) or
- Antidyskinetics (medicine for Parkinson's disease or other conditions affecting control of muscles) or
- Antihistamines or
- Antipsychotics (medicine for mental illness) or
- Buclizine (e.g., Bucladin) or
- Cimetidine (e.g., Tagamet) or
- Cyclizine (e.g., Marezine) or
- Cyclobenzaprine (e.g., Flexeril) or
- Disopyramide (e.g., Norpace) or
- Famotidine (e.g., Pepcid) or
- Flavoxate (e.g., Urispas) or
- Ipratropium (e.g., Atrovent) or
- Meclizine (e.g., Antivert) or
- Methylphenidate (e.g., Ritalin) or
- Nizatidine (e.g., Axid) or
- Omeprazole (e.g., Prilosec) or
- Orphenadrine (e.g., Norflex) or
- Oxybutynin (e.g., Ditropan) or
- Procainamide (e.g., Pronestyl) or
- Promethazine (e.g., Phenergan) or

- Quinidine (e.g., Quinidex) or
- Ranitidine (e.g., Zantac) or
- Sucralfate (e.g., Carafate) or
- Trimeprazine (e.g., Temaril)—Use of these medicines may decrease the effects of itraconazole and ketoconazole; these medicines should be taken at least 2 hours after itraconazole or ketoconazole
- Antidiabetic agents, oral (chlorpropamide [e.g., Diabinese], glipizide [e.g., Glucotrol], glyburide [e.g., DiaBeta, Micronase], tolbutamide [e.g., Orinase]) or
- Cyclosporine (e.g., Sandimmune) or
- Digoxin (e.g., Lanoxin) or
- Warfarin (e.g., Coumadin)—Fluconazole may increase the effects of these medicines, which may increase the chance of side effects
- Astemizole (e.g., Hismanal) or
- Terfenadine (e.g., Seldane)—These medications should not be taken with itraconazole or ketoconazole; these azole antifungals may increase the chance of serious side effects of astemizole or terfenadine
- Carbamazepine (e.g., Tegretol) or
- Isoniazid or
- Rifampin (e.g., Rifadin)—These medicines may decrease the effects of azole antifungals
- Cisapride (e.g., Propulsid)—Cisapride should not be taken with oral itraconazole, oral ketoconazole, or miconazole injection; these azole antifungals may increase the chance of serious side effects of cisapride
- Didanosine (e.g., ddI, Videx)—Use of didanosine with itraconazole or ketoconazole may decrease the effects of both itraconazole and ketoconazole, as well as didanosine. Itraconazole and ketoconazole should be taken at least 2 hours before or 2 hours after didanosine is given
- Phenytoin (e.g., Dilantin)—Use of phenytoin with azole antifungals may increase the effects of the azole antifungals, increase side effects of azole antifungals affecting the liver, and increase the chance of phenytoin side effects

Other medical problems—The presence of other medical problems may affect the use of azole antifungals. Make sure you tell your doctor if you have any other medical problems, especially:

- Achlorhydria (absence of stomach acid) or
- Hypochlorhydria (decreased amount of stomach acid)—Itraconazole and ketoconazole may not be absorbed from the stomach as well in patients who have low levels of or no stomach acid
- Alcohol abuse (or history of) or
- Liver disease—Alcohol abuse or liver disease may increase the chance of side effects caused by azole antifungals
- Kidney disease—The effects of fluconazole may be increased in patients with kidney disease

---

Proper Use of This Medicine

Itraconazole and ketoconazole should be taken with a meal or a snack.

For patients taking the *oral liquid form of ketoconazole:*

- Use a specially marked measuring spoon or other device to measure each dose accurately. The average household teaspoon may not hold the right amount of liquid.

If you have achlorhydria (absence of stomach acid) or hypochlorhydria (decreased amount of stomach acid), and you are taking itraconazole or ketoconazole, your doctor may want you to take your medicine with an acidic drink. You may dissolve your medicine in cola or seltzer water and drink the solution, or your may take your medicine with a glass of cola or seltzer water. Your doctor may suggest that you dissolve each capsule or tablet in a teaspoonful of weak hydrochloric acid solution to help you absorb the medicine better. Your health care professional can prepare the solution for you. After you dissolve the tablet in the acid solution, add this mixture to a small amount (1 or 2 teaspoonfuls) of water in a glass. Drink the mixture through a plastic or glass drinking straw. Place the straw behind your teeth, as far back in your mouth as you can. This will keep the acid from harming your teeth.

Be sure to drink all the liquid to get the full dose of medicine. Next, swish around in your mouth about ½ glass of water and then swallow it. This will help wash away any acid that may remain in your mouth or on your teeth.

To help clear up your infection completely, *it is very important that you keep taking this medicine for the full time of treatment,* even if your symptoms begin to clear up or you begin to feel better after a few days. Since fungus infections may be very slow to clear up, you may have to continue taking this medicine every day for as long as 6 months to a year or more. Some fungus infections never clear up completely and require continuous treatment. If you stop taking this medicine too soon, your symptoms may return.

This medicine works best when there is a constant amount in the blood. *To help keep the amount constant, do not miss any doses. Also, it is best to take each dose at the same time every day.* If you need help in planning the best time to take your medicine, check with your health care professional.

Dosing—The dose of azole antifungals may be different for different patients. *Follow your doctor's orders or the directions on the label.* The following information includes only the average doses of azole antifungals. Your dose of fluconazole may be different if you have kidney disease. *If your dose is different, do not change it* unless your doctor tells you to do so.

The number of capsules, tablets, or the amount of oral suspension that you take depends on the strength of the medicine. Also, *the number of doses you take each day, the time allowed between doses, and the length of time you take the medicine depend on the medical problem for which you are taking azole antifungals.*

For fluconazole

- For fungus infections:

—For *oral* dosage form (oral suspension and tablets):

• Adults and teenagers—200 to 400 milligrams (mg) on the first day, then 100 to 400 mg once a day for weeks or months, depending on the medical problem being treated. A vaginal yeast infection is treated with a single dose of 150 mg.

• Children up to 14 years of age—Dose must be determined by your doctor.

—For *injection* dosage form:

• Adults and teenagers—200 to 400 mg on the first day, then 100 to 400 mg once a day, injected into a vein, for weeks or months, depending on the medical problem being treated.

• Children up to 14 years of age—Dose must be determined by your doctor.

For itraconazole

• For fungus infections:

—For *oral* dosage form (capsules):

• Adults and teenagers—200 milligrams (mg) once a day, which may be increased up to 400 mg once a day for weeks or months, depending on the medical problem being treated.

• Children up to 16 years of age—Dose must be determined by your doctor.

For ketoconazole

• For fungus infections:

—For *oral* dosage form (oral suspension and tablets):

• Adults and teenagers—200 to 400 milligrams (mg) once a day for weeks or months, depending on the medical problem being treated.

• Children up to 2 years of age—Dose must be determined by your doctor.

• Children over 2 years of age—3.3 to 6.6 mg

per kilogram (kg) (1.5 to 3 mg per pound) of body weight once a day for weeks or months, depending on the medical problem being treated.

For miconazole

- For fungus infections:
  —For *injection* dosage form:
    - Adults and teenagers—200 milligrams (mg) to 1.2 gram three times a day, injected into a vein, for weeks or months, depending on the medical problem being treated.
    - Children up to 1 year of age—Dose must be determined by your doctor.
    - Children 1 year of age and over—20 to 40 mg per kilogram (kg) (9.1 to 18.2 mg per pound) of body weight per day, given in two or three doses, for weeks or months, depending on the medical problem being treated.

Missed dose—If you miss a dose of this medicine, take it as soon as possible. This will help to keep a constant amount of medicine in the blood. However, if it is almost time for your next dose, skip the missed dose and go back to your regular dosing schedule. Do not double doses.

Storage—To store this medicine:

- Keep out of the reach of children.
- Store away from heat and direct light.
- Do not store the capsule or tablet form of this medicine in the bathroom, near the kitchen sink, or in other damp places. Heat or moisture may cause the medicine to break down.
- Keep the oral liquid form of this medicine from freezing.
- Do not keep outdated medicine or medicine no longer needed. Be sure that any discarded medicine is out of the reach of children.

Precautions While Using This Medicine

It is important that your doctor check your progress at regular visits. This will allow your doctor to check for any unwanted effects.

If your symptoms do not improve within a few weeks (or months for some infections), or if they become worse, check with your doctor.

*Oral itraconazole, oral ketoconazole, and miconazole injection should **not** be taken with astemizole (e.g., Hismanal), cisapride (e.g., Propulsid), or terfenadine (e.g., Seldane).* Doing so may increase the risk of serious side effects affecting the heart.

Liver problems may be more likely to occur if you drink alcoholic beverages while you are taking this medicine. Alcoholic beverages may also cause stomach pain, nausea, vomiting, headache, or flushing or redness of the face. Other alcohol-containing preparations (for example, elixirs, cough syrups, tonics) may also cause problems. These problems may occur for at least a day after you stop taking ketoconazole. Therefore, *you should not drink alcoholic beverages or use alcohol-containing preparations while you are taking this medicine and for at least a day after you stop taking it.*

If you are taking antacids, cimetidine (e.g., Tagamet), famotidine (e.g., Pepcid), nizatidine (e.g., Axid), omeprazole (e.g., Prilosec), or ranitidine (e.g., Zantac) while you are taking itraconazole or ketoconazole, take the other medicine at least 2 hours after you take itraconazole or ketoconazole. If you take these medicines at the same time that you take itraconazole or ketoconazole, they will keep your antifungal medicine from working properly.

Ketoconazole may cause your eyes to become more sensitive to light than they are normally. Wearing sunglasses and avoiding too much exposure to bright light may help lessen the discomfort.

Side Effects of This Medicine

Along with its needed effects, a medicine may cause some unwanted effects. Although not all of these effects may occur, if they do occur they may need medical attention.

Check with your doctor immediately if any of the following side effects occur:

More common

    Redness, swelling, or pain at the place of injection—for miconazole

Less common

    Fever and chills, skin rash or itching

Rare

    Dark or amber urine; fever and sore throat; loss of appetite; pale stools; reddening, blistering, peeling, or loosening of skin and mucous membranes; stomach pain; unusual bleeding or bruising; unusual tiredness or weakness; yellow eyes or skin

Other side effects may occur that usually do not need medical attention. These side effects may go away during treatment as your body adjusts to the medicine. However, check with your doctor if any of the following side effects continue or are bothersome:

Less common

    Constipation; diarrhea; dizziness; drowsiness; flushing or redness of the face or skin; headache; nausea; vomiting

Rare—for ketoconazole

    Decreased sexual ability in males; enlargement of the breasts in males; increased sensitivity of the eyes to light; menstrual irregularities

Other side effects not listed above may also occur in some patients. If you notice any other effects, check with your doctor.

ANTIHISTAMINES Systemic

Some commonly used brand names are:

In the U.S.—

Aller-Chlor[8]
AllerMax Caplets[13]
Aller-med[13]
Anxanil[16]
Atarax[16]
Banophen[13]
Banophen Caplets[13]
Beldin[13]
Belix[13]
Bena-D 10[13]
Bena-D 50[13]
Benadryl[13]
Benadryl 25[13]
Benadryl Kapseals[13]
Benahist 10[13]
Benahist 50[13]
Ben-Allergin-50[13]
Benoject-10[13]
Benoject-50[13]
Benylin Cough[13]
Bromphen[5]
Bydramine Cough[13]
Calm X[12]
Children's Dramamine[12]
Chlo-Amine[8]
Chlor-100[8]
Chlorate[8]
Chlor-Niramine[8]
Chlorphed[5]
Chlor-Pro[8]
Chlor-Pro 10[8]
Chlorspan-12[8]
Chlortab-4[8]
Chlortab-8[8]
Chlor-Trimeton[8]
Chlor-Trimeton Allergy[8]
Chlor-Trimeton Repetabs[8]
Claritin[17]
Codimal-A[5]
Compoz[13]
Conjec-B[5]

Contac 12 Hour Allergy[9]
Cophene-B[5]
Dehist[5]
Dexchlor[11]
Diamine T.D.[5]
Dimetabs[12]
Dimetane[5]
Dimetane Extentabs[5]
Dimetapp Allergy[5]
Dimetapp Allergy Liqui-Gels[5]
Dinate[12]
Diphenacen-50[13]
Diphenadryl[13]
Diphen Cough[13]
Diphenhist[13]
Diphenhist Captabs[13]
Dommanate[12]
Dormarex 2[13]
Dormin[13]
Dramamine[12]
Dramamine Chewable[12]
Dramamine Liquid[12]
Dramanate[12]
Dramocen[12]
Dramoject[12]
Dymenate[12]
E-Vista[16]
Fynex[13]
Genahist[13]
Gen-Allerate[8]
Gen-D-phen[13]
Hismanal[2]
Histaject Modified[5]
Hydramine[13]
Hydramine Cough[13]
Hydramyn[13]
Hydrate[12]
Hydroxacen[16]
Hyrexin-50[13]
Hyzine-50[16]
Marmine[12]

In the U.S. (cont'd)—

Myidil[22]
Nasahist B[5]
ND-Stat Revised[5]
Nervine Nighttime Sleep-Aid[13]
Nico-Vert[12]
Nidryl[13]
Nisaval[19]
Nolahist[18]
Noradryl[13]
Nordryl[13]
Nordryl Cough[13]
Nytol with DPH[13]
Nytol Maximum Strength[13]
Optimine[3]
Oraminic II[5]
PBZ[21]
PBZ-SR[21]
PediaCare Allergy Formula[8]
Pelamine[21]
Periactin[10]
Pfeiffer's Allergy[8]
Phendry[13]
Phendry Children's Allergy
    Medicine[13]
Phenetron[8]
Phenetron Lanacaps[8]
Poladex T.D.[11]
Polaramine[11]

Polaramine Repetabs[11]
Quiess[16]
Seldane[20]
Siladryl[13]
Silphen Cough Syrup[13]
Sleep-Eze 3[13]
Sominex Formula 2[13]
Tavist[9]
Tavist-1[9]
Tega-Vert[12]
Telachlor[8]
Teldrin[8]
Triptone Caplets[12]
Trymegen[8]
Tusstat[13]
Twilite Caplets[13]
Uni-Bent Cough[13]
Unisom Nighttime Sleep Aid[15]
Unisom SleepGels Maximum
    Strength[13]
Veltane[5]
Vertab[12]
Vistaject-25[16]
Vistaject-50[16]
Vistaril[16]
Vistazine 50[16]
Wehdryl-10[13]
Wehdryl-50[13]

In Canada—

Allerdryl[13]
Apo-Dimenhydrinate[12]
Apo-Hydroxyzine[16]
Atarax[16]
Benadryl[13]
Chlor-Tripolon[8]
Claritin[17]
Dimetane[5]
Dimetane Extentabs[5]
Dommanate[12]
Gravol[12]
Gravol L/A[12]
Hismanal[2]
Insomnal[13]
Multipax[16]
Nauseatol[12]

Novo-Dimenate[12]
Novo-Hydroxyzin[16]
Novo-Pheniram[8]
Nova-Terfendadine[20]
Optimine[3]
Periactin[10]
PMS-Dimenhydrinate[12]
Polaramine[11]
Polaramine Repetabs[11]
Pyribenzamine[21]
Reactine[7]
Seldane[20]
Seldane Caplets[20]
Tavist[9]
Travamine[12]
Traveltabs[12]

Note: For quick reference, the following antihistamines are numbered to match the corresponding brand names.

This information applies to the following medicines:

1. Acrivastine (AK-ri-vas-teen)
2. Astemizole (a-STEM-mi-zole)
3. Azatadine (a-ZA-ta-deen)
4. Bromodiphenhydramine (broe-moe-dye-fen-HYE-dra-meen)‡
5. Brompheniramine (brome-fen-EER-a-meen)‡
6. Carbinoxamine (kar-bi-NOX-a-meen)‡
7. Cetirizine (se-TI-ra-zeen)*
8. Chlorpheniramine (klor-fen-EER-a-meen)‡
9. Clemastine (KLEM-as-teen)‡
10. Cyproheptadine (si-proe-HEP-ta-deen)‡
11. Dexchlorpheniramine (dex-klor-fen-EER-a-meen)‡
12. Dimenhydrinate (dye-men-HYE-dri-nate)‡§
13. Diphenhydramine (dye-fen-HYE-dra-meen)‡§
14. Diphenylpyraline (dye-fen-il-PEER-a-leen)§
15. Doxylamine (dox-ILL-a-meen)†
16. Hydroxyzine (hye-DROX-i-zeen)‡§
17. Loratadine (lor-AT-a-deen)
18. Phenindamine (fen-IN-da-meen)†
19. Pyrilamine (peer-ILL-a-meen)†‡
20. Terfenadine (ter-FEN-a-deen)
21. Tripelennamine (tri-pel-ENN-a-meen)‡
22. Triprolidine (trye-PROE-li-deen)†‡

---

*Not commercially available in the U.S.
†Not commercially available in Canada.
‡Generic name product may also be available in the U.S.
§Generic name product may also be available in Canada.

Description

Antihistamines are used to relieve or prevent the symptoms of hay fever and other types of allergy. They work by preventing the effects of a substance called histamine, which is produced by the body. Histamine can cause itching, sneezing, runny nose, and watery eyes. Also, in some persons histamine can close up the bronchial tubes (air passages of the lungs) and make breathing difficult.

Some of the antihistamines are also used to prevent motion sickness, nausea, vomiting, and dizziness. In patients with

Parkinson's disease, diphenhydramine may be used to decrease stiffness and tremors. Also, the syrup form of diphenhydramine is used to relieve the cough due to colds or hay fever. In addition, since antihistamines may cause drowsiness as a side effect, some of them may be used to help people go to sleep.

Hydroxyzine is used in the treatment of nervous and emotional conditions to help control anxiety. It can also be used to help control anxiety and produce sleep before surgery.

Antihistamines may also be used for other conditions as determined by your doctor.

Some antihistamine preparations are available only with your doctor's prescription. Others are available without a prescription. However, your doctor may have special instructions on the proper dose of the medicine for your medical condition.

These medicines are available in the following dosage forms:

Oral

Astemizole
- Oral suspension (Canada)
- Tablets (U.S. and Canada)

Azatadine
- Tablets (U.S. and Canada)

Brompheniramine
- Capsules (U.S.)
- Elixir (U.S. and Canada)
- Tablets (U.S. and Canada)
- Extended-release tablets (U.S. and Canada)

Cetirizine
- Tablets (Canada)

Chlorpheniramine
- Extended-release capsules (U.S.)
- Syrup (U.S. and Canada)
- Tablets (U.S. and Canada)

- Chewable tablets (U.S.)
- Extended-release tablets (U.S. and Canada)

Clemastine
- Syrup (U.S. and Canada)
- Tablets (U.S. and Canada)

Cyproheptadine
- Syrup (U.S. and Canada)
- Tablets (U.S. and Canada)

Dexchlorpheniramine
- Syrup (U.S. and Canada)
- Tablets (U.S. and Canada)
- Extended-release tablets (U.S. and Canada)

Dimenhydrinate
- Capsules (U.S.)
- Extended-release capsules (Canada)
- Elixir (U.S. and Canada)
- Syrup (U.S.)
- Tablets (U.S. and Canada)
- Chewable tablets (U.S.)

Diphenhydramine
- Capsules (U.S. and Canada)
- Elixir (U.S. and Canada)
- Syrup (U.S.)
- Tablets (U.S.)

Doxylamine
- Tablets (U.S.)

Hydroxyzine
- Capsules (U.S. and Canada)
- Oral suspension (U.S.)
- Syrup (U.S. and Canada)
- Tablets (U.S.)

Loratadine
- Syrup (Canada)
- Tablets (U.S. and Canada)

Phenindamine
- Tablets (U.S.)

Pyrilamine
- Tablets (U.S.)

Terfenadine
- Oral suspension (Canada)
- Tablets (U.S. and Canada)

Tripelennamine
- Elixir (U.S.)
- Tablets (U.S. and Canada)
- Extended-release tablets (U.S.)

Triprolidine
- Syrup (U.S.)

Parenteral

Brompheniramine
- Injection (U.S.)

Chlorpheniramine
- Injection (U.S. and Canada)

Dimenhydrinate
- Injection (U.S. and Canada)

Diphenhydramine
- Injection (U.S. and Canada)

Hydroxyzine
- Injection (U.S. and Canada)

Rectal

Dimenhydrinate
- Suppositories (Canada)

Before Using This Medicine

In deciding to use a medicine, the risks of taking the medicine must be weighed against the good it will do. This is a decision you and your doctor will make. For antihistamines, the following should be considered:

Allergies—Tell your doctor if you have ever had any unusual or allergic reaction to antihistamines. Also tell your health care professional if you are allergic to any other substances, such as foods, preservatives, or dyes.

Diet—Make certain your health care professional knows if you are on a low-sodium, low-sugar, or any other special diet. Most medicines contain more than their active ingredient, and many liquid medicines contain alcohol.

Pregnancy—Most antihistamines have not been studied in pregnant women. Although these antihistamines have not been shown to cause problems in humans, studies in animals have shown that some other antihistamines, such as meclizine (e.g., Antivert) and cyclizine (e.g., Marezine), may cause birth defects.

Also, studies in animals have shown that terfenadine, when given in doses several times the human dose, lowers the birth weight and increases the risk of death of the offspring.

Cetirizine and hydroxyzine are not recommended for use in the first months of pregnancy since they have been shown to cause birth defects in animal studies when given in doses many times higher than the usual human dose. Be sure you have discussed this with your doctor.

Breast-feeding—Small amounts of antihistamines pass into the breast milk. Use is not recommended since babies are more susceptible to the side effects of antihistamines, such as unusual excitement or irritability. Also, since these medicines tend to decrease the secretions of the body, it is possible that the flow of breast milk may be reduced in some patients. It is not known yet whether astemizole, cetirizine, loratadine, and terfenadine cause these same side effects.

Children—Serious side effects, such as convulsions (seizures), are more likely to occur in younger patients and would be of greater risk to infants than to older children or adults. In general, children are more sensitive to the effects of antihistamines. Also, nightmares or unusual excitement, nervousness, restlessness, or irritability may be more likely to occur in children.

Older adults—Elderly patients are usually more sensitive to the effects of antihistamines. Confusion; difficult or painful urination; dizziness; drowsiness; feeling faint; or dryness of mouth, nose, or throat may be more likely to occur in elderly patients. Also, nightmares or unusual excitement, nervousness, restlessness, or irritability may be more likely to occur in elderly patients.

Other medicines—Although certain medicines should not be used together at all, in other cases different medicines may be used together even if an interaction might occur. In these cases, your doctor may want to change the dose, or other precautions may be necessary. When you are taking antihistamines it is especially important that your health care professional knows if you are taking any of the following:

- Anticholinergics (medicine for abdominal or stomach spasms or cramps)—Side effects, such as dryness of mouth, of antihistamines or anticholinergics may be more likely to occur

- Azithromycin (e.g., Zithromax) or
- Clarithromycin (e.g., Biaxin) or
- Erythromycin (e.g., E-Mycin) or
- Itraconazole (e.g., Sporanox) or
- Ketoconazole (e.g., Nizoral)—Use of these medicines with astemizole and terfenadine may cause heart problems, such as an irregular heartbeat; these medicines should not be used together

- Bipridil (e.g., Vascor) or
- Disopyramide (e.g., Norpace) or
- Maprotiline (e.g., Ludiomil) or
- Phenothiazines (acetophenazine [e.g., Tindal], chlorpromazine [e.g., Thorazine], fluphenazine [e.g., Prolixin], mesoridazine [e.g., Serentil], perphenazine [e.g., Trilafon], prochlorperazine [e.g., Compazine], promazine [e.g., Sparine], promethazine [e.g., Phenergan], thioridazine [e.g., Mellaril], trifluoperazine [e.g., Stelazine], triflupromazine [e.g., Vesprin], trimeprazine [e.g., Temaril]) or
- Pimozide (e.g., Orap) or
- Procainamide (e.g., Pronestyl) or
- Quinidine (e.g., Quinaglute Dura-tabs) or
- Tricyclic antidepressants (amitriptyline [e.g., Elavil], amoxapine [e.g., Asendin], clomipramine [e.g., Anafranil], desipramine [e.g., Pertofrane], doxepin [e.g., Sinequan], imipramine [e.g., Tofranil], nortriptyline [e.g., Aventyl],

protriptyline [e.g., Vivactil], trimipramine [e.g., Surmontil])—Use of these medicines with astemizole or terfenadine may increase the risk of heart rhythm problems

- Central nervous system (CNS) depressants—Effects, such as drowsiness, of CNS depressants or antihistamines may be worsened; also, taking maprotiline or tricyclic antidepressants may cause some side effects of either of these medicines, such as dryness of mouth, to become more severe
- Monoamine oxidase (MAO) inhibitors (furazolidone [e.g., Furoxone], isocarboxazid [e.g., Marplan], phenelzine [e.g., Nardil], procarbazine [e.g., Matulane], tranylcypromine [e.g., Parnate])—If you are now taking, or have taken within the past 2 weeks, any of the MAO inhibitors, the side effects of the antihistamines, such as drowsiness and dryness of mouth, may become more severe; these medicines should not be used together

Other medical problems—The presence of other medical problems may affect the use of antihistamines. Make sure you tell your doctor if you have any other medical problems, especially:

- Enlarged prostate or
- Urinary tract blockage or difficult urination—Antihistamines may make urinary problems worse
- Glaucoma—These medicines may cause a slight increase in inner eye pressure that may make the condition worse
- Heart rhythm problems (history of) or
- Low potassium blood levels—Use of astemizole or terfenadine can cause serious heart rhythm problems
- Liver disease—Higher blood levels of astemizole or terfenadine may result, which may increase the chance of heart problems

Proper Use of This Medicine

Antihistamines are used to relieve or prevent the symptoms of your medical problem. Take them only as directed. Do not take more of them and do not take them more often than recommended on the label, unless otherwise directed by your doctor. To do so may increase the chance of side effects.

Dosing—The dose of an antihistamine will be different for different patients. *Follow your doctor's orders or the directions on the label.* The following information includes only the average doses of antihistamines. *If your dose is different, do not change it* unless your doctor tells you to do so.

The number of capsules or tablets or teaspoonfuls of liquid that you take or the number of suppositories you use depends on the strength of the medicine. Also, *the number of doses you take each day and the time between doses depends on whether you are taking a short-acting or long-acting form of antihistamine.*

- For use as an antihistamine:
    - *For astemizole*
        - For *oral* dosage forms (tablets or liquid):
            —Adults and teenagers: 10 milligrams (mg) once a day.
            —Children younger than 6 years of age: 0.2 mg per kilogram (kg) (0.1 mg per pound) of body weight once a day.
            —Children 6 to 12 years of age: 5 mg once a day.
    - *For azatadine*
        - For *oral* dosage form (tablets):
            —Adults: 1 to 2 milligrams (mg) every eight to twelve hours as needed.
            —Children younger than 12 years of age: Use and dose must be determined by your doctor.
            —Children 12 years of age and older: 0.5 mg to 1 mg two times a day as needed.
    - *For brompheniramine*
        - For *regular (short-acting) oral* dosage forms (capsules, tablets, or liquid):

—Adults and teenagers: 4 milligrams (mg) every four to six hours as needed.

—Children 2 to 6 years of age: 1 mg every four to six hours as needed.

—Children 6 to 12 years of age: 2 mg every four to six hours as needed.

• For *long-acting oral* dosage form (tablets):

—Adults: 8 milligrams (mg) every eight or twelve hours, or 12 mg every twelve hours as needed.

—Children younger than 6 years of age: Use and dose must be determined by your doctor.

—Children 6 years of age and older: 8 or 12 mg every twelve hours as needed.

• For *injection* dosage form:

—Adults and teenagers: 10 milligrams (mg) injected into a muscle, under the skin, or into a vein every eight to twelve hours.

—Children younger than 12 years of age: 0.125 mg per kilogram (0.06 mg per pound) of body weight injected into a muscle, under the skin, or into a vein three or four times a day as needed.

For cetirizine

• For *oral* dosage form (tablets):

—Adults: 5 to 10 milligrams (mg) once a day.

—Children: Use and dose must be determined by your doctor.

For chlorpheniramine

• For *regular (short-acting) oral* dosage forms (tablets or liquid):

—Adults and teenagers: 4 milligrams (mg) every four to six hours as needed.

—Children younger than 6 years of age: Use and dose must be determined by your doctor.

—Children 6 to 12 years of age: 2 mg three or four times a day as needed.

• For *long-acting oral* dosage forms (capsules or tablets):

   —Adults: 8 or 12 milligrams (mg) every eight to twelve hours as needed.

   —Children younger than 12 years of age: Use and dose must be determined by your doctor.

   —Children 12 years of age and older: 8 mg every twelve hours as needed.

• For *injection* dosage form:

   —Adults: 5 to 40 milligrams (mg) injected into a muscle, into a vein, or under the skin.

   —Children: 0.0875 mg per kilogram (0.04 mg per pound) of body weight injected under the skin every six hours as needed.

For clemastine

• For *oral* dosage forms (tablets or liquid):

   —Adults and teenagers: 1.34 milligrams (mg) two times a day or 2.68 mg one to three times a day as needed.

   —Children younger than 6 years of age: Use and dose must be determined by your doctor.

   —Children 6 to 12 years of age: 0.67 to 1.34 mg two times a day.

For cyproheptadine

• For *oral* dosage forms (tablets or liquid):

   —Adults and children 14 years of age and older: 4 milligrams (mg) every eight hours. The doctor may increase the dose if needed.

   —Children 2 to 6 years of age: 2 mg every eight to twelve hours as needed.

   —Children 6 to 14 years of age: 4 mg every eight to twelve hours as needed.

For dexchlorpheniramine

• For *regular (short-acting) oral* dosage forms (tablets or liquid):

   —Adults and teenagers: 2 milligrams (mg) every four to six hours as needed.

—Children 2 to 5 years of age: 0.5 mg every four to six hours as needed.

—Children 5 to 12 years of age: 1 mg every four to six hours as needed.

• For *long-acting oral* dosage form (tablets):

—Adults: 4 or 6 milligrams (mg) every eight to twelve hours as needed.

—Children: Use and dose must be determined by your doctor.

For diphenhydramine

• For *oral* dosage forms (capsules, tablets, or liquid):

—Adults and teenagers: 25 to 50 milligrams (mg) every four to six hours as needed.

—Children younger than 6 years of age: 6.25 to 12.5 mg every four to six hours.

—Children 6 to 12 years of age: 12.5 to 25 mg every four to six hours.

• For *injection* dosage form:

—Adults: 10 to 50 milligrams (mg) injected into a muscle or into a vein.

—Children: 1.25 mg per kg (0.6 mg per pound) of body weight injected into a muscle four times a day.

For doxylamine

• For *oral* dosage form (tablets):

—Adults and teenagers: 12.5 to 25 milligrams (mg) every four to six hours as needed.

—Children younger than 6 years of age: Use and dose must be determined by your doctor.

—Children 6 to 12 years of age: 6.25 to 12.5 mg every four to six hours as needed.

For hydroxyzine

• For *oral* dosage forms (capsules, tablets, or liquid):

—Adults and teenagers: 25 to 100 milligrams (mg) three or four times a day as needed.

—Children younger than 12 years of age: 0.5 mg per kg (0.2 mg per pound) of body weight every six hours as needed.

For loratadine
• For *oral* dosage forms (tablets or liquid):
—Adults and children 10 years of age and older: 10 milligrams (mg) once a day on an empty stomach.
—Children 2 to 9 years of age: 5 mg once a day on an empty stomach.

For phenindamine
• For *oral* dosage form (tablets):
—Adults and teenagers: 25 milligrams (mg) every four to six hours as needed.
—Children younger than 6 years of age: Use and dose must be determined by your doctor.
—Children 6 to 12 years of age: 12.5 mg every four to six hours as needed.

For pyrilamine
• For *oral* dosage form (tablets):
—Adults: 25 to 50 milligrams (mg) every eight hours as needed.
—Children 2 to 6 years of age: Use and dose must be determined by your doctor.
—Children 6 years of age and older: 12.5 to 25 mg every eight hours as needed.

For terfenadine
• For *oral* dosage forms (tablets or liquid):
—Adults and teenagers: 60 milligrams (mg) every twelve hours.
—Children 3 to 6 years of age: 15 mg every twelve hours as needed.
—Children 7 to 12 years of age: 30 mg every twelve hours as needed.

For tripelennamine
• For *regular (short-acting) oral* dosage forms (tablets or liquid):

—Adults: 25 to 50 milligrams (mg) every four to six hours as needed.

—Children: 1.25 mg per kilogram (kg) (0.6 mg per pound) of body weight every six hours as needed.

• For *long-acting oral* dosage form (tablets):

—Adults: 100 milligrams (mg) every eight to twelve hours as needed.

—Children: Use and dose must be determined by your doctor.

For triprolidine

• For *oral* dosage forms (liquid):

—Adults and teenagers: 2.5 milligrams (mg) every four to six hours as needed.

—Children 4 months to 2 years of age: 0.312 mg (1/4 teaspoonful) every six to eight hours as needed.

—Children 2 to 4 years of age: 0.625 mg (1/2 teaspoonful) every six to eight hours as needed.

—Children 4 to 6 years of age: 0.937 mg (3/4 teaspoonful) every six to eight hours as needed.

—Children 6 to 12 years of age: 1.25 mg (1 teaspoonful) every six to eight hours as needed.

• For nausea, vomiting, and vertigo (only dimenhydrinate and diphenhydramine are used for vertigo):

For dimenhydrinate

• For *regular (short-acting) oral* dosage forms (capsules, tablets, or liquid):

—Adults and teenagers: 50 to 100 milligrams (mg) every four hours as needed.

—Children 2 to 6 years of age: 12.5 to 25 mg every six to eight hours as needed.

—Children 6 to 12 years of age: 25 to 50 mg every six to eight hours as needed.

- For *long-acting oral* dosage form (capsules):

  —Adults: 1 capsule (contains 25 milligrams [mg] for immediate action and 50 mg for long action) every twelve hours.

  —Children: Use and dose must be determined by your doctor.

- For *injection* dosage form:

  —Adults: 50 milligrams (mg) injected into a muscle or into a vein every four hours as needed.

  —Children: 1.25 mg per kg (0.6 mg per pound) of body weight injected into a muscle or into a vein every six hours as needed.

- For *suppository* dosage form:

  —Adults: 50 to 100 milligrams (mg) inserted into the rectum every six to eight hours as needed.

  —Children younger than 6 years of age: Use and dose must be determined by your doctor.

  —Children 6 to 8 years of age: 12.5 to 25 mg inserted into the rectum every eight to twelve hours as needed.

  —Children 8 to 12 years of age: 25 to 50 mg inserted into the rectum every eight to twelve hours as needed.

  —Children 12 years of age and older: 50 mg inserted into the rectum every eight to twelve hours as needed.

For diphenhydramine

- For *oral* dosage forms (capsules, tablets, or liquid):

  —Adults: 25 to 50 milligrams (mg) every four to six hours as needed.

  —Children: 1 to 1.5 mg per kg (0.45 to 0.7 mg per pound) of body weight every four to six hours as needed.

- For *injection* dosage form:

—Adults: 10 milligrams (mg) injected into a muscle or into a vein. Dose may be increased to 25 to 50 mg every two to three hours.

—Children: 1 to 1.5 mg per kg (0.45 to 0.68 mg per pound) of body weight injected into a muscle every six hours.

For hydroxyzine

• For *oral* dosage forms (capsules, tablets, or liquid):

—Adults: 25 to 100 milligrams (mg) three or four times a day as needed.

—Children younger than 6 years of age: 12.5 mg every six hours as needed.

—Children 6 years of age and older: 12.5 to 25 mg every six hours as needed.

• For *injection* dosage form:

—Adults: 25 to 100 milligrams (mg) injected into a muscle.

—Children: 1 mg per kg (0.45 mg per pound) of body weight injected into a muscle.

• For Parkinson's disease:

For diphenhydramine

• For *oral* dosage forms (capsules, tablets, or liquid):

—Adults: 25 milligrams (mg) three times a day when starting treatment. Your doctor may increase the dose gradually later if needed.

• For *injection* dosage form:

—Adults: 10 to 50 milligrams (mg) injected into a muscle or into a vein.

—Children: 1.25 mg per kg (0.6 mg per pound) of body weight four times a day injected into a muscle.

• For use as a sedative (to help sleep):

For diphenhydramine

• For *oral* dosage forms (capsules, tablets, or liquid):

—Adults: 50 milligrams (mg) twenty to thirty minutes before bedtime if needed.

For doxylamine
   • For *oral* dosage form (tablets):
      —Adults: 25 milligrams (mg) thirty minutes before bedtime if needed.
      —Children: Use and dose must be determined by your doctor.

For hydroxyzine
   • For *oral* dosage forms (capsules, tablets, or liquid):
      —Adults: 50 to 100 milligrams (mg).
      —Children: 0.6 mg per kg (0.3 mg per pound) of body weight.
   • For *injection* dosage form:
      —Adults: 50 milligrams (mg) injected into a muscle.

• For cough:

For diphenhydramine
   • For *oral* dosage form (liquid):
      —Adults and teenagers: 25 milligrams (mg) every four to six hours.
      —Children younger than 2 years of age: Use and dose must be determined by your doctor.
      —Children 2 to 6 years of age: 6.25 mg (1/2 teaspoonful) every four to six hours as needed.
      —Children 6 to 12 years of age: 12.5 mg (1 teaspoonful) every four to six hours as needed.

• For anxiety:

For hydroxyzine
   • For *oral* dosage forms (capsules, tablets, or liquid):
      —Adults: 50 to 100 milligrams (mg).
      —Children: 0.6 mg per kilogram (0.3 mg per pound) of body weight.

- For *injection* dosage form:
  —Adults: 50 to 100 milligrams (mg) injected into a muscle every four to six hours as needed.
  —Children: 1 mg per kilogram (0.45 mg per pound) of body weight injected into a muscle.

Missed dose—If you are taking this medicine regularly and you miss a dose, take it as soon as possible. However, if it is almost time for your next dose, skip the missed dose and go back to your regular dosing schedule. Do not double doses.

For patients *taking this medicine by mouth:*

- Antihistamines can be taken with food or a glass of water or milk to lessen stomach irritation if necessary. However, food may change the amounts of astemizole and loratadine that are absorbed. For this reason, astemizole and loratadine should be taken on an empty stomach.
- If you are taking the extended-release tablet form of this medicine, swallow the tablets whole. Do not break, crush, or chew before swallowing.

For patients taking *dimenhydrinate or diphenhydramine for motion sickness:*

- Take this medicine at least 30 minutes or, even better, 1 to 2 hours before you begin to travel.

For patients using the *suppository form of this medicine:*

- To insert suppository: First remove the foil wrapper and moisten the suppository with cold water. Lie down on your side and use your finger to push the suppository well up into the rectum. If the suppository is too soft to insert, chill the suppository in the refrigerator for 30 minutes or run cold water over it before removing the foil wrapper.

For patients using the *injection form of this medicine:*

- If you will be giving yourself the injections, make

sure you understand exactly how to give them. If you have any questions about this, check with your health care professional.

Storage—To store this medicine:

- Keep out of the reach of children, since overdose may be very dangerous in children.
- Store away from heat and direct light.
- Do not store the capsule or tablet form of this medicine in the bathroom medicine cabinet, near the kitchen sink, or in other damp places. Heat or moisture may cause the medicine to break down.
- Keep the liquid form of this medicine from freezing.
- Do not keep outdated medicine or medicine no longer needed. Be sure that any discarded medicine is out of the reach of children.

Precautions While Using This Medicine

Before you have any skin tests for allergies, tell the doctor in charge that you are taking this medicine. The results of the test may be affected by this medicine.

When taking antihistamines on a regular basis, make sure your doctor knows if you are taking large amounts of aspirin at the same time (as for arthritis or rheumatism). Effects of too much aspirin, such as ringing in the ears, may be covered up by the antihistamine.

Antihistamines will add to the effects of alcohol and other CNS depressants (medicines that slow down the nervous system, possibly causing drowsiness). Some examples of CNS depressants are sedatives, tranquilizers, or sleeping medicine; prescription pain medicine or narcotics; barbiturates; medicine for seizures; muscle relaxants; or anesthetics, including some dental anesthetics. *Check with your doctor before taking any of the above while you are using this medicine.*

This medicine may cause some people to become drowsy or less alert than they are normally. Even if taken at bedtime, it may cause some people to feel drowsy or less alert on arising. Some antihistamines are more likely to cause drowsiness than others. Drowsiness is less likely with cetirizine, and rare with astemizole, loratadine, and terfenadine. *Make sure you know how you react to the antihistamine you are taking before you drive, use machines, or do anything else that could be dangerous if you are not alert.*

Antihistamines may cause dryness of the mouth, nose, and throat. Some antihistamines are more likely to cause dryness of the mouth than others (astemizole, cetirizine, loratadine, and terfenadine, for example, rarely produce this effect). For temporary relief of mouth dryness, use sugarless candy or gum, melt bits of ice in your mouth, or use a saliva substitute. However, if your mouth continues to feel dry for more than 2 weeks, check with your medical doctor or dentist. Continuing dryness of the mouth may increase the chance of dental disease, including tooth decay, gum disease, and fungus infections.

For patients using *dimenhydrinate, diphenhydramine, or hydroxyzine:*

* This medicine controls nausea and vomiting. For this reason, it may cover up the signs of overdose caused by other medicines or the symptoms of appendicitis. This will make it difficult for your doctor to diagnose these conditions. Make sure your doctor knows that you are taking this medicine if you have other symptoms of appendicitis such as stomach or lower abdominal pain, cramping, or soreness. Also, if you think you may have taken an overdose of any medicine, tell your doctor that you are taking this medicine.

For patients using *diphenhydramine or doxylamine as a sleeping aid:*

- If you are already taking a sedative or tranquilizer, do not take this medicine without consulting your doctor first.

Side Effects of This Medicine

Along with its needed effects, a medicine may cause some unwanted effects. Although not all of these side effects may occur, if they do occur they may need medical attention.

Check with your doctor immediately if the following side effect occurs:

Less common or rare—with high doses of astemizole or terfenadine only

Fast or irregular heartbeat

Also, check with your doctor as soon as possible if any of the following side effects occur:

Less common or rare

Sore throat and fever; unusual bleeding or bruising; unusual tiredness or weakness

Symptoms of overdose

Clumsiness or unsteadiness; convulsions (seizures); drowsiness (severe); dryness of mouth, nose, or throat (severe); feeling faint; flushing or redness of face; hallucinations (seeing, hearing, or feeling things that are not there); shortness of breath or troubled breathing; trouble in sleeping

Other side effects may occur that usually do not need medical attention. These side effects may go away during treatment as your body adjusts to the medicine. However, check with your health care professional if any of the following side effects continue or are bothersome:

More common—less common with cetirizine; rare with astemizole, loratadine, and terfenadine

Drowsiness; thickening of mucus

Less common or rare

Blurred vision or any change in vision; confusion; difficult or painful urination; dizziness; dryness of mouth, nose, or throat; fast heartbeat; increased sensitivity of skin to sun; increased sweating; loss of appetite (increased appetite with astemizole, cetirizine, cyproheptadine, loratadine, and terfenadine); nightmares; ringing or buzzing in ears; skin rash; stomach upset or stomach pain (more common with pyrilamine and tripelennamine); unusual excitement, nervousness, restlessness, or irritability; weight gain (with astemizole and cyproheptadine only)

Other side effects not listed above may also occur in some patients. If you notice any other effects, check with your health care professional.

Additional Information

Once a medicine has been approved for marketing for a certain use, experience may show that it is also useful for other medical problems. Although this use is not included in product labeling, astemizole, cetirizine, loratadine, and terfenadine are used in certain patients with asthma together with asthma medicines. The antihistamine is used before and during exposure to substances that cause reactions, to prevent or reduce bronchospasm (wheezing or difficulty in breathing).

Other than the above information, there is no additional information relating to proper use, precautions, or side effects for this use.

ANTIHISTAMINES AND DECONGESTANTS   Systemic

Some commonly used brand names are:

In the U.S.—

Actagen[25]
Actifed[25]
Actifed Head Cold
   and Allergy Medicine[25]
Alamine[11]
Alersule[9]
Allent[6]
Allercon[25]
Allerest[11]
Allerest, Children's[11]
Allerest 12 Hour[11]
Allerest 12 Hour
   Caplets[11]
Allerest Maximum Strength[14]
Allerfrim[25]
Allerfrin[25]
Allergy Cold[25]
Allergy Formula Sinutab[18]
Allergy Relief Medicine[11]
Allerphed[25]
Amaril D[13]
Amaril D Spantab[13]
Ami-Drix[18]
Anamine[14]
Anamine T.D.[14]
Anaplex[14]
Anaplex S.R.[14]
Aprodrine[25]
A.R.M. Maximum
   Strength Caplets[11]
Atrohist Pediatric[15]
Atrohist Sprinkle[5]
Benadryl Decongestant[19]
Benylin Decongestant[19]
Brexin L.A.[14]
Brofed[6]
Bromaline[4]
Bromanate[4]

Bromatap[4]
Bromatapp[4]
Bromfed[6]
Bromfed-PD[6]
Bromophen T.D.[3]
Bromphen[4]
Brompheril[18]
Carbiset[7]
Carbiset-TR[7]
Carbodec[7]
Carbodec TR[7]
Cardec-S[7]
Cenafed Plus[25]
Cheracol Sinus[18]
Chlorafed[14]
Chlorafed H.S. Timecelles[14]
Chlorafed Timecelles[14]
Chlordrine S.R.[14]
Chlorphedrine SR[14]
Chlor-Rest[11]
Chlor-Trimeton 4 Hour
   Relief[14]
Chlor-Trimeton 12 Hour
   Relief[14]
Codimal-L.A.[14]
Colfed-A[14]
Coltab Children's[9]
Comhist[12]
Comhist LA[12]
Condrin-LA[11]
Conex D.A.[11]
Contac 12-Hour[11]
Contac Maximum Strength
   12-Hour Caplets[11]
Cophene No.2[14]
Co-Pyronil 2[14]
Dallergy-D[9] [14]
Dallergy Jr.[6]

In the U.S. (cont'd)—

Deconamine[14]
Deconamine SR[14]
Decongestabs[13]
Dehist[11]
Demazin[11]
Demazin Repetabs[11]
Dexaphen SA[18]
Dexophed[18]
Dihistine[9]
Dimaphen[4]
Dimaphen S.A.[3]
Dimetane
  Decongestant[2]
Dimetane
  Decongestant Caplets[2]
Dimetapp[4]
Dimetapp Cold
  and Allergy[4]
Dimetapp Extentabs[4]
Dimetapp 4-Hour
  Liqui-gels Maximum
  Strength[4]
Disobrom[18]
Disophrol[18]
Disophrol Chronotabs[18]
Dorcol Children's Cold
  Formula[14]
Dristan Allergy[6]
Drixoral[6][18]
Drixoral Cold
  and Allergy[18]
Drize[11]
Duralex[14]
Dura-Tap PD[14]
Dura-Vent/A[11]
Ed A-Hist[9]
Endafed[6]
E.N.T.[4]
Fedahist[14]
Fedahist
  Decongestant[14]
Fedahist Gyrocaps[14]
Fedahist Timecaps[14]
Genac[25]
Genamin[11]

Genatap[4]
Gencold[11]
Hayfebrol[14]
Histalet[14]
Histalet Forte[16]
Histamic[13]
Histatab Plus[9]
Histatan[15]
Hista-Vadrin[10]
Histor-D[9]
12-Hour Cold[11]
Isoclor[14]
Isoclor Timesules[14]
Klerist-D[14]
Kronofed-A Jr. Kronocaps[14]
Kronofed-A Kronocaps[14]
Lodrane LD[6]
Myphetapp[4]
Naldecon[13]
Naldecon Pediatric Drops[13]
Naldecon Pediatric Syrup[13]
Naldelate[13]
Naldelate Pediatric Syrup [13]
Nalgest[13]
Nalgest Pediatric[13]
Napril[14]
Nasahist[10]
ND Clear T.D.[14]
New-Decongest
  Pediatric Syrup[13]
New-Decongestant
  Pediatric[13]
Nolamine[8]
Noraminic[11]
Normatane[3]
Novafed A[14]
Novahistine[9]
Oraminic Spancaps[11]
Ornade Spansules[11]
Par-Drix[18]
Parhist SR[11]
Partapp[4]
Partapp TD[3]
PediaCare Cold Formula[14]
Phenergan VC[22]

In the U.S. (cont'd)—

Pherazine VC[22]
Poly-Histine-D[20]
Poly-Histine-D Ped[20]
Prehist[9]
Prometh VC Plain[22]
Promethazine VC[22]
Pseudo-Chlor[14]
Pseudo-gest Plus[14]
Quadra-Hist[13]
Quadra-Hist Pediatric[13]
Resaid S.R.[11]
Rescon[11][14]
Rescon-ED[14]
Rescon JR[14]
Rhinatate[15]
Rhinolar-EX[11]
Rhinolar-EX 12[11]
Rhinosyn[14]
Rhinosyn-PD[14]
Rinade B.I.D.[14]
Rolatuss Plain[9]
Rondec[7]
Rondec Drops[7]
Rondec-TR[7]
R-Tannamine[15]
R-Tannamine Pediatric[15]
R-Tannate[15]
R-Tannate Pediatric[15]
Ru-Tuss[9]
Ru-Tuss II[11]
Ryna[14]
Rynatan[15]
Rynatan Pediatric[15]
Rynatan-S Pediatric[15]
Seldane-D[24]
Semprex-D[1]
Sinucon Pediatric
   Drops[13]
Snaplets-D[11]
Sudafed Plus[14]
Tamine S.R.[3]
Tanoral[15]
Tavist-D[17]
T-Dry[14]

T-Dry Junior[14]
Temazin Cold[11]
Touro A & H[6]
Triafed[25]
Triaminic-12[11]
Triaminic Allergy[11]
Triaminic Chewables[11]
Triaminic Cold[11]
Triaminic Oral
   Infant Drops[21]
Triaminic TR[21]
Trifed[25]
Trinalin Repetabs[1a]
Trind[11]
Tri-Nefrin
   Extra Strength[11]
Triofed[25]
Triotann[15]
Triotann Pediatric[15]
Tripalgen Cold[11]
Tri-Phen-Chlor[13]
Tri-Phen-Chlor Pediatric[13]
Tri-Phen-Chlor T.R.[13]
Triphenyl[11]
Triphenyl T.D.[21]
Triposed[25]
Tritann[15]
Tritann Pediatric[15]
Tri-Tannate[15]
Tri-Tannate Pediatric[15]
Tussanil Plain[9]
ULTRAbrom PD[6]
Uni-Decon[13]
Vanex Forte Caplets[16]
Veltap[3]
Vicks Children's
   NyQuil Allergy/Head
   Cold[14]
Vicks DayQuil
   4 Hour Allergy
   Relief[4]
Vicks DayQuil
   12 Hour Allergy
   Relief[4]

In Canada—

Actifed[25]
Benylin Cold[14]
Chlor-Tripolon
  Decongestant[11 14]
Chlor-Tripolon
  Decongestant Extra
  Strength[14]
Chlor-Tripolon
  Decongestant Repetabs[14]
Claritin Extra[19a]
Corsym[11]
Dimetapp[3]
Dimetapp Extentabs[3]

Dimetapp Oral
  Infant Drops[3]
Drixoral[18]
Drixtab[18]
NeoCitran A[19b]
Novahistex[14]
Ornade[11]
Ornade-A.F.[11]
Ornade Spansules[11]
Triaminic[11 21]
Triaminic Oral
  Infant Drops[21]
Trinalin Repetabs[1]

Note: For quick reference the following antihistamine and decongestant combinations are numbered to match the corresponding brand names.

This information applies to the following medicines:

1. Acrivastine (AK-ri-vas-teen) and Pseudoephedrine (soo-doe-e-FED-rin)
1a. Azatadine (a-ZA-ta-deen) and Pseudoephedrine
2. Brompheniramine (brome-fen-EER-a-meen) and Phenylephrine (fen-ill-EF-rin)
3. Brompheniramine, Phenylephrine, and Phenylpropanolamine (fen-ill-proe-pa-NOLE-a-meen)
4. Brompheniramine and Phenylpropanolamine
5. Brompheniramine, Phenyltoloxamine (fen-ill-toe-LOX-a-meen), and Phenylephrine
6. Brompheniramine and Pseudoephedrine
7. Carbinoxamine (kar-bi-NOX-a-meen) and Pseudoephedrine
8. Chlorpheniramine (klor-fen-EER-a-meen), Phenindamine (fen-IN-da-meen), and Phenylpropanolamine
9. Chlorpheniramine and Phenylephrine
10. Chlorpheniramine, Phenylephrine, and Phenylpropanolamine
11. Chlorpheniramine and Phenylpropanolamine
12. Chlorpheniramine, Phenyltoloxamine, and Phenylephrine
13. Chlorpheniramine, Phenyltoloxamine, Phenylephrine, and Phenylpropanolamine
14. Chlorpheniramine and Pseudoephedrine
15. Chlorpheniramine, Pyrilamine (peer-ILL-a-meen), and Phenylephrine
16. Chlorpheniramine, Pyrilamine, Phenylephrine, and Phenylpropanolamine
17. Clemastine (KLEM-as-teen) and Phenylpropanolamine
18. Dexbrompheniramine (dex-brom-fen-EER-a-meen) and Pseudoephedrine

19. Diphenhydramine (dye-fen-HYE-dra-meen) and Pseudoephedrine
19a. Loratadine (lor-AT-a-deen) and Pseudoephedrine
19b. Pheniramine (fen-EER-a-meen) and Phenylephrine
20. Pheniramine, Phenyltoloxamine, Pyrilamine, and Phenylpropanolamine
21. Pheniramine, Pyrilamine, and Phenylpropanolamine
22. Promethazine (proe-METH-a-zeen) and Phenylephrine
23. No product available
24. Terfenadine (ter-FEN-a-deen) and Pseudoephedrine
25. Triprolidine (trye-PROE-li-deen) and Pseudoephedrine

Description

Antihistamine and decongestant combinations are used to treat the nasal congestion (stuffy nose), sneezing, and runny nose caused by colds and hay fever.

Antihistamines work by preventing the effects of a substance called histamine, which is produced by the body. Histamine can cause itching, sneezing, runny nose, and watery eyes. Antihistamines contained in these combinations are: acrivastine, azatadine, brompheniramine, carbinoxamine, chlorpheniramine, clemastine, dexbrompheniramine, diphenhydramine, loratadine, pheniramine, phenyltoloxamine, promethazine, pyrilamine, terfenadine, and triprolidine.

The decongestants, such as phenylephrine, phenylpropanolamine (also known as PPA), and pseudoephedrine, produce a narrowing of blood vessels. This leads to clearing of nasal congestion, but it may also cause an increase in blood pressure in patients who have high blood pressure.

Some of these combinations are available only with your doctor's prescription. Others are available without a prescription; however, your doctor may have special instructions on the proper dose of the medicine for your medical condition. They are available in the following dosage forms:

Oral

Acrivastine and Pseudoephedrine
• Capsules (U.S.)

Azatadine and Pseudoephedrine
• Extended-release tablets (U.S. and Canada)
Brompheniramine and Phenylephrine
• Elixir (U.S.)
• Tablets (U.S.)
Brompheniramine, Phenylephrine, and Phenylpropanolamine
• Elixir (U.S. and Canada)
• Oral solution (Canada)
• Tablets (Canada)
• Extended-release tablets (U.S. and Canada)
Brompheniramine and Phenylpropanolamine
• Capsules (U.S.)
• Elixir (U.S.)
• Tablets (U.S.)
• Chewable tablets (U.S.)
• Extended-release tablets (U.S.)
Brompheniramine, Phenyltoloxamine, and Phenylephrine
• Extended-release capsules (U.S.)
Brompheniramine and Pseudoephedrine
• Extended-release capsules (U.S.)
• Elixir (U.S.)
• Syrup (U.S.)
• Tablets (U.S.)
Carbinoxamine and Pseudoephedrine
• Oral solution (U.S.)
• Syrup (U.S.)
• Tablets (U.S.)
• Extended-release tablets (U.S.)
Chlorpheniramine, Phenindamine, and Phenylpropanolamine
• Extended-release tablets (U.S.)
Chlorpheniramine and Phenylephrine
• Extended-release capsules (U.S.)
• Elixir (U.S.)
• Oral solution (U.S.)
• Syrup (U.S.)
• Tablets (U.S.)
• Chewable tablets (U.S.)
Chlorpheniramine, Phenylephrine, and Phenylpropanolamine

- Extended-release capsules (U.S.)
- Tablets (U.S.)

Chlorpheniramine and Phenylpropanolamine
- Extended-release capsules (U.S. and Canada)
- Granules (U.S.)
- Oral solution (U.S. and Canada)
- Extended-release oral suspension (Canada)
- Syrup (U.S. and Canada)
- Tablets (U.S.)
- Chewable tablets (U.S.)
- Extended-release tablets (U.S.)

Chlorpheniramine, Phenyltoloxamine, and Phenylephrine
- Extended-release capsules (U.S.)
- Tablets (U.S.)

Chlorpheniramine, Phenyltoloxamine, Phenylephrine, and Phenylpropanolamine
- Extended-release capsules (U.S.)
- Oral solution (U.S.)
- Syrup (U.S.)
- Extended-release tablets (U.S.)

Chlorpheniramine and Pseudoephedrine
- Capsules (U.S. and Canada)
- Extended-release capsules (U.S. and Canada)
- Oral solution (U.S.)
- Syrup (U.S.)
- Tablets (U.S. and Canada)
- Extended-release tablets (U.S. and Canada)

Chlorpheniramine, Pyrilamine, and Phenylephrine
- Oral suspension (U.S.)
- Tablets (U.S.)
- Extended-release tablets (U.S.)

Chlorpheniramine, Pyrilamine, Phenylephrine, and Phenylpropanolamine
- Tablets (U.S.)

Clemastine and Phenylpropanolamine
- Extended-release tablets (U.S.)

Dexbrompheniramine and Pseudoephedrine
- Extended-release capsules (Canada)
- Syrup (Canada)
- Tablets (U.S.)
- Extended-release tablets (U.S. and Canada)

Diphenhydramine and Pseudoephedrine
* Capsules (U.S.)
* Oral solution (U.S.)
* Tablets (U.S.)

Loratadine and Pseudoephedrine
* Tablets (Canada)

Pheniramine and Phenylephrine
* Oral solution (Canada)

Pheniramine, Phenyltoloxamine, Pyrilamine, and Phenyl-
propanolamine
* Extended-release capsules (U.S.)
* Elixir (U.S.)

Pheniramine, Pyrilamine, and Phenylpropanolamine
* Oral solution (U.S. and Canada)
* Extended-release tablets (U.S. and Canada)

Promethazine and Phenylephrine
* Syrup (U.S.)

Terfenadine and Pseudoephedrine
* Extended-release tablets (U.S.)

Triprolidine and Pseudoephedrine
* Capsules (U.S.)
* Syrup (U.S. and Canada)
* Tablets (U.S. and Canada)

Before Using This Medicine

If you are taking this medicine without a prescription,
carefully read and follow any precautions on the label. For
antihistamine and decongestant combinations, the following should be considered:

Allergies—Tell your doctor if you have ever had any unusual or allergic reaction to antihistamines or to amphet-
amine, dextroamphetamine (e.g., Dexedrine), ephedrine
(e.g., Ephed II), epinephrine (e.g., Adrenalin), isoproter-
nol (e.g., Isuprel), metaproterenol (e.g., Alupent), metham-
phetamine (e.g., Desoxyn), norepinephrine (e.g.,
Levophed), phenylephrine (e.g., Neo-Synephrine), pseudo-

ephedrine (e.g., Sudafed), PPA (e.g., Dexatrim), or terbutaline (e.g., Brethine).

Pregnancy—The occasional use of antihistamine and decongestant combinations is not likely to cause problems in the fetus or in the newborn baby. However, when these medicines are used at higher doses and/or for a long time, the chance that problems might occur may increase. For the individual ingredients of these combinations, the following apply:

- *Alcohol*—Some of these combination medicines contain alcohol. Too much use of alcohol during pregnancy may cause birth defects.

- *Antihistamines*—Antihistamines have not been shown to cause problems in humans.

- *Phenylephrine*—Studies on birth defects have not been done in either humans or animals with phenylephrine.

- *Phenylpropanolamine*—Studies on birth defects have not been done in either humans or animals with phenylpropanolamine. However, it seems that women who take phenylpropanolamine in the weeks following delivery are more likely to suffer mental or mood changes.

- *Promethazine*—Phenothiazines, such as promethazine (contained in some of these combination medicines [e.g., Phenergan-D]), have been shown to cause jaundice and muscle tremors in a few newborn infants whose mothers received phenothiazines during pregnancy. Also, the newborn baby may have blood clotting problems if promethazine is taken by the mother within 2 weeks before delivery.

- *Pseudoephedrine*—Studies on birth defects with pseudoephedrine have not been done in humans. In animal studies pseudoephedrine did not cause birth defects but did cause a decrease in average weight, length, and rate of bone formation in the animal fetus when administered in high doses.

Breast-feeding—Small amounts of antihistamines and decongestants pass into the breast milk. Use is not recommended since the chances are greater for this medicine to cause side effects, such as unusual excitement or irritability, in the nursing baby. Also, since antihistamines tend to decrease the secretions of the body, it is possible that the flow of breast milk may be reduced in some patients. It is not known yet whether loratadine or terfenadine causes these same side effects.

Children—Very young children are usually more sensitive to the effects of this medicine. Increases in blood pressure, nightmares or unusual excitement, nervousness, restlessness, or irritability may be more likely to occur in children. Also, mental changes may be more likely to occur in young children taking combination medicines that contain phenylpropanolamine. *Before giving any of these combination medicines to a child, check the package label very carefully. Some of these medicines are too strong for use in children.* If you are not certain whether a specific product can be given to a child, or if you have any questions about the amount to give, check with your health care professional.

Older adults—Confusion, difficult and painful urination, dizziness, drowsiness, dryness of mouth, or convulsions (seizures) may be more likely to occur in the elderly, who are usually more sensitive to the effects of this medicine. Also, nightmares or unusual excitement, nervousness, restlessness, or irritability may be more likely to occur in elderly patients.

Other medicines—Although certain medicines should not be used together at all, in other cases different medicines may be used together even if an interaction might occur. In these cases, your doctor may want to change the dose, or other precautions may be necessary. When you are taking antihistamines it is especially important that your health care professional know if you are taking any of the following:

- Anticholinergics (medicine for abdominal or stomach spasms or cramps)—Side effects, such as dryness of mouth, of antihistamines or anticholinergics may be more likely to occur
- Azithromycin (e.g., Zithromax) or
- Clarithromycin (e.g., Biaxin) or
- Erythromycin (e.g., E-Mycin) or
- Itraconazole (e.g., Sporanox) or
- Ketoconazole (e.g., Nizoral)—Use of these medicines with the terfenadine-containing combination may cause heart problems, such as an irregular heartbeat; these medicines should not be used together
- Central nervous system (CNS) depressants—Effects, such as drowsiness, of CNS depressants or antihistamines may be worsened
- Maprotiline (e.g., Ludiomil) or
- Tricyclic antidepressants (amitriptyline [e.g., Elavil], amoxapine [e.g., Asendin], clomipramine [e.g., Anafranil], desipramine [e.g., Pertofrane], doxepin [e.g., Sinequan], imipramine [e.g., Tofranil], nortriptyline [e.g., Aventyl], protriptyline [e.g., Vivactil], trimipramine [e.g., Surmontil])—Effects, such as drowsiness, of CNS depressants or antihistamines may be worsened; also, taking these medicines together may cause some of their side effects, such as dryness of mouth, to become more severe
- Monoamine oxidase (MAO) inhibitors (furazolidone [e.g., Furoxone], isocarboxazid [e.g., Marplan], phenelzine [e.g., Nardil], procarbazine [e.g., Matulane], selegiline [e.g., Eldepryl], tranylcypromine [e.g., Parnate])—If you are now taking, or have taken within the past 2 weeks, any of the MAO inhibitors, the side effects of the antihistamines may become more severe; these medicines should not be used together
- Rauwolfia alkaloids (alseroxylon [e.g., Rauwiloid], deserpidine [e.g., Harmonyl], rauwolfia serpentina [e.g., Rau-

dixin], reserpine [e.g., Serpasil])—These medicines may increase or decrease the effect of the decongestant

Also, if you are taking one of the combinations containing phenylpropanolamine or pseudoephedrine and are also taking:

- Amantadine (e.g., Symmetrel) or
- Amphetamines or
- Appetite suppressants (diet pills), except fenfluramine (e.g., Pondimin) or
- Caffeine (e.g., NoDoz) or
- Chlophedianol (e.g., Ulone) or
- Medicine for asthma or other breathing problems or
- Medicine for colds, sinus problems, or hay fever or other allergies (including nose drops or sprays) or
- Methylphenidate (e.g., Ritalin) or
- Nabilone (e.g., Cesamet) or
- Pemoline (e.g., Cylert)—Using any of these medicines to-gether with an antihistamine and decongestant combination may cause excessive stimulant side effects, such as diffi-culty in sleeping, heart rate problems, nervousness, and irritability
- Beta-adrenergic blocking agents (acebutolol [e.g., Sectral], atenolol [e.g., Tenormin], betaxolol [e.g., Kerlone], bis-oprolol [e.g., Zebeta], carteolol [e.g., Cartrol], labetalol [e.g., Normodyne], metoprolol [e.g., Lopressor], nadolol [e.g., Corgard], oxprenolol [e.g., Trasicor], penbutolol [e.g., Levatol], pindolol [e.g., Visken], propanolol [e.g., Inderal], sotalol [e.g., Sotacor], timolol [e.g., Bloca-dren])—Using any of these medicines together with an antihistamine and decongestant combination may cause high blood pressure and heart problems (e.g., unusually slow heartbeat)

Other medical problems—The presence of other medical problems may affect the use of antihistamine and decon-gestant combinations. Make sure you tell your doctor if you have any other medical problems, especially:

- Diabetes mellitus (sugar diabetes)—The decongestant in this medicine may put diabetic patients at a greater risk of having heart or blood vessel disease

- Enlarged prostate or
- Urinary tract blockage or difficult urination—Some of the effects of antihistamines may make urinary problems worse
- Glaucoma—A slight increase in inner eye pressure may occur
- Heart or blood vessel disease or
- High blood pressure—The decongestant in this medicine may cause the blood pressure to increase and may also speed up the heart rate
- Liver disease—Higher blood levels of terfenadine may result, which may increase the chance of heart problems (for terfenadine-containing combination only)
- Overactive thyroid—If the overactive thyroid has caused a fast heart rate, the decongestant in this medicine may cause the heart rate to speed up further

---

Proper Use of This Medicine

Take this medicine only as directed. Do not take more of it and do not take it more often than recommended on the label, unless otherwise directed by your doctor. To do so may increase the chance of side effects.

If this medicine irritates your stomach, you may take it with food or a glass of water or milk, to lessen the irritation.

For patients *taking the extended-release capsule or tablet form of this medicine:*

- Swallow it whole.
- Do not crush, break, or chew before swallowing.
- If the capsule is too large to swallow, you may mix the contents of the capsule with applesauce, jelly, honey, or syrup and swallow without chewing.

Dosing—There is a large variety of antihistamine and decongestant combination products on the market. Some products are for use in adults only, while others may be used in children. If you have any questions about this, check with your health care professional.

The dose of antihistamines and decongestants will be different for different products. The number of capsules or tablets or teaspoonfuls of liquid or granules that you take depends on the strengths of the medicines. Also, *the number of doses you take each day and the time between doses depends on whether you are taking a short-acting or long-acting form of antihistamine and decongestant. Follow your doctor's orders if this medicine was prescribed. Or, follow the directions on the box if you are buying this medicine without a prescription.*

Missed dose—If you are taking this medicine regularly and you miss a dose, take it as soon as possible. However, if it is almost time for your next dose, skip the missed dose and go back to your regular dosing schedule. Do not double doses.

Storage—To store this medicine:

- Keep out of the reach of children.
- Store away from heat and direct light.
- Do not store in the bathroom, near the kitchen sink, or in other damp places. Heat or moisture may cause the medicine to break down.
- Keep the liquid form of this medicine from freezing.
- Do not keep outdated medicine or medicine no longer needed. Be sure that any discarded medicine is out of the reach of children.

Precautions While Using This Medicine

Before you have any skin tests for allergies, tell the doctor in charge that you are taking this medicine. The results of the test may be affected by the antihistamine in this medicine.

When taking antihistamines (contained in this combination medicine) on a regular basis, make sure your doctor knows if you are taking large amounts of aspirin at the same time (as for arthritis or rheumatism). Effects of too much aspirin, such as ringing in the ears, may be covered up by the antihistamine.

The antihistamine in this medicine will add to the effects of alcohol and other CNS depressants (medicines that slow down the nervous system, possibly causing drowsiness). Some examples of CNS depressants are other antihistamines or medicine for hay fever, other allergies, or colds; sedatives, tranquilizers, or sleeping medicine; prescription pain medicine or narcotics; barbiturates; medicine for seizures; muscle relaxants; or anesthetics, including some dental anesthetics. *Check with your doctor before taking any of the above while you are taking this medicine.*

The antihistamine in this medicine may cause some people to become drowsy, dizzy, or less alert than they are normally. *Some antihistamines are more likely to cause drowsiness than others (loratadine and terfenadine, for example, rarely produce this effect). Make sure you know how you react before you drive, use machines, or do anything else that could be dangerous if you are dizzy or are not alert.*

The decongestant in this medicine may add to the central nervous system (CNS) stimulant and other effects of phenylpropanolamine (PPA)-containing diet aids. *Do not use medicines for diet or appetite control while taking this medicine unless you have checked with your doctor.*

The decongestant in this medicine may cause some people to be nervous or restless or to have trouble in sleeping. If you have trouble in sleeping, *take the last dose of this medicine for each day a few hours before bedtime.* If you have any questions about this, check with your doctor.

Antihistamines may cause dryness of the mouth, nose, and throat. Some antihistamines are more likely to cause dryness of the mouth than others (loratadine and terfenadine, for example, rarely produce this effect). For temporary relief, use sugarless candy or gum, melt bits of ice in your mouth, or use a saliva substitute. However, if your mouth continues to feel dry for more than 2 weeks, check with your dentist. Continuing dryness of the mouth may increase the chance of dental disease, including tooth decay, gum disease, and fungus infections.

For patients *using promethazine-containing medicine:*
- This medicine controls nausea and vomiting. For this reason, it may cover up the signs of overdose caused by other medicines or the symptoms of intestinal blockage. This will make it difficult for your doctor to diagnose these conditions. Make sure your doctor knows that you are taking this medicine if you have other symptoms such as stomach or lower abdominal pain, cramping, or soreness. Also, if you think you may have taken an overdose of any medicine, tell your doctor that you are taking this medicine.

Side Effects of This Medicine

Along with its needed effects, a medicine may cause some unwanted effects. Although serious side effects occur rarely when this medicine is taken as recommended, they may be more likely to occur if:
- too much medicine is taken.
- it is taken in large doses.
- it is taken for a long period of time.

Get emergency help immediately if any of the following symptoms of overdose occur:

Clumsiness or unsteadiness; convulsions (seizures); drowsiness (severe); dryness of mouth, nose, or throat (severe); flushing or redness of face; hallucinations (seeing, hearing, or feeling things that are not there); headache (continuing); shortness of breath or troubled breathing; slow, fast, or irregular heartbeat; trouble in sleeping

For promethazine only

Muscle spasms (especially of neck and back); restlessness; shuffling walk; tic-like (jerky) movements of head and face; trembling and shaking of hands

Also, check with your doctor as soon as possible if any of the following side effects occur:

Rare

Mood or mental changes; sore throat and fever; tightness in chest; unusual bleeding or bruising; unusual tiredness or weakness

Other side effects may occur that usually do not need medical attention. These side effects may go away during treatment as your body adjusts to the medicine. However, check with your health care professional if any of the following side effects continue or are bothersome:

More common—rare with loratadine- or terfenadine–containing combination

Drowsiness; thickening of the bronchial secretions

Less common—more common with high doses

Blurred vision; confusion; difficult or painful urination; dizziness; dryness of mouth, nose, or throat; headache; loss of appetite; nightmares; pounding heartbeat; ringing or buzzing in ears; skin rash; stomach upset or pain (more common with pyrilamine and tripelennamine); unusual excitement, nervousness, restlessness, or irritability

Other side effects not listed above may also occur in some patients. If you notice any other effects, check with your doctor.

ANTIHISTAMINES, PHENOTHIAZINE-DERIVATIVE
Systemic

Some commonly used brand names are:

In the U.S.—

Anergan 25[2]	Promacot[2]
Anergan 50[2]	Pro-Med 50[2]
Antinaus 50[2]	Promet[2]
Pentazine[2]	Prorex-25[2]
Phenazine 25[2]	Prorex-50[2]
Phenazine 50[2]	Prothazine[2]
Phencen-50[2]	Prothazine Plain[2]
Phenergan[2]	Shogan[2]
Phenergan Fortis[2]	Tacaryl[1]
Phenergan Plain[2]	Temaril[3]
Phenerzine[2]	V-Gan-25[2]
Phenoject-50[2]	V-Gan-50[2]
Pro-50[2]	

In Canada—

Histantil[2]	Phenergan[2]
Panectyl[3]	

Another commonly used name for trimeprazine is alimemazine.

Note: For quick reference, the following antihistamines are numbered to match the corresponding brand names.

This information applies to the following medicines:

1. Methdilazine (meth-DILL-a-zeen)†
2. Promethazine (proe-METH-a-zeen)‡§
3. Trimeprazine (trye-MEP-ra-zeen)‡

---

†Not commercially available in Canada.
‡Generic name product may also be available in the U.S.
§Generic name product may also be available in Canada.

Description

Phenothiazine (FEE-noe-THYE-a-zeen)-derivative antihistamines are used to relieve or prevent the symptoms of hay fever and other types of allergy. They work by preventing the effects of a substance called histamine, which is produced by the body. Histamine can cause itching, sneezing, runny nose, and watery eyes. Also, in some persons histamine can close up the bronchial tubes (air passages of the lungs) and make breathing difficult.

Some of these antihistamines are also used to prevent motion sickness, nausea, vomiting, and dizziness. In addition, some of them may be used to help people go to sleep and control their anxiety before or after surgery.

Phenothiazine-derivative antihistamines may also be used for other conditions as determined by your doctor.

In the U.S. these antihistamines are available only with your doctor's prescription. In Canada some are available without a prescription. However, your doctor may have special instructions on the proper dose of the medicine for your medical condition.

These medicines are available in the following dosage forms:

Oral

Methdilazine
- Syrup (U.S.)
- Tablets (U.S.)
- Chewable tablets (U.S.)

Promethazine
- Syrup (U.S. and Canada)
- Tablets (U.S. and Canada)

Trimeprazine
- Extended-release capsules (U.S.)
- Syrup (U.S. and Canada)
- Tablets (U.S. and Canada)

Parenteral

Promethazine
- Injection (U.S. and Canada)

Rectal

Promethazine
- Suppositories (U.S.)

Before Using This Medicine

In deciding to use a medicine, the risks of taking the medicine must be weighed against the good it will do. This is a decision you and your doctor will make. For phenothiazine-derivative antihistamines, the following should be considered:

Allergies—Tell your doctor if you have ever had any unusual or allergic reaction to these medicines or to phenothiazines. Also tell your health care professional if you are allergic to any other substances, such as foods, preservatives, or dyes.

Pregnancy—Methdilazine, promethazine, and trimeprazine have not been studied in pregnant women. In animal studies, promethazine has not been shown to cause birth defects. However, other phenothiazine medicines caused jaundice and muscle tremors in a few newborn babies whose mothers received these medicines during pregnancy. Also, the newborn baby may have blood clotting problems if promethazine is taken by the mother within two weeks before delivery.

Breast-feeding—Small amounts of antihistamines pass into the breast milk. Use by nursing mothers is not recommended since babies are more sensitive to the side effects of antihistamines, such as unusual excitement or irritability. Also, with the use of phenothiazine-derivative antihistamines there is the chance that the nursing baby may be more at risk of having difficulty in breathing while sleeping or of the sudden infant death syndrome (SIDS). However, more studies are needed to confirm this.

In addition, since these medicines tend to decrease the secretions of the body, it is possible that the flow of breast milk may be reduced in some patients.

Children—Serious side effects, such as convulsions (seizures), are more likely to occur in younger patients and would be of greater risk to infants than to older children or adults. In general, children are more sensitive to the effects of antihistamines. Also, nightmares or unusual excitement, nervousness, restlessness, or irritability may be more likely to occur in children. *The use of phenothiazine-derivative antihistamines is not recommended in children who have a history of difficulty in breathing while sleeping, or a family history of sudden infant death syndrome (SIDS).*

Children who show signs of Reye's syndrome should not be given phenothiazine-derivative antihistamines, especially by injection. Uncontrolled movements that may occur with phenothiazine-derivative antihistamines may be mistakenly confused with symptoms of Reye's syndrome.

Adolescents—Adolescents who show signs of Reye's syndrome should not be given phenothiazine-derivative antihistamines, especially by injection. Uncontrolled movements that may occur with phenothiazine-derivative antihistamines may be mistakenly confused with symptoms of Reye's syndrome.

Older adults—Elderly patients are especially sensitive to the effects of antihistamines. Confusion; difficult or painful urination; dizziness; drowsiness; feeling faint; or dryness of the mouth, nose, or throat may be more likely to occur in elderly patients. Also, nightmares or unusual excitement, nervousness, restlessness, or irritability may be more likely to occur in elderly patients. In addition, uncontrolled movements may be more likely to occur in elderly patients taking phenothiazine-derivative antihistamines.

Other medicines—Although certain medicines should not be used together at all, in other cases two different medicines may be used together even if an interaction might occur. In these cases, your doctor may want to change the dose, or other precautions may be necessary. When taking phenothiazine-derivative antihistamines, it is especially important that your health care professional know if you are taking/receiving any of the following:

- Amoxapine (e.g., Asendin) or
- Antipsychotics (medicine for mental illness) or
- Methyldopa (e.g., Aldomet) or
- Metoclopramide (e.g., Reglan) or
- Metyrosine (e.g., Demser) or
- Pemoline (e.g., Cylert) or
- Pimozide (e.g., Orap) or
- Rauwolfia alkaloids (alseroxylon [e.g., Rauwiloid], deserpidine [e.g., Harmonyl], rauwolfia serpentina [e.g., Raudixin], reserpine [e.g., Serpasil])—Side effects of these medicines, such as uncontrolled body movements, may become more severe and frequent if they are used together with phenothiazine-derivative antihistamines

- Anticholinergics (medicine for abdominal or stomach spasms or cramps)—Side effects of phenothiazine-derivative antihistamines or anticholinergics, such as dryness of mouth, may be more likely to occur

- Central nervous system (CNS) depressants (medicines that cause drowsiness) or
- Maprotiline or
- Tricyclic antidepressants (medicine for depression)—Effects of CNS depressants or antihistamines, such as drowsiness, may become more severe; also, taking maprotiline or tricyclic antidepressants may cause some side effects of antihistamines, such as dryness of mouth, to become more severe

- Contrast agent, injected into spinal canal—If you are having an x-ray test of the head, spinal canal, or nervous system for which you are going to receive an injection into the spinal canal, phenothiazine-derivative antihistamines may increase the chance of seizures; stop taking any phenothiazine-derivative antihistamine 48 hours before the test and do not start taking it until 24 hours after the test

- Levodopa—When used together with phenothiazine-derivative antihistamines, the levodopa may not work as it should

- Monoamine oxidase (MAO) inhibitors (furazolidone [e.g., Furoxone], isocarboxazid [e.g., Marplan], phenelzine [e.g., Nardil], procarbazine [e.g., Matulane], selgiline [e.g., Eldepryl], tranylcypromine [e.g., Parnate])—If you are now taking or have taken within the past 2 weeks any of the MAO inhibitors, the side effects of the phenothiazine-derivative antihistamines may become more severe; these medicines should not be used together

Other medical problems—The presence of other medical problems may affect the use of antihistamines. Make sure you tell your doctor if you have any other medical problems, especially:

- Blood disease or
- Heart or blood vessel disease—These medicines may cause more serious conditions to develop
- Enlarged prostate or
- Urinary tract blockage or difficult urination—Phenothiazine-derivative antihistamines may cause urinary problems to become worse
- Epilepsy—Phenothiazine-derivative antihistamines, especially promethazine given by injection, may increase the chance of seizures
- Glaucoma—These medicines may cause a slight increase in inner eye pressure that may worsen the condition
- Jaundice—Phenothiazine-derivative antihistamines may make the condition worse
- Liver disease—Phenothiazine-derivative antihistamines may build up in the body, which may increase the chance of side effects such as muscle spasms
- Reye's syndrome—Phenothiazine-derivative antihistamines, especially promethazine given by injection, may increase the chance of uncontrolled movements

---

Proper Use of This Medicine

Antihistamines are used to relieve or prevent the symptoms of your medical problem. Take them only as directed. Do not take more of them and do not take them more often than recommended on the label, unless otherwise directed by your doctor. To do so may increase the chance of side effects.

For patients *taking this medicine by mouth:*
- Antihistamines can be taken with food or a glass of water or milk to lessen stomach irritation if necessary.
- If you are taking the *extended-release capsule* form of this medicine, swallow it whole. Do not break, crush, or chew before swallowing.

For patients taking *promethazine for motion sickness:*
- Take this medicine 30 minutes to 1 hour before you begin to travel.

For patients using the *suppository form of this medicine:*
- To insert suppository: First remove the foil wrapper and moisten the suppository with cold water. Lie down on your side and use your finger to push the suppository well up into the rectum. If the suppository is too soft to insert, chill the suppository in the refrigerator for 30 minutes or run cold water over it before removing the foil wrapper.

For patients using the *injection form of this medicine:*
- If you will be giving yourself the injections, make sure you understand exactly how to give them. If you have any questions about this, check with your health care professional.

Dosing—The dose of an antihistamine will be different for different patients. *Follow your doctor's orders or the directions on the label.* The following information includes only the average doses of antihistamines. *If your dose is different, do not change it* unless your doctor tells you to do so.

The number of capsules or tablets or teaspoonfuls of liquid that you take depends on the strength of the medicine. Also, *the number of doses you take each day and the time between doses depends on whether you are taking a short-acting or long-acting form of antihistamine.*

For methdilazine

- For *regular (short-acting) oral* dosage forms (tablets or liquid):

    —For allergy symptoms:

    • Adults and teenagers—8 milligrams (mg) every six to twelve hours as needed.

    • Children younger than 3 years of age—Use and dose must be determined by your doctor.

    • Children 3 to 12 years of age—4 mg every six to twelve hours as needed.

For promethazine

- For *regular (short-acting) oral* dosage forms (tablets or liquid):

    —For allergy symptoms:

    • Adults and teenagers—10 to 12.5 mg four times a day before meals and at bedtime; or 25 mg at bedtime as needed.

    • Children younger than 2 years of age—Use and dose must be determined by your doctor.

    • Children 2 years of age and older—Your doctor will determine dose based on the weight and/or size of the child. Children usually are given 5 to 12.5 mg three times a day or 25 mg at bedtime as needed.

    —For nausea and vomiting:

    • Adults and teenagers—25 mg for the first dose, then 10 to 25 mg every four to six hours if needed.

    • Children younger than 2 years of age—Use and dose must be determined by your doctor.

    • Children 2 years of age and older—Your doctor will determine dose based on the weight and/or size of the child. Children usually are given 10 to 25 mg every four to six hours as needed.

—For prevention of motion sickness:

• Adults and teenagers—25 mg taken one-half to one hour before traveling. The dose may be repeated eight to twelve hours later if needed.

• Children younger than 2 years of age—Use and dose must be determined by your doctor.

• Children 2 years of age and older—Your doctor will determine dose based on the weight and/or size of the child. Children usually are given 10 to 25 mg one-half to one hour before traveling. The dose may be repeated eight to twelve hours later if needed.

—For vertigo (dizziness):

• Adults and teenagers—25 mg two times a day as needed.

• Children younger than 2 years of age—Use and dose must be determined by your doctor.

• Children 2 years of age and older—Your doctor will determine dose based on the weight and/or size of the child. Children usually are given 10 to 25 mg two times a day as needed.

—For use as a sedative:

• Adults and teenagers—25 to 50 mg.

• Children younger than 2 years of age—Use and dose must be determined by your doctor.

• Children 2 years of age and older—Your doctor will determine dose based on the weight and/or size of the child. Children usually are given 10 to 25 mg.

• For *injection* dosage form:

—For allergy symptoms:

• Adults and teenagers—25 mg injected into a muscle or into a vein.

• Children younger than 2 years of age—Use and dose must be determined by your doctor.

• Children 2 years of age and older—Your doctor will determine dose based on the weight and/or size of the child. Children usually are given 6.25 to 12.5 mg injected into a muscle three times a day or 25 mg at bedtime as needed.

—For nausea and vomiting:

• Adults and teenagers—12.5 to 25 mg injected into a muscle or into a vein every four hours as needed.

• Children younger than 2 years of age—Use and dose must be determined by your doctor.

• Children 2 years of age and older—Your doctor will determine dose based on the weight and/or size of the child. Children usually are given 12.5 to 25 mg injected into a muscle every four to six hours as needed.

—For use as a sedative:

• Adults and teenagers—25 to 50 mg injected into a muscle or into a vein.

• Children younger than 2 years of age—Use and dose must be determined by your doctor.

• Children 2 years of age and older—Your doctor will determine dose based on the weight and/or size of the child. Children usually are given 12.5 to 25 mg injected into a muscle.

• For *suppository* dosage form:

—For allergy symptoms:

• Adults and teenagers—25 mg inserted in rectum. Another 25-mg suppository may be inserted two hours later if needed.

• Children younger than 2 years of age—Use and dose must be determined by your doctor.

• Children 2 years of age and older—Your doctor

will determine dose based on the weight and/or size of the child. Children usually are given 6.25 to 12.5 mg inserted into the rectum three times a day or 25 mg at bedtime as needed.

—For nausea and vomiting:

• Adults and teenagers—25 mg inserted into the rectum for the first dose, then 12.5 to 25 mg every four to six hours if needed.

• Children younger than 2 years of age—Use and dose must be determined by your doctor.

• Children 2 years of age and older—Your doctor will determine dose based on the weight and/or size of the child. Children usually are given 12.5 to 25 mg inserted into the rectum every four to six hours as needed.

—For vertigo (dizziness):

• Adults and teenagers—25 mg inserted into the rectum, two times a day as needed.

• Children younger than 2 years of age—Use and dose must be determined by your doctor.

• Children 2 years of age and older—Your doctor will determine dose based on the weight and/or size of the child. Children usually are given 12.5 to 25 mg inserted into the rectum two times a day as needed.

—For use as a sedative:

• Adults and teenagers—25 to 50 mg inserted into the rectum.

• Children younger than 2 years of age—Use and dose must be determined by your doctor.

• Children 2 years of age and older—Your doctor will determine dose based on the weight and/or size of the child. Children usually are given 12.5 to 25 mg inserted into the rectum.

For trimeprazine

- For *regular (short-acting) oral* dosage forms (tablets or liquid):
  —For allergy symptoms:
    - Adults and teenagers—2.5 mg four times a day as needed.
    - Children younger than 2 years of age—Use and dose must be determined by your doctor.
    - Children 2 to 3 years of age—1.25 mg at bedtime or three times a day as needed.
    - Children 3 to 12 years of age—2.5 mg at bedtime or three times a day as needed.

- For *long-acting oral* dosage forms (extended-release capsules):
  —For allergy symptoms:
    - Adults and teenagers—5 mg every twelve hours as needed.
    - Children younger than 6 years of age—Use and dose must be determined by your doctor.
    - Children 6 to 12 years of age—5 mg once a day as needed.

Missed dose—If you are taking this medicine regularly and you miss a dose, take it as soon as possible. However, if it is almost time for your next dose, skip the missed dose and go back to your regular dosing schedule. Do not double doses.

Storage—To store this medicine:
- Keep out of the reach of children, since overdose may be very dangerous in children.
- Store away from heat and direct light.
- Do not store the capsule or tablet form of this medicine in the bathroom medicine cabinet, near the kitchen sink, or in other damp places. Heat or moisture may cause the medicine to break down.

- Keep the liquid form of this medicine from freezing.
- Do not keep outdated medicine or medicine no longer needed. Be sure that any discarded medicine is out of the reach of children.

Precautions While Using This Medicine

Tell the doctor in charge that you are taking this medicine before you have any skin tests for allergies. The results of the tests may be affected by this medicine.

When taking phenothiazine-derivative antihistamines on a regular basis, make sure your doctor knows if you are taking large amounts of aspirin at the same time (as for arthritis or rheumatism). Effects of too much aspirin, such as ringing in the ears, may be covered up by the antihistamine.

Phenothiazine-derivative antihistamines will add to the effects of alcohol and other CNS depressants (medicines that slow down the nervous system, possibly causing drowsiness). Some examples of CNS depressants are sedatives, tranquilizers, or sleeping medicine; prescription pain medicine or narcotics; barbiturates; medicine for seizures; muscle relaxants; or anesthetics, including some dental anesthetics. *Check with your doctor before taking any of the above while you are using this medicine.*

This medicine may cause some people to become drowsy or less alert than they are normally. Even if taken at bedtime, it may cause some people to feel drowsy or less alert on arising. *Make sure you know how you react to the phenothiazine-derivative antihistamine you are taking before you drive, use machines, or do anything else that could be dangerous if you are not alert.*

Phenothiazine-derivative antihistamines may cause dryness of the mouth, nose, and throat. For temporary relief of mouth dryness, use sugarless candy or gum, melt bits of ice in your mouth, or use a saliva substitute. However, if your mouth continues to feel dry for more than 2 weeks, check with your medical doctor or dentist. Continuing dryness of the mouth may increase the chance of dental disease, including tooth decay, gum disease, and fungus infections.

This medicine controls nausea and vomiting. For this reason, it may cover up some of the signs of overdose caused by other medicines or the symptoms of appendicitis. This will make it difficult for your doctor to diagnose these conditions. Make sure your doctor knows that you are taking this medicine if you have other symptoms of appendicitis such as stomach or lower abdominal pain, cramping, or soreness. Also, if you think you may have taken an overdose of any medicine, tell your doctor that you are taking this medicine.

Side Effects of This Medicine

Along with its needed effects, a medicine may cause some unwanted effects. Although not all of these side effects may occur, if they do occur they may need medical attention.

Check with your doctor as soon as possible if any of the following side effects occur:

Less common or rare

> Sore throat and fever; unusual bleeding or bruising; unusual tiredness or weakness

Symptoms of overdose

> Clumsiness or unsteadiness; convulsions (seizures); drowsiness (severe); dryness of mouth, nose, or throat (severe); feeling faint; flushing or redness of face; hallucinations (seeing, hearing, or feeling things that are not there); muscle spasms (especially of neck and

> back); restlessness; shortness of breath or troubled breathing; shuffling walk; tic-like (jerky) movements of head and face; trembling and shaking of hands; trouble in sleeping

Other side effects may occur that usually do not need medical attention. These side effects may go away during treatment as your body adjusts to the medicine. However, check with your health care professional if any of the following side effects continue or are bothersome:

More common

> Drowsiness (less common with methdilazine); thickening of mucus

Less common or rare

> Blurred vision or any change in vision; burning or stinging of rectum (with rectal suppository); confusion; difficult or painful urination; dizziness; dryness of mouth, nose, or throat; fast heartbeat; feeling faint; increased sensitivity of skin to sun; increased sweating; loss of appetite; nightmares; ringing or buzzing in ears; skin rash; unusual excitement, nervousness, restlessness, or irritability

Other side effects not listed above may also occur in some patients. If you notice any other effects, check with your health care professional.

AZITHROMYCIN Systemic

A commonly used brand name in the U.S. and Canada is Zithromax.

Description

Azithromycin (az-ith-roe-MYE-sin) is used to treat bacterial infections in many different parts of the body. It works by killing bacteria or preventing their growth. However, this medicine will not work for colds, flu, or other virus infections. Azithromycin may be used for other problems as determined by your doctor.

Azithromycin is available only with your doctor's prescription, in the following dosage form:

Oral

• Capsules (U.S. and Canada)

Before Using This Medicine

In deciding to use a medicine, the risks of taking the medicine must be weighed against the good it will do. This is a decision you and your doctor will make. For azithromycin, the following should be considered:

Allergies—Tell your doctor if you have ever had any unusual or allergic reaction to azithromycin or to any related medicines such as erythromycin. Also tell your health care professional if you are allergic to any other substances, such as foods, preservatives, or dyes.

Pregnancy—Azithromycin has not been studied in pregnant women. However, azithromycin has not been shown to cause birth defects or other problems in animal studies.

Breast-feeding—It is not known whether azithromycin passes into breast milk. Although most medicines pass into breast milk in small amounts, many of them may be used safely while breast-feeding. Mothers who are taking this medicine and who wish to breast-feed should discuss this with their doctor.

Children—This medicine has been tested in a limited number of children up to the age of 16. In effective doses, the medicine has not been shown to cause different side effects or problems than it does in adults.

Older adults—This medicine has been tested in a limited number of elderly patients and has not been shown to cause different side effects or problems in older people than it does in younger adults.

Other medicines—Although certain medicines should not be used together at all, in other cases two different medicines may be used together even if an interaction might occur. In these cases, your doctor may want to change the dose, or other precautions may be necessary. When you are taking azithromycin, it is especially important that your health care professional know if you are taking any of the following:

- Antacids, aluminum- and magnesium-containing—Antacids may decrease the amount of azithromycin in the blood, which may decrease its effects. To avoid problems, azithromycin should be taken at least 1 hour before or at least 2 hours after antacids

Other medical problems—The presence of other medical problems may affect the use of azithromycin. Make sure you tell your doctor if you have any other medical problems, especially:

- Liver disease—Patients with severe liver disease may have an increased chance of side effects

Proper Use of This Medicine

Azithromycin should be taken at least one hour before or at least 2 hours after meals. Taking azithromycin with food may decrease the amount of medicine that gets into your blood and keep the medicine from working properly.

To help clear up your infection completely, *keep taking azithromycin for the full time of treatment,* even if you begin to feel better after a few days. If you stop taking this medicine too soon, your symptoms may return.

Dosing—The dose of azithromycin will be different for different patients. *Follow your doctor's orders or the directions on the label*. The following information includes only the average doses of azithromycin. *If your dose is* *different, do not change it* unless your doctor tells you to do so.

The number of capsules that you take depends on the medical problem for which you are taking azithromycin.

- For *oral* dosage form (capsules):

    —For bronchitis, strep throat, pneumonia, and skin infections:

    - Adults and children 16 years of age and older— 500 milligrams (mg) on the first day, then 250 mg once a day on the second through fifth days.
    - Children up to 16 years of age—Use and dose must be determined by your doctor.

    —For chlamydia infections:

    - Adults and children 16 years of age and older— 1000 mg taken once as a single dose.
    - Children up to 16 years of age—Use and dose must be determined by your doctor.

Missed dose—If you miss a dose of this medicine, take it as soon as possible. However, if it is almost time for your next dose, skip the missed dose and go back to your regular dosing schedule. Do not double doses.

Storage—To store this medicine:

- Keep out of the reach of children.
- Store away from heat and direct light.
- Do not store in the bathroom, near the kitchen sink, or in other damp places. Heat or moisture may cause the medicine to break down.
- Do not keep outdated medicine or medicine no longer needed. Be sure that any discarded medicine is out of the reach of children.

Precautions While Using This Medicine

If your symptoms do not improve within a few days, or if they become worse, check with your doctor.

Side Effects of This Medicine

Along with its needed effects, a medicine may cause some unwanted effects. Although not all of these side effects may occur, if they do occur they may need medical attention.

Stop taking this medicine and get emergency help immediately if any of the following side effects occur:

   Rare

   Difficulty in breathing; fever; joint pain; skin rash; swelling of face, mouth, neck, hands, and feet

Other side effects may occur that usually do not need medical attention. These side effects may go away during treatment as your body adjusts to the medicine. However, check with your doctor if any of the following side effects continue or are bothersome:

   Less common

   Diarrhea; nausea; stomach pain or discomfort; vomiting

   Rare

   Dizziness; headache

Other side effects not listed above may also occur in some patients. If you notice any other effects, check with your doctor.

Additional Information

Once a medicine has been approved for marketing for a certain use, experience may show that it is also useful for other medical problems. Although this use is not included in product labeling, azithromycin is used in certain patients with the following medical condition:

• Mycoplasmal pneumonia

Other than the above information, there is no additional information relating to proper use, precautions, or side effects for this use.

BENZODIAZEPINES   Systemic

Some commonly used brand names are:

In the U.S.—

Alprazolam Intensol[1]	Lorazepam Intensol[11]
Ativan[11]	Paxipam[9]
Centrax[14]	Poxi[3]
Dalmane[8]	ProSom[7]
Diazepam Intensol[6]	Restoril[16]
Doral[15]	Serax[13]
D-Val[6]	Tranxene-SD[5]
Gen-XENE[5]	Tranxene T-Tab[5]
Halcion[17]	Valium[6]
Klonopin[4]	Valrelease[6]
Libritabs[3]	Xanax[1]
Librium[3]	Zetran[6]

In Canada—

Apo-Alpraz[1]	Novoflupam[8]
Apo-Chlordiazepoxide[3]	Novo-Lorazem[11]
Apo-Clorazepate[5]	Novopoxide[3]
Apo-Diazepam[6]	Novo-Triolam[17]
Apo-Flurazepam[8]	Novoxapam[13]
Apo-Lorazepam[11]	Nu-Alpraz[1]
Apo-Oxazepam[13]	Nu-Loraz[11]
Apo-Triazo[17]	Nu-Triazo[17]
Ativan[11]	PMS-Diazepam[6]
Dalmane[8]	Restoril[16]
Diazemuls[6]	Rivotril[4]
Gen-Triazolam[17]	Serax[13]
Halcion[17]	Solium[3]
Lectopam[2]	Somnol[8]
Librium[3]	Syn-Clonazepam[4]
Loftran[10]	Tranxene[5]
Mogadon[12]	Valium[6]
Novo-Alprazol[1]	Vivol[6]
Novo-Clopate[5]	Xanax[1]
Novodipam[6]	Xanax TS[1]

Note: For quick reference, the following benzodiazepines are numbered to match the corresponding brand names.

This information applies to the following medicines:

1. Alprazolam (al-PRAZ-oh-lam)‡§
2. Bromazepam (broe-MA-ze-pam)*
3. Chlordiazepoxide (klor-dye-az-e-POX-ide)‡
4. Clonazepam (kloe-NA-ze-pam)
5. Clorazepate (klor-AZ-e-pate)‡
6. Diazepam (dye-AZ-e-pam)‡
7. Estazolam (ess-TA-zoe-lam)†
8. Flurazepam (flure-AZ-e-pam)‡
9. Halazepam (hal-AZ-e-pam)†
10. Ketazolam (kee-TAY-zoe-lam)*
11. Lorazepam (lor-AZ-e-pam)‡
12. Nitrazepam (nye-TRA-ze-pam)*
13. Oxazepam (ox-AZ-e-pam)‡
14. Prazepam (PRAZ-e-pam)†‡
15. Quazepam (KWA-ze-pam)†
16. Temazepam (tem-AZ-e-pam)‡
17. Triazolam (trye-AY-zoe-lam)§

*Not commercially available in the U.S.
†Not commercially available in Canada.
‡Generic name product may also be available in the U.S.
§Generic name product may also be available in Canada.

Description

Benzodiazepines (ben-zoe-dye-AZ-e-peens) belong to the group of medicines called central nervous system (CNS) depressants (medicines that slow down the nervous system).

Some benzodiazepines are used to relieve nervousness or tension. Others are used in the treatment of insomnia (trouble in sleeping). However, if used regularly (for example, every day) for insomnia, they are usually not effective for more than a few weeks.

One of the benzodiazepines, diazepam, is also used to help relax muscles or relieve muscle spasm. Another benzodiazepine, alprazolam, is also used in the treatment of panic disorder. Clonazepam, clorazepate, and diazepam are also used to treat certain convulsive (seizure) disorders, such as epilepsy. The benzodiazepines may also be used for other conditions as determined by your doctor.

Benzodiazepines should not be used for nervousness or tension caused by the stress of everyday life.

These medicines are available only with your doctor's prescription, in the following dosage forms:

Oral

Alprazolam
- Oral solution (U.S.)
- Tablets (U.S. and Canada)

Bromazepam
- Tablets (Canada)

Chlordiazepoxide
- Capsules (U.S. and Canada)
- Tablets (U.S.)

Clonazepam
- Tablets (U.S. and Canada)

Clorazepate
- Capsules (U.S. and Canada)
- Tablets (U.S.)

Diazepam
- Extended-release capsules (U.S.)
- Oral solution (U.S. and Canada)
- Tablets (U.S. and Canada)

Estazolam
- Tablets (U.S.)

Flurazepam
- Capsules (U.S. and Canada)
- Tablets (Canada)

Halazepam
- Tablets (U.S.)

Ketazolam
- Capsules (Canada)

Lorazepam
- Oral solution (U.S.)
- Tablets (U.S. and Canada)
- Sublingual tablets (Canada)

Nitrazepam
- Tablets (Canada)

Oxazepam
- Capsules (U.S.)
- Tablets (U.S. and Canada)

Prazepam
- Capsules (U.S.)
- Tablets (U.S.)

Quazepam
- Tablets (U.S.)

Temazepam
- Capsules (U.S. and Canada)
- Tablets (U.S.)

Triazolam
- Tablets (U.S. and Canada)

Parenteral

Chlordiazepoxide
- Injection (U.S. and Canada)

Diazepam
- Injection (U.S. and Canada)

Lorazepam
- Injection (U.S. and Canada)

Rectal

Diazepam
- For rectal solution (U.S. and Canada)

Before Using This Medicine

In deciding to use a medicine, the risks of taking the medicine must be weighed against the good it will do. This is a decision you and your doctor will make. For benzodiazepines, the following should be considered:

Allergies—Tell your doctor if you have ever had any unusual or allergic reaction to benzodiazepines. Also tell your health care professional if you are allergic to any other substances, such as foods, preservatives, or dyes.

Pregnancy—Chlordiazepoxide and diazepam have been reported to increase the chance of birth defects when used during the first 3 months of pregnancy. Although similar problems have not been reported with the other benzodiazepines, the chance always exists since all of the benzodiazepines are related.

Studies in animals have shown that clonazepam, lorazepam, and temazepam cause birth defects or other problems, including death of the animal fetus.

Too much use of benzodiazepines during pregnancy may cause the baby to become dependent on the medicine. This may lead to withdrawal side effects after birth. Also, use of benzodiazepines during pregnancy, especially during the last weeks, may cause drowsiness, slow heartbeat, shortness of breath, or troubled breathing in the newborn infant.

Benzodiazepines given just before or during labor may cause weakness in the newborn infant. When diazepam is given in high doses (especially by injection) within 15 hours before delivery, it may cause breathing problems, muscle weakness, difficulty in feeding, and body temperature problems in the newborn infant.

Breast-feeding—Benzodiazepines may pass into the breast milk and cause drowsiness, slow heartbeat, shortness of breath, or troubled breathing in nursing babies of mothers taking this medicine.

Children—Most of the side effects of these medicines are more likely to occur in children, especially the very young. These patients are usually more sensitive than adults to the effects of benzodiazepines.

When clonazepam is used for long periods of time in children, it may cause unwanted effects on physical and mental growth. These effects may not be noticed until many years later. Before this medicine is given to children for long periods of time, you should discuss its use with your child's doctor.

Older adults—Most of the side effects of these medicines are more likely to occur in the elderly, who are usually more sensitive to the effects of benzodiazepines.

Taking benzodiazepines for trouble in sleeping may cause more daytime drowsiness in elderly patients than in younger adults. In addition, falls and related injuries may be more likely to occur in elderly patients taking benzodiazepines.

Other medicines—Although certain medicines should not be used together at all, in other cases two different medicines may be used together even if an interaction might occur. In these cases, your doctor may want to change the dose, or other precautions may be necessary. When you are taking or receiving benzodiazepines it is especially important that your health care professional know if you are taking any of the following:

- Central nervous system (CNS) depressants (medicine that causes drowsiness)—The CNS depressant effects of either these medicines or benzodiazepines may be increased; your doctor may want to change the dose of either or both medicines

Other medical problems—The presence of other medical problems may affect the use of benzodiazepines. Make sure you tell your doctor if you have any other medical problems, especially:

- Alcohol abuse (or history of) or
- Drug abuse or dependence (or history of)—Dependence on benzodiazepines may develop
- Brain disease—CNS depression and other side effects of benzodiazepines may be more likely to occur
- Difficulty in swallowing (in children) or
- Emphysema, asthma, bronchitis, or other chronic lung disease or
- Glaucoma or
- Hyperactivity or
- Mental depression or
- Mental illness (severe) or
- Myasthenia gravis or
- Porphyria or
- Sleep apnea (temporarily stopping of breathing during sleep)—Benzodiazepines may make the condition worse

- Epilepsy or history of seizures—Although clonazepam and diazepam are used in treating epilepsy, starting or suddenly stopping treatment with these medicines may increase seizures
- Kidney or liver disease—Higher blood levels of benzodiazepines may result, increasing the chance of side effects

---

Proper Use of This Medicine

For patients taking *diazepam extended-release capsules:*

- Swallow capsules whole.
- Do not crush, break, or chew the capsules before swallowing.

For patients taking *lorazepam oral solution:*

- Each dose may be diluted with water, soda or soda-like beverages, or semisolid food, such as applesauce or pudding.

For patients taking *lorazepam sublingual tablets:*

- Do not chew or swallow the tablet. This medicine is meant to be absorbed through the lining of the mouth. Place the tablet under your tongue (sublingual) and let it slowly dissolve there. Do not swallow for at least 2 minutes.

Take this medicine only as directed by your doctor. Do not take more of it, do not take it more often, and do not take it for a longer time than your doctor ordered. If too much is taken, it may become habit-forming (causing mental or physical dependence).

If you think this medicine is not working properly after you have taken it for a few weeks, *do not increase the dose*. Instead, check with your doctor.

For patients taking this medicine *for epilepsy or other seizure disorder:*

- *In order for this medicine to control your seizures, it must be taken every day in regularly spaced doses as ordered by your doctor*. This is necessary to keep a constant amount of the medicine in the blood. To help keep the amount constant, do not miss any doses.

For patients taking this medicine *for insomnia:*

- *Do not take this medicine when your schedule does not permit you to get a full night's sleep (7 to 8 hours)*. If you must wake up before this, you may continue to feel drowsy and may experience memory problems, because the effects of the medicine have not had time to wear off.

For patients taking *flurazepam:*

- *When you begin to take this medicine, your sleeping problem will improve somewhat the first night. However, 2 or 3 nights may pass before you receive the full effects of this medicine.*

Dosing—The dose of benzodiazepines will be different for different patients. *Follow your doctor's orders or the directions on the label*. The following information includes only the average doses of benzodiazepines. *If your dose is different, do not change it* unless your doctor tells you to do so.

The number of capsules or tablets, or the amount of solution that you take, or the number of injections you receive, depends on the strength of the medicine. Also, *the number of doses you take each day, the time allowed between doses, and the length of time you take the medicine depend on the medical problem for which you are taking benzodiazepines.*

For alprazolam

- For *oral* dosage form (solution or tablets):
  —For anxiety:

• Adults—At first, 0.25 to 0.5 milligrams (mg) three times a day. Your doctor may increase your dose if needed. However, the dose is usually not more than 4 mg a day.

• Children up to 18 years of age—Use and dose must be determined by your doctor.

• Older adults—At first, 0.25 mg two to three times a day. Your doctor may increase your dose if needed.

—For panic disorder:

• Adults—At first, 0.5 mg three times a day. Your doctor may increase your dose if needed. However, the dose is usually not more than 10 mg a day.

• Children up to 18 years of age—Use and dose must be determined by your doctor.

For bromazepam

• For *oral* dosage form (tablets):

—For anxiety:

• Adults—6 to 30 milligrams (mg) a day, taken in smaller doses during the day.

• Children up to 18 years of age—Use and dose must be determined by your doctor.

• Older adults—At first, up to 3 mg a day. Your doctor may change your dose if needed.

For chlordiazepoxide

• For *oral* dosage form (capsules or tablets):

—For anxiety:

• Adults—5 to 25 milligrams (mg) three or four times a day.

• Children 6 years of age and over—5 mg two to four times a day. Your doctor may increase your dose if needed.

• Children up to 6 years of age—Use and dose must be determined by your doctor.

• Older adults—At first, 5 mg two to four times a day. Your doctor may increase your dose if needed.

—For sedation during withdrawal from alcohol:

• Adults—At first, 50 to 100 mg, repeated if needed. However, the dose is usually not more than 400 mg a day.

• Children—Use and dose must be determined by your doctor.

• For *injection* dosage form:

—For anxiety:

• Adults—At first, 50 to 100 mg, injected into a muscle or vein. Then, if needed, 25 to 50 mg three or four times a day.

• Teenagers—25 to 50 mg, injected into a muscle or vein.

• Children up to 12 years of age—Use and dose must be determined by your doctor.

• Older adults—25 to 50 mg, injected into a muscle or vein.

—For sedation during withdrawal from alcohol:

• Adults—At first, 50 to 100 mg, injected into a muscle or vein. If needed, the dose may be repeated in two to four hours.

• Children—Use and dose must be determined by your doctor.

For clonazepam

• For *oral* dosage form (tablets):

—For control of seizures:

• Adults—At first, 0.5 milligrams (mg) three times a day. Your doctor may increase your dose if needed. However, the dose is usually not more than 20 mg a day.

• Infants and children up to 10 years of age—

Dose is based on weight and must be determined by your doctor.

For clorazepate

• For *oral* dosage form (capsules or tablets):

—For anxiety:

• Adults and teenagers—7.5 to 15 milligrams (mg) two to four times a day. Or your doctor may want you to start by taking 15 mg at bedtime.

• Children up to 12 years of age—Use and dose must be determined by your doctor.

• Older adults—At first, 3.75 to 15 mg a day. Your doctor may increase your dose if needed.

—For sedation during withdrawal from alcohol:

• Adults and teenagers—At first, 30 mg. Your doctor will set up a schedule that will gradually reduce your dose.

• Children up to 12 years of age—Use and dose must be determined by your doctor.

—For control of seizures:

• Adults and teenagers—At first, up to 7.5 mg taken three times a day. Your doctor may increase your dose if needed. However, the dose is usually not more than 90 mg a day.

• Children 9 to 12 years of age—At first, 7.5 mg two times a day. Your doctor may increase your dose if needed. However, the dose is usually not more than 60 mg a day.

• Children up to 9 years of age—Use and dose must be determined by your doctor.

For diazepam

• For *oral* dosage form (extended-release capsules):

—For anxiety:

• Adults—15 to 30 milligrams (mg) once a day.

• Children 6 months of age and over—15 mg once a day.

- Children up to 6 months of age—Use is not recommended.
- Older adults—15 mg once a day.

—For relaxing muscles:

- Adults—15 to 30 mg once a day.
- Children 6 months of age and over—15 mg once a day.
- Children up to 6 months of age—Use is not recommended.
- Older adults—15 mg once a day.

- For *oral* dosage form (solution or tablets):

—For anxiety:

- Adults—2 to 10 mg two to four times a day.
- Children 6 months of age and over—Dose is based on body weight or size and must be determined by your doctor.
- Children up to 6 months of age—Use is not recommended.
- Older adults—2 to 2.5 mg one or two times a day. Your doctor may increase your dose if needed.

—For sedation during withdrawal from alcohol:

- Adults—At first, 10 mg three or four times a day. Your doctor will set up a schedule that will gradually decrease your dose.
- Children—Use and dose must be determined by your doctor.

—For control of seizures:

- Adults—2 to 10 mg taken two to four times a day.
- Children 6 months of age and over—Dose is based on body weight or size and must be determined by your doctor.

• Children up to 6 months of age—Use is not recommended.

• Older adults—2 to 2.5 mg one or two times a day. Your doctor may increase your dose if needed.

—For relaxing muscles:

• Adults—2 to 10 mg three or four times a day.

• Children 6 months of age and over—Dose is based on body weight or size and must be determined by your doctor.

• Children up to 6 months of age—Use is not recommended.

• Older adults—2 to 2.5 mg one or two times a day. Your doctor may increase your dose if needed.

• For *injection* dosage form:

—For anxiety:

• Adults—2 to 10 mg, injected into a muscle or vein.

• Children—Use and dose must be determined by your doctor.

• For older adults—2 to 5 mg, injected into a muscle or vein.

—For sedation during withdrawal from alcohol:

• Adults—At first, 10 mg injected into a muscle or vein. If needed, 5 to 10 mg may be given three or four hours later.

• Children—Use and dose must be determined by your doctor.

—For sedation before surgery or other procedures:

• Adults—5 to 20 mg, injected into a muscle or vein.

• Children—Use and dose must be determined by your doctor.

- Older adults—2 to 5 mg, injected into a muscle or vein.

—For control of seizures:

- Adults—At first, 5 to 10 mg, usually injected into a vein. If needed, the dose may be repeated.

- Children 5 years of age and older—At first, 1 mg injected into a vein every two to five minutes. The dose may need to be repeated.

- Infants over 30 days of age and children up to 5 years of age—At first, 0.2 to 0.5 mg injected into a vein every two to five minutes. The dose may need to be repeated.

- Newborns and infants up to 30 days of age: Use and dose must be determined by your doctor.

- Older adults—2 to 5 mg, injected into a muscle or vein.

—For relaxing muscle spasms:

- Adults—At first, 5 to 10 mg injected into a muscle or vein. The dose may be repeated in three or four hours.

- Children: Use and dose must be determined by your doctor.

- Older adults—2 to 5 mg, injected into a muscle or vein.

—For relaxing muscles in tetanus:

- Adults—At first, 5 to 10 mg injected into a muscle or vein. Your doctor may increase your dose if needed.

- Children 5 years of age and older—5 to 10 mg, injected into a muscle or vein. The dose may be repeated every three to four hours if needed.

- Infants over 30 days of age and children up to 5 years of age—1 to 2 mg, injected into a muscle or vein. The dose may be repeated every three to four hours if needed.

• Newborns and infants up to 30 days of age: Use and dose must be determined by your doctor.

• For *rectal* dosage form (solution):

—For control of seizures:

• Adults and teenagers—Dose is based on body weight and must be determined by your doctor.

• Children—Dose is based on body weight and must be determined by your doctor.

For estazolam

• For *oral* dosage form (tablets):

—For trouble in sleeping:

• Adults—1 milligram (mg) at bedtime.

• Children up to 18 years of age—Use and dose must be determined by your doctor.

For flurazepam

• For *oral* dosage form (capsules or tablets):

—For trouble in sleeping:

• Adults—15 or 30 milligrams (mg) at bedtime.

• Children up to 15 years of age—Use and dose must be determined by your doctor.

• Older adults—At first, 15 mg at bedtime. Your doctor may increase your dose if needed.

For halazepam

• For *oral* dosage form (tablets):

—For anxiety:

• Adults—20 to 40 milligrams (mg) three or four times a day.

• Children up to 18 years of age—Use and dose must be determined by your doctor.

• Older adults—20 mg one or two times a day.

For ketazolam

• For *oral* dosage form (capsules):

—For anxiety:

- Adults—15 milligrams (mg) one or two times a day. Your doctor may increase your dose if needed.

- Children up to 18 years of age—Use and dose must be determined by your doctor.

- Infants—Use is not recommended.

- Older adults—15 mg once a day.

For lorazepam

- For *oral* dosage form (solution or tablets):

  —For anxiety:

  - Adults—1 to 3 milligrams (mg) two or three times a day.

  - Children up to 12 years of age—Use and dose must be determined by your doctor.

  - Older adults—0.5 to 2 mg a day, taken in smaller doses during the day.

  —For trouble in sleeping:

  - Adults—2 to 4 mg taken at bedtime.

  - Children up to 12 years of age—Use and dose must be determined by your doctor.

- For *sublingual tablet* dosage form:

  —For anxiety:

  - Adults—2 to 3 mg a day, in smaller doses placed under the tongue during the day. Your doctor may increase your dose if needed. However, the dose is usually not more than 6 mg a day.

  - Children 6 to 18 years of age—Use and dose must be determined by your doctor.

  - Children up to 6 years of age—Use is not recommended.

  - Older adults—At first, 0.5 mg a day. Your doctor may increase your dose if needed.

  —For sedation before surgery:

• Adults—Dose is based on body weight and is usually 0.05 mg per kilogram (0.023 mg per pound) of body weight, placed under the tongue, one to two hours before surgery. The dose is usually not more than 4 mg.

• Children—Use and dose must be determined by your doctor.

• For *injection* dosage form:

—For sedation before surgery or other procedures:

• Adults—Dose is based on body weight and will be determined by your doctor. However, the dose is usually not more than 4 mg, injected into a muscle or vein.

• Children up to 18 years of age—Use and dose must be determined by your doctor.

For nitrazepam

• For *oral* dosage form (tablets):

—For trouble in sleeping:

• Adults—5 to 10 milligrams (mg) at bedtime.

• Children—Use and dose must be determined by your doctor.

• Older adults—At first, 2.5 mg taken at bedtime. Your doctor may increase your dose if needed.

—For control of seizures:

• Children up to 30 kilograms (66 pounds) of body weight—Dose is based on body weight and is usually 0.3 to 1 mg per kilogram (0.14 to 0.45 mg per pound) of body weight per day, taken in smaller doses three times during the day. Your doctor may increase your dose if needed.

For oxazepam

• For *oral* dosage form (capsules or tablets):

—For anxiety:

• Adults—10 to 30 milligrams (mg) three or four times a day.

- Children 6 to 12 years of age—Use and dose must be determined by your doctor.

- Children up to 6 years of age—Use is not recommended.

- Older adults—At first, 10 mg three times a day. Your doctor may increase your dose if needed. However, the dose is usually not more than 15 mg taken four times a day.

—For sedation during withdrawal from alcohol:

- Adults—15 to 30 mg three or four times a day.

- Children—Use and dose must be determined by your doctor.

For prazepam

- For *oral* dosage form (capsules or tablets):

—For anxiety:

- Adults—10 milligrams (mg) three times a day, or 20 to 40 mg taken at bedtime.

- Children—Use and dose must be determined by your doctor.

- Older adults—At first, 10 to 15 mg a day, taken in smaller doses during the day. Your doctor may increase your dose if needed.

For quazepam

- For *oral* dosage form (tablets):

—For trouble in sleeping:

- Adults—7.5 to 15 milligrams (mg) taken at bedtime.

- Children up to 18 years of age—Use and dose must be determined by your doctor.

For temazepam

- For *oral* dosage form (capsules or tablets):

—For trouble in sleeping:

- Adults—15 milligrams (mg) taken at bedtime.

  • Children up to 18 years of age—Use and dose must be determined by your doctor.
  • Older adults—At first, 7.5 mg at bedtime. Your doctor may increase your dose if needed.

For triazolam

  • For *oral* dosage form (tablets):
    —For trouble in sleeping:
      • Adults—125 to 250 micrograms (mcg) taken at bedtime.
      • Children up to 18 years of age—Use and dose must be determined by your doctor.
      • Older adults—At first, 125 mcg at bedtime. Your doctor may increase your dose if needed.

Missed dose—If you are taking this medicine regularly (for example, every day as for epilepsy) and you miss a dose, take it right away if you remember within an hour or so of the missed dose. However, if you do not remember until later, skip the missed dose and go back to your regular dosing schedule. Do not double doses.

Storage—To store this medicine:

  • Keep out of the reach of children. Overdose of benzodiazepines may be especially dangerous in children.
  • Store away from heat and direct light.
  • Do not store the capsule or tablet form of this medicine in the bathroom, near the kitchen sink, or in other damp places. Heat or moisture may cause the medicine to break down.
  • Keep the liquid form of this medicine from freezing.
  • Do not keep outdated medicine or medicine no longer needed. Be sure that any discarded medicine is out of the reach of children.

Precautions While Using This Medicine

If you will be *taking this medicine regularly for a long time:*

- Your doctor should check your progress at regular visits to make sure that this medicine does not cause unwanted effects. If you are taking clonazepam, this is also important during the first few months of treatment.

- If you are taking this medicine for nervousness or tension or for panic disorder, check with your doctor at least every 4 months to make sure you need to continue taking this medicine.

- If you are taking estazolam, flurazepam, quazepam, temazepam, or triazolam for insomnia (trouble in sleeping), and you think you need this medicine for more than 7 to 10 days, be sure to discuss it with your doctor. Insomnia that lasts longer than this may be a sign of another medical problem.

If you will be taking this medicine in large doses or for a long time, do not stop taking it without first checking with your doctor. Your doctor may want you to reduce gradually the amount you are taking before stopping completely. Stopping this medicine suddenly may cause withdrawal side effects. Also, if you are taking this medicine for epilepsy or another seizure disorder, stopping this medicine suddenly may cause seizures.

For patients taking this medicine *for epilepsy or another seizure disorder:*

- Your doctor may want you to carry a medical identification card or bracelet stating that you are taking this medicine.

This medicine will add to the effects of alcohol and other CNS depressants (medicines that slow down the nervous system, possibly causing drowsiness). Some examples of CNS depressants are antihistamines or medicine for hay fever, other allergies, or colds; sedatives, tranquilizers, or sleeping medicine; prescription pain medicine or narcotics; barbiturates; medicine for seizures; muscle relaxants; or anesthetics, including some dental anesthetics. This effect may last for a few days after you stop taking this medicine. *Check with your doctor before taking any of the above while you are taking this medicine.*

If you think you or someone else may have taken an overdose of this medicine, get emergency help at once. Taking an overdose of a benzodiazepine or taking alcohol or other CNS depressants with the benzodiazepine may lead to unconsciousness and possibly death. Some signs of an overdose are continuing slurred speech or confusion, severe drowsiness, severe weakness, and staggering.

Before you have any medical tests, tell the medical doctor in charge that you are taking this medicine. The results of the metyrapone test may be affected by chlordiazepoxide.

If you develop any unusual and strange thoughts or behavior while you are taking this medicine, be sure to discuss it with your doctor. Some changes that have occurred in people taking this medicine are like those seen in people who drink alcohol and then act in a manner that is not normal. Other changes may be more unusual and extreme, such as confusion, agitation, and hallucinations (seeing, hearing, or feeling things that are not there).

This medicine may cause some people, especially older persons, to become drowsy, dizzy, lightheaded, clumsy or unsteady, or less alert than they are normally. Even if taken at bedtime, it may cause some people to feel drowsy or less alert on arising. *Make sure you know how you react to this medicine before you drive, use machines, or do anything else that could be dangerous if you are dizzy or are not alert.*

If you have been taking this medicine for insomnia, you may have difficulty sleeping (rebound insomnia) for the first few nights after you stop taking the medicine.

Side Effects of This Medicine

Along with its needed effects, a medicine may cause some unwanted effects. Although not all of these side effects may occur, if they do occur they may need medical attention.

Check with your doctor as soon as possible if any of the following side effects occur:

Less common or rare

> Behavior problems, including difficulty in concentrating and outbursts of anger; confusion or mental depression; convulsions (seizures); hallucinations (seeing, hearing, or feeling things that are not there); hypotension (low blood pressure); impaired memory—may be more common with triazolam; muscle weakness; skin rash or itching; sore throat, fever, and chills; trouble in sleeping; ulcers or sores in mouth or throat (continuing); uncontrolled movements of body, including the eyes; unusual bleeding or bruising; unusual excitement, nervousness, or irritability; unusual tiredness or weakness (severe); yellow eyes or skin

Symptoms of overdose

> Confusion (continuing); drowsiness (severe); shakiness; slow heartbeat, shortness of breath, or troubled breathing; slow reflexes; slurred speech (continuing); staggering; weakness (severe)

Other side effects may occur that usually do not need medical attention. These side effects may go away during treatment as your body adjusts to the medicine. However, check with your doctor if any of the following side effects continue or are bothersome:

More common

> Clumsiness or unsteadiness; dizziness or lightheadedness; drowsiness; slurred speech

Less common or rare

> Abdominal or stomach cramps or pain; blurred vision or other changes in vision; changes in sexual drive or per-

formance; constipation; diarrhea; dryness of mouth or increased thirst; false sense of well-being; fast or pounding heartbeat; headache; increased bronchial secretions or watering of mouth; muscle spasm; nausea or vomiting; problems with urination; trembling; unusual tiredness or weakness

Not all of the side effects listed above have been reported for each of these medicines, but they have been reported for at least one of them. All of the benzodiazepines are similar, so any of the above side effects may occur with any of these medicines.

For patients having *chlordiazepoxide, diazepam, or lorazepam injected:*

- Check with your doctor if there is redness, swelling, or pain at the place of injection.

After you stop using this medicine, your body may need time to adjust. If you took this medicine in high doses or for a long time, this may take up to 3 weeks. During this period of time check with your doctor if you notice any of the following side effects:

More common

   Irritability; nervousness; trouble in sleeping

Less common

   Abdominal or stomach cramps; confusion; fast or pounding heartbeat; increased sense of hearing; increased sensitivity to touch and pain; increased sweating; loss of sense of reality; mental depression; muscle cramps; nausea or vomiting; sensitivity of eyes to light; tingling, burning, or prickly sensations; trembling

Rare

   Confusion as to time, place, or person; convulsions (seizures); feelings of suspicion or distrust; hallucinations (seeing, hearing, or feeling things that are not there)

Other side effects not listed above may also occur in some patients. If you notice any other effects, check with your doctor.

Additional Information

Once a medicine has been approved for marketing for a certain use, experience may show that it is also useful for other medical problems. Although these uses are not included in product labeling, some of the benzodiazepines are used in certain patients with the following medical conditions:

- Nausea and vomiting caused by cancer chemotherapy
- Tension headache
- Tremors

Other than the above information, there is no additional information relating to proper use, precautions, or side effects for these uses.

BETA-ADRENERGIC BLOCKING AGENTS   Systemic

Some commonly used brand names are:

In the U.S.—

Betapace[13]	Lopressor[7]
Blocadren[14]	Normodyne[6]
Cartrol[5]	Sectral[1]
Corgard[8]	Tenormin[2]
Inderal[12]	Toprol-XL[7]
Inderal LA[12]	Trandate[6]
Kerlone[3]	Visken[11]
Levatol[10]	Zebeta[4]

In Canada—

Apo-Atenolol[2]	Detensol[12]
Apo-Metoprolol[7]	Inderal[12]
Apo-Metoprolol (Type L)[7]	Inderal LA[12]
Apo-Propranolol[12]	Lopresor[7]
Apo-Timol[14]	Lopresor SR[7]
Betaloc[7]	Monitan[1]
Betaloc Durules[7]	Novo-Atenol[2]
Blocadren[14]	Novometoprol[7]
Corgard[8]	Novo-Pindol[11]

In Canada (cont'd)—

Novo-Timol[14]	Syn-Nadolol[8]
Novopranol[12]	Syn-Pindolol[11]
pms Propranolol[12]	Tenormin[2]
Sectral[1]	Trandate[6]
Slow-Trasicor[9]	Trasicor[9]
Sotacor[13]	Visken[11]

Note: For quick reference, the following beta-adrenergic blocking agents are numbered to match the corresponding brand names.

This information applies to the following medicines:

1. Acebutolol (a-se-BYOO-toe-lole)
2. Atenolol (a-TEN-oh-lole)‡
3. Betaxolol (be-TAX-oh-lol)†
4. Bisoprolol (bis-OH-proe-lol)†
5. Carteolol (KAR-tee-oh-lole)†
6. Labetalol (la-BET-a-lole)
7. Metoprolol (me-TOE-proe-lole)§
8. Nadolol (NAY-doe-lole)§
9. Oxprenolol (ox-PREN-oh-lole)*
10. Penbutolol (pen-BYOO-toe-lole)†
11. Pindolol (PIN-doe-lole)
12. Propranolol (proe-PRAN-oh-lole)‡§
13. Sotalol (SOE-ta-lole)
14. Timolol (TIM-oh-lole)‡

---

*Not commercially available in the U.S.
†Not commercially available in Canada.
‡Generic name product may also be available in the U.S.
§Generic name product may also be available in Canada.

Description

This group of medicines is known as beta-adrenergic blocking agents, beta-blocking agents, or, more commonly, beta-blockers. Beta-blockers are used in the treatment of high blood pressure (hypertension). Some beta-blockers are also used to relieve angina (chest pain) and in heart attack patients to help prevent additional heart attacks. Beta-blockers are also used to correct irregular heartbeat, prevent migraine headaches, and treat tremors. They may also be used for other conditions as determined by your doctor.

Beta-blockers work by affecting the response to some nerve impulses in certain parts of the body. As a result, they decrease the heart's need for blood and oxygen by reducing its workload. They also help the heart to beat more regularly.

Beta-adrenergic blocking agents are available only with your doctor's prescription, in the following dosage forms:

Oral

Acebutolol
- Capsules (U.S.)
- Tablets (Canada)

Atenolol
- Tablets (U.S. and Canada)

Betaxolol
- Tablets (U.S.)

Bisoprolol
- Tablets (U.S.)

Carteolol
- Tablets (U.S.)

Labetalol
- Tablets (U.S. and Canada)

Metoprolol
- Tablets (U.S. and Canada)
- Extended-release tablets (U.S. and Canada)

Nadolol
- Tablets (U.S. and Canada)

Oxprenolol
- Tablets (Canada)
- Extended-release tablets (Canada)

Penbutolol
- Tablets (U.S.)

Pindolol
- Tablets (U.S. and Canada)

Propranolol
- Extended-release capsules (U.S. and Canada)
- Oral solution (U.S.)
- Tablets (U.S. and Canada)

Sotalol
- Tablets (U.S. and Canada)

Timolol
  • Tablets (U.S. and Canada)

Parenteral

Atenolol
  • Injection (U.S.)

Labetalol
  • Injection (U.S. and Canada)

Metoprolol
  • Injection (U.S. and Canada)

Propranolol
  • Injection (U.S. and Canada)

Before Using This Medicine

In deciding to use a medicine, the risks of taking the medicine must be weighed against the good it will do. This is a decision you and your doctor will make. For the beta-blockers, the following should be considered:

Allergies—Tell your doctor if you have ever had any unusual or allergic reaction to the beta-blocker medicine prescribed. Also tell your health care professional if you are allergic to any other substances, such as foods, preservatives, or dyes.

Pregnancy—Use of some beta-blockers during pregnancy has been associated with low blood sugar, breathing problems, a lower heart rate, and low blood pressure in the newborn infant. Other reports have not shown unwanted effects on the newborn infant. Animal studies have shown some beta-blockers to cause problems in pregnancy when used in doses many times the usual human dose. Before taking any of these medicines, make sure your doctor knows if you are pregnant or if you may become pregnant.

Breast-feeding—It is not known whether bisoprolol, carteolol, or penbutolol passes into breast milk. All other beta-blockers pass into breast milk. Problems such as slow heartbeat, low blood pressure, and trouble in breathing have been reported in nursing babies. Mothers who are taking beta-blockers and who wish to breast-feed should discuss this with their doctor.

Children—Some of these medicines have been used in children and, in effective doses, have not been shown to cause different side effects or problems in children than they do in adults.

Older adults—Some side effects are more likely to occur in the elderly, who are usually more sensitive to the effects of beta-blockers. Also, beta-blockers may reduce tolerance to cold temperatures in elderly patients.

Other medicines—Although certain medicines should not be used together at all, in other cases two different medicines may be used together even if an interaction might occur. In these cases, your doctor may want to change the dose, or other precautions may be necessary. When you are taking or receiving a beta-blocker it is especially important that your health care professional know if you are taking any of the following:

- Allergen immunotherapy (allergy shots) or
- Allergen extracts for skin testing—Beta-blockers may increase the risk of serious allergic reaction to these medicines
- Aminophylline (e.g., Somophyllin) or
- Caffeine (e.g., NoDoz) or
- Dyphylline (e.g., Lufyllin) or
- Oxtriphylline (e.g., Choledyl) or
- Theophylline (e.g., Somophyllin-T)—The effects of both these medicines and beta-blockers may be blocked; in addition, theophylline levels in the body may be increased, especially in patients who smoke
- Antidiabetics, oral (diabetes medicine you take by mouth) or
- Insulin—There is an increased risk of hyperglycemia (high blood sugar); beta-blockers may cover up certain symptoms of hypoglycemia (low blood sugar) such as increases

in pulse rate and blood pressure, and may make the hypoglycemia last longer

- Calcium channel blockers (bepridil [e.g., Bepadin], diltiazem [e.g., Cardizem], felodipine [e.g., Plendil], flunarizine [e.g., Sibelium], isradipine [e.g., DynaCirc], nicardipine [e.g., Cardene], nifedipine [e.g., Procardia], nimodipine [e.g., Nimotop], verapamil [e.g., Calan]) or
- Clonidine (e.g., Catapres) or
- Guanabenz (e.g., Wytensin)—Effects on blood pressure may be increased. In addition, unwanted effects may occur if clonidine, guanabenz, or a beta-blocker is stopped suddenly after use together. Unwanted effects on the heart may occur when beta-blockers are used with calcium channel blockers
- Cocaine—Cocaine may block the effects of beta-blockers; in addition, there is an increased risk of high blood pressure, fast heartbeat, and possibly heart problems if you use cocaine while taking a beta-blocker
- Monoamine oxidase (MAO) inhibitors (furazolidone [e.g., Furoxone], isocarboxazid [e.g., Marplan], phenelzine [e.g., Nardil], procarbazine [e.g., Matulane], selegiline [e.g., Eldepryl], tranylcypromine [e.g., Parnate])—Taking beta-blockers while you are taking or within 2 weeks of taking monoamine oxidase (MAO) inhibitors may cause severe high blood pressure

Other medical problems—The presence of other medical problems may affect the use of the beta blockers. Make sure you tell your doctor if you have any other medical problems, especially:

- Allergy, history of (asthma, eczema, hay fever, hives), or
- Bronchitis or
- Emphysema—Severity and duration of allergic reactions to other substances may be increased; in addition, beta-blockers can increase trouble in breathing
- Bradycardia (unusually slow heartbeat) or
- Heart or blood vessel disease—There is a risk of further decreased heart function; also, if treatment is stopped suddenly, unwanted effects may occur
- Diabetes mellitus (sugar diabetes)—Beta-blockers may

cause hyperglycemia (high blood sugar) and circulation problems; in addition, if your diabetes medicine causes your blood sugar to be too low, beta-blockers may cover up some of the symptoms (fast heartbeat), although they will not cover up other symptoms such as dizziness or sweating

- Kidney disease or
- Liver disease—Effects of beta-blockers may be increased because of slower removal from the body
- Mental depression (or history of)—May be increased by beta-blockers
- Myasthenia gravis or
- Psoriasis—Beta-blockers may make these conditions worse
- Overactive thyroid—Stopping beta-blockers suddenly may increase symptoms; beta-blockers may cover up fast heartbeat, which is a sign of overactive thyroid

---

Proper Use of This Medicine

For patients taking the *extended-release capsule or tablet* form of this medicine:

- Swallow the capsule or tablet whole.
- Do not crush, break (except metoprolol succinate extended-release tablets, which may be broken in half), or chew before swallowing.

For patients taking the *concentrated oral solution* form of *propranolol:*

- This medicine is to be taken by mouth even though it comes in a dropper bottle. The amount you should take is to be measured only with the specially marked dropper.
- Mix the medicine with some water, juice, or a carbonated drink. After drinking all the liquid containing the medicine, rinse the glass with a little more liquid and drink that also, to make sure you get all the medicine.

If you prefer, you may mix this medicine with apple-sauce or pudding instead.

- Mix the medicine immediately before you are going to take it. Throw away any mixed medicine that you do not take immediately. Do not save medicine that has been mixed.

Ask your doctor about checking your pulse rate before and after taking beta-blocking agents. Then, while you are taking this medicine, check your pulse regularly. If it is much slower than your usual rate (or less than 50 beats per minute), check with your doctor. A pulse rate that is too slow may cause circulation problems.

To help you remember to take your medicine, try to get into the habit of taking it at the same time each day.

For patients taking this medicine *for high blood pressure:*

- In addition to the use of the medicine your doctor has prescribed, treatment for your high blood pressure may include weight control and care in the types of foods you eat, especially foods high in sodium. Your doctor will tell you which of these are most important for you. You should check with your doctor before changing your diet.

- Many patients who have high blood pressure will not notice any signs of the problem. In fact, many may feel normal. However, if high blood pressure is not treated, it can cause serious problems such as heart failure, blood vessel disease, stroke, or kidney disease.

- Remember that this medicine will not cure your high blood pressure but it does help control it. It is very important that you *take your medicine exactly as directed*, even if you feel well. You must continue to take it as directed if you expect to lower your blood pressure and keep it down. *You may have to take high blood pressure medicine for the rest of your life.*

Also, it is very important to keep your appointments with your doctor, even if you feel well.

Dosing—The dose of beta-blocker will be different for different patients. *Follow your doctor's orders or the directions on the label.* The following information includes only the average doses. *If your dose is different, do not change it* unless your doctor tells you to do so.

The number of capsules or tablets or teaspoonfuls of solution that you take depends on the strength of the medicine. Also, *the number of doses you take each day, the time allowed between doses, and the length of time you take the medicine depend on the medical problem for which you are taking the beta-blocker.*

For acebutolol

- For *oral* dosage forms (capsules and tablets):
  —For angina (chest pain) or irregular heartbeat:
  - Adults—200 milligrams (mg) two times a day. The dose may be increased up to a total of 1200 mg a day.
  - Children—Dose must be determined by your doctor.
  —For high blood pressure:
  - Adults—200 to 800 mg a day as a single dose or divided into two daily doses.
  - Children—Dose must be determined by your doctor.

For atenolol

- For *oral* dosage form (tablets):
  —For angina (chest pain):
  - Adults—50 to 100 mg once a day.
  —For high blood pressure:
  - Adults—25 to 100 mg once a day.
  - Children—Dose must be determined by your doctor.

　—For treatment after a heart attack:

　　• Adults—50 mg ten minutes after the last intravenous dose, followed by another 50 mg twelve hours later. Then 100 mg once a day or 50 mg two times a day for six to nine days or until discharge from hospital.

　• For *injection* dosage form:

　　—For treatment of heart attacks:

　　　• Adults—5 mg given over 5 minutes. The dose is repeated ten minutes later.

For betaxolol

　• For *oral* dosage form (tablets):

　　—For high blood pressure:

　　　• Adults—10 mg once a day. Your doctor may double your dose after seven to fourteen days.

　　　• Children—Dose must be determined by your doctor.

For bisoprolol

　• For *oral* dosage form (tablets):

　　—For high blood pressure:

　　　• Adults—5 to 10 mg once a day.

　　　• Children—Dose must be determined by your doctor.

For carteolol

　• For *oral* dosage form (tablets):

　　—For high blood pressure:

　　　• Adults—2.5 to 10 mg once a day.

　　　• Children—Dose must be determined by your doctor.

For labetalol

　• For *oral* dosage form (tablets):

　　—For high blood pressure:

　　　• Adults—100 to 400 mg two times a day.

• Children—Dose must be determined by your doctor.

• For *injection* dosage form:
  —For high blood pressure:

  • Adults—20 mg injected slowly over two minutes with additional injections of 40 and 80 mg given every ten minutes if needed, up to a total of 300 mg; may be given instead as an infusion at a rate of 2 mg per minute to a total dose of 50 to 300 mg.

  • Children—Dose must be determined by your doctor.

For metoprolol

• For *regular (short-acting) oral* dosage form (tablets):
  —For high blood pressure or angina (chest pain):

  • Adults—100 to 450 mg a day, taken as a single dose or in divided doses.

  • Children—Dose must be determined by your doctor.

  —For treatment after a heart attack:

  • Adults—50 mg every six hours starting fifteen minutes after last intravenous dose. Then 100 mg two times a day for three months to 1 year.

• For *long-acting oral* dosage forms (extended-release tablets):
  —For high blood pressure or angina (chest pain):

  • Adults—Up to 400 mg once a day.

  • Children—Dose must be determined by your doctor.

• For *injection* dosage form:
  —For treatment of a heart attack:

  • Adults—5 mg every two minutes for three doses.

For nadolol
- For *oral* dosage form (tablets):
  —For angina (chest pain):
    - Adults—40 to 240 mg once a day.
  —For high blood pressure:
    - Adults—40 to 320 mg once a day.
    - Children—Dose must be determined by your doctor.

For oxprenolol
- For *regular (short-acting) oral* dosage form (tablets):
  —For high blood pressure:
    - Adults—20 mg three times a day. Your doctor may increase your dose up to 480 mg a day.
    - Children—Dose must be determined by your doctor.
- For *long-acting oral* dosage form (extended-release tablets):
  —For high blood pressure:
    - Adults—80 to 160 mg once a day.
    - Children—Dose must be determined by your doctor.

For penbutolol
- For *oral* dosage form (tablets):
  —For high blood pressure:
    - Adults—20 mg once a day.
    - Children—Dose must be determined by your doctor.

For pindolol
- For *oral* dosage form (tablets):
  —For high blood pressure:
    - Adults—5 mg two times a day. Your doctor may increase your dose up to 60 mg a day.

• Children—Dose must be determined by your doctor.

For propranolol

• For *regular (short-acting) oral* dosage forms (tablets and oral solution):

—For angina (chest pain):

• Adults—80 to 320 mg a day taken in two, three, or four divided doses.

—For irregular heartbeat:

• Adults—10 to 30 mg three or four times a day.

• Children—500 micrograms (0.5 mg) to 4 mg per kilogram of body weight a day taken in divided doses.

—For high blood pressure:

• Adults—40 mg two times a day. Your doctor may increase your dose up to 640 mg a day.

• Children—500 micrograms (0.5 mg) to 4 mg per kilogram of body weight a day taken in divided doses.

—For diseased heart muscle (cardiomyopathy):

• Adults—20 to 40 mg three or four times a day.

—For treatment after a heart attack:

• Adults—180 to 240 mg a day taken in divided doses.

—For treating pheochromocytoma:

• Adults—30 to 160 mg a day taken in divided doses.

—For preventing migraine headaches:

• Adults—20 mg four times a day. Your doctor may increase your dose up to 240 mg a day.

—For trembling:

• Adults—40 mg two times a day. Your doctor may increase your dose up to 320 mg a day.

- For *long-acting oral* dosage form (extended-release capsules):
    - —For high blood pressure:
        - Adults—80 to 160 mg once a day. Doses up to 640 mg once a day may be needed in some patients.
    - —For angina (chest pain):
        - Adults—80 to 320 mg once a day.
    - —For preventing migraine headaches:
        - Adults—80 to 240 mg once a day.
- For *injection* dosage form:
    - —For irregular heartbeat:
        - Adults—1 to 3 mg given at a rate not greater than 1 mg per minute. Dose may be repeated after two minutes and again after four hours if needed.
        - Children—10 to 100 micrograms (0.01 to 0.1 mg) per kilogram of body weight given intravenously every six to eight hours.

For sotalol

- For *oral* dosage form (tablets):
    - —For irregular heartbeat:
        - Adults—80 mg two times a day. Your doctor may increase your dose up to 320 mg per day taken in two or three divided doses.
        - Children—Dose must be determined by your doctor.

For timolol

- For *oral* dosage form (tablets):
    - —For high blood pressure:
        - Adults—10 mg two times a day. Your doctor may increase your dose up 60 mg per day taken as a single dose or in divided doses.
        - Children—Dose must be determined by your doctor.

—For treatment after a heart attack:
  • Adults—10 mg two times a day.
—For preventing migraine headaches:
  • Adults—10 mg two times a day. Your doctor
    may increase your dose up to 30 mg once a day
    or in divided doses.

Missed dose—Do not miss any doses. This is especially
important when you are taking only one dose per day.
Some conditions may become worse if this medicine is
not taken regularly.

If you do miss a dose of this medicine, take it as soon as
possible. However, if it is within 4 hours of your next
dose (8 hours when using atenolol, betaxolol, bisoprolol,
carteolol, labetalol, nadolol, penbutolol, sotalol, or extended-release [long-acting] metoprolol, oxprenolol, or
propranolol), skip the missed dose and go back to your
regular dosing schedule. Do not double doses.

Storage—To store this medicine:
  • Keep out of the reach of children.
  • Store away from heat and direct light.
  • Do not store in the bathroom, near the kitchen sink,
    or in other damp places. Heat or moisture may cause
    the medicine to break down.
  • Do not keep outdated medicine or medicine no longer
    needed. Be sure that any discarded medicine is out
    of the reach of children.

Precautions While Using This Medicine

It is important that your doctor check your progress at
regular visits. This is to make sure the medicine is working
for you and to allow the dosage to be changed if needed.

*Do not stop taking this medicine without first checking
with your doctor.* Your doctor may want you to reduce

gradually the amount you are taking before stopping completely. Some conditions may become worse when the medicine is stopped suddenly, and the danger of heart attack is increased in some patients.

Make sure that you have enough medicine on hand to last through weekends, holidays, or vacations. You may want to carry an extra written prescription in your billfold or purse in case of an emergency. You can then have it filled if you run out of medicine while you are away from home.

Your doctor may want you to carry medical identification stating that you are taking this medicine.

Before having any kind of surgery (including dental surgery) or emergency treatment, tell the medical doctor or dentist in charge that you are taking this medicine.

For *diabetic patients:*

- *This medicine may cause your blood sugar levels to rise.* Also, *this medicine may cover up signs of hypoglycemia (low blood sugar),* such as change in pulse rate.

This medicine may cause some people to become dizzy, drowsy, or lightheaded. *Make sure you know how you react to this medicine before you drive, use machines, or do anything else that could be dangerous if you are dizzy or are not alert.* If the problem continues or gets worse, check with your doctor.

Beta-blockers may make you more sensitive to cold temperatures, especially if you have blood circulation problems. Beta-blockers tend to decrease blood circulation in the skin, fingers, and toes. Dress warmly during cold weather and be careful during prolonged exposure to cold, such as in winter sports.

Chest pain resulting from exercise or physical exertion is usually reduced or prevented by this medicine. This may tempt a patient to be overly active. *Make sure you discuss with your doctor a safe amount of exercise for your medical problem.*

Before you have any medical tests, tell the doctor in charge that you are taking this medicine. The results of some tests may be affected by this medicine.

Before you have any allergy shots, tell the doctor in charge that you are taking a beta-blocker. Beta-blockers may cause you to have a serious reaction to the allergy shot.

For patients with *allergies to foods, medicines, or insect stings:*

- There is a chance that this medicine will cause allergic reactions to be worse and harder to treat. If you have a severe allergic reaction while you are being treated with this medicine, check with a doctor right away so that it can be treated. Be sure to tell the doctor that you are taking a beta-blocker.

For patients taking this medicine *for high blood pressure:*

- *Do not take other medicines unless they have been discussed with your doctor.* This especially includes over-the-counter (nonprescription) medicines for appetite control, asthma, colds, cough, hay fever, or sinus problems since they may tend to increase your blood pressure.

For patients taking *labetalol by mouth:*

- *Dizziness, lightheadedness, or fainting may occur, especially when you get up from a lying or sitting position.* This is more likely to occur when you first start taking labetalol or when the dose is increased. *Getting up slowly may help.* When you get up from lying down, sit on the edge of the bed with your feet dangling for 1 to 2 minutes. Then stand up slowly. If the problem continues or gets worse, check with your doctor.
- The dizziness, lightheadedness, or fainting is also

more likely to occur if you drink alcohol, stand for long periods of time, or exercise, or if the weather is hot. *While you are taking this medicine, be careful to limit the amount of alcohol you drink. Also, use extra care during exercise or hot weather or if you must stand for long periods of time.*

For patients receiving *labetalol by injection:*

• It is very important that you lie down flat while receiving labetalol and for up to 3 hours afterward. If you try to get up too soon, you may become dizzy or faint. *Do not try to sit or stand until your doctor or nurse tells you to do so.*

Side Effects of This Medicine

Along with its needed effects, a medicine may cause some unwanted effects. Although not all of these side effects may occur, if they do occur they may need medical attention.

Check with your doctor as soon as possible if any of the following side effects occur:

Less common

Breathing difficulty and/or wheezing; cold hands and feet; mental depression; shortness of breath; slow heartbeat (especially less than 50 beats per minute); swelling of ankles, feet, and/or lower legs

Rare

Back pain or joint pain; chest pain; confusion (especially in elderly); dark urine—for acebutolol, bisoprolol, or labetalol; dizziness or lightheadedness when getting up from a lying or sitting position; fever and sore throat; hallucinations (seeing, hearing, or feeling things that are not there); irregular heartbeat; red, scaling, or crusted skin; skin rash; unusual bleeding and bruising; yellow eyes or skin—for acebutolol, bisoprolol, or labetalol

Signs and symptoms of overdose (in the order in which they may occur)

Slow heartbeat; dizziness (severe) or fainting; fast or irregular heartbeat; difficulty in breathing; bluish-colored fingernails or palms of hands; convulsions (seizures)

Other side effects may occur that usually do not need medical attention. These side effects may go away during treatment as your body adjusts to the medicine. However, check with your doctor if any of the following side effects continue or are bothersome:

More common

Decreased sexual ability; dizziness or lightheadedness; drowsiness (slight); trouble in sleeping; unusual tiredness or weakness

Less common or rare

Anxiety and/or nervousness; changes in taste—for labetalol only; constipation; diarrhea; dry, sore eyes; frequent urination—for acebutolol and carteolol only; itching of skin; nausea or vomiting; nightmares and vivid dreams; numbness and/or tingling of fingers and/or toes; numbness and/or tingling of skin, especially on scalp—for labetalol only; stomach discomfort; stuffy nose

Although not all of the side effects listed above have been reported for all of these medicines, they have been reported for at least one of them. Since all of the beta-adrenergic blocking agents are very similar, any of the above side effects may occur with any of these medicines. However, they may be more or less common with some agents than with others.

After you have been taking a beta-blocker for a while, it may cause unpleasant or even harmful effects if you stop taking it too suddenly. After you stop taking this medicine or while you are gradually reducing the amount you are taking, check with your doctor right away if any of the following occur:

Chest pain; fast or irregular heartbeat; general feeling of discomfort or illness or weakness; headache; shortness of breath (sudden); sweating; trembling

For patients taking *labetalol:*

- You may notice a tingling feeling on your scalp when you first begin to take labetalol. This is to be expected and usually goes away after you have been taking labetalol for a while.

Other side effects not listed above may also occur in some patients. If you notice any other effects, check with your doctor.

Additional Information

Once a medicine has been approved for marketing for a certain use, experience may show that it is also useful for other medical problems. Although these uses are not included in product labeling, some beta-blockers are used in certain patients with the following medical conditions:

- Glaucoma
- Neuroleptic-induced akathisia (restlessness or the need to keep moving caused by some medicines used to treat nervousness or mental and emotional disorders)

Other than the above information, there is no additional information relating to proper use, precautions, or side effects for these uses.

BRONCHODILATORS, ADRENERGIC Inhalation

Some commonly used brand names are:

In the U.S.—

Adrenalin Chloride[3]	Arm-a-Med Isoetharine[5]
Airet[1]	Arm-a-Med Metaproterenol[7]
Alupent[7]	AsthmaHaler Mist[3]

In the U.S. (cont'd)—

AsthmaNefrin[10]
Brethaire[11]
Bronitin Mist[3]
Bronkaid Mist[3]
Bronkometer[5]
Bronkosol[5]
Dey-Lute Isoetharine S/F[5]
Dey-Lute Metaproterenol[7]
Isuprel[6]
Isuprel Mistometer[6]
Maxair[8]
Medihaler-Epi[3]
Medihaler-Iso[6]

Metaprel[7]
microNefrin[10]
Nephron[10]
Primatene Mist[3]
Primatene Mist Suspension[3]
Proventil[1]
S-2[10]
Tornalate[2]
Vaponefrin[10]
Ventolin[1]
Ventolin Nebules[1]
Ventolin Rotacaps[1]

In Canada—

Alupent[7]
Berotec[4]
Bricanyl[11]
Bronkaid Mistometer[3]
Gen-Salbutamol[1]
Isuprel[6]
Isuprel Mistometer[6]
Medihaler-Epi[3]

Novo-Salmol[1]
Pro-Air[9]
Vaponefrin[10]
Ventodisk[1]
Ventolin[1]
Ventolin Nebules P.F.[1]
Ventolin Rotacaps[1]

Other commonly used names are:
Salbutamol[1]
Orciprenaline[7]

Note: For quick reference, the following adrenergic bronchodilators are numbered to match the corresponding brand names.

This information applies to the following medicines:

1. Albuterol (al-BYOO-ter-ole)‡§
2. Bitolterol (bye-TOLE-ter-ole)†
3. Epinephrine (ep-i-NEF-rin)‡
4. Fenoterol (fen-OH-ter-ole)*
5. Isoetharine (eye-soe-ETH-a-reen)†‡
6. Isoproterenol (eye-soe-proe-TER-e-nole)‡
7. Metaproterenol (met-a-proe-TER-e-nole)‡
8. Pirbuterol (peer-BYOO-ter-ole)†
9. Procaterol (proe-KAY-ter-ole)*
10. Racepinephrine (race-ep-i-NEF-rin)
11. Terbutaline (ter-BYOO-ta-leen)

---

*Not commercially available in the U.S.
†Not commercially available in Canada.
‡Generic name product may also be available in the U.S.
§Generic name product may also be available in Canada.

Description

Adrenergic bronchodilators are medicines that open up the bronchial tubes (air passages) of the lungs. They are taken by oral inhalation to treat the symptoms of bronchial asthma, chronic bronchitis, emphysema, and other lung diseases. They relieve cough, wheezing, shortness of breath, and troubled breathing by increasing the flow of air through the bronchial tubes.

Some of these medicines are also taken by oral inhalation to prevent bronchospasm (wheezing or difficulty in breathing) caused by exercise. In addition, some of these medicines are taken by oral inhalation to prevent attacks of bronchial asthma and bronchospasm. Also, racepinephrine may be used in the treatment of croup.

All of these medicines, except some epinephrine preparations, are available only with your doctor's prescription. Although some of the epinephrine preparations are available without a prescription, your doctor may have special instructions on the proper dose of epinephrine for your medical condition.

These medicines are available in the following dosage forms:

Inhalation

Albuterol
- Capsules for inhalation (U.S. and Canada)
- Inhalation aerosol (U.S. and Canada)
- Inhalation solution (U.S. and Canada)

Bitolterol
- Inhalation aerosol (U.S.)

Epinephrine
- Inhalation aerosol (U.S. and Canada)
- Inhalation solution (U.S.)

Fenoterol
- Inhalation aerosol (Canada)
- Inhalation solution (Canada)

Isoetharine
- Inhalation aerosol (U.S.)
- Inhalation solution (U.S.)

Isoproterenol
- Inhalation aerosol (U.S. and Canada)
- Inhalation solution (U.S. and Canada)

Metaproterenol
- Inhalation aerosol (U.S. and Canada)
- Inhalation solution (U.S. and Canada)

Pirbuterol
- Inhalation aerosol (U.S.)

Procaterol
- Inhalation aerosol (Canada)

Racepinephrine
- Inhalation solution (U.S. and Canada)

Terbutaline
- Inhalation aerosol (U.S. and Canada)

Before Using This Medicine

In deciding to use a medicine, the risks of taking the medicine must be weighed against the good it will do. This is a decision you and your doctor will make. For inhalation adrenergic bronchodilators, the following should be considered:

Allergies—Tell your doctor if you have ever had any unusual or allergic reaction to albuterol, bitolterol, epinephrine, fenoterol, isoetharine, isoproterenol, metaproterenol, pirbuterol, procaterol, racepinephrine, terbutaline, or other inhalation medicines. Also tell your health care professional if you are allergic to any other substances, such as foods, preservatives, or dyes.

Pregnancy—
- *For albuterol, bitolterol, and metaproterenol:* Albuterol, bitolterol, and metaproterenol have not been studied in pregnant women. However, studies in animals have shown that albuterol, bitolterol, and meta-

proterenol cause birth defects when given in doses many times the usual human inhalation dose.

- *For epinephrine and racepinephrine:* Epinephrine and racepinephrine have not been studied in pregnant women. However, studies in animals have shown that epinephrine causes birth defects when given in doses many times the usual human inhalation dose. Use of epinephrine or racepinephrine during pregnancy may decrease the supply of oxygen to the fetus.

- *For fenoterol:* Fenoterol has not been shown to cause birth defects or other problems in humans.

- *For isoetharine and isoproterenol:* Studies on birth defects with isoetharine or isoproterenol have not been done in either humans or animals.

- *For pirbuterol:* Pirbuterol has not been studied in pregnant women. However, in some animal studies, pirbuterol has been shown to cause miscarriage and death of the animal fetus when given in doses many times the usual human inhalation dose.

- *For procaterol:* Procaterol has not been studied in pregnant women.

- *For terbutaline:* Terbutaline has not been studied in pregnant women. It has not been shown to cause birth defects in animal studies when given in doses many times the human inhalation dose. However, terbutaline may delay labor.

Breast-feeding—

- *For albuterol, bitolterol, fenoterol, isoetharine, isoproterenol, metaproterenol, pirbuterol, and procaterol:* It is not known whether albuterol, bitolterol, fenoterol, isoetharine, isoproterenol, metaproterenol, pirbuterol, or procaterol passes into the breast milk. Although most medicines pass into breast milk in small amounts, many of them may be used safely while breast-feeding. Mothers who are taking this medicine and who wish to breast-feed should discuss this with their doctor.

- *For epinephrine and racepinephrine:* Epinephrine passes into the breast milk. Epinephrine and racepinephrine may cause unwanted side effects in babies of mothers using epinephrine or racepinephrine.

- *For terbutaline:* Terbutaline passes into the breast milk. Although most medicines pass into breast milk in small amounts, many of them may be used safely while breast-feeding. Mothers who are taking this medicine and who wish to breast-feed should discuss this with their doctor.

Children—Although there is no specific information comparing use of albuterol, bitolterol, fenoterol, isoetharine, isoproterenol, metaproterenol, pirbuterol, procaterol, racepinephrine, or terbutaline in children with use in other age groups, these medicines are not expected to cause different side effects or problems in children than they do in adults.

Infants and children may be especially sensitive to the effects of epinephrine. Fainting has occurred after epinephrine was given to children with asthma.

Older adults—Many medicines have not been studied specifically in older people. Therefore, it may not be known whether they work exactly the same way they do in younger adults or if they cause different side effects or problems in older people. There is no specific information comparing use of inhalation adrenergic bronchodilators in the elderly.

Other medicines—Although certain medicines should not be used together at all, in other cases two different medicines may be used together even if an interaction might occur. In these cases, your doctor may want to change the dose, or other precautions may be necessary. When you are using inhalation adrenergic bronchodilators, it is especially important that your health care professional know if you are taking any of the following:

- Beta-blockers (acebutolol [e.g., Sectral], atenolol [e.g., Tenormin], betaxolol [e.g., Betoptic, Kerlone], bisoprolol [e.g., Zebeta], carteolol [e.g., Cartrol], labetalol [e.g., Normodyne], levobunolol [e.g., Betagan], metoprolol [e.g., Lopressor], nadolol [e.g., Corgard], oxprenolol [e.g., Trasicor], penbutolol [e.g., Levatol], pindolol [e.g., Visken], propranolol [e.g., Inderal], sotalol [e.g., Sotacor], timolol [e.g., Blocadren, Timoptic])—These medicines may prevent the adrenergic bronchodilators from working properly
- Cocaine or
- Ergoloid mesylates (e.g., Hydergine) or
- Ergotamine (e.g., Gynergen) or
- Maprotiline (e.g., Ludiomil) or
- Tricyclic antidepressants (medicine for depression)—The effects of these medicines on the heart and blood vessels may be increased
- Digitalis glycosides (heart medicine)—The chance of irregular heartbeat may be increased
- Monoamine oxidase (MAO) inhibitors (furazolidone [e.g., Furoxone], isocarboxazid [e.g., Marplan], phenelzine [e.g., Nardil], procarbazine [e.g., Matulane], tranylcypromine [e.g., Parnate])—Using adrenergic bronchodilators while you are taking or within 2 weeks of taking monoamine oxidase (MAO) inhibitors may increase the effects of MAO inhibitors

Other medical problems—The presence of other medical problems may affect the use of inhalation adrenergic bronchodilators. Make sure you tell your doctor if you have any other medical problems, especially:

- Brain damage
- Convulsions (seizures) (or history of)
- Diabetes mellitus (sugar diabetes)—Adrenergic bronchodilators may make the condition worse; your doctor may need to change the dose of your diabetes medicine
- Heart or blood vessel disease or

- High blood pressure—Adrenergic bronchodilators may make the condition worse
- Mental disease—Epinephrine may make the condition worse
- Overactive thyroid—The chance of side effects may be increased
- Parkinson's disease—Epinephrine may temporarily increase certain symptoms of Parkinson's disease, such as rigidity and tremor

---

Proper Use of This Medicine

For patients using *epinephrine, isoetharine, isoproterenol, or racepinephrine:*

- Do not use if the solution turns pinkish to brownish in color or if it becomes cloudy.

Some epinephrine preparations are available without a doctor's prescription. However, *do not use this medicine without a doctor's prescription, unless your medical problem has been diagnosed as asthma by a doctor.*

Some of these preparations may come with patient directions. Read them carefully before using this medicine.

If you are using this medicine in a nebulizer or in a combination nebulizer and respirator, make sure you understand exactly how to use it. If you have any questions about this, check with your health care professional.

For patients using the *inhalation aerosol* form of this medicine:

- *Keep spray away from the eyes because it may cause irritation.*
- *Do not take more than 2 inhalations of this medicine at any one time,* unless otherwise directed by your doctor. Allow 1 to 2 minutes after the first inhalation to make certain that a second inhalation is necessary.

• Save your applicator. Refill units of this medicine may be available.

Use this medicine only as directed. Do not use more of it and do not use it more often than recommended on the label, unless otherwise directed by your doctor. To do so may increase the chance of serious side effects. Inhalation aerosol medicines have been reported to cause death when too much of the medicine was used.

Dosing—The dose of these medicines will be different for different patients. *Follow your doctor's orders or the directions on the label.* The following information includes only the average doses of these medicines. *If your dose is different, do not change it* unless your doctor tells you to do so.

The number of inhalations or the amount of medicine that you use depends on the strength of the medicine. Also, *the number of doses you take each day, the time allowed between doses, and the length of time you take the medicine depend on the medical problem for which you are taking the adrenergic bronchodilator.*

For albuterol

• For *inhalation aerosol* dosage form:

  —For symptoms of bronchial asthma, chronic bronchitis, emphysema, or other lung disease:

  • Adults and children 12 years of age and older—180 or 200 micrograms (mcg) (2 puffs) every four to six hours.

  • Children up to 12 years of age—Dose must be determined by your doctor.

  —For prevention of bronchospasm (wheezing or difficulty in breathing) caused by exercise:

  • Adults and children 12 years of age and older—180 or 200 mcg (2 puffs) fifteen minutes before exercise.

       • Children up to 12 years of age—Dose must be determined by your doctor.

   • For *inhalation solution* dosage form:

    —For symptoms of bronchial asthma, chronic bronchitis, emphysema, or other lung disease:

      • Adults and children 12 years of age and older—1.25 to 5 milligrams (mg) of albuterol in 2 to 5 milliliters (mL) or more of sterile 0.9% sodium chloride solution or sterile water for inhalation, depending on the product. This medicine is usually used in a combination nebulizer and respirator and is taken by inhalation three or four times a day every four to six hours if needed. However, your doctor may use other inhalation methods to give you this medicine.

      • Children up to 12 years of age—Dose must be determined by your doctor.

   • For *capsules for inhalation* dosage form:

    —For symptoms of bronchial asthma, chronic bronchitis, emphysema, or other lung disease:

      • Adults and children 12 years of age and older—200 or 400 mcg taken by inhalation every four to six hours.

      • Children up to 12 years of age—Dose must be determined by your doctor.

    —For bronchospasm (wheezing or difficulty in breathing) caused by exercise:

      • Adults and children 12 years of age and older—200 mcg taken by inhalation fifteen minutes before exercise.

      • Children up to 12 years of age—Dose must be determined by your doctor.

For bitolterol

   • For *inhalation aerosol* dosage form:

    —For prevention of symptoms of bronchial asthma,

chronic bronchitis, emphysema, or other lung disease:

- Adults and children 12 years of age and older— 740 micrograms (mcg) (2 puffs) every eight hours.

- Children up to 12 years of age—Dose must be determined by your doctor.

—For treatment of symptoms of bronchial asthma, chronic bronchitis, emphysema, or other lung disease:

- Adults and children 12 years of age and older— At first, 740 mcg (2 puffs), allowing one to three minutes between each puff. This dose may be followed by another dose of 370 mcg (1 puff), if needed. However, the dose taken each day should not be more than 740 mcg (2 puffs) every four hours or 1.11 milligrams (mg) (3 puffs) every six hours.

- Children up to 12 years of age—Dose must be determined by your doctor.

For epinephrine

- For symptoms of bronchial asthma, chronic bronchitis, emphysema, or other lung disease:

    —For *inhalation aerosol* dosage form:

    - Adults and children 4 years of age and older— 200 to 275 micrograms (mcg) (1 puff). The dose may be repeated after one to two minutes, if needed. Doses should be taken at least three hours apart.

    - Children up to 4 years of age—Dose must be determined by your doctor.

    —For *inhalation solution* dosage form:

    - Adults and children 6 years of age and older— This medicine should be used in a nebulizer as directed. The usual dose is 1 puff of a 1% solution. The dose may be repeated, if necessary, after one or two minutes as needed.

• Children up to 6 years of age—Dose must be determined by your doctor.

For epinephrine bitartrate

• For *inhalation aerosol* dosage form:

—For symptoms of bronchial asthma, chronic bronchitis, emphysema, or other lung disease:

• Adults and children 4 years of age and older—160 micrograms (mcg) (1 puff) of epinephrine. The dose may be repeated after one minute, if needed. Doses should be taken at least three hours apart.

• Children up to 4 years of age—Dose must be determined by your doctor.

For fenoterol

• For *inhalation aerosol* dosage form:

—For symptoms of bronchial asthma, chronic bronchitis, emphysema, or other lung disease:

• Adults and children 12 years of age and older—200 or 400 micrograms (mcg) (1 or 2 puffs), repeated up to four times a day if needed. This medicine should not be taken more often than every four hours.

• Children up to 12 years of age—Dose must be determined by your doctor.

• For *inhalation solution* dosage form:

—For symptoms of bronchial asthma, chronic bronchitis, emphysema, or other lung disease:

• Adults and children 12 years of age and older—This medicine is usually used in a nebulizer and is taken by inhalation. However, your doctor may use other inhalation methods to give you this medicine. The usual dose is 500 mcg to 1 milligram (mg) as a 0.1% solution, diluted to 5 milliliters (mL) with 0.9% sodium chloride solution. The total amount of this solution should be inhaled over a period of ten to fifteen minutes. The dose may be repeated every six hours if needed.

• Children up to 12 years of age—Dose must be determined by your doctor.

For isoetharine

• For *inhalation solution* dosage form:

—For symptoms of bronchial asthma, chronic bronchitis, emphysema, or other lung disease:

• Adults—This medicine is usually used in a nebulizer and is taken by inhalation. However, your doctor may use other inhalation methods to give you this medicine. The amount of medicine you use and whether it requires dilution depend on the product ordered by your doctor. This medicine usually should not be used more often than every four hours.

• Children—Dose must be determined by your doctor.

For isoetharine mesylate

• For *inhalation aerosol* dosage form:

—For symptoms of bronchial asthma, chronic bronchitis, emphysema, or other lung disease:

• Adults—340 micrograms (mcg) (1 puff), repeated after one to two minutes if needed. This dose may be repeated every four hours as necessary.

• Children—Dose must be determined by your doctor.

For isoproterenol

• For *inhalation solution* dosage form:

—For symptoms of bronchial asthma, chronic bronchitis, emphysema, or other lung disease:

• Adults and children—This medicine is usually used in a nebulizer and is taken by inhalation. However, your doctor may use other inhalation methods to give you this medicine. The usual dose is 6 to 12 puffs of a 0.25% solution, repeated every fifteen minutes, if needed, for three doses. No more than eight treatments should be taken in twenty-four hours. Or,

—For severe bronchial asthma or asthma attack:

• Adults—This medicine is usually used in a nebulizer and is taken by inhalation. However, your doctor may use other inhalation methods to give you this medicine. The usual dose is 5 to 15 deep puffs of a 0.5% solution or 3 to 7 deep puffs of a 1% solution, repeated once after five to ten minutes if needed. This dose may be taken up to five times a day if necessary.

• Children—This medicine is usually used in a nebulizer and is taken by inhalation. However, your doctor may use other inhalation methods to give you this medicine. The usual dose is 5 to 15 deep puffs of a 0.5% solution, repeated once after five to ten minutes if needed. This dose may be taken up to five times a day if necessary.

—For bronchospasm (wheezing or difficulty in breathing) in chronic lung disease:

• Adults—This medicine is usually used in a nebulizer and is taken by inhalation. However, your doctor may use other inhalation methods to give you this medicine. The usual dose of this medicine when used in a nebulizer is 5 to 15 deep inhalations of a 0.5% solution or 3 to 7 deep inhalations of a 1% solution. This dose should not be taken more often than every three to four hours.

• Children—This medicine is usually used in a nebulizer and is taken by inhalation. However, your doctor may use other inhalation methods to give you this medicine. The usual dose of this medicine when used in a nebulizer is 5 to 15 deep inhalations of a 0.5% solution. This dose should not be taken more often than every three to four hours.

For isoproterenol hydrochloride

• For *inhalation aerosol* dosage form:

—For severe bronchial asthma or asthma attack:

• Adults and children—120 to 131 micrograms (mcg) (1 puff), repeated after one to five minutes if needed. This dose is taken four to six times a day.

—For symptoms of bronchial asthma, chronic bronchitis, emphysema, or other lung disease:

• Adults and children—120 to 131 mcg (1 puff) taken not more often than once every three to four hours.

For isoproterenol sulfate

• For *inhalation aerosol* dosage form:

—For symptoms of bronchial asthma, chronic bronchitis, emphysema, or other lung disease:

• Adults and children—75 or 80 micrograms (mcg) (1 puff), repeated after two to five minutes if needed. This dose is taken four to six times a day.

For metaproterenol

• For *inhalation aerosol* dosage form:

—For symptoms of bronchial asthma, chronic bronchitis, emphysema, or other lung disease:

       • Adults and children 12 years of age and older—1.3 to 2.25 milligrams (mg) (2 or 3 puffs) every three to four hours. The total dose should not be more than 9 mg (12 puffs) a day.

       • Children up to 12 years of age—Use is not recommended.

   • For *inhalation solution* dosage form:

     —For attacks of bronchospasm (wheezing or difficulty in breathing):

       • Adults and children 12 years of age and older—This medicine is usually used in a nebulizer and is taken by inhalation. However, your doctor may use other inhalation methods to give you this medicine. The usual dose of this medicine when used in a nebulizer is 10 puffs of a 0.4 to 0.6% solution. This medicine should not be used more often than every four hours.

       • Children up to 12 years of age—Dose must be determined by your doctor.

     —For symptoms of bronchial asthma, chronic bronchitis, emphysema, or other lung disease:

       • Adults and children 12 years of age and older—This medicine is usually used in a nebulizer and is taken by inhalation. However, your doctor may use other inhalation methods to give you this medicine. The usual dose of this medicine when used in a nebulizer is 10 puffs of a 0.4 to 0.6% solution. This medicine should not be used more often than three or four times a day.

       • Children up to 12 years of age—Dose must be determined by your doctor.

For pirbuterol

   • For *inhalation aerosol* dosage form:

     —For symptoms of bronchial asthma, chronic bronchitis, emphysema, or other lung disease:

• Adults and children 12 years of age and older—200 or 400 micrograms (mcg) (1 or 2 puffs) every four to six hours. The total dose should not be more than 2.4 milligrams (mg) (12 puffs) a day.

• Children up to 12 years of age—Dose must be determined by your doctor.

For procaterol

• For *inhalation aerosol* dosage form:

—For symptoms of bronchial asthma, chronic bronchitis, emphysema, or other lung disease:

• Adults and children 12 years of age and older—20 micrograms (mcg) (2 puffs) three times a day.

• Children up to 12 years of age—Dose must be determined by your doctor.

—For bronchospasm (wheezing or difficulty in breathing) caused by exercise:

• Adults and children 12 years of age and older—20 mcg (2 puffs) taken at least fifteen minutes before exercise.

• Children up to 12 years of age—Dose must be determined by your doctor.

For racepinephrine

• For *inhalation solution* dosage form:

—For symptoms of bronchial asthma, chronic bronchitis, emphysema, or other lung disease:

• Adults and children 4 years of age and older—

—For solution used in a nebulizer: 2 or 3 puffs of a 2.25% solution, followed in five minutes by 2 or 3 more puffs if needed. This dose may be taken four to six times a day.

—For solution used in a combination nebulizer and respirator: 5 mL of a 0.1% solution used for a period of fifteen minutes every three to four hours.

- Children up to 4 years of age—Dose must be determined by your doctor.

For terbutaline
- For *inhalation aerosol* dosage form:
  —For symptoms of bronchial asthma, chronic bronchitis, emphysema, or other lung disease:
  - Adults and children 12 years of age and older—200 to 500 micrograms (mcg) (1 or 2 puffs) every four to six hours. If 2 puffs are taken, allow sixty seconds between puffs.
  - Children up to 12 years of age—Dose must be determined by your doctor.

Missed dose—If you are using this medicine regularly and you miss a dose, use it as soon as possible. Then use any remaining doses for that day at regularly spaced intervals. Do not double doses.

Storage—To store this medicine:
- Keep out of the reach of children.
- Store away from heat.
- Store the solution form of this medicine away from direct light. Store the inhalation aerosol form of this medicine away from direct sunlight.
- Keep the medicine from freezing.
- Do not puncture, break, or burn the inhalation aerosol container, even if it is empty.
- Do not keep outdated medicine or medicine no longer needed. Be sure that any discarded medicine is out of the reach of children.

Precautions While Using This Medicine

If you still have trouble breathing after using this medicine, or if your condition becomes worse, check with your doctor at once.

For *diabetic patients* using *epinephrine:*

- This medicine may cause your blood sugar levels to rise. If you notice a change in the results of your blood or urine sugar tests or if you have any questions, check with your doctor.

For patients using the *aerosol form* of this medicine:

- If you are also using the inhalation aerosol form of a corticosteroid (cortisone-like medicine, such as beclomethasone, dexamethasone, flunisolide, or triamcinolone) or ipratropium, *use the adrenergic bronchodilator inhalation aerosol first and then wait about 5 minutes before using the corticosteroid or ipratropium inhalation aerosol,* unless otherwise directed by your doctor. This will help the corticosteroid or ipratropium inhalation aerosol to reach the passages of the lungs (bronchioles) after the adrenergic bronchodilator inhalation aerosol opens them.

For patients using *albuterol inhalation aerosol:*

- If you use all of the medicine in one canister (container) in less than 2 weeks, check with your doctor. You may be using too much of the medicine.

Dryness of the mouth and throat may occur after use of this medicine. Rinsing the mouth with water after each dose may help prevent the dryness.

Some of these preparations may contain sulfites as a preservative. Sulfites may cause an allergic reaction in some people. *If you know that you are allergic to sulfites, do not use this medicine until you have carefully read the label or checked with your health care professional to make sure the medicine does not contain sulfites.* Signs of an allergic reaction to sulfites include bluish coloration of skin; severe dizziness or feeling faint; continuing flushing or redness of face or skin; increased wheezing or difficulty in breathing; skin rash, hives, or itching; or swelling of face, lips, or eyelids. *If any of these signs occur, check with your doctor immediately.*

Side Effects of This Medicine

In some animal studies, albuterol and terbutaline were shown to increase the chance of benign (not cancerous) tumors. Terbutaline was also shown to increase the chance of ovarian cysts. The doses given were many times the inhalation dose of albuterol and the oral dose of terbutaline given to humans. It is not known if albuterol or terbutaline increases the chance of tumors in humans, or if terbutaline increases the chance of ovarian cysts in humans.

Along with its needed effects, a medicine may cause some unwanted effects. Although not all of these side effects may occur, if they do occur they may need medical attention.

Check with your doctor immediately if any of the following side effects occur:

> Bluish coloration of skin; dizziness (severe) or feeling faint; flushing or redness of face or skin (continuing); increased wheezing or difficulty in breathing; skin rash, hives, or itching; swelling of face, lips, or eyelids

Check with your doctor as soon as possible if any of the following side effects occur:

Rare

> Chest discomfort or pain; irregular heartbeat; numbness in hands or feet; unusual bruising

With high doses

> Hallucinations (seeing, hearing, or feeling things that are not there)

Symptoms of overdose

> Chest discomfort or pain (continuing or severe); chills or fever; convulsions (seizures); dizziness or lightheadedness (continuing or severe); fast or slow heartbeat (continuing); headache (continuing or severe); increase

or decrease in blood pressure (severe); irregular or pounding heartbeat (continuing or severe); muscle cramps (severe); nausea or vomiting (continuing or severe); shortness of breath or troubled breathing (severe); trembling (severe); unusual anxiety, nervousness, or restlessness; unusually large pupils or blurred vision; unusual paleness and coldness of skin; weakness (severe)

Other side effects may occur that usually do not need medical attention. These side effects may go away during treatment as your body adjusts to the medicine. However, check with your doctor if any of the following side effects continue or are bothersome:

More common

Nervousness or restlessness; trembling

Less common

Coughing or other bronchial irritation; dizziness or lightheadedness; drowsiness; dryness or irritation of mouth or throat; fast or pounding heartbeat; flushing or redness of face or skin; headache; increased sweating; increase in blood pressure; muscle cramps or twitching; nausea or vomiting; trouble in sleeping; unusual paleness; weakness

Not all of the side effects listed above have been reported for each of these medicines, but they have been reported for at least one of them. All of the adrenergic bronchodilators are similar, so any of the above side effects may occur with any of these medicines.

While you are using albuterol, bitolterol, fenoterol, metaproterenol, or terbutaline, you may notice an unusual or unpleasant taste. Also, pirbuterol may cause changes in smell or taste. These effects may be expected and will go away when you stop using the medicine.

Isoproterenol may cause the saliva to turn pinkish to red. This is to be expected while you are using this medicine.

Other side effects not listed above may also occur in some patients. If you notice any other effects, check with your doctor.

BRONCHODILATORS, ADRENERGIC Oral/Injection

Some commonly used brand names are:

In the U.S.—

Adrenalin Chloride Solution[3]	Isuprel Glossets[6]
Alupent[7]	Metaprel[7]
Ana-Guard[3]	Prometa[7]
Brethine[8]	Proventil[1]
Bricanyl[8]	Proventil Repetabs[1]
Bronkephrine[4]	Sus-Phrine[3]
EpiPen Auto-Injector[3]	Ventolin[1]
EpiPen Jr. Auto-Injector[3]	Volmax[1]
Isuprel[6]	

In Canada—

Adrenalin[3]	EpiPen Jr. Auto-Injector[3]
Alupent[7]	Isuprel[6]
Berotec[5]	Novo-Salmol[1]
Bricanyl[8]	Ventolin[1]
EpiPen Auto-Injector[3]	Volmax[1]

Other commonly used names are:
Salbutamol[1]
Orciprenaline[7]

Note: For quick reference the following adrenergic bronchodilators are numbered to match the corresponding brand names.

This information applies to the following medicines:

1. Albuterol (al-BYOO-ter-ole)‡
2. Ephedrine (e-FED-rin)‡§
3. Epinephrine (ep-i-NEF-rin)‡§
4. Ethylnorepinephrine (ETH-il-nor-ep-i-NEF-rin)†
5. Fenoterol (fen-OH-ter-ole)*
6. Isoproterenol (eye-soe-proe-TER-e-nole)‡
7. Metaproterenol (met-a-proe-TER-e-nole)‡
8. Terbutaline (ter-BYOO-ta-leen)

---

*Not commercially available in the U.S.
†Not commercially available in Canada.
‡Generic name product may also be available in the U.S.
§Generic name product may also be available in Canada.

Description

Adrenergic bronchodilators are medicines that open up the bronchial tubes (air passages) of the lungs. They are used to treat the symptoms of bronchial asthma, chronic bronchitis, emphysema, and other lung diseases. They relieve cough, wheezing, shortness of breath, and troubled breathing by increasing the flow of air through the bronchial tubes.

Ephedrine may also be used for the relief of nasal congestion in hay fever or other allergies. In addition, ephedrine may be used in the treatment of narcolepsy (uncontrolled desire for sleep or sudden attacks of sleep) and certain types of mental depression.

Epinephrine injection (not including the auto-injector or the sterile suspension) may be used in eye surgery to stop bleeding, reduce congestion, and dilate the pupil. It may also be applied topically to the skin or mucous membranes to stop bleeding.

Epinephrine injection (including the auto-injector but not the sterile suspension) is used in the emergency treatment of allergic reactions to insect stings, medicines, foods, or other substances. It relieves skin rash, hives, and itching; wheezing; and swelling of the lips, eyelids, tongue, and inside of nose.

Adrenergic bronchodilators may be used for other conditions as determined by your doctor.

Ephedrine capsules are available without a prescription. However, your doctor may have special instructions on the proper dose of ephedrine for your medical condition.

All of the other adrenergic bronchodilators are available only with your doctor's prescription.

These medicines are available in the following dosage forms:

Oral

Albuterol
- Oral solution (Canada)
- Syrup (U.S.)
- Tablets (U.S. and Canada)
- Extended-release tablets (U.S. and Canada)

Ephedrine
- Capsules (U.S.)

Fenoterol
- Tablets (Canada)

Isoproterenol
- Tablets (U.S.)

Metaproterenol
- Syrup (U.S. and Canada)
- Tablets (U.S. and Canada)

Terbutaline
- Tablets (U.S. and Canada)

Parenteral

Albuterol
- Injection (Canada)

Ephedrine
- Injection (U.S. and Canada)

Epinephrine
- Injection (U.S. and Canada)

Ethylnorepinephrine
- Injection (U.S.)

Isoproterenol
- Injection (U.S. and Canada)

Terbutaline
- Injection (U.S.)

Before Using This Medicine

In deciding to use a medicine, the risks of taking the medicine must be weighed against the good it will do. This is a decision you and your doctor will make. For adrenergic bronchodilators taken by mouth or given by injection, the following should be considered:

Allergies—Tell your doctor if you have ever had any unusual or allergic reaction to albuterol, ephedrine, epinephrine, ethylnorepinephrine, fenoterol, isoproterenol, metaproterenol, or terbutaline. Also tell your health care professional if you are allergic to any other substances, such as foods, preservatives, or dyes.

Pregnancy—

- *For albuterol:* Albuterol has not been studied in pregnant women. However, studies in animals have shown that albuterol causes birth defects when given in doses many times the usual human dose. In addition, although albuterol has been reported to delay preterm labor when taken by mouth, it has not been shown to stop preterm labor or prevent labor at term.

- *For ephedrine:* Studies on birth defects with ephedrine have not been done in either humans or animals. When ephedrine is used just before or during labor, its effects on the newborn infant or on the growth and development of the child are not known.

- *For epinephrine:* Epinephrine has not been studied in pregnant women. However, studies in animals have shown that epinephrine causes birth defects when given in doses many times the usual human dose. Also, use of epinephrine during pregnancy may decrease the supply of oxygen to the fetus. Epinephrine is not recommended for use during labor since it may delay the second stage of labor. In addition, high doses of epinephrine that decrease contractions of the uterus may result in excessive bleeding when used during labor and delivery.

- *For ethylnorepinephrine and isoproterenol:* Studies on birth defects with ethylnorepinephrine or isoproterenol have not been done in either humans or animals.

- *For fenoterol:* Fenoterol has not been shown to cause birth defects or other problems in humans.

- *For metaproterenol:* Metaproterenol has not been

studied in pregnant women. However, studies in animals have shown that metaproterenol causes birth defects when given in doses many times the usual human dose. Also, studies in animals have shown that metaproterenol causes death of the animal fetus when given in doses many times the usual human dose.

- *For terbutaline:* Terbutaline has not been studied in pregnant women. It has not been shown to cause birth defects in animal studies when given in doses many times the usual human dose. However, terbutaline given by injection during pregnancy has been reported to cause an unusually fast heartbeat in the fetus. Although terbutaline is used to delay preterm labor, it may also delay labor at term.

Breast-feeding—

- *For albuterol, fenoterol, isoproterenol, and metaproterenol:* It is not known whether albuterol, fenoterol, isoproterenol, or metaproterenol passes into the breast milk. Although most medicines pass into breast milk in small amounts, many of them may be used safely while breast-feeding. Mothers who are taking this medicine and who wish to breast-feed should discuss this with their doctor.

- *For ephedrine and epinephrine:* Ephedrine and epinephrine pass into the breast milk and may cause unwanted side effects in babies of mothers using ephedrine or epinephrine.

- *For terbutaline:* Terbutabline passes into the breast milk. Although most medicines pass into breast milk in small amounts, many of them may be used safely while breast-feeding. Mothers who are taking this medicine and who wish to breast-feed should discuss this with their doctor.

Children—Although there is no specific information comparing use of albuterol, ethylnorepinephrine, fenoterol, isoproterenol, metaproterenol, or terbutaline in children with use in other age groups, these medicines are not expected to cause different side effects or problems in children than they do in adults.

Infants may be especially sensitive to the effects of ephedrine.

Infants and children may be especially sensitive to the effects of epinephrine. Fainting has occurred after epinephrine was given to children with asthma.

Older adults—Many medicines have not been studied specifically in older people. Therefore, it may not be known whether they work exactly the same way they do in younger adults or if they cause different side effects or problems in older people. There is no specific information comparing use of adrenergic bronchodilators in the elderly with use in other age groups.

Other medicines—Although certain medicines should not be used together at all, in other cases two different medicines may be used together even if an interaction might occur. In these cases, your doctor may want to change the dose, or other precautions may be necessary. When you are taking adrenergic bronchodilators, it is especially important that your health care professional know if you are taking any of the following:

- Beta-blockers (acebutolol [e.g., Sectral], atenolol [e.g., Tenormin], betaxolol [e.g., Betoptic, Kerlone], bisoprolol [e.g., Zebeta], carteolol [e.g., Cartrol], labetalol [e.g., Normodyne], levobunolol [e.g., Betagan], metoprolol [e.g., Lopressor], nadolol [e.g., Corgard], oxprenolol [e.g., Trasicor], penbutolol [e.g., Levatol], pindolol [e.g., Visken], propranolol [e.g., Inderal], sotalol [e.g., Sotacor], timolol [e.g., Blocadren, Timoptic])—These medicines may prevent the adrenergic bronchodilators from working properly
- Cocaine or
- Ergoloid mesylates (e.g., Hydergine) or
- Ergotamine (e.g., Gynergen) or

- Maprotiline (e.g., Ludiomil) or
- Tricyclic antidepressants (medicine for depression)—The effects of these medicines on the heart and blood vessels may be increased
- Digitalis glycosides (heart medicine)—The chance of irregular heartbeat may be increased
- Monoamine oxidase (MAO) inhibitors (furazolidone [e.g., Furoxone], isocarboxazid [e.g., Marplan], phenelzine [e.g., Nardil], procarbazine [e.g., Matulane], tranylcypromine [e.g., Parnate])—Taking adrenergic bronchodilators while you are taking or within 2 weeks of taking monoamine oxidase (MAO) inhibitors may increase the effects of MAO inhibitors

Other medical problems—The presence of other medical problems may affect the use of adrenergic bronchodilators. Make sure you tell your doctor if you have any other medical problems, especially:

- Brain damage
- Convulsions (seizures) (history of)
- Diabetes mellitus (sugar diabetes)—Adrenergic bronchodilators may make the condition worse; your doctor may need to change the dose of your diabetes medicine
- Enlarged prostate—Ephedrine may make the condition worse
- Heart or blood vessel disease or
- High blood pressure—Adrenergic bronchodilators may make the condition worse
- Mental disease—Epinephrine may make the condition worse
- Overactive thyroid—The chance of side effects may be increased
- Parkinson's disease—Epinephrine may temporarily increase certain symptoms of Parkinson's disease, such as rigidity and tremor

---

Proper Use of This Medicine

For patients taking *albuterol extended-release tablets:*
- Swallow the tablet whole.

• Do not crush, break, or chew before swallowing.

For patients taking *ephedrine:*

• Ephedrine may cause trouble in sleeping. To help prevent this, *take the last dose of ephedrine for each day a few hours before bedtime.* If you have any questions about this, check with your doctor.

For patients taking *isoproterenol sublingual tablets*:

• Do not chew or swallow the tablet. This medicine is meant to be absorbed through the lining of the mouth. Place the tablet under your tongue (sublingual) and let it slowly dissolve there. Do not swallow until the tablet has dissolved completely.

For patients using the *injection* form of this medicine:

• Do not use the epinephrine solution or suspension if it turns pinkish to brownish in color or if the solution becomes cloudy.

• *Use this medicine only for the conditions for which it was prescribed by your doctor.*

• Keep this medicine ready for use at all times. Also, keep the telephone numbers for your doctor and the nearest hospital emergency room readily available.

• Check the expiration date on the injection regularly. Replace the medicine before that date.

• This medicine is for injection only. If you will be giving yourself the injections, make sure you understand exactly how to give them. If you have any questions about this, check with your doctor.

For patients using *epinephrine injection* for an *allergic reaction emergency*:

• If an allergic reaction as described by your doctor occurs, *use the epinephrine injection immediately.*

• Notify your doctor immediately or go to the nearest hospital emergency room. If you have used the epinephrine injection, be sure to tell your doctor.

- If you have been stung by an insect, remove the insect's stinger with your fingernails, if possible. Be careful not to squeeze, pinch, or push it deeper into the skin. Ice packs or sodium bicarbonate (baking soda) soaks, if available, may then be applied to the area stung.

- If you are using the epinephrine auto-injector (automatic injection device):

    —It is important that you do not remove the safety cap on the auto-injector until you are ready to use it. This prevents accidental activation of the device during storage and handling.

    —Epinephrine auto-injector comes with patient directions. Read them carefully before you actually need to use this medicine. Then, when an emergency arises, you will know how to inject the epinephrine.

    —To use the epinephrine auto-injector:

    - Remove the gray safety cap.
    - Place the black tip on the thigh, at a right angle to the leg.
    - Press hard into the thigh until the auto-injector functions. Hold in place for several seconds. Then remove the auto-injector and discard.
    - Massage the injection area for 10 seconds.

Use this medicine only as directed. Do not use more of it and do not use it more often than your doctor ordered, or more than recommended on the label unless otherwise directed by your doctor. To do so may increase the chance of side effects.

Dosing—The dose of these medicines will be different for different patients. *Follow your doctor's orders or the directions on the label.* The following information includes only the average doses of these medicines. *If your dose is different, do not change it* unless your doctor tells you to do so.

The number of capsules or tablets, teaspoonfuls of solution or syrup, or amount of injection that you take depends on the strength of the medicine. Also, *the number of doses you take each day, the time allowed between doses, and the length of time you take the medicine depend on the medical problem for which you are taking the adrenergic bronchodilator.*

For albuterol

- For symptoms of bronchial asthma, chronic bronchitis, emphysema, or other lung disease:

  —For *solution* dosage form:

    - Adults—2 to 4 milligrams (mg) of albuterol three or four times a day.

    - Children 6 to 12 years of age—2 mg of albuterol three or four times a day.

    - Children 2 to 6 years of age—Dose is based on body weight and must be determined by your doctor. The usual dose is 100 micrograms (mcg) of albuterol per kilogram (kg) (45 mcg per pound) of body weight three or four times a day.

    - Children up to 2 years of age—Dose must be determined by your doctor.

  —For *syrup* dosage form:

    - Adults and children 14 years of age and older—At first, 2 to 6 mg of albuterol three or four times a day. Then your doctor may increase your dose, if needed, up to 8 mg four times a day.

    - Children 6 to 14 years of age—At first, 2 mg of albuterol three or four times a day. Then your doctor may increase your dose, if needed, up to 24 mg a day taken in divided doses.

    - Children 2 to 6 years of age—Dose is based on body weight and must be determined by your doctor. At first, the usual dose is 100 mcg of albuterol per kg (45 mcg per pound) of body weight. Then your doctor may increase your dose, if needed, up to 200 mcg per kg (90 mcg per pound) of body weight. However, the dose should not be more than 4 mg three times a day.

• Children up to 2 years of age—Dose must be determined by your doctor.

—For *tablet* dosage form:

• Older adults—At first, 2 mg of albuterol three or four times a day. Then your doctor may increase your dose, if needed, up to 8 mg three or four times a day.

• Adults and children 12 years of age and older—At first, 2 to 6 mg of albuterol three or four times a day. Then your doctor may increase your dose, if needed, up to 8 mg four times a day.

• Children 6 to 12 years of age—At first, 2 mg of albuterol three or four times a day. Then your doctor may increase your dose, if needed, up to 24 mg a day taken in divided doses.

• Children up to 6 years of age—Dose must be determined by your doctor.

—For *extended-release tablet* dosage form:

• Adults and children 12 years of age and older—4 or 8 mg of albuterol every twelve hours.

• Children up to 12 years of age—Dose must be determined by your doctor.

—For *injection* dosage form:

• Dose is usually based on body weight and must be determined by your doctor. Depending on your condition, this medicine is injected into either a muscle or vein or injected slowly into a vein over a period of time.

    —Adults:

         • The usual dose injected into a muscle is 8 mcg of albuterol per kg (3.6 mcg per pound) of body weight every four hours as needed, up to a total dose of 2 mg a day.

• The usual dose injected into a vein is 4 mcg per kg (1.8 mcg per pound) of body weight, given over a period of two to five minutes. The dose may be repeated after fifteen minutes, if needed, up to a total dose of 1 mg a day.

• When albuterol is injected slowly into a vein, it is given at a rate of 5 mcg per minute. Your doctor may increase the rate to 10 mcg per minute and then 20 mcg per minute every fifteen to thirty minutes, if needed.

—Children: Dose must be determined by your doctor.

For ephedrine

• For *capsule* dosage form:

—For nasal congestion, narcolepsy (uncontrolled desire for sleep), or symptoms of bronchial asthma, chronic bronchitis, emphysema, or other lung disease:

• Adults—25 or 50 milligrams (mg) every three or four hours, if needed.

• Children—Dose is based on body weight or size and must be determined by your doctor. The usual dose is 3 mg per kg (1.3 mg per pound) of body weight a day. This dose is divided into four to six doses.

• For *injection* dosage form:

—For symptoms of bronchial asthma, chronic bronchitis, emphysema, or other lung disease:

• Adults—12.5 to 25 mg injected into a muscle, a vein, or under the skin. Your doctor may give you another dose, if needed.

• Children—Dose is based on body weight and must be determined by your doctor. The usual dose is 3 mg per kg (1.3 mg per pound) of body weight a day. This dose is divided into four to six doses.

For epinephrine

• For *injection* dosage form:

—For symptoms of bronchial asthma, chronic bronchitis, emphysema, or other lung disease:

• Adults and teenagers—200 to 500 micrograms (mcg) injected under the skin. The dose may be repeated every twenty minutes to four hours as needed. Your doctor may increase your dose up to 1 mg a dose, if needed.

• Children—Dose is based on body weight or size and must be determined by your doctor. The usual dose is 10 mcg per kilogram (kg) (4.5 mcg per pound) of body weight, up to 500 mcg a dose. The dose may be repeated every fifteen minutes for two doses, then every four hours as needed.

—For allergic reactions:

• Adults—At first, 200 to 500 mcg injected into a muscle or under the skin. Then the dose may be repeated every ten to fifteen minutes as needed. Your doctor may increase your dose up to 1 mg a dose, if needed.

• Children—Dose is based on body weight or size and must be determined by your doctor. The usual dose is 10 mcg per kg (4.5 mcg per pound) of body weight, up to 500 mcg a dose. The dose may be repeated every fifteen minutes for two doses, then every four hours as needed.

• For *sterile suspension (injection)* dosage form:

—For symptoms of bronchial asthma, chronic bronchitis, emphysema, or other lung disease:

• Adults—At first, 500 mcg injected under the

skin. Then 500 mcg to 1.5 milligrams (mg) injected no more often than every six hours as needed.

• Children—Dose is based on body weight or size and must be determined by your doctor. The usual dose is 25 mcg per kg (11 mcg per pound) of body weight. The dose may be repeated, if needed, but not more often than every six hours.

For *ethylnorepinephrine*

• For *injection* dosage form:

—For symptoms of bronchial asthma, chronic bronchitis, emphysema, or other lung disease:

• Adults—1 to 2 milligrams (mg) injected into a muscle or under the skin.

• Children—200 micrograms (mcg) to 1 mg injected into a muscle or under the skin.

For *fenoterol*

• For *tablet* dosage form:

—For symptoms of bronchial asthma, chronic bronchitis, emphysema, or other lung disease:

• Adults and children 12 years of age and older— At first, 2.5 milligrams (mg) two times a day. Then your doctor may increase your dose up to 5 mg three times a day, if needed. However, the medicine should not be taken more often than every six hours.

• Children up to 12 years of age—Dose must be determined by your doctor.

For *isoproterenol*

• For *tablet* dosage form:

—For symptoms of bronchial asthma, chronic bronchitis, emphysema, or other lung disease:

• Adults—10 to 15 milligrams (mg) dissolved under the tongue three or four times a day.

• Children—5 to 10 mg dissolved under the tongue three times a day.

For metaproterenol

• For *oral* dosage form (syrup or tablets):

—For symptoms of bronchial asthma, chronic bronchitis, emphysema, or other lung disease:

• Adults and children 9 years of age and older or weighing 27 kilograms (kg) (59 pounds) or more—20 milligrams (mg) three or four times a day.

• Children 6 to 9 years of age and older or weighing up to 27 kg (59 pounds)—10 mg three or four times a day.

• Children up to 6 years of age—Dose must be determined by your doctor.

For terbutaline

• For symptoms of bronchial asthma, chronic bronchitis, emphysema, or other lung disease:

—For *tablet* dosage form:

• Adults—2.5 to 5 milligrams (mg) three times a day, taken about every six hours.

• Children 12 to 15 years of age—2.5 mg three times a day, taken about every six hours.

• Children up to 12 years of age—Dose must be determined by your doctor.

—For *injection* dosage form:

• Adults—250 micrograms (mcg) injected under the skin. The dose may be repeated after fifteen to thirty minutes, if needed. However, not more than 500 mcg should be taken within a four-hour period.

• Children up to 12 years of age—Dose must be determined by your doctor.

Missed dose—If you are using this medicine regularly and you miss a dose, use it as soon as possible. Then use any remaining doses for that day at regularly spaced intervals. Do not double doses.

Storage—To store this medicine:

- Keep out of the reach of children.
- Store away from heat and direct light.
- Do not store the capsule or tablet form of this medicine in the bathroom, near the kitchen sink, or in other damp places. Heat or moisture may cause the medicine to break down.
- Keep the injection or syrup form of this medicine from freezing.
- Store the suspension form of epinephrine injection in the refrigerator.
- Do not keep outdated medicine or medicine no longer needed. Be sure that any discarded medicine is out of the reach of children.

Precautions While Using This Medicine

If after using this medicine for asthma or other breathing problems you still have trouble breathing, or if your condition becomes worse, check with your doctor at once.

For *diabetic patients* using *epinephrine:*

- This medicine may cause your blood sugar levels to rise. If you notice a change in the results of your blood or urine sugar tests or if you have any questions, check with your doctor.

For patients using *epinephrine injection* (including the auto-injector but not the sterile suspension) or *ethylnorepinephrine injection:*

- Some of the injection preparations may contain sulfites as a preservative. Sulfites may cause an allergic reaction in some people. If you know that you are allergic to sulfites, carefully read the label on the injection or check with your health care professional to find out if the injection contains sulfites.

- Although epinephrine injection may contain sulfites, it is still used to treat serious allergic reactions or other emergency conditions because other medicines may not work properly in a life-threatening situation.

- If you have any questions about when or whether you should use an epinephrine injection that contains sulfites, check with your doctor.

- Signs of an allergic reaction to sulfites include bluish coloration of skin; severe dizziness or feeling faint; continuing flushing or redness of face or skin; increased wheezing or difficulty in breathing; skin rash, hives, or itching; or swelling of face, lips, or eyelids. *If any of these signs occur, check with your doctor immediately.*

Side Effects of This Medicine

In some animal studies, albuterol and terbutaline were shown to increase the chance of benign (not cancerous) tumors. Terbutaline was also shown to increase the chance of ovarian cysts. The doses given were many times the oral dose of albuterol or terbutaline given to humans. It is not known if albuterol or terbutaline increases the chance of tumors in humans, or if terbutaline increases the chance of ovarian cysts in humans.

Along with its needed effects, a medicine may cause some unwanted effects. Although not all of these side effects may occur, if they do occur they may need medical attention.

Check with your doctor immediately if any of the following side effects occur:

Bluish coloration of skin; dizziness (severe) or feeling faint;

flushing or redness of face or skin (continuing); increased wheezing or difficulty in breathing; skin rash, hives, or itching; swelling of face, lips, or eyelids

Check with your doctor as soon as possible if any of the following side effects occur:

Rare

Chest discomfort or pain; irregular heartbeat

With high doses

Hallucinations (seeing, hearing, or feeling things that are not there); mood or mental changes (reported for ephedrine only)

Symptoms of overdose

Bluish coloration of skin; chest discomfort or pain (continuing or severe); chills or fever; convulsions (seizures); dizziness or lightheadedness (continuing or severe); fast or slow heartbeat (continuing); headache (continuing or severe); increase or decrease in blood pressure (severe); irregular or pounding heartbeat (continuing or severe); muscle cramps (severe); nausea or vomiting (continuing or severe); shortness of breath or troubled breathing (severe); trembling (severe); unusual anxiety, nervousness, or restlessness; unusually large pupils or blurred vision; unusual paleness and coldness of skin; weakness (severe)

Other side effects may occur that usually do not need medical attention. These side effects may go away during treatment as your body adjusts to the medicine. However, check with your doctor if any of the following side effects continue or are bothersome:

More common

Nervousness or restlessness; trembling

Less common

Difficult or painful urination; dizziness or lightheadedness; drowsiness; fast or pounding heartbeat; flushing or redness of face or skin; headache; heartburn; increased sweating; increase in blood pressure; loss of appetite;

muscle cramps or twitching; nausea or vomiting; trouble in sleeping; unusual paleness; weakness

Not all of the side effects listed above have been reported for each of these medicines, but they have been reported for at least one of them. All of the adrenergic bronchodilators are similar, so any of the above side effects may occur with any of these medicines.

While you are using albuterol, fenoterol, metaproterenol, or terbutaline, you may notice an unusual or unpleasant taste. This may be expected and will go away when you stop using the medicine.

Isoproterenol sublingual (under-the-tongue) tablets may cause the saliva to turn pinkish to red. This is to be expected while you are using this medicine.

Other side effects not listed above may also occur in some patients. If you notice any other effects, check with your doctor.

Additional Information

Once a medicine has been approved for marketing for a certain use, experience may show that it is also useful for other medical problems. Although these uses are not included in product labeling, some of the adrenergic bronchodilators are used in certain patients with the following medical conditions:

- Premature labor (terbutaline)
- Urticaria (hives) (ephedrine)
- Hemorrhage (bleeding) of gums and teeth (epinephrine)
- Priapism (prolonged abnormal erection of penis) (epinephrine)

Other than the above information, there is no additional information relating to proper use, precautions, or side effects for these uses.

BRONCHODILATORS, XANTHINE-DERIVATIVE
Systemic

Some commonly used brand names are:

In the U.S.—

Aerolate III[4]	Solu-Phyllin[4]
Aerolate Jr.[4]	Theo-24[4]
Aerolate Sr.[4]	Theo 250[4]
Aquaphyllin[4]	Theobid Duracaps[4]
Asmalix[4]	Theobid Jr. Duracaps[4]
Bronkodyl[4]	Theochron[4]
Choledyl Delayed-release[3]	Theoclear-80[4]
Choledyl SA[3]	Theoclear L.A.-130[4]
Dilor[2]	Theoclear L.A.-260[4]
Dilor-400[2]	Theo-Dur[4]
Dyflex-200[2]	Theo-Dur Sprinkle[4]
Elixomin[4]	Theolair[4]
Elixophyllin[4]	Theolair-SR[4]
Elixophyllin SR[4]	Theomar[4]
Lanophyllin[4]	Theo-Sav[4]
Lufyllin[2]	Theospan-SR[4]
Lufyllin-400[2]	Theostat 80[4]
Neothylline[2]	Theo-Time[4]
Phyllocontin[1]	Theovent Long-Acting[4]
Quibron-T Dividose[4]	Theo-X[4]
Quibron-T/SR Dividose[4]	T-Phyl[4]
Respbid[4]	Truphylline[1]
Slo-bid Gyrocaps[4]	Truxophyllin[4]
Slo-Phyllin[4]	Uniphyl[4]
Slo-Phyllin Gyrocaps[4]	

In Canada—

Apo-Oxtriphylline[3]	
Choledyl[3]	Quibron-T/SR[4]
Choledyl SA[3]	Slo-Bid[4]
Novotriphyl[3]	Somophyllin-12[4]
Phyllocontin[1]	Theochron[4]
Phyllocontin-350[1]	Theo-Dur[4]
PMS-Oxtriphylline[3]	Theolair[4]
PMS Theophylline[4]	Theolair-SR[4]
Pulmophylline[4]	Theo-SR[4]
	Uniphyl[4]

Note: For quick reference, the following xanthine-derivative bronchodilators are numbered to match the corresponding brand names.

This information applies to the following medicines:

1. Aminophylline (am-in-OFF-i-lin)‡§
2. Dyphylline (DYE-fi-lin)†‡
3. Oxtriphylline (ox-TRYE-fi-lin)‡
4. Theophylline (thee-OFF-i-lin)‡§

---

†Not commercially available in Canada.
‡Generic name product may also be available in the U.S.
§Generic name product may also be available in Canada.

Description

Xanthine-derivative bronchodilators are used to treat and/or prevent the symptoms of bronchial asthma, chronic bronchitis, and emphysema. These medicines relieve cough, wheezing, shortness of breath, and troubled breathing. They work by opening up the bronchial tubes (air passages of the lungs) and increasing the flow of air through them.

Aminophylline and theophylline may also be used for other conditions as determined by your doctor.

The oral liquid, uncoated or chewable tablet, and capsule dosage forms of xanthine-derivative bronchodilators may be used for treatment of the acute attack and for chronic (long-term) treatment. The enteric-coated tablet and extended-release dosage forms are usually used only for chronic treatment. Sometimes, aminophylline rectal suppositories may be used but they generally are not recommended because of possible poor absorption.

These medicines are available only with your doctor's prescription, in the following dosage forms:

Oral

   Aminophylline
- Oral solution (U.S.)
- Tablets (U.S. and Canada)
- Enteric-coated tablets (U.S.)
- Extended-release tablets (U.S. and Canada)

Dyphylline
- Elixir (U.S.)
- Tablets (U.S.)

Oxtriphylline
- Oral solution (U.S. and Canada)
- Syrup (U.S. and Canada)
- Tablets (U.S. and Canada)
- Delayed-release tablets (U.S.)
- Extended-release tablets (U.S. and Canada)

Theophylline
- Capsules (U.S.)
- Extended-release capsules (U.S. and Canada)
- Elixir (U.S. and Canada)
- Oral solution (U.S. and Canada)
- Syrup (U.S.)
- Tablets (U.S. and Canada)
- Extended-release tablets (U.S. and Canada)

Parenteral

Aminophylline
- Injection (U.S. and Canada)

Aminophylline and Sodium Chloride
- Injection (U.S.)

Dyphylline
- Injection (U.S.)

Theophylline in Dextrose
- Injection (U.S. and Canada)

Rectal

Aminophylline
- Suppositories (U.S.)

Before Using This Medicine

In deciding to use a medicine, the risks of taking the medicine must be weighed against the good it will do. This is a decision you and your doctor will make. For xanthine-derivative bronchodilators, the following should be considered:

Allergies—Tell your doctor if you have ever had any unusual or allergic reaction to aminophylline, caffeine, dyphylline, ethylenediamine (contained in aminophylline), oxtriphylline, theobromine, or theophylline. Also tell your health care professional if you are allergic to any other substances, such as foods, preservatives, or dyes.

Diet—Make certain your health care professional knows if you are on any special diet, such as a low-sodium or low-sugar diet or a high-protein, low-carbohydrate or low-protein, high-carbohydrate diet.

Avoid eating or drinking large amounts of caffeine-containing foods or beverages, such as chocolate, cocoa, tea, coffee, and cola drinks, because they may increase the central nervous system (CNS) stimulant effects of the xanthine-derivative bronchodilators.

Also, eating charcoal broiled foods every day while taking aminophylline, oxtriphylline, or theophylline may keep these medicines from working properly.

Pregnancy—Studies on birth defects have not been done in humans. However, some studies in animals have shown that theophylline (including aminophylline and oxtriphylline) causes birth defects when given in doses many times the human dose. Also, use of aminophylline, oxtriphylline, or theophylline during pregnancy may cause unwanted effects such as fast heartbeat, jitteriness, irritability, gagging, vomiting, and breathing problems in the newborn infant. Studies on birth defects with dyphylline have not been done in either humans or animals.

Breast-feeding—Theophylline passes into the breast milk and may cause irritability, fretfulness, or trouble in sleeping in nursing babies of mothers taking aminophylline, oxtriphylline, or theophylline. Although dyphylline passes into the breast milk, it has not been reported to cause problems in nursing babies.

Children—The side effects of xanthine-derivative bronchodilators are more likely to occur in newborn infants,

who are usually more sensitive to the effects of these
medicines.

Older adults—The side effects of xanthine-derivative
bronchodilators are more likely to occur in elderly patients,
who are usually more sensitive than younger adults to the
effects of these medicines.

Other medicines—Although certain medicines should not
be used together at all, in other cases two different medicines may be used together even if an interaction might
occur. In these cases, your doctor may want to change the
dose, or other precautions may be necessary. When you
are taking xanthine-derivative bronchodilators, it is especially important that your health care professional know if
you are taking any of the following:

- Beta-blockers (acebutolol [e.g., Sectral], atenolol [e.g., Te-
  normin], betaxolol [e.g., Kerlone], bisoprolol [e.g., Zebeta],
  carteolol [e.g., Cartrol], labetalol [e.g., Normodyne], metoprolol [e.g., Lopressor], nadolol [e.g., Corgard], oxprenolol
  [e.g., Trasicor], penbutolol [e.g., Levatol], pindolol [e.g.,
  Visken], propranolol [e.g., Inderal], sotalol [e.g., Sotacor],
  timolol [e.g., Blocadren])—Use of these medicines with
  xanthine-derivative bronchodilators may prevent either the
  beta-blocker or the bronchodilator from working properly
- Cimetidine (e.g., Tagamet) or
- Ciprofloxacin or
- Erythromycin (e.g., E-Mycin) or
- Nicotine chewing gum (e.g., Nicorette) or
- Norfloxacin or
- Ranitidine (e.g., Zantac) or
- Troleandomycin (e.g., TAO)—These medicines may in-
  crease the effects of aminophylline, oxtriphylline, or
  theophylline
- Corticosteroids (cortisone-like medicines)—Use of these
  medicines with aminophylline and sodium chloride injec-
  tion may result in too much sodium in the blood
- Phenytoin (e.g., Dilantin)—The effects of phenytoin may be
  decreased by aminophylline, oxtriphylline, or theophylline
- Smoking tobacco or marijuana—If you smoke or have

smoked tobacco or marijuana regularly within the last 2 years, the amount of medicine you need may vary, depending on how much and how recently you have smoked

Other medical problems—The presence of other medical problems may affect the use of xanthine-derivative bronchodilators. Make sure you tell your doctor if you have any other medical problems, especially:

- Alcohol abuse (or history of) or
- Fever or
- Liver disease or
- Respiratory infections, such as influenza (flu)—The effects of aminophylline, oxtriphylline, or theophylline may be increased
- Diarrhea—The absorption of xanthine-derivative bronchodilators, especially the extended-release dosage forms, may be decreased; therefore, the effects of these medicines may be decreased
- Enlarged prostate or
- Heart disease or
- High blood pressure or
- Stomach ulcer (or history of) or other stomach problems—Xanthine-derivative bronchodilators may make the condition worse
- Fibrocystic breast disease—Symptoms of this disease may be increased by xanthine-derivative bronchodilators
- Kidney disease—The effects of dyphylline may be increased
- Overactive thyroid—The effects of aminophylline, oxtriphylline, or theophylline may be decreased

---

Proper Use of This Medicine

For patients *taking this medicine by mouth:*

- If you are taking the *capsule, tablet, liquid, or extended-release (not including the once-a-day capsule or tablet) form* of this medicine, *it works best when taken with a glass of water on an empty stomach* (either 30 minutes to 1 hour before meals or 2 hours after meals). That way the medicine will get into the blood sooner. However, in some cases your doctor may want you to take this medicine with meals or right after meals to lessen stomach upset. If you have any questions about how you should be taking this medicine, check with your doctor.

- If you are taking the *once-a-day capsule or tablet form* of this medicine, *some products are to be taken each morning after fasting overnight and at least 1 hour before eating. However, other products are to be taken in the morning or evening with or without food. Be sure you understand exactly how to take the medicine prescribed for you.* Try to take the medicine about the same time each day.

- There are several different forms of xanthine-derivative bronchodilator capsules and tablets. If you are taking:

    —enteric-coated or delayed-release tablets, swallow the tablets whole. Do not crush, break, or chew before swallowing.

    —extended-release capsules, swallow the capsule whole. Do not crush, break, or chew before swallowing.

    —extended-release tablets, swallow the tablets whole. Do not break (unless tablet is scored for breaking), crush, or chew before swallowing.

Use this medicine only as directed by your doctor. Do not use more of it, do not use it more often, and do not use it for a longer time than your doctor ordered. To do so may increase the chance of serious side effects.

In order for this medicine to help your medical problem, it must be taken every day in regularly spaced doses as ordered by your doctor. This is necessary to keep a constant amount of this medicine in the blood. To help keep the amount constant, do not miss any doses.

Dosing—When you are taking aminophylline, dyphylline, oxtriphylline, or theophylline, it is very important that you get the exact amount of medicine that you need. The dose of these medicines will be different for different patients. Your doctor will determine the proper dose of the xanthine-derivative bronchodilator for you. *Follow your doctor's orders or the directions on the label.*

After you begin taking aminophylline, oxtriphylline, or theophylline, it is very important that your doctor check your blood level of theophylline at regular times to find out if your dose of aminophylline, oxtriphylline, or theophylline needs to be changed. *Do not change your dose of aminophylline, dyphylline, oxtriphylline, or theophylline* unless your doctor tells you to do so.

The number of capsules or tablets or teaspoonfuls of solution or syrup that you take depends on the strength of the medicine. Also, the number of doses you take each day and the time beween doses depend on whether you are taking a short-acting or a long-acting form of aminophylline, dyphylline, oxtriphylline, or theophylline.

Missed dose—If you miss a dose of this medicine, take it as soon as possible. However, if it is almost time for your next dose, skip the missed dose and go back to your regular dosing schedule. Do not double doses.

Storage—To store this medicine:
* Keep out of the reach of children.
* Store away from heat and direct light.
* Do not store the capsule or tablet form of this medicine in the bathroom, near the kitchen sink, or in other damp places. Heat or moisture may cause the medicine to break down.
* Keep the liquid form of this medicine from freezing.

- Do not keep outdated medicine or medicine no longer needed. Be sure that any discarded medicine is out of the reach of children.

Precautions While Using This Medicine

Your doctor should check your progress at regular visits, especially for the first few weeks after you begin using this medicine. A blood test may be taken to help your doctor decide whether the dose of this medicine should be changed.

Do not change brands or dosage forms of this medicine without first checking with your doctor. Different products may not work the same way. If you refill your medicine and it looks different, check with your pharmacist.

This medicine may add to the central nervous system (CNS) stimulant effects of caffeine-containing foods or beverages such as chocolate, cocoa, tea, coffee, and cola drinks. *Avoid eating or drinking large amounts of these foods or beverages while using this medicine.* If you have any questions about this, check with your doctor.

For patients using *aminophylline, oxtriphylline, or the-ophylline*:

- Do not eat charcoal-broiled foods every day while using this medicine since these foods may keep the medicine from working properly.

- *Check with your doctor at once if you develop symptoms of influenza (flu) or a fever* since either of these may increase the chance of side effects with this medicine.

- Also, *check with your doctor if diarrhea occurs* because the dose of this medicine may need to be changed.

Side Effects of This Medicine

Along with its needed effects, a medicine may cause some unwanted effects. Although not all of these side effects may occur, if they do occur they may need medical attention.

Check with your doctor as soon as possible if any of the following side effects occur:

Less common
  Heartburn and/or vomiting

Rare
  Skin rash or hives (with aminophylline only)

Symptoms of overdose
  Bloody or black, tarry stools; confusion or change in behavior; convulsions (seizures); diarrhea; dizziness or lightheadedness; fast breathing; fast, pounding, or irregular heartbeat; flushing or redness of face; headache; increased urination; irritability; loss of appetite; muscle twitching; nausea (continuing or severe) or vomiting; stomach cramps or pain; trembling; trouble in sleeping; unusual tiredness or weakness; vomiting blood or material that looks like coffee grounds

Other side effects may occur that usually do not need medical attention. These side effects may go away during treatment as your body adjusts to the medicine. However, check with your doctor if any of the following side effects continue or are bothersome:

More common
  Nausea; nervousness or restlessness

Other side effects not listed above may also occur in some patients. If you notice any other effects, check with your doctor.

Additional Information

Once a medicine has been approved for marketing for a certain use, experience may show that it is also useful for

other medical problems. Although this use is not included in product labeling, aminophylline and theophylline are used in certain patients with the following medical condition:

- Apnea (breathing problem) in newborns

Other than the above information, there is no additional information relating to proper use, precautions, or side effects for this use.

BUPROPION   Systemic†

A commonly used brand name in the U.S. is Wellbutrin.
Another commonly used name is amfebutamone.

†Not commercially available in Canada.

Description

Bupropion (byoo-PROE-pee-on) is used to relieve mental depression.

This medicine is available only with your doctor's prescription, in the following dosage form:

Oral
- Tablets (U.S.)

Before Using This Medicine

In deciding to use a medicine, the risks of taking the medicine must be weighed against the good it will do. This is a decision you and your doctor will make. For bupropion, the following should be considered:

Allergies—Tell your doctor if you have ever had any unusual or allergic reaction to bupropion. Also tell your health care professional if you are allergic to any other substances, such as foods, preservatives, or dyes.

Pregnancy—Studies have not been done in pregnant women. However, bupropion has not been reported to cause birth defects or other problems in animal studies.

Breast-feeding—Bupropion passes into breast milk. Because it may cause unwanted effects in nursing babies, use of bupropion is not recommended during breast-feeding.

Children—Studies on this medicine have been done only in adult patients, and there is no specific information comparing use of bupropion in children with use in other age groups.

Older adults—This medicine has been tested in a limited number of patients 60 years of age and older and has not been shown to cause different side effects or problems in older people than it does in younger adults.

Other medicines—Although certain medicines should not be used together at all, in other cases two different medicines may be used together even if an interaction might occur. In these cases, your doctor may want to change the dose, or other precautions may be necessary. When you are taking bupropion, it is especially important that your health care professional know if you are taking any of the following:

- Alcohol or
- Antipsychotics (medicine for mental illness) or
- Fluoxetine (e.g., Prozac) or
- Lithium (e.g., Lithane) or
- Maprotiline (e.g., Ludiomil) or
- Trazodone (e.g., Desyrel) or
- Tricyclic antidepressants (amitriptyline [e.g., Elavil], amoxapine [e.g., Asendin], clomipramine [e.g., Anafranil], desipramine [e.g., Pertofrane], doxepin [e.g., Sinequan], imipramine [e.g., Tofranil], nortriptyline [e.g., Aventyl], protriptyline [e.g., Vivactil], trimipramine [e.g., Surmon-

til])—Using these medicines with bupropion may increase
the risk of seizures

- Monoamine oxidase (MAO) inhibitors (furazolidone [e.g.,
  Furoxone], isocarboxazid [e.g., Marplan], phenelzine [e.g.,
  Nardil], procarbazine [e.g., Matulane], selegiline [e.g., El-
  depryl], tranylcypromine [e.g., Parnate])—Taking bupropion while you are taking or within 2 weeks of taking MAO
  inhibitors may increase the chance of side effects; at least
  14 days should be allowed between stopping treatment
  with one medicine and starting treatment with the other

Other medical problems—The presence of other medical
problems may affect the use of bupropion. Make sure you
tell your doctor if you have any other medical problems,
especially:

- Anorexia nervosa or
- Brain tumor or
- Bulimia or
- Head injury, history of, or
- Seizure disorder—The risk of seizures may be increased
  when bupropion is taken by patients with these conditions
- Bipolar disorder (manic-depressive illness) or
- Other nervous, mental, or emotional conditions—Bupropion
  may make the condition worse
- Heart attack (recent) or heart disease—Bupropion may
  cause unwanted effects on the heart
- Kidney disease or
- Liver disease—Higher blood levels of bupropion may re-
  sult, increasing the chance of side effects

Proper Use of This Medicine

Use bupropion only as directed by your doctor. Do not
use more of it, do not use it more often, and do not use
it for a longer time than your doctor ordered. To do so
may increase the chance of side effects.

To lessen stomach upset, this medicine may be taken with
food, unless your doctor has told you to take it on an
empty stomach.

Usually this medicine must be taken for several weeks before you feel better. Your doctor should check your progress at regular visits.

Dosing—The dose of bupropion will be different for different patients. *Follow your doctor's orders or the directions on the label.* The following information includes only the average doses of bupropion. *If your dose is different, do not change it* unless your doctor tells you to do so.

The number of tablets that you take depends on the strength of the medicine. Also, *the number of doses you take each day, the time allowed between doses, and the length of time you take the medicine depend on the medical problem for which you are taking bupropion.*

- For *oral* dosage form (tablets):
    —For depression:
    - Adults—At first, 100 milligrams (mg) twice a day. Your doctor may increase your dose as needed. However, the dose is usually not more than 450 mg a day.
    - Children—Use and dose must be determined by your doctor.

Missed dose—If you miss a dose of this medicine, take it as soon as possible. However, if it is within 4 hours of your next dose, skip the missed dose and go back to your regular dosing schedule. Do not double doses.

Storage—To store this medicine:
- Keep out of the reach of children.
- Store away from heat and direct light.
- Do not store in the bathroom, near the kitchen sink, or in other damp places. Heat or moisture may cause the medicine to break down.
- Do not keep outdated medicine or medicine no longer needed. Be sure that any discarded medicine is out of the reach of children.

Precautions While Using This Medicine

Your doctor should check your progress at regular visits, especially during the first few months of treatment with this medicine. The amount of bupropion you take may have to be changed often to meet the needs of your condition and to help avoid unwanted effects.

If you have been taking this medicine regularly, do not stop taking it without first checking with your doctor. Your doctor may want you to reduce gradually the amount you are taking before stopping completely. This will help reduce the possibility of side effects.

Drinking of alcoholic beverages should be limited or avoided, if possible, while taking bupropion. This will help prevent unwanted effects.

This medicine may cause some people to feel a false sense of well-being, or to become drowsy, dizzy, or less alert than they are normally. *Make sure you know how you react to this medicine before you drive, use machines, or do anything else that could be dangerous if you are dizzy or are not alert and clearheaded.*

Side Effects of This Medicine

Along with its needed effects, a medicine may cause some unwanted effects. Although not all of these side effects may occur, if they do occur they may need medical attention.

Check with your doctor as soon as possible if any of the following side effects occur:

> *More common*
>> Agitation or excitement; anxiety; confusion; fast or irregular heartbeat; headache (severe); restlessness; trouble in sleeping

Less common

Hallucinations; skin rash

Rare

Fainting; seizures (convulsions), especially with higher doses

Other side effects may occur that usually do not need medical attention. These side effects may go away during treatment as your body adjusts to the medicine. However, check with your doctor if any of the following side effects continue or are bothersome:

More common

Constipation; decrease in appetite; dizziness; dryness of mouth; increased sweating; nausea or vomiting; tremor; weight loss (unusual)

Less common

Blurred vision; difficulty concentrating; drowsiness; fever or chills; hostility or anger; tiredness; sleep disturbances; unusual feeling of well-being

Other side effects not listed above may also occur in some patients. If you notice any other effects, check with your doctor.

BUSPIRONE   Systemic

A commonly used brand name in the U.S. and Canada is BuSpar.

Description

Buspirone (byoo-SPYE-rone) is used to treat certain anxiety disorders or to relieve the symptoms of anxiety. However, buspirone is usually not used for anxiety or tension caused by the stress of everyday life.

It is not known exactly how buspirone works to relieve the symptoms of anxiety.

Buspirone is available only with your doctor's prescription, in the following dosage form:

Oral

- Tablets (U.S. and Canada)

Before Using This Medicine

In deciding to use a medicine, the risks of taking the medicine must be weighed against the good it will do. This is a decision you and your doctor will make. For buspirone, the following should be considered:

Allergies—Tell your doctor if you have ever had any unusual or allergic reaction to buspirone. Also tell your health care professional if you are allergic to any other substances, such as foods, preservatives, or dyes.

Pregnancy—Buspirone has not been studied in pregnant women. However, buspirone has not been shown to cause birth defects or other problems in animal studies.

Breast-feeding—It is not known whether buspirone passes into the breast milk of humans.

Children—Studies on this medicine have been done only in adult patients, and there is no specific information comparing use of buspirone in children up to 18 years of age with use in other age groups.

Older adults—This medicine has been tested and has not been shown to cause different side effects or problems in older people than it does in younger adults.

Other medicines—Although certain medicines should not be used together at all, in other cases 2 different medicines may be used together even if an interaction might occur. In these cases, your doctor may want to change the dose, or other precautions may be necessary. When you are taking buspirone, it is especially important that your health care professional know if you are taking any of the following:

- Monoamine oxidase (MAO) inhibitors (furazolidone [e.g., Furoxone], isocarboxazid [e.g., Marplan], phenelzine [e.g., Nardil], procarbazine [e.g., Matulane], selegiline at doses more than 10 mg a day [e.g., Eldepryl], tranylcypromine [e.g., Parnate])—Taking buspirone while you are taking or within 2 weeks of taking monoamine oxidase (MAO) inhibitors may cause high blood pressure

Other medical problems—The presence of other medical problems may affect the use of buspirone. Make sure you tell your doctor if you have any other medical problems, especially:

- Drug abuse or dependence (history of)—There is a possibility that buspirone could become habit-forming, causing mental or physical dependence
- Kidney disease or
- Liver disease—The effects of buspirone may be increased, which may increase the chance of side effects

---

Proper Use of This Medicine

Take buspirone only as directed by your doctor. Do not take more of it, do not take it more often, and do not take it for a longer time than your doctor ordered. To do so may increase the chance of unwanted effects.

After you begin taking buspirone, 1 to 2 weeks may pass before you feel the full effects of this medicine.

Dosing—The dose of buspirone will be different for different patients. *Follow your doctor's orders or the directions on the label.* The following information includes only the average doses of buspirone. *If your dose is different, do not change it* unless your doctor tells you to do so.

The number of tablets that you take depends on the strength of the medicine. Also, *the number of doses you take each day, the time allowed between doses, and the length of time you take the medicine depend on the medical problem for which you are taking buspirone.*

- For *oral* dosage forms (tablets):

    —Adults: To start, 5 milligrams three times a day. Your doctor may increase your dose by 5 milligrams a day every few days if needed. However, the dose is usually not more than 60 milligrams a day.

    —Children up to 18 years of age: Dose must be determined by the doctor.

Missed dose—If you are taking this medicine regularly and you miss a dose, take it as soon as possible. However, if it is almost time for your next dose, skip the missed dose and go back to your regular dosing schedule. Do not double doses.

Storage—To store this medicine:

- Keep out of the reach of children.
- Store away from heat and direct light.
- Do not store in the bathroom, near the kitchen sink, or in other damp places. Heat or moisture may cause the medicine to break down.
- Do not keep outdated medicine or medicine no longer needed. Be sure that any discarded medicine is out of the reach of children.

Precautions While Using This Medicine

If you will be using buspirone regularly for a long time, your doctor should check your progress at regular visits to make sure the medicine does not cause unwanted effects.

Buspirone, when taken with alcohol or other CNS depressants (medicines that slow down the nervous system, possibly causing drowsiness), may increase the chance of drowsiness. Some examples of CNS depressants are antihistamines or medicine for hay fever, other allergies, or colds; sedatives, tranquilizers, or sleeping medicine; prescription pain medicine or narcotics; barbiturates; medicine for seizures; muscle relaxants; or anesthetics, including some dental anesthetics. Check with your doctor before taking any of the above while you are taking this medicine.

Buspirone may cause some people to become dizzy, lightheaded, drowsy, or less alert than they are normally. *Make sure you know how you react to this medicine before you drive, use machines, or do anything else that could be dangerous if you are dizzy or are not alert.*

If you think you or someone else may have taken an overdose of buspirone, get emergency help at once. Some symptoms of an overdose are severe dizziness or drowsiness; severe stomach upset, including nausea or vomiting; or unusually small pupils.

Side Effects of This Medicine

Along with its needed effects, a medicine may cause some unwanted effects. Although not all of these side effects may occur, if they do occur they may need medical attention.

Check with your doctor as soon as possible if any of the following side effects occur:

Rare

Chest pain; confusion or mental depression; fast or pounding heartbeat; muscle weakness; numbness, tingling, pain, or weakness in hands or feet; sore throat or fever; uncontrolled movements of the body

Symptoms of overdose

Dizziness (severe); drowsiness (severe); stomach upset, including nausea or vomiting (severe); unusually small pupils

Other side effects may occur that usually do not need medical attention. These side effects may go away during treatment as your body adjusts to the medicine. However, check with your doctor if any of the following side effects continue or are bothersome:

More common

Dizziness or lightheadedness; headache; nausea; restlessness, nervousness, or unusual excitement

Less common or rare

Blurred vision; decreased concentration; drowsiness (more common with doses of more than 20 mg per day); dryness of mouth; muscle pain, spasms, cramps, or stiffness; ringing in the ears; stomach upset; trouble in sleeping, nightmares, or vivid dreams; unusual tiredness or weakness

Other side effects not listed above may also occur in some patients. If you notice any other effects, check with your doctor.

BUTALBITAL AND ASPIRIN Systemic

Some commonly used brand names are:

In the U.S.—

Axotal[1]	Isobutyl[2]
Butalgen[2]	Isolin[2]
Fiorgen[2]	Isollyl[2]
Fiorinal[2]	Laniroif[2]
Fiormor[2]	Lanorinal[2]
Fortabs[2]	Marnal[2]
Isobutal[2]	Vibutal[2]

In Canada—

Fiorinal[2]	Tecnal[2]

Other commonly used names for the butalbital, aspirin, and caffeine combination medicine are butalbital-AC and butalbital compound.

Note: For quick reference, the following medicines are numbered to match the corresponding brand names.

This information applies to the following medicines:

1. For Butalbital and Aspirin†
2. For Butalbital, Aspirin#, and Caffeine‡

---

†Not commercially available in Canada.
‡Generic name product may also be available in the U.S.
#In Canada, *Aspirin* is a brand name. Acetylsalicylic acid is the generic name in Canada. ASA, a synonym for acetylsalicylic acid, is the term that commonly appears on Canadian product labels.

Description

Butalbital (byoo-TAL-bi-tal) and aspirin (AS-pir-in) combination is a pain reliever and relaxant. It is used to treat tension headaches. Butalbital belongs to the group of medicines called barbiturates (bar-BI-tyoo-rates). Barbiturates act in the central nervous system (CNS) to produce their effects.

When you use butalbital for a long time, your body may get used to it so that larger amounts are needed to produce the same effects. This is called tolerance to the medicine. Also, butalbital may become habit-forming (causing mental or physical dependence) when it is used for a long time or in large doses. Physical dependence may lead to withdrawal side effects when you stop taking the medicine. In patients who get headaches, the first symptom of withdrawal may be new (rebound) headaches.

Some of these medicines also contain caffeine (kaf-EEN). Caffeine may help to relieve headaches. However, caffeine can also cause physical dependence when it is used for a long time. This may lead to withdrawal (rebound) headaches when you stop taking it.

Butalbital and aspirin combination is sometimes also used for other kinds of headaches or other kinds of pain, as determined by your doctor.

Butalbital and aspirin combination is available only with your doctor's prescription, in the following dosage forms:

Oral

Butalbital and Aspirin
• Tablets (U.S.)
Butalbital, Aspirin, and Caffeine
• Capsules (U.S. and Canada)
• Tablets (U.S. and Canada)

Before Using This Medicine

In deciding to use a medicine, the risks of taking the medicine must be weighed against the good it will do. This is a decision you and your doctor will make. For butalbital and aspirin combinations, the following should be considered:

Allergies—Tell your doctor if you have ever had any unusual or allergic reaction to butalbital or other barbiturates; aspirin or other salicylates, including methyl salicylate (oil of wintergreen); caffeine; or any of the following medicines:

Diclofenac (e.g., Voltaren)
Diflunisal (e.g., Dolobid)
Etodolac (e.g., Lodine)
Fenoprofen (e.g., Nalfon)
Floctafenine (e.g., Idarac)
Flurbiprofen, oral (e.g., Ansaid)
Ibuprofen (e.g., Motrin)
Indomethacin (e.g., Indocin)
Ketoprofen (e.g., Orudis)
Ketorolac (e.g., Toradol)
Meclofenamate (e.g., Meclomen)
Mefenamic acid (e.g., Ponstel)
Nabumetone (e.g., Relafen)
Naproxen (e.g., Naprosyn)
Oxaprozin (e.g., Daypro)
Oxyphenbutazone (e.g., Tandearil)
Phenylbutazone (e.g., Butazolidin)
Piroxicam (e.g., Feldene)
Sulindac (e.g., Clinoril)
Suprofen (e.g., Suprol)

Tenoxicam (e.g., Mobiflex)
Tiaprofenic acid (e.g., Surgam)
Tolmetin (e.g., Tolectin)
Zomepirac (e.g., Zomax)

Also tell your health care professional if you are allergic to any other substances, such as foods, preservatives, or dyes.

Pregnancy—

- *For butalbital:* Barbiturates such as butalbital have been shown to increase the chance of birth defects in humans. Also, one study in humans has suggested that barbiturates taken during pregnancy may increase the chance of brain tumors in the baby. Butalbital may cause breathing problems in the newborn baby if taken just before or during delivery.

- *For aspirin:* Although studies in humans have not shown that aspirin causes birth defects, it has caused birth defects in animal studies.

  Do not take aspirin during the last 3 months of pregnancy unless it has been ordered by your doctor. Some reports have suggested that use of aspirin late in pregnancy may cause a decrease in the newborn's weight and possible death of the fetus or newborn baby. However, the mothers in these reports had been taking much larger amounts of aspirin than are usually recommended. Studies of mothers taking aspirin in the doses that are usually recommended did not show these unwanted effects.

  There is a chance that regular use of aspirin late in pregnancy may cause unwanted effects on the heart or blood flow in the fetus or in the newborn baby. Also, use of aspirin during the last 2 weeks of pregnancy may cause bleeding problems in the fetus before or during delivery or in the newborn baby. In addition, too much use of aspirin during the last 3 months of pregnancy may increase the length of pregnancy, prolong labor, cause other problems during delivery, or cause severe bleeding in the mother before, during, or after delivery.

- *For caffeine:* Studies in humans have not shown that caffeine causes birth defects. However, use of large amounts of caffeine during pregnancy may cause problems with the heart rhythm and the growth of the fetus. Also, studies in animals have shown that caffeine causes birth defects when given in very large doses (amounts equal to the amount in 12 to 24 cups of coffee a day).

Breast-feeding—Although this combination medicine has not been reported to cause problems, the chance always exists, especially if the medicine is taken for a long time or in large amounts.

- *For butalbital:* Barbiturates such as butalbital pass into the breast milk and may cause drowsiness, unusually slow heartbeat, shortness of breath, or troubled breathing in nursing babies.
- *For aspirin:* Aspirin passes into the breast milk. However, taking aspirin in the amounts present in these combination medicines has not been reported to cause problems in nursing babies.
- *For caffeine:* The caffeine in some of these combination medicines passes into the breast milk in small amounts. Taking caffeine in the amounts present in these medicines has not been reported to cause problems in nursing babies. However, studies have shown that nursing babies may appear jittery and have trouble in sleeping when their mothers drink large amounts of caffeine-containing beverages. Therefore, breast-feeding mothers who use caffeine-containing medicines should probably limit the amount of caffeine they take in from other medicines or from beverages.

Children—

- *For butalbital:* Although barbiturates such as butalbital often cause drowsiness, some children become excited after taking them.

- *For aspirin: Do not give a medicine containing aspirin to a child with fever or other symptoms of a virus infection, especially flu or chickenpox, without first discussing its use with your child's doctor.* This is very important because aspirin may cause a serious illness called Reye's syndrome in children with fever caused by a virus infection, especially flu or chickenpox. Children who do not have a virus infection may also be more sensitive to the effects of aspirin, especially if they have a fever or have lost large amounts of body fluid because of vomiting, diarrhea, or sweating. This may increase the chance of side effects during treatment.

- *For caffeine:* There is no specific information comparing use of caffeine in children up to 12 years of age with use in other age groups. However, caffeine is not expected to cause different side effects or problems in children than it does in adults.

Teenagers—*Teenagers with fever or other symptoms of a virus infection, especially flu or chickenpox, should check with a doctor before taking this medicine.* The aspirin in this combination medicine may cause a serious illness called Reye's syndrome in teenagers with fever caused by a virus infection, especially flu or chickenpox.

Older adults—

- *For butalbital:* Confusion, depression, or excitement may be especially likely to occur in elderly patients, who are usually more sensitive than younger adults to the effects of butalbital.

- *For aspirin:* Elderly patients are more sensitive than younger adults to the effects of aspirin. This may increase the chance of side effects during treatment.

- *For caffeine:* Many medicines have not been studied specifically in older people. Therefore, it may not be

known whether they work exactly the same way they
do in younger adults or if they cause different side
effects or problems in older people. There is no specific information comparing use of caffeine in the
elderly with use in other age groups.

Other medicines—Although certain medicines should not
be used together at all, in other cases two different medicines may be used together even if an interaction might
occur. In these cases, your doctor may want to change the
dose, or other precautions may be necessary. When you
are taking a butalbital and aspirin combination, it is especially important that your health care professional know if
you are taking any of the following:

- Antacids, large amounts taken regularly, especially calcium-
  and/or magnesium-containing antacids or sodium bicarbonate (baking soda), or
- Urinary alkalizers (medicine that makes the urine less acid,
  such as acetazolamide [e.g., Diamox], dichlorphenamide
  [e.g., Daranide], methazolamide [e.g., Neptazane], potassium or sodium citrate and/or citric acid)—These medicines may cause aspirin to be removed from the body
  faster than usual, which may shorten the time that aspirin
  is effective; acetazolamide, dichlorphenamide, and methazolamide may also increase the chance of side effects
  when taken together with aspirin
- Anticoagulants (blood thinners) or
- Heparin—Use of these medicines together with aspirin may
  increase the chance of bleeding; also, butalbital may cause
  anticoagulants to be less effective
- Antidepressants, tricyclic (amitriptyline [e.g., Elavil], amoxapine [e.g., Asendin], clomipramine [e.g., Anafranil], desipramine [e.g., Pertofrane], doxepin [e.g., Sinequan],
  imipramine [e.g., Tofranil], nortriptyline [e.g., Aventyl],
  protriptyline [e.g., Vivactil], trimipramine [e.g., Surmon-
  til]) or
- Central nervous system (CNS) depressants (medicines that
  often cause drowsiness)—These medicines may add to the
  effects of butalbital and increase the chance of drowsiness
  or other side effects

- Carbamazepine (e.g., Tegretol) or
- Contraceptives, oral (birth control pills), containing estrogen or
- Corticosteroids (cortisone-like medicines) or
- Corticotropin (e.g., ACTH)—Butalbital may make these medicines less effective
- Divalproex (e.g., Depakote) or
- Methotrexate (e.g., Folex, Mexate) or
- Valproic acid (e.g., Depakene) or
- Vancomycin (e.g., Vancocin)—The chance of serious side effects may be increased
- Probenecid (e.g., Benemid) or
- Sulfinpyrazone (e.g., Anturane)—Aspirin can keep these medicines from working properly for treating gout

Other medical problems—The presence of other medical problems may affect the use of butalbital and aspirin combinations. Make sure you tell your doctor if you have any other medical problems, especially:

- Alcohol abuse (or history of) or
- Drug abuse or dependence (or history of)—Dependence on butalbital may develop
- Asthma, especially if occurring together with other allergies and nasal polyps (or history of), or
- Emphysema or other chronic lung disease or
- Hyperactivity (in children) or
- Kidney disease or
- Liver disease—The chance of serious side effects may be increased
- Diabetes mellitus (sugar diabetes) or
- Mental depression or
- Overactive thyroid or
- Porphyria (or history of)—Butalbital may make these conditions worse
- Gout—Aspirin can make this condition worse and can also lessen the effects of some medicines used to treat gout
- Heart disease (severe)—The caffeine in some of these combination medicines can make some kinds of heart disease worse
- Hemophilia or other bleeding problems or

- Vitamin K deficiency—Aspirin increases the chance of serious bleeding
- Stomach ulcer, especially with a history of bleeding, or other stomach problems—Aspirin can make your condition worse

---

Proper Use of This Medicine

Take this medicine with food or a full glass (8 ounces) of water to lessen stomach irritation.

Do not take this medicine if it has a strong vinegar-like odor. This odor means the aspirin in it is breaking down. If you have any questions about this, check with your health care professional.

Take this medicine only as directed by your doctor. Do not take more of it, do not take it more often, and do not take it for a longer time than your doctor ordered. If butalbital and aspirin combination is taken regularly (for example, every day), it may become habit-forming (causing mental or physical dependence). The caffeine in some butalbital and aspirin combinations can also increase the chance of dependence. Dependence is especially likely to occur in patients who take this medicine to relieve frequent headaches. Taking too much of this combination medicine can also lead to stomach problems or to other medical problems.

This medicine will relieve a headache best if you *take it as soon as the headache begins*. If you get warning signs of a migraine, take this medicine as soon as you are sure that the migraine is coming. This may even stop the headache pain from occurring. *Lying down in a quiet, dark room for a while after taking the medicine also helps to relieve headaches.*

People who get a lot of headaches may need to take a different medicine to help prevent headaches. *It is im-

portant that you follow your doctor's directions about taking the other medicine, even if your headaches continue to occur. Headache-preventing medicines may take several weeks to start working. Even after they do start working, your headaches may not go away completely. However, your headaches should occur less often, and they should be less severe and easier to relieve than before. This will reduce the amount of headache relievers that you need. If you do not notice any improvement after several weeks of headache-preventing treatment, check with your doctor.

Dosing—The dose of butalbital and aspirin combination medicines will be different for different patients. *Follow your doctor's orders or the directions on the label.* The following information includes only the average doses of the medicine. *If your dose is different, do not change it* unless your doctor tells you to do so.

For Butalbital and Aspirin combination
- For *oral* dosage form (tablets):
  —For tension headaches:
    • Adults—One tablet every four hours as needed. You should not take more than six tablets a day.
    • Children—Dose must be determined by your doctor.

For Butalbital, Aspirin, and Caffeine combination
- For *oral* dosage forms (capsules or tablets):
  —For tension headaches:
    • Adults—One or 2 capsules or tablets every four hours as needed. You should not take more than six capsules or tablets a day.
    • Children—Dose must be determined by your doctor.

Missed dose—If your doctor has ordered you to take this medicine according to a regular schedule and you miss a dose, take it as soon as you remember. However, if it is almost time for your next dose, skip the missed dose and go back to your regular dosing schedule. Do not double doses.

Storage—To store this medicine:

- Keep out of the reach of children. Overdose is especially dangerous in young children.
- Store away from heat and direct light.
- Do not store this medicine in the bathroom, near the kitchen sink, or in other damp places. Heat or moisture may cause the medicine to break down.
- Do not keep outdated medicine or medicine no longer needed. Be sure that any discarded medicine is out of the reach of children.

Precautions While Using This Medicine

Check with your doctor:

- If the medicine stops working as well as it did when you first started using it. This may mean that you are in danger of becoming dependent on the medicine. *Do not try to get better pain relief by increasing the dose.*
- *If you are having headaches more often than you did before you started using this medicine.* This is especially important if a new headache occurs within 1 day after you took your last dose of headache medicine, headaches begin to occur every day, or a headache continues for several days in a row. This may mean that you are dependent on the headache medicine. *Continuing to take this medicine will cause even more headaches later on.* Your doctor can give you advice on how to relieve the headaches.

Check the labels of all nonprescription (over-the-counter [OTC]) and prescription medicines you now take. If any contain a barbiturate, aspirin, or other salicylates, includ-

ing diflunisal, check with your health care professional.
Taking them together with this medicine may cause an overdose.

The butalbital in this medicine will add to the effects of alcohol and other CNS depressants (medicines that slow down the nervous system, possibly causing drowsiness). Some examples of CNS depressants are antihistamines or medicine for hay fever, other allergies, or colds; sedatives, tranquilizers, or sleeping medicine; other prescription pain medicine or narcotics; other barbiturates; medicine for seizures; muscle relaxants; or anesthetics, including some dental anesthetics. Also, stomach problems may be more likely to occur if you drink alcoholic beverages while you are taking aspirin. Therefore, *do not drink alcoholic beverages, and check with your doctor before taking any of the medicines listed above, while you are using this medicine.*

This medicine may cause some people to become drowsy, dizzy, or lightheaded. *Make sure you know how you react to this medicine before you drive, use machines, or do anything else that could be dangerous if you are dizzy or are not alert and clearheaded.*

Before having any kind of surgery (including dental surgery) or emergency treatment, tell the medical doctor or dentist in charge that you are taking this medicine. Serious side effects may occur if your medical doctor or dentist gives you certain other medicines without knowing that you have taken butalbital.

Do not take this medicine for 5 days before any planned surgery, including dental surgery, unless otherwise directed by your medical doctor or dentist. Taking aspirin during this time may cause bleeding problems.

Before you have any medical tests, tell the person in charge that you are taking this medicine. Caffeine (present in some butalbital and aspirin combinations) interferes with the results of certain tests that use dipyridamole (e.g.,

Persantine) to help show how well blood is flowing to your heart. Caffeine should not be taken for 8 to 12 hours before the test. The results of some other tests may also be affected by butalbital and aspirin combinations.

If you have been taking large amounts of this medicine, or if you have been taking it regularly for several weeks or more, *do not suddenly stop using it without first checking with your doctor.* Your doctor may want you to reduce gradually the amount you are taking before stopping completely, to lessen the chance of withdrawal side effects.

If you think you or anyone else may have taken an overdose of this medicine, get emergency help at once. Taking an overdose of this medicine or taking alcohol or CNS depressants with this medicine may lead to unconsciousness or death. Symptoms of overdose of this medicine include convulsions (seizures); hearing loss; confusion; ringing or buzzing in the ears; severe excitement, nervousness, or restlessness; severe dizziness; severe drowsiness; shortness of breath or troubled breathing; and severe weakness.

Side Effects of This Medicine

Along with its needed effects, a medicine may cause some unwanted effects. Although not all of these side effects may occur, if they do occur they may need medical attention.

The following side effects may mean that a serious allergic reaction is occurring. Check with your doctor or get emergency help immediately if they occur, especially if several of them occur at the same time.

Less common or rare

Bluish discoloration or flushing or redness of skin (occurring together with other effects listed in this section); coughing, shortness of breath, troubled breathing, tightness in chest, or wheezing; difficulty in swallowing; dizziness or feeling faint (severe); hive-like swellings (large) on eyelids, face, lips, or tongue; skin rash, itching, or hives; stuffy nose (occurring together with other effects listed in this section)

Also check with your doctor immediately if any of the following side effects occur, especially if several of them occur together:

Rare

Bleeding or crusting sores on lips; chest pain; fever with or without chills; red, thickened, or scaly skin; sores, ulcers, or white spots in mouth (painful); sore throat (unexplained); tenderness, burning, or peeling of skin

Symptoms of overdose

Anxiety, confusion, excitement, irritability, nervousness, restlessness, or trouble in sleeping (severe, especially with products containing caffeine); convulsions (seizures, with products containing caffeine); diarrhea (severe or continuing); dizziness, lightheadedness, drowsiness, or weakness (severe); frequent urination (for products containing caffeine); hallucinations (seeing, hearing, or feeling things that are not there); increased sensitivity to touch or pain (for products containing caffeine); increased thirst; muscle trembling or twitching (for products containing caffeine); nausea or vomiting (severe or continuing), sometimes with blood; ringing or buzzing in ears (continuing) or hearing loss; seeing flashes of ''zig-zag'' lights (for products containing caffeine); slow, fast, or irregular heartbeat; slow, fast, irregular, or troubled breathing; slurred speech; staggering; stomach pain (severe); uncontrollable flapping movements of the hands, especially in elderly patients; unusual movements of the eyes; vision problems

Also, check with your doctor as soon as possible if any of the following side effects occur:

Less common or rare

Bloody or black, tarry stools; bloody urine; confusion or

mental depression; muscle cramps or pain; pinpoint red spots on skin; swollen or painful glands; unusual bleeding or bruising; unusual excitement (mild)

Other side effects may occur that usually do not need medical attention. These side effects may go away during treatment as your body adjusts to the medicine. However, check with your doctor if any of the following side effects continue or are bothersome:

More common

Bloated or "gassy" feeling; dizziness or lightheadedness (mild); drowsiness (mild); heartburn or indigestion; nausea, vomiting, or stomach pain (occurring without other symptoms of overdose)

Other side effects not listed above may also occur in some patients. If you notice any other effects, check with your doctor.

CALCIUM CHANNEL BLOCKING AGENTS   Systemic

Some commonly used brand names are:

In the U.S.—

Adalat[7]	DynaCirc[5]
Adalat CC[7]	Isoptin[9]
Bepadin[1]	Isoptin SR[9]
Calan[9]	Nimotop[8]
Calan SR[9]	Plendil[3]
Cardene[6]	Procardia[7]
Cardizem[2]	Procardia XL[7]
Cardizem CD[2]	Vascor[1]
Cardizem SR[2]	Verelan[9]
Dilacor-XR[2]	

In Canada—

Adalat[7]	Apo-Verap[9]
Adalat FT[7]	Cardene[6]
Adalat P.A.[7]	Cardizem[2]
Apo-Diltiaz[2]	Cardizem SR[2]
Apo-Nifed[7]	Isoptin[9]

In Canada (cont'd)—

Isoptin SR[9]
Nimotop[8]
Novo-Diltazem[2]
Novo-Nifedin[7]
Novo-Veramil[9]
Nu-Diltiaz[2]

Nu-Nifed[7]
Nu-Verap[9]
Plendil[3]
Renedil[3]
Sibelium[4]
Syn-Diltiazem[2]

Note: For quick reference, the following calcium channel blocking agents are numbered to match the corresponding brand names.

This information applies to the following medicines:

1. Bepridil (BE-pri-dil)†
2. Diltiazem (dil-TYE-a-zem)§
3. Felodipine (fe-LOE-di-peen)
4. Flunarizine (floo-NAR-i-zeen)*
5. Isradipine (is-RA-di-peen)†
6. Nicardipine (nye-KAR-de-peen)
7. Nifedipine (nye-FED-i-peen)‡
8. Nimodipine (nye-MOE-di-peen)
9. Verapamil (ver-AP-a-mil)‡§

---

*Not commercially available in the U.S.
†Not commercially available in Canada.
‡Generic name product may also be available in the U.S.
§Generic name product may also be available in Canada.

Description

Bepridil, diltiazem, felodipine, flunarizine, isradipine, nicardipine, nifedipine, nimodipine, and verapamil belong to the group of medicines called calcium channel blockers.

Calcium channel blocking agents affect the movement of calcium into the cells of the heart and blood vessels. As a result, they relax blood vessels and increase the supply of blood and oxygen to the heart while reducing its workload.

Some of the calcium channel blocking agents are used to relieve and control angina pectoris (chest pain).

Some are also used to treat high blood pressure (hypertension). High blood pressure adds to the workload of the heart and arteries. If it continues for a long time, the heart and arteries may not function properly. This can damage the blood vessels of the brain, heart, and kidneys, resulting in a stroke, heart failure, or kidney failure. High blood pressure may also increase the risk of heart attacks. These problems may be less likely to occur if blood pressure is controlled.

Flunarizine is used to prevent migraine headaches.

Nimodipine is used to prevent and treat problems caused by a burst blood vessel in the head (also known as a ruptured aneurysm or subarachnoid hemorrhage).

Other calcium channel blocking agents may also be used for these and other conditions as determined by your doctor.

These medicines are available only with your doctor's prescription, in the following dosage forms:

> *Oral*
>> Bepridil
>>> • Tablets (U.S.)
>> Diltiazem
>>> • Extended-release capsules (U.S. and Canada)
>>> • Tablets (U.S. and Canada)
>> Felodipine
>>> • Extended-release tablets (U.S. and Canada)
>> Flunarizine
>>> • Capsules (Canada)
>> Isradipine
>>> • Capsules (U.S.)
>> Nicardipine
>>> • Capsules (U.S. and Canada)
>> Nifedipine
>>> • Capsules (U.S. and Canada)
>>> • Tablets (Canada)
>>> • Extended-release tablets (U.S. and Canada)
>> Nimodipine
>>> • Capsules (U.S. and Canada)
>> Verapamil
>>> • Extended-release capsules (U.S.)
>>> • Tablets (U.S. and Canada)
>>> • Extended-release tablets (U.S. and Canada)

Parenteral
Diltiazem
- Injection (U.S.)
Verapamil
- Injection (U.S. and Canada)

Before Using This Medicine

In deciding to use a medicine, the risks of taking the medicine must be weighed against the good it will do. This is a decision you and your doctor will make. For the calcium channel blocking agents, the following should be considered:

Allergies—Tell your doctor if you have ever had any unusual or allergic reaction to bepridil, diltiazem, felodipine, flunarizine, isradipine, nicardipine, nifedipine, nimodipine, or verapamil. Also tell your health care professional if you are allergic to any other substances, such as foods, preservatives, or dyes.

Pregnancy—Calcium channel blockers have not been studied in pregnant women. However, studies in animals have shown that large doses of calcium channel blockers cause birth defects, prolonged pregnancy, poor bone development, and stillbirth.

Breast-feeding—Although bepridil, diltiazem, nifedipine, verapamil, and possibly other calcium channel blockers pass into breast milk, they have not been reported to cause problems in nursing babies.

Children—Although there is no specific information comparing use of this medicine in children with use in other age groups, it is not expected to cause different side effects or problems in children than it does in adults.

Older adults—Elderly people may be especially sensitive to the effects of calcium channel blockers. This may increase the chance of side effects during treatment.

Other medicines—Although certain medicines should not be used together at all, in other cases two different medicines may be used together even if an interaction might occur. In these cases, your doctor may want to change the dose, or other precautions may be necessary. When taking calcium channel blockers it is especially important that your health care professional know if you are taking any of the following:

- Acetazolamide (e.g., Diamox) or
- Amphotericin B by injection (e.g., Fungizone) or
- Corticosteroids (cortisone-like medicine) or
- Dichlorphenamide (e.g., Daranide) or
- Diuretics (water pills) or
- Methazolamide (e.g., Naptazane)—These medicines can cause hypokalemia (low levels of potassium in the body), which can increase the unwanted effects of bepridil
- Beta-blockers (acebutolol [e.g., Sectral], atenolol [e.g., Tenormin], betaxolol [e.g., Kerlone], carteolol [e.g., Cartrol], labetalol [e.g., Normodyne], metoprolol [e.g., Lopressor], nadolol [e.g., Corgard], oxprenolol [e.g., Trasicor], penbutolol [e.g., Levatol], pindolol [e.g., Visken], propranolol [e.g., Inderal], sotalol [e.g., Sotacor], timolol [e.g., Blocadren])—Effects of both may be increased. In addition, unwanted effects may occur if a calcium channel blocker or a beta-blocker is stopped suddenly after use together
- Carbamazepine (e.g., Tegretol) or
- Cyclosporine (e.g., Sandimmune) or
- Procainamide (e.g., Pronestyl) or
- Quinidine (e.g., Quinidex)—Effects of these medicines may be increased if they are used with some calcium channel blockers
- Digitalis glycosides (heart medicine)—Effects of these medicines may be increased if they are used with some calcium channel blockers
- Disopyramide (e.g., Norpace)—Effects of some calcium channel blockers on the heart may be increased

Also, tell your health care professional if you are using any of the following medicines in the eye:

- Betaxolol (e.g., Betoptic) or
- Levobunolol (e.g., Betagan) or

- Metipranolol (e.g., OptiPranolol) or
- Timolol (e.g., Timoptic)—Effects on the heart and blood pressure may be increased

Other medical problems—The presence of other medical problems may affect the use of the calcium channel blockers. Make sure you tell your doctor if you have any other medical problems, especially:

- Heart rhythm problems (history of)—Bepridil can cause serious heart rhythm problems
- Kidney disease or
- Liver disease—Effects of the calcium channel blocker may be increased
- Mental depression (history of)—Flunarizine may cause mental depression
- Parkinson's disease or similar problems—Flunarizine can cause parkinsonian-like effects
- Other heart or blood vessel disorders—Calcium channel blockers may make some heart conditions worse

---

Proper Use of This Medicine

Take this medicine exactly as directed even if you feel well and do not notice any signs of chest pain. Do not take more of this medicine and do not take it more often than your doctor ordered. Do not miss any doses.

For patients taking *bepridil:*

- If this medicine causes upset stomach, it can be taken with meals or at bedtime.

For patients taking *diltiazem extended-release capsules:*

- Swallow the capsule whole, without crushing or chewing it.
- *Do not change to another brand without checking with your physician.* Different brands have different doses. If you refill your medicine and it looks different, check with your pharmacist.

For patients taking *nifedipine or verapamil extended-release capsules:*
- Swallow the capsule whole, without crushing or chewing it.

For patients taking *regular nifedipine or extended-release felodipine or nifedipine tablets:*
- Swallow the tablet whole, without breaking, crushing, or chewing it.
- If you are taking *Procardia XL*, you may sometimes notice what looks like a tablet in your stool. That is just the empty shell that is left after the medicine has been absorbed into your body.

For patients taking *verapamil extended-release tablets:*
- Swallow the tablet whole, without crushing or chewing it. However, if your doctor tells you to, you may break the tablet in half.
- Take the medicine with food or milk.

For patients taking this medicine *for high blood pressure:*
- In addition to the use of the medicine your doctor has prescribed, appropriate treatment for your high blood pressure may include weight control and care in the types of food you eat, especially foods high in sodium (salt). Your doctor will tell you which factors are most important for you. You should check with your doctor before changing your diet.
- Many patients who have high blood pressure will not notice any signs of the problem. In fact, many may feel normal. It is very important that you *take your medicine exactly as directed* and that you keep your appointments with your doctor even if you feel well.
- Remember that this medicine will not cure your high blood pressure but it does help control it. Therefore, you must continue to take it as directed if you expect to lower your blood pressure and keep it down. *You*

may have to take high blood pressure medicine for the rest of your life. If high blood pressure is not treated, it can cause serious problems such as heart failure, blood vessel disease, stroke, or kidney disease.

Dosing—The dose of these medicines will be different for different patients. *Follow your doctor's orders or the directions on the label.* The following information includes only the average doses of these medicines. *If your dose is different, do not change it* unless your doctor tells you to do so.

The number of capsules or tablets that you take depends on the strength of the medicine. Also, *the number of doses you take each day, the time allowed between doses, and the length of time you take the medicine depend on the medical problem for which you are taking calcium channel blocking agents.*

For bepridil

• For *oral* dosage form (tablets):

—For angina (chest pain):

• Adults—200 to 300 milligrams (mg) once a day.

• Children—Use and dose must be determined by your doctor.

For diltiazem

• For *long-acting oral* dosage form (extended-release capsules):

—For high blood pressure:

• Adults and teenagers—

—For *Cardizem CD* or *Dilacor-XR:* 180 to 240 milligrams (mg) once a day.

—For *Cardizem SR:* 60 to 120 mg two times a day.

• Children—Dose must be determined by your doctor.

- For *regular (short-acting) oral* dosage form (tablets):
    - —For angina (chest pain):
        - Adults and teenagers—30 mg three or four times a day. Your doctor may gradually increase your dose as needed.
        - Children—Dose must be determined by your doctor.
- For *injection* dosage form:
    - —For arrhythmias (irregular heartbeat):
        - Adults and teenagers—Dose is based on body weight and must be determined by your doctor.
        - Children—Use and dose must be determined by your doctor.

For felodipine

- For *long-acting oral* dosage form (extended-release tablets):
    - —For high blood pressure:
        - Adults—5 to 10 milligrams (mg) once a day.
        - Children—Use and dose must be determined by your doctor.
    - —For angina (chest pain):
        - Adults—10 mg once a day.
        - Children—Use and dose must be determined by your doctor.

For flunarizine

- For *oral* dosage form (capsules):
    - —To prevent headaches:
        - Adults—10 milligrams (mg) once a day in the evening.
        - Children—Dose must be determined by your doctor.

For isradipine

- For *oral* dosage form (capsules):

—For high blood pressure:

- Adults—2.5 milligrams (mg) two times a day. Your doctor may increase your dose as needed.
- Children—Use and dose must be determined by your doctor.

For nicardipine

- For *oral* dosage form (capsules):

  —For high blood pressure or angina (chest pain):

  - Adults and teenagers—20 milligrams (mg) three times a day.
  - Children—Dose must be determined by your doctor.

For nifedipine

- For *regular (short-acting) oral* dosage form (capsules or tablets):

  —For high blood pressure or angina (chest pain):

  - Adults and teenagers—10 milligrams (mg) three times a day. Your doctor may increase your dose as needed.
  - Children—Dose must be determined by your doctor.

- For *long-acting oral* dosage form (extended-release tablets):

  —For high blood pressure or angina (chest pain):

  - Adults and teenagers—

    —For *Adalat CC* or *Procardia XL:* 30 or 60 mg once a day. Your doctor may increase your dose as needed.

    —For *Adalat P.A.:* 20 mg two times a day. Your doctor may increase your dose as needed.

  - Children—Dose must be determined by your doctor.

For nimodipine

- For *oral* dosage form (capsules):

—To treat a burst blood vessel in the head:

- Adults—60 milligrams (mg) every four hours.
- Children—Dose must be determined by your doctor.

For verapamil

- For *regular (short-acting) oral* dosage form (tablets):

—For angina (chest pain), arrhythmias (irregular heartbeat), or high blood pressure:

- Adults and teenagers—40 to 120 milligrams (mg) three times a day. Your doctor may increase your dose as needed.
- Children—Dose is based on body weight and must be determined by your doctor. The usual dose is 4 to 8 mg per kilogram (kg) (1.82 to 3.64 mg per pound) of body weight a day. This is divided into smaller doses.

- For *long-acting oral* dosage form (extended-release capsules):

—For high blood pressure:

- Adults and teenagers—240 to 480 mg once a day.
- Children—Dose must be determined by your doctor.

- For *long-acting oral* dosage form (extended-release tablets):

—For high blood pressure:

- Adults and teenagers—120 mg once a day to 240 mg every twelve hours.
- Children—Dose must be determined by your doctor.

- For *injection* dosage form:

—For arrhythmias (irregular heartbeat):

- Adults—5 to 10 mg slowly injected into a vein. The dose may be repeated after thirty minutes.

- Children—Dose is based on body weight and must be determined by your doctor.

    —Infants up to 1 year of age: 100 to 200 micrograms (mcg) per kg (45.5 to 90.9 mcg per pound) of body weight injected slowly into a vein. The dose may be repeated after thirty minutes.

    —Children 1 to 15 years of age: 100 to 300 mcg per kg (45.5 to 136.4 mcg per pound) of body weight injected slowly into a vein. The dose may be repeated after thirty minutes.

Missed dose—If you miss a dose of this medicine, take it as soon as possible. However, if it is almost time for your next dose, skip the missed dose and go back to your regular dosing schedule. Do not double doses.

Storage—To store this medicine:

- Keep out of the reach of children.
- Store away from heat and direct light.
- Do not store in the bathroom, near the kitchen sink, or in other damp places. Heat or moisture may cause the medicine to break down.
- Do not keep outdated medicine or medicine no longer needed. Be sure that any discarded medicine is out of the reach of children.

Precautions While Using This Medicine

It is important that your doctor check your progress at regular visits. This will allow your doctor to make sure the medicine is working properly and to change the dosage if needed.

If you have been using this medicine regularly for several weeks, do not suddenly stop using it. Stopping suddenly may bring on your previous problem. Check with your doctor for the best way to reduce gradually the amount you are taking before stopping completely.

Chest pain resulting from exercise or physical exertion is usually reduced or prevented by this medicine. This may tempt you to be overly active. *Make sure you discuss with your doctor a safe amount of exercise for your medical problem.*

After taking a dose of this medicine you may get a headache that lasts for a short time. This effect is more common if you are taking felodipine, isradipine, or nifedipine. This should become less noticeable after you have taken this medicine for a while. If this effect continues or if the headaches are severe, check with your doctor.

In some patients, tenderness, swelling, or bleeding of the gums may appear soon after treatment with this medicine is started. Brushing and flossing your teeth carefully and regularly and massaging your gums may help prevent this. *See your dentist regularly to have your teeth cleaned. Check with your medical doctor or dentist if you have any questions about how to take care of your teeth and gums, or if you notice any tenderness, swelling, or bleeding of your gums.*

For patients taking *bepridil, diltiazem,* or *verapamil:*

- *Ask your doctor how to count your pulse rate. Then, while you are taking this medicine, check your pulse regularly.* If it is much slower than your usual rate, or less than 50 beats per minute, check with your doctor. A pulse rate that is too slow may cause circulation problems.

For patients taking *flunarizine:*

- This medicine may cause some people to become drowsy or less alert than they are normally. This is more likely to happen when you begin to take it or when you increase the amount of medicine you are taking. *Make sure you know how you react to this medicine before you drive, use machines, or do anything else that could be dangerous if you are not alert.*

For patients taking this medicine *for high blood pressure:*

- *Do not take other medicines unless they have been discussed with your doctor.* This especially includes over-the-counter (nonprescription) medicines for appetite control, asthma, colds, cough, hay fever, or sinus problems, since they may tend to increase your blood pressure.

Side Effects of This Medicine

Along with its needed effects, a medicine may cause some unwanted effects. Although not all of these side effects may occur, if they do occur they may need medical attention.

Not all of the side effects listed below have been reported for each of these medicines, but they have been reported for at least one of them. Since many of the effects of calcium channel blockers are similar, some of these side effects may occur with any of these medicines. However, they may be more common with some of these medicines than with others.

Check with your doctor as soon as possible if any of the following side effects occurs:

Less common

Breathing difficulty, coughing, or wheezing; irregular or fast, pounding heartbeat; skin rash; slow heartbeat (less than 50 beats per minute—bepridil, diltiazem, and verapamil only); swelling of ankles, feet, or lower legs (more common with felodipine and nifedipine)

For flunarizine only—less common

Loss of balance control; mask-like face; mental depression; shuffling walk; stiffness of arms or legs; trembling and shaking of hands and fingers; trouble in speaking or swallowing

Rare

> Bleeding, tender, or swollen gums; chest pain (may appear about 30 minutes after medicine is taken); fainting; painful, swollen joints (for nifedipine only); trouble in seeing (for nifedipine only)

For flunarizine and verapamil only—rare

> Unusual secretion of milk

Other side effects may occur that usually do not need medical attention. These side effects may go away during treatment as your body adjusts to the medicine. However, check with your doctor if any of the following side effects continue or are bothersome:

More common

> Drowsiness (for flunarizine only); increased appetite and/or weight gain (for flunarizine only)

Less common

> Constipation; diarrhea; dizziness or lightheadedness (more common with bepridil and nifedipine); dryness of mouth (for flunarizine only); flushing and feeling of warmth (more common with nicardipine and nifedipine); headache (more common with felodipine, isradipine, and nifedipine); nausea (more common with bepridil and nifedipine); unusual tiredness or weakness

Other side effects not listed above may also occur in some patients. If you notice any other effects, check with your doctor.

Additional Information

Once a medicine has been approved for marketing for a certain use, experience may show that it is also useful for other medical problems. Although these uses are not included in product labeling, calcium channel blockers are used in certain patients with the following medical conditions:

- Hypertrophic cardiomyopathy (a heart condition) (verapamil)

- Raynaud's phenomenon (circulation problems) (nicardipine and nifedipine)

Other than the above information, there is no additional information relating to proper use, precautions, or side effects for these uses.

CARBAMAZEPINE   Systemic

Some commonly used brand names are:

In the U.S.—
Epitol
Tegretol
Generic name product may also be available.

In Canada—
Apo-Carbamazepine   Tegretol Chewtabs
Novocarbamaz   Tegretol CR
Tegretol

Description

Carbamazepine (kar-ba-MAZ-e-peen) is used to control some types of seizures in the treatment of epilepsy. It is also used to relieve pain due to trigeminal neuralgia (tic douloureux). It should not be used for other, more common aches or pains.

Carbamazepine may also be used for other conditions as determined by your doctor.

This medicine is available only with your doctor's prescription, in the following dosage forms:

Oral

- Suspension (U.S.)
- Tablets (U.S. and Canada)
- Chewable tablets (U.S. and Canada)
- Extended-release tablets (Canada)

Before Using This Medicine

In deciding to use a medicine, the risks of taking the medicine must be weighed against the good it will do. This is a decision you and your doctor will make. For carbamazepine, the following should be considered:

Allergies—Tell your doctor if you have ever had any unusual or allergic reaction to carbamazepine or to any of the tricyclic antidepressants, such as amitriptyline, amoxapine, clomipramine, desipramine, doxepin, imipramine, nortriptyline, protriptyline, or trimipramine. Also tell your health care professional if you are allergic to any other substances, such as foods, preservatives, or dyes.

Pregnancy—Carbamazepine has not been studied in pregnant women. However, there have been reports of babies having low birth weight, small head size, skull and facial defects, underdeveloped fingernails, and delays in growth when their mothers had taken carbamazepine in high doses during pregnancy. In addition, birth defects have been reported in some babies when the mothers took other medicines for epilepsy during pregnancy. Also, studies in animals have shown that carbamazepine causes birth defects when given in large doses. Therefore, the use of carbamazepine during pregnancy should be discussed with your doctor.

Breast-feeding—Carbamazepine passes into the breast milk, and in some cases the baby may receive enough of it to cause unwanted effects. In animal studies, carbamazepine has affected the growth and appearance of the nursing babies.

Children—Behavior changes are more likely to occur in children.

Older adults—Confusion; restlessness and nervousness; irregular, pounding, or unusually slow heartbeat; and chest pain may be especially likely to occur in elderly patients, who are usually more sensitive than younger adults to the effects of carbamazepine.

Other medicines—Although certain medicines should not be used together at all, in other cases two different medicines may be used together even if an interaction might occur. In these cases, your doctor may want to change the dose, or other precautions may be necessary. When you are taking carbamazepine, it is especially important that your health care professional know if you are taking any of the following:

- Anticoagulants (blood thinners)—The effects of anticoagulants may be decreased; monitoring of blood clotting time may be necessary during and after carbamazepine treatment
- Cimetidine (e.g., Tagamet)—Blood levels of carbamazepine may be increased, leading to an increase in serious side effects
- Clarithromycin (e.g., Biaxin)—Blood levels of carbamazepine may be increased, increasing the risk of unwanted effects
- Corticosteroids (cortisone-like medicine)—The effects of corticosteroids may be decreased
- Diltiazem (e.g., Cardizem) or
- Erythromycin (e.g., E-Mycin, Erythrocin, Ilosone) or
- Propoxyphene (e.g., Darvon) or
- Verapamil (e.g., Calan)—Blood levels of carbamazepine may be increased; these medicines should not be used with carbamazepine
- Estrogens (female hormones) or
- Quinidine or
- Oral contraceptives (birth control pills) containing estrogen—The effects of these medicines may be decreased; use of a nonhormonal method of birth control or an oral contraceptive containing only a progestin may be necessary
- Isoniazid (e.g., INH)—The risk of serious side effects may be increased
- Monoamine oxidase (MAO) inhibitors (furazolidone [e.g., Furoxone], isocarboxazid [e.g., Marplan], phenelzine [e.g.,

Nardil], procarbazine [e.g., Matulane], selegiline [e.g., Eldepryl], tranylcypromine [e.g., Parnate])—Taking carbamazepine while you are taking or within 2 weeks of taking monoamine oxidase (MAO) inhibitors may cause sudden high body temperature, extremely high blood pressure, and severe convulsions; at least 14 days should be allowed between stopping treatment with one medicine and starting treatment with the other

- Other anticonvulsants (seizure medicine)—The effects of these medicines may be decreased; in addition, if these medicines and carbamazepine are used together during pregnancy, the risk of birth defects may be increased

- Tricyclic antidepressants (amitriptyline [e.g., Elavil], amoxapine [e.g., Asendin], clomipramine [e.g., Anafranil], desipramine [e.g., Pertofrane], doxepin [e.g., Sinequan], imipramine [e.g., Tofranil], nortriptyline [e.g., Aventyl], protriptyline [e.g., Vivactil], trimipramine [e.g., Surmontil])—Central nervous system depressant effects of carbamazepine may be increased while the anticonvulsant effects of carbamazepine may be decreased; seizures may occur more frequently

Other medical problems—The presence of other medical problems may affect the use of carbamazepine. Make sure you tell your doctor if you have any other medical problems, especially:

- Alcohol abuse (or history of) —Drinking alcohol may decrease the effectiveness of carbamazepine

- Anemia or other blood problems or
- Behavioral problems or
- Glaucoma or
- Heart or blood vessel disease or
- Problems with urination—Carbamazepine may make the condition worse

- Diabetes mellitus (sugar diabetes)—Carbamazepine may cause increased urine glucose levels

- Kidney disease or
- Liver disease—Higher blood levels of carbamazepine may result, increasing the chance of side effects

Proper Use of This Medicine

Carbamazepine should be taken with meals to lessen the chance of stomach upset (nausea and vomiting).

It is very important that you take this medicine exactly as directed by your doctor to obtain the best results and lessen the chance of serious side effects. Do not take more of it, do not take it more often, and do not take it for a longer time than your doctor ordered.

If you are taking this medicine for pain relief:

- Carbamazepine is *not* an ordinary pain reliever. It should be used only when a doctor prescribes it for certain kinds of pain. *Do not take carbamazepine for any other aches or pains.*

If you are taking this medicine for epilepsy:

- *Do not suddenly stop taking this medicine without first checking with your doctor.* To keep your seizures under control, it is usually best to gradually reduce the amount of carbamazepine you are taking before stopping completely.

Dosing—The dose of carbamazepine will be different for different patients. *Follow your doctor's orders or the directions on the label.* The following information includes only the average doses of carbamazepine. *If your dose is different, do not change it,* unless your doctor tells you to do so.

The number of tablets or teaspoonfuls of suspension that you take depends on the strength of the medicine. Also, *the number of doses you take each day, the time allowed between doses, and the length of time you take the medicine depend on the medical problem for which you are taking carbamazepine.*

- For *oral* dosage form (suspension):

—For epilepsy:

• Adults and teenagers—At first, 100 milligrams (mg) taken up to four times a day. Your doctor may increase your dose if needed. However, the dose is usually not more than 1200 mg a day.

• Children 6 to 12 years of age—At first, 50 mg taken four times a day. Your doctor may increase your dose if needed. However, the dose is usually not more than 1000 mg a day.

• Children up to 6 years of age—Dose is based on weight and will be determined by your doctor.

—For trigeminal neuralgia:

• Adults and teenagers—At first, 50 mg four times a day. Your doctor may increase your dose if needed. However, the dose is usually not more than 1200 mg a day.

• Children—Use and dose must be determined by your doctor.

• For *oral* dosage form (tablets and chewable tablets):

—For epilepsy:

• Adults and teenagers—At first, 200 mg taken two times a day. Your doctor may increase your dose if needed. However, the dose is usually not more than 1200 mg a day.

• Children 6 to 12 years of age—At first, 100 mg taken two times a day. Your doctor may increase your dose if needed. However, the dose is usually not more than 1000 mg a day.

• Children up to 6 years of age—Dose is based on weight and will be determined by your doctor.

—For trigeminal neuralgia:

• Adults and teenagers—At first, 100 mg taken two times a day. Your doctor may increase your dose if needed. However, the dose is usually not more than 1200 mg a day.

- Children—Use and dose must be determined by your doctor.
- For *oral extended-release tablet* dosage form:
  —For epilepsy:
  - Adults and teenagers—At first, 100 to 200 mg taken one or two times a day with meals. Your doctor may increase your dose if needed. However, the dose is usually not more than 1200 mg a day.
  - Children 6 to 12 years of age—At first, 100 mg taken in smaller doses during the day. Your doctor may increase your dose if needed. However, the dose is usually not more than 1000 mg a day.
  - Children up to 6 years of age—Use and dose must be determined by your doctor.
  —For trigeminal neuralgia:
  - Adults and teenagers—At first, 100 mg taken two times a day. Your doctor may increase your dose if needed. However, the dose is usually not more than 1200 mg a day.
  - Children—Use and dose must be determined by your doctor.

Missed dose—If you miss a dose of this medicine, take it as soon as possible. However, if it is almost time for your next dose, skip the missed dose and go back to your regular dosing schedule. Do not double doses. However, if you miss more than one dose a day, check with your doctor.

Storage—To store this medicine:
- Keep out of the reach of children.
- Store away from heat and direct light.
- *Do not store the tablet forms of carbamazepine in the bathroom, near the kitchen sink, or in other damp places. Heat or moisture may cause the medicine to break down and become less effective.*

- Keep the liquid form of this medicine from freezing.
- Do not keep outdated medicine or medicine no longer needed. Be sure that any discarded medicine is out of the reach of children.

Precautions While Using This Medicine

It is very important that your doctor check your progress at regular visits. Your doctor may want to have certain tests done to see if you are receiving the right amount of medicine or if certain side effects may be occurring without your knowing it. Also, the amount of medicine you are taking may have to be changed often.

This medicine will add to the effects of alcohol and other CNS depressants (medicines that cause drowsiness). Some examples of CNS depressants are antihistamines or medicine for hay fever, other allergies, or colds; sedatives, tranquilizers, or sleeping medicine; prescription pain medicine or narcotics; barbiturates; medicine for seizures; muscle relaxants; or anesthetics, including some dental anesthetics. *Check with your doctor before taking any of the above while you are using this medicine.*

This medicine may cause some people to become drowsy, dizzy, lightheaded, or less alert than they are normally, especially when they are starting treatment or increasing the dose. It may also cause blurred or double vision, weakness, or loss of muscle control in some people. *Make sure you know how you react to this medicine before you drive, use machines, or do anything else that could be dangerous if you are not alert and well-coordinated or able to see well.*

Some people who take carbamazepine may become more sensitive to sunlight than they are normally. Exposure to sunlight, even for brief periods of time, may cause a skin rash, itching, redness or other discoloration of the skin, or a severe sunburn. When you begin taking this medicine:

- Stay out of direct sunlight, especially between the hours of 10:00 a.m. and 3:00 p.m., if possible.
- Wear protective clothing, including a hat. Also, wear sunglasses.
- Apply a sun block product that has a skin protection factor (SPF) of at least 15. Some patients may require a product with a higher SPF number, especially if they have a fair complexion. If you have any questions about this, check with your health care professional.
- Apply a sun block lipstick that has an SPF of at least 15 to protect your lips.
- Do not use a sunlamp or tanning bed or booth.

If you have a severe reaction from the sun, check with your doctor.

Oral contraceptives (birth control pills) containing estrogen may not work properly if you take them while you are taking carbamazepine. Unplanned pregnancies may occur. You should use a different or additional means of birth control while you are taking carbamazepine. If you have any questions about this, check with your health care professional.

For diabetic patients:

- Carbamazepine may affect urine sugar levels. While you are using this medicine, be especially careful when testing for sugar in your urine. If you notice a change in the results of your urine sugar tests or have any questions about this, check with your doctor.

Before having any medical tests, tell the medical doctor in charge that you are taking this medicine. The results of some pregnancy tests and the metyrapone test may be affected by this medicine.

Before having any kind of surgery, dental treatment, or emergency treatment, tell the medical doctor or dentist in charge that you are taking this medicine. Taking carbamazepine together with medicines that are used during surgery or dental or emergency treatments may increase the CNS depressant effects.

Your doctor may want you to carry a medical identification card or bracelet stating that you are taking this medicine.

Side Effects of This Medicine

Along with its needed effects, a medicine may cause some unwanted effects. Although not all of these side effects may occur, if they do occur they may need medical attention.

Check with your doctor immediately if any of the following side effects occur:

> *Rare*
>
> > Black, tarry stools; blood in urine or stools; bone or joint pain; cough or hoarseness; darkening of urine; lower back or side pain; nosebleeds or other unusual bleeding or bruising; painful or difficult urination; pain, tenderness, swelling, or bluish color in leg or foot; pale stools; pinpoint red spots on skin; shortness of breath or cough; sores, ulcers, or white spots on lips or in the mouth; sore throat, chills, and fever; swollen or painful glands; unusual tiredness or weakness; wheezing, tightness in chest, or troubled breathing; yellow eyes or skin
>
> *Symptoms of overdose*
>
> > Body spasm in which head and heels are bent backward and body is bowed forward; clumsiness or unsteadiness; convulsions (seizures)—especially in small children; dizziness (severe) or fainting; drowsiness (severe); fast or irregular heartbeat; high or low blood pressure (hypertension or hypotension); irregular, slow,

or shallow breathing; large pupils; nausea or vomiting (severe); overactive reflexes followed by underactive reflexes; poor control in body movements (for example, when reaching or stepping); sudden decrease in amount of urine; trembling, twitching, or abnormal body movements

In addition, check with your doctor as soon as possible if any of the following side effects occur:

More common

Blurred vision or double vision; continuous back-and-forth eye movements

Less common

Behavioral changes (especially in children); confusion, agitation, or hostility (especially in the elderly); diarrhea (severe); headache (continuing); increase in seizures; nausea and vomiting (severe); skin rash, hives, or itching; unusual drowsiness

Rare

Chest pain; difficulty in speaking or slurred speech; fainting; frequent urination; irregular, pounding, or unusually slow heartbeat; mental depression with restlessness and nervousness or other mood or mental changes; muscle or stomach cramps; numbness, tingling, pain, or weakness in hands and feet; rapid weight gain; rigidity; ringing, buzzing, or other unexplained sounds in the ears; sudden decrease in amount of urine; swelling of face, hands, feet, or lower legs; trembling; uncontrolled body movements; visual hallucinations (seeing things that are not there)

Other side effects may occur that usually do not need medical attention. These side effects may go away during treatment as your body adjusts to the medicine. However, check with your doctor if any of the following side effects continue or are bothersome:

More common

Clumsiness or unsteadiness; dizziness (mild); drowsiness (mild); lightheadedness; nausea or vomiting (mild)

Less common or rare

Aching joints or muscles; constipation; diarrhea; dryness of mouth; headache; increased sensitivity of skin to sunlight (skin rash, itching, redness or other discoloration of skin, or severe sunburn); increased sweating; irritation or soreness of tongue or mouth; loss of appetite; loss of hair; muscle or abdominal cramps; sexual problems in males; stomach pain or discomfort

Other side effects not listed above may also occur in some patients. If you notice any other effects, check with your doctor.

Additional Information

Once a medicine has been approved for marketing for a certain use, experience may show that it is also useful for other medical problems. Although these uses are not included in product labeling, carbamazepine is used in certain patients with the following medical conditions:

- Neurogenic pain (a type of continuing pain)
- Bipolar disorder (manic-depressive illness)
- Central partial diabetes insipidus (water diabetes)
- Alcohol withdrawal
- Psychotic disorders (severe mental illness)

Other than the above information, there is no additional information relating to proper use, precautions, or side effects for these uses.

CEPHALOSPORINS   Systemic

Some commonly used brand names are:

In the U.S.—

Ancef[4]	Cefanex[18]
Ceclor[1]	Cefizox[15]
Cefadyl[20]	Cefobid[8]

In the U.S. (cont'd)—

Cefotan[10]

Ceftin[17]

Cefzil[13]

Ceptaz[14]

Claforan[9]

C-Lexin[18]

Duricef[2]

Fortaz[14]

Keflex[18]

Keflin[19]

Keftab[18]

Kefurox[17]

Kefzol[4]

Mandol[3]

Mefoxin[11]

Monocid[7]

Rocephin[16]

Suprax[5]

Tazicef[14]

Tazidime[14]

Ultracef[2]

Vantin[12]

Velosef[21]

Zefazone[6]

Zinacef[17]

Zolicef[4]

In Canada—

Ancef[4]

Apo-Cephalex[18]

Ceclor[1]

Cefizox[15]

Cefobid[8]

Cefotan[10]

Ceftin[17]

Ceptaz[14]

Claforan[9]

Duricef[2]

Fortaz[14]

Gen-Cefazolin[4]

Keflex[18]

Keflin[19]

Kefurox[17]

Kefzol[4]

Mandol[3]

Mefoxin[11]

Novo-Lexin[18]

Nu-Cephalex[18]

Rocephin[16]

Suprax[5]

Tazidime[14]

Velosef[21]

Zinacef[17]

Note: For quick reference, the following cephalosporins are numbered to match the corresponding brand names.

This information applies to the following medicines:

1. Cefaclor (SEF-a-klor)
2. Cefadroxil (sef-a-DROX-ill)‡
3. Cefamandole (sef-a-MAN-dole)
4. Cefazolin (sef-A-zoe-lin)‡
5. Cefixime (sef-IX-eem)
6. Cefmetazole (sef-MET-a-zole)†
7. Cefonicid (se-FON-i-sid)†
8. Cefoperazone (sef-oh-PER-a-zone)
9. Cefotaxime (sef-oh-TAKS-eem)
10. Cefotetan (sef-oh-TEE-tan)
11. Cefoxitin (se-FOX-i-tin)
12. Cefpodoxime (sef-pode-OX-eem)†
13. Cefprozil (sef-PROE-zil)†
14. Ceftazidime (sef-TAY-zi-deem)

15. Ceftizoxime (sef-ti-ZOX-eem)
16. Ceftriaxone (sef-try-AX-one)
17. Cefuroxime (se-fyoor-OX-eem)
18. Cephalexin (sef-a-LEX-in)‡
19. Cephalothin (sef-A-loe-thin)‡
20. Cephapirin (sef-a-PYE-rin)†‡
21. Cephradine (SEF-ra-deen)‡

---

†Not commercially available in Canada.
‡Generic name product may also be available in the U.S.

Description

Cephalosporins (sef-a-loe-SPOR-ins) are used in the treatment of infections caused by bacteria. They work by killing bacteria or preventing their growth.

Cephalosporins are used to treat infections in many different parts of the body. They are sometimes given with other antibiotics. Some cephalosporins are also given by injection to prevent infections before, during, and after surgery. However, cephalosporins will not work for colds, flu, or other virus infections.

Cephalosporins are available only with your doctor's prescription, in the following dosage forms:

Oral

Cefaclor
- Capsules (U.S. and Canada)
- Oral suspension (U.S. and Canada)

Cefadroxil
- Capsules (U.S. and Canada)
- Oral suspension (U.S.)
- Tablets (U.S.)

Cefixime
- Oral suspension (U.S. and Canada)
- Tablets (U.S. and Canada)

Cefpodoxime
- Oral suspension (U.S.)
- Tablets (U.S.)

Cefprozil
- Oral suspension (U.S.)

- Tablets (U.S.)

Cefuroxime
- Tablets (U.S. and Canada)

Cephalexin
- Capsules (U.S. and Canada)
- Oral suspension (U.S. and Canada)
- Tablets (U.S. and Canada)

Cephradine
- Capsules (U.S. and Canada)
- Oral suspension (U.S.)

Parenteral

Cefamandole
- Injection (U.S. and Canada)

Cefazolin
- Injection (U.S. and Canada)

Cefmetazole
- Injection (U.S.)

Cefonicid
- Injection (U.S.)

Cefoperazone
- Injection (U.S. and Canada)

Cefotaxime
- Injection (U.S. and Canada)

Cefotetan
- Injection (U.S. and Canada)

Cefoxitin
- Injection (U.S. and Canada)

Ceftazidime
- Injection (U.S. and Canada)

Ceftizoxime
- Injection (U.S. and Canada)

Ceftriaxone
- Injection (U.S. and Canada)

Cefuroxime
- Injection (U.S. and Canada)

Cephalothin
- Injection (U.S. and Canada)

Cephapirin
- Injection (U.S.)

Cephradine
- Injection (U.S.)

Before Using This Medicine

In deciding to use a medicine, the risks of taking the medicine must be weighed against the good it will do. This is a decision you and your doctor will make. For the cephalosporins, the following should be considered:

Allergies—Tell your doctor if you have ever had any unusual or allergic reaction to any of the cephalosporins, penicillins, penicillin-like medicines, or penicillamine. Also tell your health care professional if you are allergic to any other substances, such as foods, preservatives, or dyes.

Pregnancy—Studies have not been done in humans. However, most cephalosporins have not been reported to cause birth defects or other problems in animal studies. Studies in rabbits have shown that cefoxitin may increase the risk of miscarriages and cause other problems.

Breast-feeding—Most cephalosporins pass into human breast milk, usually in small amounts. However, cephalosporins have not been reported to cause problems in nursing babies.

Children—Many cephalosporins have been tested in children and, in effective doses, have not been shown to cause different side effects or problems than they do in adults. However, there are some cephalosporins that have not been tested in children up to 1 year of age.

Older adults—Cephalosporins have been used in the elderly, and they are not expected to cause different side effects or problems in older people than they do in younger adults.

Other medicines—Although certain medicines should not be used together at all, in other cases two different medicines may be used together even if an interaction might occur. In these cases, your doctor may want to change the dose, or other precautions may be necessary. When you

are taking a cephalosporin, it is especially important that your health care professional know if you are taking any of the following:

- Alcohol and alcohol-containing medicine (cefamandole, cefmetazole, cefoperazone, and cefotetan only)—Using alcohol and these cephalosporins together may cause abdominal or stomach cramps, nausea, vomiting, headache, dizziness or lightheadedness, shortness of breath, sweating, or facial flushing; this reaction usually begins within 15 to 30 minutes after alcohol is consumed and usually goes away over several hours
- Anticoagulants (blood thinners) or
- Carbenicillin by injection (e.g., Geopen) or
- Dipyridamole (e.g., Persantine) or
- Divalproex (e.g., Depakote) or
- Heparin (e.g., Panheprin) or
- Pentoxifylline (e.g., Trental) or
- Plicamycin (e.g., Mithracin) or
- Sulfinpyrazone (e.g., Anturane) or
- Ticarcillin (e.g., Ticar) or
- Thrombolytic agents or
- Valproic acid (e.g., Depakene)—Any of these medicines may increase the chance of bleeding, especially when used with cefamandole, cefmetazole, cefoperazone, or cefotetan
- Probenecid (e.g., Benemid) (except cefoperazone, ceftazidime, or ceftriaxone)—Probenecid increases the blood level of many cephalosporins. Although probenecid may be given with a cephalosporin by your doctor purposely to increase the blood level to treat some infections, in other cases this effect may be unwanted and may increase the chance of side effects

Other medical problems—The presence of other medical problems may affect the use of cephalosporins. Make sure you tell your doctor if you have any other medical problems, especially:

- Bleeding problems, history of (cefamandole, cefmetazole, cefoperazone, and cefotetan only)—These medicines may increase the chance of bleeding
- Kidney disease—Some cephalosporins need to be given at a lower dose to people with kidney disease. Also, cephalothin, especially, may increase the chance of kidney damage

- Liver disease (cefoperazone only)—Cefoperazone needs to be given at a lower dose to people with liver and kidney disease
- Phenylketonuria—Cefprozil oral suspension contains phenylalanine
- Stomach or intestinal disease, history of (especially colitis, including colitis caused by antibiotics, or enteritis)—Cephalosporins may cause colitis in some patients

---

Proper Use of This Medicine

Cephalosporins may be taken on a full or empty stomach. If this medicine upsets your stomach, it may help to take it with food.

Cefuroxime axetil tablets and cefpodoxime should be taken with food to increase absorption of the medicine.

For patients taking the *oral liquid* form of this medicine:

- This medicine is to be taken by mouth even if it comes in a dropper bottle. If this medicine does not come in a dropper bottle, use a specially marked measuring spoon or other device to measure each dose accurately. The average household teaspoon may not hold the right amount of liquid.
- Do not use after the expiration date on the label since the medicine may not work properly after that date. Check with your pharmacist if you have any questions about this.

For patients unable to swallow *cefuroxime axetil tablets* whole ask your doctor for suggestions.

To help clear up your infection completely, *keep taking this medicine for the full time of treatment,* even if you begin to feel better after a few days. *If you have a "strep" infection, you should keep taking this medicine for at least 10 days. This is especially important in "strep" infections since serious heart or kidney problems could develop later* if your infection is not cleared up completely. Also, if you stop taking this medicine too soon, your symptoms may return.

This medicine works best when there is a constant amount in the blood or urine. *To help keep the amount constant, do not miss any doses. Also, it is best to take the doses at evenly spaced times, day and night.* For example, if you are to take 4 doses a day, the doses should be spaced about 6 hours apart. If this interferes with your sleep or other daily activities, or if you need help in planning the best times to take your medicine, check with your health care professional.

Dosing—The dose of these medicines will be different for different patients. *Follow your doctor's orders or the directions on the label.* The following information includes only the average doses of these medicines. Your dose may be different if you have kidney disease. *If your dose is different, do not change it* unless your doctor tells you to do so.

The number of capsules or tablets or teaspoonfuls of suspension that you take depends on the strength of the medicine. Also, *the number of doses you take each day, the time allowed between doses, and the length of time you take the medicine depend on the medical problem for which you are taking a cephalosporin.*

For cefaclor

• For bacterial infections

—For *oral* dosage form (capsules or oral suspension):

• Adults and teenagers—250 to 500 milligrams (mg) every eight hours.

• Infants and children 1 month of age and older—6.7 to 13.4 mg per kilogram (kg) (3 to 6 mg per pound) of body weight every eight hours, or 10 to 20 mg per kg (4.5 to 9 mg per pound) of body weight every twelve hours.

For cefadroxil

- For bacterial infections

    —For *oral* dosage form (capsules, tablets, or oral suspension):

    • Adults and teenagers—500 milligrams (mg) every twelve hours, or 1 to 2 grams once a day.

    • Children—15 mg per kilogram (kg) (6.8 mg per pound) of body weight every twelve hours, or 30 mg per kg (13.6 mg per pound) of body weight once a day.

For cefamandole

- For bacterial infections

    —For *injection* dosage form:

    • Adults and teenagers—500 milligrams (mg) to 2 grams every four to eight hours, injected into a muscle or vein.

    • Infants and children 1 month of age and older—8.3 to 33.3 mg per kilogram (kg) (3.8 to 15.1 mg per pound) of body weight every four to eight hours, injected into a muscle or vein.

For cefazolin

- For bacterial infections

    —For *injection* dosage form:

    • Adults and teenagers—250 milligrams (mg) to 1.5 grams every six to eight hours, injected into a vein.

    • Infants and children 1 month of age and older—6.25 to 25 mg per kilogram (kg) (2.8 to 11.4 mg per pound) of body weight every six hours, or 8.3 to 33.3 mg per kg (3.8 to 15.1 mg per pound) of body weight every eight hours, injected into a vein.

For cefixime
- For bacterial infections
  - —For *oral* dosage form (tablets or oral suspension):
    - Adults and teenagers—200 milligrams (mg) every twelve hours, or 400 mg once a day. Gonorrhea is treated with a single, oral dose of 400 mg.
    - Children 6 months of age to 12 years of age— 4 mg per kilogram (kg) (1.8 mg per pound) of body weight every twelve hours, or 8 mg per kg (3.6 mg per pound) of body weight once a day.

For cefmetazole
- For bacterial infections
  - —For *injection* dosage form:
    - Adults and teenagers—2 grams every six to twelve hours, injected into a vein, for five to fourteen days. Gonorrhea is treated with a single dose of 1 gram, injected into the muscle, along with a single, oral 1 gram dose of probenecid.
    - Children—Dose must be determined by your doctor.

For cefonicid
- For bacterial infections
  - —For *injection* dosage form:
    - Adults and teenagers—500 milligrams (mg) to 1 gram every twenty-four hours, injected into a vein or muscle.
    - Children—Dose must be determined by your doctor.

For cefoperazone
- For bacterial infections
  - —For *injection* dosage form:
    - Adults and teenagers—1 to 6 grams every twelve hours, or 2 to 4 grams every eight hours, injected into a vein.

• Children—Dose must be determined by your doctor.

For cefotaxime

• For bacterial infections

—For *injection* dosage form:

• Adults and teenagers—1 to 2 grams every four to twelve hours. Gonorrhea is usually treated with a single dose of 250 milligrams (mg), injected into a muscle.

• Newborns up to 1 week of age—50 mg per kilogram (kg) (22.7 mg per pound) of body weight every twelve hours, injected into a vein.

• Newborns 1 to 4 weeks of age—50 mg per kg (22.7 mg per pound) of body weight every eight hours, injected into a vein.

• Infants and children up to 50 kg of body weight (110 pounds)—8.3 to 30 mg per kg (3.8 to 13.6 mg per pound) of body weight every four hours, or 12.5 to 45 mg per kg (5.7 to 20.4 mg per pound) of body weight every six hours, injected into a vein.

• Children over 50 kg of body weight (110 pounds)—1 to 2 grams every four to twelve hours.

For cefotetan

• For bacterial infections

—For *injection* dosage form:

• Adults and teenagers—1 to 3 grams every twelve hours, injected into a vein or muscle.

• Children—Dose must be determined by your doctor.

For cefoxitin

• For bacterial infections

—For *injection* dosage form:

• Adults and teenagers—1 to 3 grams every four

to eight hours, injected into a vein. Gonorrhea is treated with a single dose of 2 grams, injected into a muscle, and given along with a single, oral 1 gram dose of probenecid.

• Infants and children 3 months of age and over—13.3 to 26.7 milligrams (mg) per kilogram (kg) (6 to 12 mg per pound) of body weight every four hours, or 20 to 40 mg per kg (9 to 18 mg per pound) of body weight every six hours.

For cefpodoxime

• For bacterial infections

—For *oral* dosage forms (tablets or oral suspension):

• Adults and teenagers—100 to 400 milligrams (mg) every twelve hours for seven to fourteen days. Gonorrhea is treated with a single, oral dose of 200 mg.

• Infants and children 6 months to 12 years of age—5 mg per kilogram (kg) (2.3 mg per pound) of body weight every twelve hours for ten days.

• Infants up to 6 months of age—Dose must be determined by your doctor.

For cefprozil

• For bacterial infections

—For *oral* dosage forms (tablets or oral suspension):

• Adults and teenagers—250 to 500 milligrams (mg) every twelve to twenty-four hours for ten days.

• Children 2 to 12 years of age—7.5 mg per kilogram (kg) (3.4 mg per pound) of body weight every twelve hours for ten days.

• Infants and children 6 months to 12 years of age—15 mg per kg (6.8 mg per pound) of body weight every twelve hours for ten days.

For ceftazidime

• For bacterial infections

—For *injection* dosage form:

• Adults and teenagers—500 milligrams (mg) to 2 grams every eight to twelve hours.

• Newborns up to 4 weeks of age—30 mg per kilogram (kg) (13.6 mg per pound) of body weight every twelve hours, injected into a vein.

• Infants and children 1 month to 12 years of age—30 mg to 50 mg per kg (13.6 to 22.7 mg per pound) of body weight every eight hours, injected into a vein.

For ceftizoxime

• For bacterial infections

—For *injection* dosage form:

• Adults and teenagers—1 to 4 grams every eight to twelve hours injected into a vein.

• Infants and children 6 months of age and older—50 milligrams (mg) per kilogram (kg) (22.7 mg per pound) of body weight every six to eight hours, injected into a vein.

For ceftriaxone

• For bacterial infections

—For *injection* dosage form:

• Adults and teenagers—1 to 2 grams every twenty-four hours, or 500 milligrams (mg) to 1 gram every twelve hours, injected into a vein or muscle. Gonorrhea is treated with a single 250 mg dose injected into a muscle.

• Infants and children—25 to 50 mg per kilogram (kg) (11.4 to 22.7 mg per pound) of body weight every twelve hours, or 50 to 75 mg per kg (22.7 to 34.1 mg per pound) of body weight once a day, injected into a vein. Meningitis is treated with an initial dose of 100 mg per kg, then, 100 mg per kg once a day injected into a vein.

For cefuroxime

- For bacterial infections

    —For *oral* dosage form (tablets):

    - Adults and teenagers—125 to 500 milligrams (mg) every twelve hours. Gonorrhea is treated with a single, oral 1 gram dose.

    - Children up to 12 years of age—125 mg every twelve hours.

    —For *injection* dosage form:

    - Adults and teenagers—750 mg to 1.5 grams every eight hours injected into a vein or a muscle. Gonorrhea is treated with a single dose of 1.5 grams, injected into a muscle; the total 1.5-gram dose is divided into two doses and injected into muscles at two separate places on the body, and given along with a single oral 1 gram dose of probenecid.

    - Newborns—10 to 33.3 mg per kilogram (kg) (4.5 to 15.1 mg per pound) of body weight every eight hours, or 15 to 50 mg per kg (6.8 to 22.7 mg per pound) of body weight every twelve hours, injected into a muscle or a vein.

    - Infants and children 3 months of age and over—16.7 to 33.3 mg per kg (7.6 to 15.1 mg per pound) of body weight every eight hours, injected into a muscle or a vein.

For cephalexin

- For bacterial infections

    —For *oral* dosage form (capsules, oral suspension, or tablets):

    - Adults and teenagers—250 to 500 milligrams (mg) every six to twelve hours.

    - Children—6.25 to 25 mg per kilogram (kg) (1.6 to 11.4 mg per pound) of body weight every six hours, or 12.5 to 50 mg per kg (5.7 to 22.7 mg per pound) of body weight every twelve hours.

For cephalothin

• For bacterial infections

—For *injection* dosage form:

• Adults and teenagers—500 milligrams (mg) to 2 grams every four to six hours, injected into a vein.

• Children—13.3 to 26.6 mg per kilogram (kg) (6 to 12 mg per pound) of body weight every four hours, or 20 to 40 mg per kg (9.1 to 18.2 mg per pound) of body weight every six hours, injected into a vein.

For cephapirin

• For bacterial infections

—For *injection* dosage form:

• Adults and teenagers—500 milligrams (mg) to 1 gram every four to six hours, injected into a muscle or a vein.

• Infants and children 3 months of age and over—10 to 20 mg per kilogram (kg) (4.5 to 9.1 mg per pound) of body weight every six hours, injected into a muscle or a vein.

For cephradine

• For bacterial infections

—For *oral* dosage forms (capsules or oral suspension):

• Adults and teenagers—250 to 500 milligrams (mg) every six hours, or 500 mg to 1 gram every twelve hours.

• Children—6.25 to 25 mg per kilogram (kg) (2.8 to 11.4 mg per pound) of body weight every six hours.

—For *injection* dosage form:

• Adults and teenagers—500 mg to 1 gram every six hours, injected into a muscle or a vein.

> • Children 1 year of age and over—12.5 to 25 mg
> per kg (5.7 to 11.4 mg per pound) of body weight
> every six hours, injected into a muscle or a vein.

Missed dose—If you miss a dose of this medicine, take it as soon as possible. This will help to keep a constant amount of medicine in the blood or urine. However, if it is almost time for your next dose, skip the missed dose and go back to your regular dosing schedule. Do not double doses.

Storage—To store this medicine:

- Keep out of the reach of children.
- Store away from heat and direct light.
- Do not store the capsule or tablet form of this medicine in the bathroom, near the kitchen sink, or in other damp places. Heat or moisture may cause the medicine to break down.
- Store the oral liquid form of most cephalosporins in the refrigerator because heat will cause this medicine to break down. However, keep the medicine from freezing. Follow the directions on the label. Cefixime oral suspension (Suprax) does not need to be refrigerated.
- Do not keep outdated medicine or medicine no longer needed. Be sure that any discarded medicine is out of the reach of children.

Precautions While Using This Medicine

If your symptoms do not improve within a few days, or if they become worse, check with your doctor.

For diabetic patients:

- *This medicine may cause false test results with some urine sugar tests.* Check with your doctor before changing your diet or the dosage of your diabetes medicine.

For patients with phenylketonuria (PKU):

- Cefprozil oral suspension contains phenylalanine. Check with your doctor before taking this medicine.

In some patients, cephalosporins may cause diarrhea:

- Severe diarrhea may be a sign of a serious side effect. *Do not take any diarrhea medicine without first checking with your doctor.* Diarrhea medicines may make your diarrhea worse or make it last longer.

- For mild diarrhea, diarrhea medicine containing kaolin or attapulgite (e.g., Kaopectate tablets, Diasorb) may be taken. However, other kinds of diarrhea medicine should not be taken. They may make your diarrhea worse or make it last longer.

- If you have any questions about this or if mild diarrhea continues or gets worse, check with your health care professional.

For patients receiving *cefamandole, cefmetazole, cefoperazone, or cefotetan by injection:*

- Drinking alcoholic beverages or taking other alcohol-containing preparations (for example, elixirs, cough syrups, tonics, or injections of alcohol) while receiving these medicines may cause problems. The problems may occur if you consume alcohol even several days after you stop taking the cephalosporin. Drinking alcoholic beverages may result in increased side effects such as abdominal or stomach cramps, nausea, vomiting, headache, fainting, fast or irregular heartbeat, difficult breathing, sweating, or redness of the face or skin. These effects usually start within 15 to 30 minutes after you drink alcohol and may not go away for up to several hours. Therefore, *you should not drink alcoholic beverages or take other alcohol-*

containing preparations while you are receiving these medicines and for several days after stopping them.

Side Effects of This Medicine

Along with its needed effects, a medicine may cause some unwanted effects. Although not all of these side effects may occur, if they do occur they may need medical attention.

Check with your doctor immediately if any of the following side effects occur:

Less common or rare

Abdominal or stomach cramps and pain (severe); fever; watery and severe diarrhea, which may also be bloody; (these side effects may also occur up to several weeks after you stop taking this medicine); unusual bleeding or bruising (more common for cefamandole, cefmetazole, cefoperazone, and cefotetan)

Rare

Blistering, peeling, or loosening of skin; convulsions (seizures); decrease in urine output; dizziness or lightheadedness; joint pain; loss of appetite; pain, redness, and swelling at place of injection; skin rash, itching, redness, or swelling; trouble in breathing; unusual tiredness or weakness; yellowing of the eyes or skin

Other side effects may occur that usually do not need medical attention. These side effects may go away during treatment as your body adjusts to the medicine. However, check with your doctor if any of the following side effects continue or are bothersome:

More common (less common with some cephalosporins)

Diarrhea (mild); nausea and vomiting; sore mouth or tongue; stomach cramps (mild)

Less common or rare

Vaginal itching or discharge

Other side effects not listed above may also occur in some patients. If you notice any other effects, check with your doctor.

CHOLESTYRAMINE   Oral

Some commonly used brand names in the U.S. and Canada are Questran and Questran Light.

Description

Cholestyramine (koe-less-TEAR-a-meen) is used to lower high cholesterol levels in the blood. This may help prevent medical problems caused by cholesterol clogging the blood vessels. Cholestyramine is also used to remove substances called bile acids from your body. With some liver problems, there is too much bile acid in your body and this can cause severe itching.

Cholestyramine works by attaching to certain substances in the intestine. Since cholestyramine is not absorbed into the body, these substances also pass out of the body without being absorbed.

Cholestyramine may also be used for other conditions as determined by your doctor.

Cholestyramine is available only with your doctor's prescription, in the following dosage form:

Oral
• Powder (U.S. and Canada)

Before Using This Medicine

In deciding to use a medicine, the risks of taking the medicine must be weighed against the good it will do.

This is a decision you and your doctor will make. For cholestyramine, the following should be considered:

Allergies—Tell your doctor if you have ever had any unusual or allergic reaction to cholestyramine. Also tell your health care professional if you are allergic to any other substances, such as foods, preservatives, or dyes.

Pregnancy—Cholestyramine is not absorbed into the body and is not likely to cause problems. However, it may reduce absorption of vitamins into the body. Ask your doctor whether you need to take extra vitamins.

Breast-feeding—Cholestyramine is not absorbed into the body and is not likely to cause problems. However, the reduced absorption of vitamins by the mother may affect the nursing infant.

Children—This medicine has been tested in a limited number of children. In effective doses, the medicine has not been shown to cause different side effects or problems than it does in adults.

Older adults—Side effects may be more likely to occur in patients over 60 years of age, who are usually more sensitive to the effects of cholestyramine.

Other medicines—Although certain medicines should not be used together at all, in other cases two different medicines may be used together even if an interaction might occur. In these cases, your doctor may want to change the dose, or other precautions may be necessary. When you are taking cholestyramine it is especially important that your health care professional know if you are taking any of the following:

- Anticoagulants (blood thinners)—The effects of the anticoagulant may be changed and this may increase the chance of bleeding.
- Digitalis glycosides (heart medicine) or
- Diuretics (water pills) or

- Penicillin G, taken by mouth or
- Phenylbutazone or
- Propranolol (e.g., Inderal) or
- Tetracyclines, taken by mouth (medicine for infection) or
- Thyroid hormones or
- Vancomycin, taken by mouth—Cholestyramine may prevent these medicines from working properly

Other medical problems—The presence of other medical problems may affect the use of cholestyramine. Make sure you tell your doctor if you have any other medical problems, especially:

- Bleeding problems or
- Constipation or
- Gallstones or
- Heart or blood vessel disease or
- Hemorrhoids or
- Stomach ulcer or other stomach problems or
- Underactive thyroid—Cholestyramine may make these conditions worse
- Kidney disease—There is an increased risk of developing electrolyte problems (problems in the blood)
- Phenylketonuria—Phenylalanine in aspartame is included in the sugar-free brand of cholestyramine and should be avoided. Aspartame can cause problems in people with phenylketonuria. Therefore, it is best if you avoid using the sugar-free product.

Proper Use of This Medicine

Take this medicine exactly as directed by your doctor. Try not to miss any doses and do not take more medicine than your doctor ordered.

This medicine should never be taken in its dry form, since it could cause you to choke. Instead, always mix as follows:

- Place the medicine in 2 ounces of any beverage and mix thoroughly. Then add an additional 2 to 4 ounces of beverage and again mix thoroughly (it will not dissolve) before drinking. After drinking all the liquid containing the medicine, rinse the glass with a little more liquid and drink that also, to make sure you get all the medicine.

- You may also mix this medicine with milk in hot or regular breakfast cereals, or in thin soups such as tomato or chicken noodle soup. Or you may add it to some pulpy fruits such as crushed pineapple, pears, peaches, or fruit cocktail.

For patients taking this medicine *for high cholesterol:*

- Importance of diet—Before prescribing medicine for your condition, your doctor will probably try to control your condition by prescribing a personal diet for you. Such a diet may be low in fats, sugars, and/ or cholesterol. Many people are able to control their condition by carefully following their doctor's orders for proper diet and exercise. Medicine is prescribed only when additional help is needed. *Follow carefully the special diet your doctor gave you,* since the medicine is effective only when a schedule of diet and exercise is properly followed.

- Also, this medicine is less effective if you are greatly overweight. It may be very important for you to go on a reducing diet. However, check with your doctor before going on any diet.

- Remember that this medicine will not cure your cholesterol problem but it will help control it. Therefore, you must continue to take it as directed if you expect to lower your cholesterol level.

Dosing—The dose of cholestyramine will be different for different patients. *Follow your doctor's orders or the directions on the label.* The following information includes only the average doses of cholestyramine. *If your dose is different, do not change it* unless your doctor tells you to do so.

- For *oral* dosage form (powder for oral suspension):
  —For high cholesterol or pruritis (itching) related to biliary obstruction:
    • Adults—At first, 4 grams one or two times a day before meals. Then, your doctor may increase your dose to 8 to 24 grams a day. This is divided into two to six doses.
    • Children—At first, 4 grams a day. This is divided into two doses and taken before meals. Then, your doctor may increase your dose to 8 to 24 grams a day. This is divided into two or more doses.

Missed dose—If you miss a dose of this medicine, take it as soon as possible. Then go back to your regular dosing schedule. However, if it is almost time for your next dose, skip the missed dose and go back to your regular dosing schedule. Do not double doses.

Storage—To store this medicine:
- Keep out of the reach of children.
- Store away from heat and direct light.
- Do not store in the bathroom, near the kitchen sink, or in other damp places. Heat or moisture may cause the medicine to break down.
- Do not keep outdated medicine or medicine no longer needed. Be sure that any discarded medicine is out of the reach of children.

Precautions While Using This Medicine

It is very important that your doctor check your progress at regular visits. This will allow your doctor to see if the medicine is working properly and to decide if you should continue to take it.

Do not take any other medicine unless prescribed by your doctor since cholestyramine may change the effect of other medicines.

Do not stop taking this medicine without first checking with your doctor. When you stop taking this medicine, your blood cholesterol levels may increase again. Your doctor may want you to follow a special diet to help prevent this from happening.

Side Effects of This Medicine

In some animal studies, cholestyramine was found to cause tumors. It is not known whether cholestyramine causes tumors in humans.

Along with its needed effects, a medicine may cause some unwanted effects. Although not all of these side effects may occur, if they do occur they may need medical attention.

Check with your doctor immediately if any of the following side effects occur:

Rare

Black, tarry stools; stomach pain (severe) with nausea and vomiting

Check with your doctor as soon as possible if any of the following side effects occur:

More common

Constipation

Rare

Loss of weight (sudden)

Other side effects may occur that usually do not need medical attention. These side effects may go away during treatment as your body adjusts to the medicine. However, check with your doctor if any of the following side effects continue or are bothersome:

More common

Heartburn or indigestion; nausea or vomiting; stomach pain

Less common
   Belching; bloating; diarrhea; dizziness; headache

Other side effects not listed above may also occur in some patients. If you notice any other effects, check with your doctor.

Additional Information

Once a medicine has been approved for marketing for a certain use, experience may show that it is also useful for other medical problems. Although these uses are not included in product labeling, cholestyramine is used in certain patients with the following medical conditions:
   • Digitalis glycoside overdose
   • Excess oxalate in the urine

Other than the above information, there is no additional information relating to proper use, precautions, or side effects for these uses.

CISAPRIDE   Systemic

Some commonly used brand names are:

In the U.S.—
   Propulsid
In Canada—
   Prepulsid

Description

Cisapride (SIS-a-pride) is a medicine that increases the movements or contractions of the stomach and intestines. It is used to treat symptoms such as heartburn caused by a backward flow of stomach acid into the esophagus.

Cisapride is available only with your doctor's prescription. It is available in the following dosage forms:

Oral

- Oral suspension (Canada)
- Tablets (U.S. and Canada)

Before Using This Medicine

In deciding to use a medicine, the risks of taking the medicine must be weighed against the good it will do. This is a decision you and your doctor will make. For cisapride, the following should be considered:

Allergies—Tell your doctor if you have ever had any unusual or allergic reaction to cisapride. Also tell your health care professional if you are allergic to any other substances, such as foods, preservatives, or dyes.

Pregnancy—Cisapride has not been studied in pregnant women. However, studies in animals have shown that cisapride causes harm to the fetus. Before taking this medicine, make sure your doctor knows if you are pregnant or if you may become pregnant.

Breast-feeding—Although cisapride passes into the breast milk, it has not been shown to cause problems in nursing babies.

Children—This medicine has been tested in a limited number of children. In effective doses, the medicine has not been shown to cause different side effects or problems than it does in adults.

Older adults—Elderly people are especially sensitive to the effects of cisapride. Cisapride stays in the body longer so the dose may be different than in younger people.

Other medicines—Although certain medicines should not be used together at all, in other cases two different medicines may be used together even if an interaction might occur. In these cases, your doctor may want to change the dose, or other precautions may be necessary. When you are taking cisapride, it is especially important that your health care professional know if you are taking any of the following:

- Amantadine (e.g., Symmetrel) or
- Anticholinergics (medicine for abdominal or stomach spasms or cramps) or
- Antidepressants (medicine for depression) or
- Antidyskinetics (medicine for Parkinson's disease or other conditions affecting control of muscles) or
- Antihistamines or
- Antipsychotics (medicine for mental illness) or
- Buclizine (e.g., Bucladin) or
- Carbamazepine (e.g., Tegretol) or
- Cyclizine (e.g., Marezine) or
- Cyclobenzaprine (e.g., Flexeril) or
- Disopyramide (e.g., Norpace) or
- Flavoxate (e.g., Urispas) or
- Ipratropium (e.g., Atrovent) or
- Meclizine (e.g., Antivert) or
- Methylphenidate (e.g., Ritalin) or
- Orphenadrine (e.g., Norflex) or
- Oxybutynin (e.g., Ditropen) or
- Procainamide (e.g., Pronestyl) or
- Promethazine (e.g., Phenergan) or
- Quinidine (e.g., Quinidex) or
- Trimeprazine (e.g., Temaril)—Cisapride may decrease the absorption of these medicines and cause them to be less effective
- Itraconazole (e.g., Sporanox) or
- Ketoconazole (e.g., Nizoral) or
- Miconazole (e.g., Monistat i.v.) or
- Troleandomycin (e.g., Tao)—These medicines may increase the chance of serious side effects and should not be taken with cisapride

Other medical problems—The presence of other medical problems may affect the use of cisapride. Make sure you tell your doctor if you have any other medical problems, especially:

- Abdominal or stomach bleeding or
- Intestinal blockage—Cisapride may make these conditions worse
- Epilepsy or history of seizures—Cisapride has been reported to cause seizures in patients with a history of seizures
- Kidney disease or
- Liver disease—Higher blood levels of cisapride may result and a smaller dose may be needed

Proper Use of This Medicine

Take this medicine 15 minutes before meals and at bedtime with a beverage, unless otherwise directed by your doctor.

Dosing—The dose of cisapride will be different for different patients. *Follow your doctor's orders or the directions on the label.* The following information includes only the average doses of cisapride. *If your dose is different, do not change it* unless your doctor tells you to do so.

- For *oral* dosage forms (tablets and solution):

  —For heartburn caused by gastroesophageal reflux:

  • Adults and children 12 years of age and older: 5 to 20 milligrams (mg) of cisapride two to four times a day. Cisapride should be taken fifteen minutes before meals and at bedtime.

  • Children up to 12 years of age: Dose is based on body weight and must be determined by your doctor. The dose is usually 0.15 to 0.3 mg of cisapride per kilogram (0.07 to 0.14 mg per pound) of body weight three to four times a day, fifteen minutes before meals.

Missed dose—If you miss a dose of this medicine, take it as soon as possible. However, if it is almost time for your next dose, skip the missed dose and go back to your regular dosing schedule. Do not double doses.

Storage—To store this medicine:

- Keep out of the reach of children.
- Store away from heat and direct light.
- Do not store in the bathroom, near the kitchen sink, or in other damp places. Heat or moisture may cause the medicine to break down.
- Keep the medicine from freezing. Do not refrigerate.
- Do not keep outdated medicine or medicine no longer needed. Be sure that any discarded medicine is out of the reach of children.

Precautions While Using This Medicine

This medicine may cause your body to absorb alcohol more quickly than you normally would. Therefore, you may notice the effects sooner. *Check with your doctor before drinking alcohol while you are using this medicine.*

This medicine may cause some people to become drowsy or less alert than they are normally. *Make sure you know how you react to this medicine before you drive, use machines, or do anything else that could be dangerous if you are dizzy or are not alert.*

Side Effects of This Medicine

Along with its needed effects, a medicine may cause some unwanted effects. Although not all of these side effects may occur, if they do occur they may need medical attention.

Check with your doctor immediately if the following side effect occurs:

Rare
    Seizures

Note: Seizures have occurred only in patients with a history of seizures.

Other side effects may occur that usually do not need medical attention. These side effects may go away during treatment as your body adjusts to the medicine. However, check with your doctor if any of the following side effects continue or are bothersome:

Less common

Abdominal cramping, constipation, diarrhea, drowsiness, headache, nausea, unusual tiredness or weakness

Other side effects not listed above may also occur in some patients. If you notice any other effects, check with your doctor.

Additional Information

Once a medicine has been approved for marketing for a certain use, experience may show that it is also useful for other medical problems. Although this use is not included in product labeling, cisapride is used in certain patients with the following medical condition:

• Gastroparesis (stomach condition)

Other than the above information, there is no additional information relating to proper use, precautions, or side effects for this use.

CLARITHROMYCIN Systemic

A commonly used brand name in the U.S. and Canada is Biaxin.

Description

Clarithromycin (kla-RITH-roe-mye-sin) is used to treat bacterial infections in many different parts of the body. It works by killing bacteria or preventing their growth. It is also used to treat *Mycobacterium avium* complex (MAC) infection. However, this medicine will not work for colds, flu, or other virus infections. Clarithromycin may be used for other problems as determined by your doctor.

Clarithromycin is available only with your doctor's prescription, in the following dosage forms:

Oral
- Oral suspension (U.S.)
- Tablets (U.S. and Canada)

Before Using This Medicine

In deciding to use a medicine, the risks of taking the medicine must be weighed against the good it will do. This is a decision you and your doctor will make. For clarithromycin, the following should be considered:

Allergies—Tell your doctor if you have ever had any unusual or allergic reaction to clarithromycin or to any related medicines, such as erythromycin. Also tell your health care professional if you are allergic to any other substances, such as foods, preservatives, or dyes.

Pregnancy—Clarithromycin has not been studied in pregnant women. However, studies in animals have shown that clarithromycin causes birth defects and other problems. Before taking this medicine, make sure your doctor knows if you are pregnant or if you may become pregnant.

Breast-feeding—Clarithromycin passes into breast milk.

Children—Studies on this medicine have not been done in children up to 6 months of age. In effective doses, the medicine has not been shown to cause different side effects or problems in children over the age of 6 months than it does in adults.

Older adults—This medicine has been tested in a limited number of elderly patients and has not been shown to cause different side effects or problems in older people than it does in younger adults.

Other medicines—Although certain medicines should not be used together at all, in other cases two different medicines may be used together even if an interaction might occur. In these cases, your doctor may want to change the dose, or other precautions may be necessary. When you are taking clarithromycin, it is especially important that your health care professional know if you are taking any of the following:

- Carbamazepine (e.g., Tegretol) or
- Terfenadine (e.g., Seldane) or
- Theophylline (e.g., Theodur, Slo-Bid)—Clarithromycin may increase the chance of side effects of these medicines
- Rifabutin (e.g., Mycobutin)—Rifabutin may decrease the amount of clarithromycin in the blood
- Zidovudine (e.g., Retrovir)—Clarithromycin may decrease the amount of zidovudine in the blood

Other medical problems—The presence of other medical problems may affect the use of clarithromycin. Make sure you tell your doctor if you have any other medical problems, especially:

- Kidney disease—Patients with severe kidney disease may have an increased chance of side effects

---

Proper Use of This Medicine

Clarithromycin may be taken with meals or milk or on an empty stomach.

To help clear up your infection completely, *keep taking clarithromycin for the full time of treatment,* even if you begin to feel better after a few days. If you stop taking this medicine too soon, your symptoms may return.

If you are using *clarithromycin oral suspension*, use a specially marked measuring spoon or other device to measure each dose accurately. The average household teaspoon may not hold the right amount of liquid.

Dosing—The dose of clarithromycin will be different for different patients. *Follow your doctor's orders or the directions on the label*. The following information includes only the average doses of clarithromycin. Your dose may be different if you have kidney disease. *If your dose is different, do not change it* unless your doctor tells you to do so:

The number of tablets or teaspoonfuls of suspension that you take depends on the strength of the medicine.

- For *oral* dosage forms (suspension and tablets):
  —For bacterial infections:
    - Adults and teenagers—250 to 500 milligrams (mg) every twelve hours for seven to fourteen days.
    - Children 6 months of age and older—Use and dose must be determined by your doctor. However, 7.5 mg per kilogram (kg) (3.4 mg per pound) of body weight every twelve hours has been used.
  —For treatment of *Mycobacterium avium* complex (MAC):
    - Adults and teenagers—500 mg every twelve hours.
    - Children 6 months of age and older—7.5 mg per kg (3.4 mg per pound) of body weight, up to 500 mg, every twelve hours.

Missed dose—If you miss a dose of this medicine, take it as soon as possible. However, if it is almost time for your next dose, skip the missed dose and go back to your regular dosing schedule. Do not double doses.

Storage—To store this medicine:
* Keep out of the reach of children.
* Store away from heat and direct light.
* Do not store in the bathroom, near the kitchen sink, or in other damp places. Heat or moisture may cause the medicine to break down.
* Do not keep outdated medicine or medicine no longer needed. Be sure that any discarded medicine is out of the reach of children.

Precautions While Using This Medicine

If your symptoms do not improve within a few days, or if they become worse, check with your doctor.

Side Effects of This Medicine

Along with its needed effects, a medicine may cause some unwanted effects. Although neither of these side effects may occur, if they do occur they may need medical attention. Check with your doctor as soon as possible if either of the following side effects occur:

Rare

Unusual bleeding or bruising

Other side effects may occur that usually do not need medical attention. These side effects may go away during treatment as your body adjusts to the medicine. However, check with your doctor if any of the following side effects continue or are bothersome:

Less common

Abnormal taste; diarrhea; headache; nausea; stomach pain or discomfort; vomiting

Other side effects not listed above may also occur in some patients. If you notice any other effects, check with your doctor.

Additional Information

Once a medicine has been approved for marketing for a certain use, experience may show that it is also useful for other medical problems. Although this use is not included in product labeling, clarithromycin is used in certain patients with the following medical condition:

- Legionnaires' disease

Other than the above information, there is no additional information relating to proper use, precautions, or side effects for this use.

CLINDAMYCIN   Systemic

Some commonly used brand names are:

In the U.S.
    Cleocin
    Cleocin Pediatric
    Generic name product may also be available.

In Canada
    Dalacin C   Dalacin C Phosphate
    Dalacin C Palmitate

Description

Clindamycin (klin-da-MYE-sin) is used to treat bacterial infections. It will not work for colds, flu, or other virus infections.

Clindamycin is available only with your doctor's prescription, in the following dosage forms:

Oral

- Capsules (U.S. and Canada)
- Oral solution (U.S. and Canada)

Parenteral

- Injection (U.S. and Canada)

Before Using This Medicine

In deciding to use a medicine, the risks of taking the medicine must be weighed against the good it will do. This is a decision you and your doctor will make. For clindamycin, the following should be considered:

Allergies—Tell your doctor if you have ever had any unusual or allergic reaction to clindamycin, lincomycin, or doxorubicin. Also tell your health care professional if you are allergic to any other substances, such as foods, preservatives, or dyes.

Pregnancy—Clindamycin has not been reported to cause birth defects or other problems in humans.

Breast-feeding—Clindamycin passes into the breast milk. However, clindamycin has not been reported to cause problems in nursing babies.

Children—This medicine has been tested in children and, in effective doses, has not been reported to cause different side effects or problems than it does in adults.

Older adults—Many medicines have not been studied specifically in older people. Therefore, it may not be known whether they work exactly the same way they do in younger adults or if they cause different side effects or problems in older people. There is no specific information comparing use of clindamycin in the elderly with use in other age groups.

Other medicines—Although certain medicines should not be used together at all, in other cases two different medicines may be used together even if an interaction might occur. In these cases, your doctor may want to change the dose, or other precautions may be necessary. When you are taking clindamycin, it is especially important that your health care professional know if you are taking any of the following:

- Chloramphenicol (e.g., Chloromycetin) or
- Diarrhea medicine containing kaolin or attapulgite or
- Erythromycins (medicine for infection)—Taking these medicines along with clindamycin may decrease the effects
  of clindamycin

Other medical problems—The presence of other medical
problems may affect the use of clindamycin. Make sure
you tell your doctor if you have any other medical problems, especially:

- Kidney disease (severe) or
- Liver disease (severe)—Severe kidney or liver disease may
  increase blood levels of this medicine, increasing the
  chance of side effects
- Stomach or intestinal disease, history of (especially colitis,
  including colitis caused by antibiotics, or enteritis)—Patients with a history of stomach or intestinal disease may
  have an increased chance of side effects

Proper Use of This Medicine

For patients taking the *capsule form* of clindamycin:

- *The capsule form of clindamycin should be taken with
  a full glass (8 ounces) of water or with meals* to
  prevent irritation of the esophagus (tube between the
  throat and stomach).

For patients taking the *oral liquid form* of clindamycin:

- Use a specially marked measuring spoon or other device to measure each dose accurately. The average
  household teaspoon may not hold the right amount
  of liquid.
- Do not use after the expiration date on the label. The
  medicine may not work properly after this date.
  Check with your pharmacist if you have any questions about this.

To help clear up your infection completely, *keep taking
this medicine for the full time of treatment,* even if you

begin to feel better after a few days. *If you have a "strep" infection, you should keep taking this medicine for at least 10 days. This is especially important in "strep" infections. Serious heart problems could develop later* if your infection is not cleared up completely. Also, if you stop taking this medicine too soon, your symptoms may return.

This medicine works best when there is a constant amount in the blood. *To help keep the amount constant, do not miss any doses. Also, it is best to take each dose at evenly spaced times day and night.* For example, if you are to take 4 doses a day, doses should be spaced about 6 hours apart. If this interferes with your sleep or other daily activities, or if you need help in planning the best times to take your medicine, check with your health care professional.

Dosing—The dose of clindamycin will be different for different patients. *Follow your doctor's orders or the directions on the label.* The following information includes only the average doses of clindamycin. *If your dose is different, do not change it* unless your doctor tells you to do so.

The number of capsules or teaspoonfuls of solution that you take depends on the strength of the medicine. Also, *the number of doses you take each day, the time allowed between doses, and the length of time you take the medicine depend on the medical problem for which you are taking clindamycin.*

• For bacterial infection:

—For *oral* dosage forms (capsules and solution):

    • Adults and teenagers—150 to 300 milligrams (mg) every six hours.

    • Children—

        —Infants up to 1 month of age: Use and dose must be determined by your doctor.

        —Infants and children 1 month of age and older: Dose is based on body weight. The usual dose is 2 to 5 mg per kilogram (kg) (0.9 to 2.3 mg per pound) of body weight every six hours; or 2.7 to 6.7 mg per kg (1.2 to 3.0 mg per pound) of body weight every eight hours.

—For *injection* dosage form:

• Adults and teenagers—300 to 600 mg every six to eight hours injected into a muscle or vein; or 900 mg every eight hours injected into a muscle or vein.

• Children—

—Infants up to 1 month of age: Dose is based on body weight. The usual dose is 3.75 to 5 mg per kg (1.7 to 2.3 mg per pound) of body weight every six hours injected into a muscle or vein; or 5 to 6.7 mg per kg (2.3 to 3.0 mg per pound) of body weight every eight hours injected into a muscle or vein.

—Infants and children 1 month of age and older: Dose is based on body weight. The usual dose is 3.75 to 10 mg per kg (1.7 to 4.5 mg per pound) of body weight every six hours injected into a muscle or vein; or 5 to 13.3 mg per kg (2.3 to 6.0 mg per pound) of body weight every eight hours injected into a muscle or vein.

Missed dose—If you miss a dose of this medicine, take it as soon as possible. This will help to keep a constant amount of medicine in the blood. However, if it is almost time for your next dose, skip the missed dose and go back to your regular dosing schedule. Do not double doses.

Storage—To store this medicine:

• Keep out of the reach of children.

• Store away from heat and direct light.

• Do not store the capsule form of this medicine in the bathroom, near the kitchen sink, or in other damp places. Heat or moisture may cause the medicine to break down.

- Do not refrigerate the oral liquid form of clindamycin. If chilled, the liquid may thicken and be difficult to pour. Follow the directions on the label.

- Do not keep outdated medicine or medicine no longer needed. Be sure that any discarded medicine is out of the reach of children.

Precautions While Using This Medicine

It is important that your doctor check your progress at regular visits.

If your symptoms do not improve within a few days, or if they become worse, check with your doctor.

In some patients, clindamycin may cause diarrhea.

- Severe diarrhea may be a sign of a serious side effect. *Do not take any diarrhea medicine without first checking with your doctor.* Diarrhea medicines, such as loperamide (Imodium A-D) or diphenoxylate and atropine (Lomotil), may make your diarrhea worse or make it last longer.

- For mild diarrhea, diarrhea medicine containing attapulgite (e.g., Kaopectate tablets, Diasorb) may be taken. However, attapulgite may keep clindamycin from being absorbed into the body. Therefore, these diarrhea medicines should be taken at least 2 hours before or 3 to 4 hours after you take clindamycin by mouth.

- If you have any questions about this or if mild diarrhea continues or gets worse, check with your health care professional.

Before having surgery (including dental surgery) with a general anesthetic, tell the medical doctor or dentist in charge that you are taking clindamycin.

Side Effects of This Medicine

Along with its needed effects, a medicine may cause some unwanted effects. Although not all of these side effects may occur, if they do occur they may need medical attention.

Check with your doctor immediately if any of the following side effects occur:

> *More common*
>> Abdominal or stomach cramps and pain (severe); abdominal tenderness; diarrhea (watery and severe), which may also be bloody; fever (side effects may also occur up to several weeks after you stop taking this medicine)

> *Less common*
>> Sore throat and fever; skin rash, redness, and itching; unusual bleeding or bruising

Other side effects may occur that usually do not need medical attention. These side effects may go away during treatment as your body adjusts to the medicine. However, check with your doctor if any of the following side effects continue or are bothersome:

> *More common*
>> Diarrhea (mild); nausea and vomiting; stomach pain

> *Less common*
>> Itching of rectal or genital (sex organ) areas

Other side effects not listed above may also occur in some patients. If you notice any other effects, check with your doctor.

CLONIDINE   Systemic

Some commonly used brand names are:

In the U.S.—
   Catapres
   Catapres-TTS
   Generic name product may also be available.

In Canada—
   Catapres
   Dixarit

Description

Clonidine (KLOE-ni-deen) belongs to the general class of medicines called antihypertensives. It is used to treat high blood pressure (hypertension).

High blood pressure adds to the workload of the heart and arteries. If it continues for a long time, the heart and arteries may not function properly. This can damage the blood vessels of the brain, heart, and kidneys, resulting in a stroke, heart failure, or kidney failure. Hypertension may also increase the risk of heart attacks. These problems may be less likely to occur if blood pressure is controlled.

Clonidine works by controlling nerve impulses along certain nerve pathways. As a result, it relaxes blood vessels so that blood passes through them more easily. This helps to lower blood pressure.

Clonidine may also be used for other conditions as determined by your doctor.

Clonidine is available only with your doctor's prescription, in the following dosage forms:

   Oral
   • Tablets (U.S. and Canada)
   Transdermal
   • Skin patch (U.S.)

Before Using This Medicine

In deciding to use a medicine, the risks of taking the medicine must be weighed against the good it will do. This is a decision you and your doctor will make. For clonidine, the following should be considered:

Allergies—Tell your doctor if you have ever had any unusual or allergic reaction to clonidine. Also tell your health care professional if you are allergic to any other substance, such as foods, preservatives, or dyes.

Pregnancy—Clonidine has not been studied in pregnant women. However, studies in animals have shown that clonidine causes harmful effects in the fetus, but not birth defects.

Breast-feeding—Although clonidine passes into breast milk, it has not been reported to cause problems in nursing babies.

Children—Children may be more sensitive than adults to clonidine. Clonidine overdose has been reported when children accidentally took this medicine.

Older adults—Dizziness or faintness may be more likely to occur in the elderly, who are more sensitive than younger adults to the effects of clonidine.

Other medicines—Although certain medicines should not be used together at all, in other cases two different medicines may be used together even if an interaction might occur. In these cases, your doctor may want to change the dose, or other precautions may be necessary. When you are taking clonidine, it is especially important that your health care professional know if you are taking any of the following:
  • Beta-blockers (acebutolol [e.g., Sectral], atenolol [e.g., Tenormin], betaxolol [e.g., Kerlone], carteolol [e.g., Cartrol], labetalol [e.g., Normodyne], metoprolol [e.g., Lopressor],

nadolol [e.g., Corgard], oxprenolol [e.g., Trasicor], penbutolol [e.g., Levatol], pindolol [e.g., Visken], propranolol [e.g., Inderal], sotalol [e.g., Sotacor], timolol [e.g., Blocadren])—These medicines may increase the risk of harmful effects when clonidine treatment is stopped suddenly

- Tricyclic antidepressants (amitriptyline [e.g., Elavil], amoxapine [e.g., Asendin], clomipramine [e.g., Anafranil], desipramine [e.g., Pertofrane], doxepin [e.g., Sinequan], imipramine [e.g., Tofranil], nortriptyline [e.g., Aventyl], protriptyline [e.g., Vivactil], trimipramine [e.g., Surmontil])—These medicines may decrease clonidine's effects on blood pressure

Other medical problems—The presence of other medical problems may affect the use of clonidine. Make sure you tell your doctor if you have any other medical problems, especially:

- Heart or blood vessel disease—Clonidine may make these conditions worse
- Irritated or scraped skin (with transdermal system [skin patch] only)—The effects of clonidine may be increased if the skin patch is placed on an area of scraped or irritated skin because more medicine is absorbed into the body
- Kidney disease—Effects of clonidine may be increased because of slower removal of clonidine from the body
- Mental depression (history of) or
- Raynaud's syndrome—Clonidine may make these conditions worse
- Polyarteritis nodosa or
- Scleroderma or
- Systemic lupus erythematosus (SLE)—with transdermal system (skin patch) only—Effects of clonidine may be decreased because absorption of this medicine into the body is blocked

---

Proper Use of This Medicine

For patients taking this medicine *for high blood pressure:*

- In addition to the use of the medicine your doctor

has prescribed, treatment for your high blood pressure
may include weight control and care in the types of
foods you eat, especially foods high in sodium. Your
doctor will tell you which of these are most important
for you. You should check with your doctor before
changing your diet.

- Many patients who have high blood pressure will not
notice any signs of the problem. In fact, many may
feel normal. It is very important that you *take your
medicine exactly as directed* and that you keep your
appointments with your doctor even if you feel well.

- Remember that this medicine will not cure your high
blood pressure but it does help control it. Therefore,
you must continue to use it as directed if you expect
to lower your blood pressure and keep it down. *You
may have to take high blood pressure medicine for
the rest of your life*. If high blood pressure is not
treated, it can cause serious problems such as heart
failure, blood vessel disease, stroke, or kidney
disease.

For patients using the *transdermal system (skin patch)*:

- *Use this medicine exactly as directed by your doctor.*
It will work only if applied correctly. *This medicine
usually comes with patient instructions. Read them
carefully before using.*

- Do not try to trim or cut the adhesive patch to adjust
the dosage. Check with your doctor if you think the
medicine is not working as it should.

- Apply the patch to a clean, dry area of skin on your
upper arm or chest. Choose an area with little or no
hair and free of scars, cuts, or irritation.

- The system should stay in place even during showering, bathing, or swimming. If the patch becomes
loose, cover it with the extra adhesive overlay provided. Apply a new patch if the first one becomes
too loose or falls off.

- Each dose is best applied to a different area of skin to prevent skin problems or other irritation.

- After removing a used patch, fold the patch in half with the sticky sides together. Make sure to dispose of it out of the reach of children.

To help you remember to use your medicine, try to get into the habit of using it at regular times. If you are taking the tablets, take them at the same time each day. If you are using the transdermal system (skin patch), try to change it at the same time and day of the week.

Dosing—The dose of clonidine will be different for different patients. *Follow your doctor's orders or the directions on the label.* The following information includes only the average doses of clonidine used for the treatment of high blood pressure. *If your dose is different, do not change it* unless your doctor tells you to do so:

- For *oral* dosage form (tablets):

  —For high blood pressure:

    • Adults—100 mcg (0.1 mg) two times a day. Your doctor may increase your dose up to 200 mcg (0.2 mg) to 600 mcg (0.6 mg) a day taken in divided doses.

    • Children—Use and dose must be determined by your doctor.

- For *transdermal* dosage form (skin patch):

  —For high blood pressure:

    • Adults—One transdermal dosage system (skin patch) applied once a week.

    • Children—Use and dose must be determined by your doctor.

Missed dose—If you miss a dose of this medicine, take it or use it as soon as possible. Then go back to your regular dosing schedule. *If you miss 2 or more doses of the tablets in a row or if you miss changing the transder-*

mal patch for 3 or more days, check with your doctor right away. If your body goes without this medicine for too long, your blood pressure may go up to a dangerously high level and some unpleasant effects may occur.

Storage—To store this medicine:
- Keep out of the reach of children.
- Store away from heat and direct light.
- Do not store in the bathroom, near the kitchen sink, or in other damp places. Heat or moisture may cause the medicine to break down.
- Do not keep outdated medicine or medicine no longer needed. Be sure that any discarded medicine is out of the reach of children.

Precautions While Using This Medicine

It is important that your doctor check your progress at regular visits to make sure that this medicine is working properly.

Check with your doctor before you stop using this medicine. Your doctor may want you to reduce gradually the amount you are using before stopping completely.

Make sure that you have enough clonidine on hand to last through weekends, holidays, or vacations. You should not miss any doses. You may want to ask your doctor for another written prescription for clonidine to carry in your wallet or purse. You can then have it filled if you run out of medicine when you are away from home.

For patients taking this medicine *for high blood pressure:*
- *Do not take other medicines unless they have been discussed with your doctor.* This especially includes over-the-counter (nonprescription) medicines for appetite control, asthma, colds, cough, hay fever, or

sinus problems, since they may tend to increase your blood pressure.

Clonidine will add to the effects of alcohol and other CNS depressants (medicines that slow down the nervous system, possibly causing drowsiness). Some examples of CNS depressants are antihistamines or medicine for hay fever, other allergies, or colds; sedatives, tranquilizers, or sleeping medicine; prescription pain medicine or narcotics; barbiturates; medicine for seizures; muscle relaxants; or anesthetics, including some dental anesthetics. *Check with your doctor before taking any of the above while you are using this medicine.*

Clonidine may cause some people to become drowsy or less alert than they are normally. This is more likely to happen when you begin to take it or when you increase the amount of medicine you are taking. *Make sure you know how you react to this medicine before you drive, use machines, or do anything else that could be dangerous if you are not alert.*

Before having any kind of surgery (including dental surgery) or emergency treatment, *tell the medical doctor or dentist in charge that you are using this medicine.*

Dizziness, lightheadedness, or fainting may occur after you take this medicine, especially when you get up from a lying or sitting position. Getting up slowly may help, but if the problem continues or gets worse, check with your doctor.

The dizziness, lightheadedness, or fainting is also more likely to occur if you drink alcohol, stand for long periods of time, exercise, or if the weather is hot. While you are taking clonidine, be careful to limit the amount of alcohol you drink. Also, use extra care during exercise or hot weather or if you must stand for a long time.

Clonidine may cause dryness of the mouth. For temporary relief, use sugarless candy or gum, melt bits of ice in your mouth, or use a saliva substitute. However, if your mouth continues to feel dry for more than 2 weeks, check with your medical doctor or dentist. Continuing dryness of the mouth may increase the chance of dental disease, including tooth decay, gum disease, and fungus infections.

Side Effects of This Medicine

Along with its needed effects, a medicine may cause some unwanted effects. Although not all of these side effects may occur, if they do occur they may need medical attention.

Check with your doctor immediately if any of the following side effects occur:

> *Signs and symptoms of overdose*
> > Difficulty in breathing; dizziness (extreme) or faintness; pinpoint pupils of eyes; slow heartbeat; unusual tiredness or weakness (extreme)

Check with your doctor as soon as possible if any of the following side effects occur:

> *More common—with transdermal system (skin patch) only*
> > Itching or redness of skin

> *Less common*
> > Mental depression; swelling of feet and lower legs

> *Rare*
> > Paleness or cold feeling in fingertips and toes; vivid dreams or nightmares

Other side effects may occur that usually do not need medical attention. These side effects may go away during treatment as your body adjusts to the medicine. However, check with your doctor if any of the following side effects continue or are bothersome:

> *More common*
> > Constipation; dizziness; drowsiness; dryness of mouth; unusual tiredness or weakness

Less common

Darkening of skin—with transdermal system (skin patch) only; decreased sexual ability; dizziness, lightheadedness, or fainting, especially when getting up from a lying or sitting position; dry, itching, or burning eyes; loss of appetite; nausea or vomiting; nervousness

After you have been using this medicine for a while, it may cause unpleasant or even harmful effects if you stop taking it too suddenly. After you stop taking this medicine, *check with your doctor immediately* if any of the following occur:

Anxiety or tenseness; chest pain; fast or pounding heartbeat; headache; increased salivation; nausea; nervousness; restlessness; shaking or trembling of hands and fingers; stomach cramps; sweating; trouble in sleeping; vomiting

Other side effects not listed above may also occur in some patients. If you notice any other effects, check with your doctor.

Additional Information

Once a medicine has been approved for marketing for a certain use, experience may show that it is also useful for other medical problems. Although this use is not included in product labeling, clonidine is used in certain patients with the following medical conditions:

- Migraine headache
- Symptoms associated with menopause or menstrual discomfort
- Symptoms of withdrawal associated with alcohol, nicotine, or narcotics
- Gilles de la Tourette's syndrome

Other than the above information, there is no additional information relating to proper use, precautions, or side effects for these uses.

CLOZAPINE   Systemic

Some commonly used brand names are:

In the U.S. and Canada—
    Clozaril

Other—
    Leponex

Description

Clozapine (KLOE-za-peen) is used to treat schizophrenia in patients who have not been helped by or are unable to take other medicines.

Clozapine is only available from pharmacies that agree to participate with your doctor in a plan to monitor your blood tests. You will need to have blood tests done every week, and you will receive a 7-day supply of clozapine only if the results of your blood tests show that it is safe for you to take this medicine.

Clozapine is available in the following dosage form:

Oral

   • Tablets (U.S. and Canada)

Before Using This Medicine

In deciding to use a medicine, the risks of taking the medicine must be weighed against the good it will do. This is a decision you and your doctor will make. For clozapine, the following should be considered:

Allergies—Tell your doctor if you have ever had any unusual or allergic reaction to clozapine. Also tell your health care professional if you are allergic to any other substance, such as foods, preservatives, or dyes.

Pregnancy—Clozapine has not been studied in pregnant women. However, clozapine has not been shown to cause birth defects or other problems in animal studies.

Breast-feeding—Clozapine may pass into breast milk and cause sedation, decreased suckling, restlessness or irritability, seizures, or heart or blood vessel problems in nursing babies.

Children—Studies on this medicine have been done only in adult patients, and there is no specific information comparing use of clozapine in children with use in other age groups.

Older adults—Many medicines have not been tested in older people. Therefore, it may not be known whether they work exactly the same way they do in younger adults. Clozapine may be more likely to cause side effects in the elderly, including dizziness and fainting, low blood pressure, and confusion or excitement.

Other medicines—Although certain medicines should not be used together at all, in other cases two different medicines may be used together even if an interaction might occur. In these cases, your doctor may want to change the dose, or other precautions may be necessary. When you are taking clozapine, it is especially important that your health care professional know if you are taking any of the following:

- Alcohol or
- Central nervous system (CNS) depressants (medicines that cause drowsiness) or
- Tricyclic antidepressants (medicine for depression)—Clozapine may cause an increase in sedation or effects on the heart, or increase the risk of seizures
- Amphotericin B by injection (e.g., Fungizone) or
- Antineoplastics (cancer medicine) or
- Antithyroid agents (medicine for overactive thyroid) or
- Azathioprine (e.g., Imuran) or
- Chlorambucil (e.g., Leukeran) or

- Chloramphenicol (e.g., Chloromycetin) or
- Colchicine or
- Cyclophosphamide (e.g., Cytoxan) or
- Flucytosine (e.g., Ancobon) or
- Interferon (e.g., Intron A, Roferon-A) or
- Mercaptopurine (e.g., Purinethol) or
- Methotrexate (e.g., Mexate) or
- Plicamycin (e.g., Mithracin) or
- Zidovudine (e.g., Retrovir)—Taking clozapine with any of these medicines may cause increased blood problems
- Lithium—Using clozapine with lithium may increase the risk of seizures, or cause confusion or body movement disorders

Other medical problems—The presence of other medical problems may affect the use of clozapine. Make sure you tell your doctor if you have any other medical problems, especially:

- Blood diseases or
- Enlarged prostate or difficult urination or
- Gastrointestinal problems or
- Heart or blood vessel problems—Clozapine may make the condition worse
- Epilepsy or other seizure disorder—Clozapine may increase the risk of seizures
- Kidney or liver disease—Higher blood levels of clozapine may occur, increasing the chance of side effects

---

Proper Use of This Medicine

Take this medicine exactly as directed. Do not take more of this medicine and do not take it more often than your doctor ordered. Do not miss any doses.

This medicine has been prescribed for your current medical problem only. It must not be given to other people or used for other problems unless you are directed to do so by your doctor.

Dosing—The dose of clozapine will be different for different patients. *Follow your doctor's orders or the directions on the label.* The following information includes only the average doses of clozapine. *If your dose is different, do not change it* unless your doctor tells you to do so.

The number of tablets that you take depends on the strength of the medicine. Also, *the number of doses you take each day, the time allowed between doses, and the length of time you take the medicine depend on your special needs.*

- For *oral* dosage form (tablets):
  —For schizophrenia:
    - Adults—At first, 25 milligrams (mg) once or twice a day. Your doctor may increase your dose as needed. However, the dose is usually not more than 900 mg a day.
    - Children up to 16 years of age—Use and dose must be determined by your doctor.

Missed dose—If you miss a dose of this medicine, take it as soon as possible. However, if it is almost time for your next dose, skip the missed dose and go back to your regular dosing schedule. Do not double doses.

Storage—To store this medicine:
- Keep out of the reach of children.
- Store away from heat and direct light.
- Do not store in the bathroom, near the kitchen sink, or in other damp places. Heat or moisture may cause the medicine to break down.
- Do not keep outdated medicine or medicine no longer needed. Be sure that any discarded medicine is out of the reach of children.

Precautions While Using This Medicine

It is important that you have your blood tests done weekly and that your doctor check your progress at regular visits.

This will allow your doctor to make sure the medicine is working properly and to change the dosage if needed.

If you have been using this medicine regularly, do not stop taking it without first checking with your doctor. Your doctor may want you to reduce gradually the amount you are taking before stopping completely.

This medicine will add to the effects of alcohol and other CNS depressants (medicines that slow down the nervous system, possibly causing drowsiness). Some examples of CNS depressants are antihistamines or medicine for hay fever, other allergies, or colds; sedatives, tranquilizers, or sleeping medicine; prescription pain medicine or narcotics; barbiturates; medicine for seizures; muscle relaxants; or anesthetics, including some dental anesthetics. *Check with your doctor before taking any of the above while you are using this medicine.*

Clozapine may cause drowsiness, blurred vision or convulsions (seizures). *Do not drive, climb, swim, operate machines or do anything else that could be dangerous* while you are taking this medicine.

Dizziness, lightheadedness, or fainting may occur, especially when you get up from a lying or sitting position. Getting up slowly may help. If this problem continues or gets worse, check with your doctor.

In some patients, clozapine may cause increased watering of the mouth. Other patients, however, may get dryness of the mouth. For temporary relief of mouth dryness, use sugarless gum or candy, melt bits of ice in your mouth, or use a saliva substitute. However, if your mouth continues to feel dry for more than 2 weeks, check with your medical doctor or dentist. Continuing dryness of the mouth may increase the chance of dental disease, including tooth decay, gum disease, and fungus infections.

Side Effects of This Medicine

Along with its needed effects, a medicine may cause some unwanted effects. Although not all of these side effects may occur, if they do occur they may need medical attention.

Check with your doctor immediately if any of the following side effects occur:

More common

Fast or irregular heartbeat; fever; low blood pressure

Less common

High blood pressure

Rare

Chills; convulsions (seizures); difficult or fast breathing; increased sweating; loss of bladder control; muscle stiffness (severe); sore throat; sores, ulcers, or white spots on lips or in mouth; unusual bleeding or bruising; unusual tiredness or weakness; unusually pale skin

Check with your doctor as soon as possible if any of the following side effects occur:

More common

Dizziness or fainting

Less common

Blurred vision; confusion; restlessness or need to keep moving; trembling; unusual anxiety, nervousness, or irritability

Rare

Absence of or decrease in movement; decreased sexual ability; difficulty in sleeping; difficulty in urinating; headache (severe or continuing); lip smacking or puckering; mental depression; puffing of cheeks; rapid or worm-like movements of tongue; uncontrolled chewing movements; uncontrolled movements of arms and legs

Symptoms of overdose

Dizziness or fainting; drowsiness (severe); fast, slow, or

irregular heartbeat; hallucinations (seeing, hearing, or feeling things that are not there); increased watering of mouth (severe); slow, irregular, or troubled breathing; unusual excitement, nervousness, or restlessness

Other side effects may occur that usually do not need medical attention. These side effects may go away during treatment as your body adjusts to the medicine. However, check with your doctor if any of the following side effects continue or are bothersome:

More common

Constipation; dizziness or lightheadedness (mild); drowsiness; headache (mild); increased watering of mouth; nausea or vomiting; unusual weight gain

Less common

Abdominal discomfort or heartburn; dryness of mouth

Other side effects not listed above may also occur in some patients. If you notice any other effects, check with your doctor.

COLESTIPOL   Oral

A commonly used brand name is:

In the U.S.—
Colestid

In Canada—
Colestid

Description

Colestipol (koe-LES-ti-pole) is used to lower high cholesterol levels in the blood. This may help prevent medical problems caused by cholesterol clogging the blood vessels.

Colestipol works by attaching to certain substances in the intestine. Since colestipol is not absorbed into the body, these substances also pass out of the body without being absorbed.

Colestipol may also be used for other conditions as determined by your doctor.

Colestipol is available only with your doctor's prescription, in the following dosage form:

Oral
- Powder (U.S. and Canada)

Before Using This Medicine

In deciding to use a medicine, the risks of taking the medicine must be weighed against the good it will do. This is a decision you and your doctor will make. For colestipol, the following should be considered:

Allergies—Tell your doctor if you have ever had any unusual or allergic reaction to colestipol. Also tell your health care professional if you are allergic to any substances, such as foods, preservatives, or dyes.

Diet—Before prescribing medicine for your condition, your doctor will probably try to control your condition by prescribing a personal diet for you. Such a diet may be low in fats, sugars, and/or cholesterol. Many people are able to control their condition by carefully following their doctor's orders for proper diet and exercise. Medicine is prescribed only when additional help is needed and is effective only when a schedule of diet and exercise is properly followed.

Also, this medicine is less effective if you are greatly overweight. It may be very important for you to go on a reducing diet. However, check with your doctor before going on any diet.

Make certain your health care professional knows if you are on a low-sodium, low-sugar, or any other special diet.

Pregnancy—Colestipol is not absorbed into the body and is not likely to cause problems. However, it may reduce absorption of vitamins into the body. Ask your doctor whether you need to take extra vitamins.

Breast-feeding—Colestipol is not absorbed into the body and is not likely to cause problems.

Children—There is no specific information comparing use of colestipol in children with use in other age groups. However, use is not recommended in children under 2 years of age since cholesterol is needed for normal development.

Older adults—Side effects may be more likely to occur in patients over 60 years of age, who are usually more sensitive to the effects of colestipol.

Other medicines—Although certain medicines should not be used together at all, in other cases two different medicines may be used together even if an interaction might occur. In these cases, your doctor may want to change the dose, or other precautions may be necessary. When you are taking colestipol it is especially important that your health care professional knows if you are taking any of the following:

- Anticoagulants (blood thinners)—The effects of the anticoagulant may be altered
- Digitalis glycosides (heart medicine) or
- Diuretics (water pills) or
- Penicillin G, taken by mouth, or
- Propranolol, taken by mouth, or
- Tetracyclines (medicine for infection), taken by mouth, or
- Thyroid hormones or
- Vancomycin, taken by mouth—Colestipol may cause these medicines to be less effective; these medicines should be taken 4 to 5 hours apart from colestipol

Other medical problems—The presence of other medical problems may affect the use of colestipol. Make sure you tell your doctor if you have any other medical problems, especially:

- Bleeding problems or
- Constipation or
- Gallstones or
- Heart or blood vessel disease or
- Hemorrhoids or
- Stomach ulcer or other stomach problems or
- Underactive thyroid—Colestipol may make these conditions worse
- Kidney disease—There is an increased risk of developing electrolyte problems
- Liver disease—Cholesterol levels may be raised

Proper Use of This Medicine

Take this medicine exactly as directed by your doctor. Try not to miss any doses and do not take more medicine than your doctor ordered.

Follow carefully the special diet your doctor gave you. This is the most important part of controlling your condition and is necessary if the medicine is to work properly.

This medicine should never be taken in its dry form, since it could cause you to choke. Instead, always mix as follows:

- Add this medicine to 3 ounces or more of water, milk, flavored drink, or your favorite juice or carbonated drink. If you use a carbonated drink, slowly mix in the powder in a large glass to prevent too much foaming. Stir until it is completely mixed (it will *not* dissolve) before drinking. After drinking all the liquid containing the medicine, rinse the glass with a little more liquid and drink that also, to make sure you get all the medicine.
- You may also mix this medicine with milk in hot or regular breakfast cereals, or in thin soups such as

tomato or chicken noodle soup. Or you may add it to some pulpy fruits such as crushed pineapple, pears, peaches, or fruit cocktail.

Dosing—The dose of colestipol will be different for different patients. *Follow your doctor's orders or the directions on the label.* The following information includes only the average doses of colestipol. *If your dose is different, do not change it* unless your doctor tells you to do so.

* For *oral* dosage form (powder for oral suspension):

　—For high cholesterol:

　　* Adults—15 to 30 grams a day. This is divided into two to four doses and taken before meals.
　　* Children—Use and dose must be determined by your doctor.

Missed dose—If you miss a dose of this medicine, take it as soon as possible. Then go back to your regular dosing schedule. However, if it is almost time for your next dose, skip the missed dose and go back to your regular dosing schedule. Do not double doses.

Storage—To store this medicine:

* Keep out of the reach of children.
* Store away from heat and direct light.
* Do not store in the bathroom, near the kitchen sink or in other damp places. Heat or moisture may cause the medicine to break down.
* Do not keep outdated medicine or medicine no longer needed. Be sure that any discarded medicine is out of the reach of children.

Precautions While Using This Medicine

It is very important that your doctor check your progress at regular visits. This will allow your doctor to see if the medicine is working properly to lower your cholesterol levels and to decide if you should continue to take it.

Do not stop taking this medicine without first checking with your doctor. When you stop taking this medicine, your blood cholesterol levels may increase again. Your doctor may want you to follow a special diet to help prevent this from happening.

Do not take any other medicine unless prescribed by your doctor since colestipol may interfere with other medicines.

Side Effects of This Medicine

Along with its needed effects, a medicine may cause some unwanted effects. Although not all of these side effects may occur, if they do occur they may need medical attention.

Check with your doctor immediately if either of the following side effects occurs:

Rare

Black, tarry stools; stomach pain (severe) with nausea and vomiting

Check with your doctor as soon as possible if either of the following side effects occurs:

More common

Constipation

Rare

Loss of weight (sudden)

Other side effects may occur that usually do not need medical attention. These side effects may go away during treatment as your body adjusts to the medicine. However, check with your doctor if any of the following side effects continue or are bothersome:

Less common

   Belching; bloating; diarrhea; dizziness; headache; nausea
     or vomiting; stomach pain

Other side effects not listed above may also occur in some
patients. If you notice any other effects, check with your
doctor.

Additional Information

Once a medicine has been approved for marketing for a
certain use, experience may show that it is also useful for
other medical problems. Although these uses are not included in product labeling, colestipol is used in certain
patients with the following medical conditions:

- Diarrhea caused by bile acids
- Digitalis glycoside overdose
- Excess oxalate in the urine
- Itching (pruritus) associated with partial biliary obstruction

Other than the above information, there is no additional
information relating to proper use, precautions, or side effects for these uses.

CORTICOSTEROIDS Inhalation

Some commonly used brand names are:

In the U.S.—

AeroBid[4]	Beclovent[1]
AeroBid-M[4]	Decadron Respihaler[3]
Azmacort[5]	Vanceril[1]

In Canada—

Azmacort[5]	Bronalide[4]
Beclodisk[1]	Pulmicort Nebuamp[2]
Becloforte[1]	Pulmicort Turbuhaler[2]
Beclovent[1]	Vanceril[1]
Beclovent Rotacaps[1]	

Other commonly used names are:
Beclomethasone dipropionate[1]   Beclometasone dipropionate[1]
Beclometasone[1]

Note: For quick reference, the following corticosteroids are numbered to match the corresponding brand names.

This information applies to the following medicines:

1. Beclomethasone (be-kloe-METH-a-sone)
2. Budesonide (byoo-DESS-oh-nide)*
3. Dexamethasone (dex-a-METH-a-sone)†
4. Flunisolide (floo-NISS-oh-lide)
5. Triamcinolone (trye-am-SIN-oh-lone)

---

*Not commercially available in the U.S.
†Not commercially available in Canada.

Description

Inhalation corticosteroids (kor-ti-koe-STER-oids) are cortisone-like medicines. They are used to help prevent the symptoms of asthma. When used regularly every day, inhalation corticosteroids decrease the number and severity of asthma attacks. However, they will not relieve an asthma attack that has already started.

Inhaled corticosteroids work by preventing certain cells in the lungs and breathing passages from releasing substances that cause asthma symptoms.

This medicine may be used with other asthma medicines, such as bronchodilators (medicines that open up narrowed breathing passages) or other corticosteroids taken by mouth.

Inhalation corticosteroids are available only with your doctor's prescription, in the following dosage forms:

Inhalation

Beclomethasone
- Aerosol (U.S. and Canada)
- Capsules for inhalation (Canada)
- Powder for inhalation (Canada)

Budesonide
- Powder for inhalation (Canada)
- Suspension for inhalation (Canada)

Dexamethasone
- Aerosol (U.S.)

Flunisolide
- Aerosol (U.S. and Canada)

Triamcinolone
- Aerosol (U.S. and Canada)

Before Using This Medicine

In deciding to use a medicine, the risks of taking the medicine must be weighed against the good it will do. This is a decision you and your doctor will make. For inhalation corticosteroids, the following should be considered:

Pregnancy—When used in regular daily doses during pregnancy to keep the mother's asthma under control, these medicines have not been reported to cause breathing problems or birth defects in the baby.

Breast-feeding—It is not known whether inhaled corticosteroids pass into breast milk. Although most medicines pass into breast milk in small amounts, many of them may be used safely while breast-feeding. Mothers who are using this medicine and who wish to breast-feed should discuss this with their doctor.

Children—Inhalation corticosteroids have been tested in children and, in low effective doses, have not been shown to cause different side effects or problems than they do in adults.

There have been a few reports of slowed growth or reduced adrenal gland function in some children using inhaled corticosteroids in recommended doses. However, poorly contolled asthma may cause slowed growth, especially when corticosteroids taken by mouth are needed often. Your doctor will want you to use the lowest possible dose of an inhaled corticosteroid that controls asthma. This will lessen the chance of an effect on growth or adrenal gland function.

Regular use of inhaled corticosteroids may allow some children to stop using or decrease the amount of corticosteroids taken by mouth. This also will reduce the risk of slowed growth or reduced adrenal function.

Children who are using inhaled corticosteroids in large doses should avoid exposure to chickenpox or measles. When a child is exposed or the disease develops, the doctor's directions should be followed carefully.

Before this medicine is given to a child, you and your child's doctor should talk about the good this medicine will do as well as the risks of using it. Follow the doctor's directions very carefully to lessen the chance that unwanted effects will occur.

Older adults—Many medicines have not been studied specifically in older people. Therefore, it may not be known whether they work exactly the same way they do in younger adults. Although there is no specific information comparing use of inhaled corticosteroids in the elderly with use in other age groups, this medicine is not expected to cause different side effects or problems in older people than it does in younger adults.

Other medicines—Although certain medicines should not be used together at all, in other cases two different medicines may be used together even if an interaction might occur. In these cases, your doctor may want to change the dose, or other precautions may be necessary. Tell your health care professional if you are taking any other prescription or nonprescription (over-the-counter [OTC]) medicine.

Other medical problems—The presence of other medical problems may affect the use of inhaled corticosteroids. Make sure you tell your doctor if you have any other medical problems, especially:

- Osteoporosis (bone disease)—Inhaled corticosteroids in high doses may make this condition worse in women who are past menopause and who are not receiving an estrogen replacement
- Tuberculosis (history of)—Use of this medicine may cause a tuberculosis infection to occur again

---

Proper Use of This Medicine

Inhaled corticosteroids will not relieve an asthma attack that has already started. However, your doctor may want you to continue taking this medicine at the usual time, even if you use another medicine to relieve the asthma attack.

Use this medicine only as directed. Do not use more of it and do not use it more often than your doctor ordered. To do so may increase the chance of side effects.

In order for this medicine to help prevent asthma attacks, it must be used every day in regularly spaced doses, as ordered by your doctor. Up to four weeks may pass before you begin to notice improvement in your condition. It may take several months before you feel the full effects of this medicine. This may not take as long if you have already been taking certain other medicines for your asthma.

Gargling and rinsing your mouth with water after each dose may help prevent hoarseness, throat irritation, and infection in the mouth. However, do not swallow the water after rinsing. Your doctor may also want you to use a spacer device to lessen these problems.

Inhaled corticosteroids are used with a special inhaler and usually come with patient directions. *Read the directions carefully before using this medicine.* If you do not understand the directions or you are not sure how to use the inhaler, ask your health care professional to show you what to do. Also, *ask your health care professional to check regularly how you use the inhaler to make sure you are using it properly.*

For patients using *beclomethasone, flunisolide, or triamcinolone inhalation aerosol:*

- When you use the inhaler for the first time, it may not deliver the right amount of medicine with the first puff. Therefore, before using the inhaler, test it to make sure it works properly.

- *To test the inhaler:*

    —Insert the metal canister firmly into the clean mouthpiece according to the manufacturer's instructions. Check to make sure the canister is placed properly into the mouthpiece.

    —Take the cover off the mouthpiece and shake the inhaler three or four times.

    —Hold the canister well away from you against a light background and press the top of the canister, spraying the medicine once into the air. If you see a fine mist, you will know the inhaler is working properly to provide the right amount of medicine when you use it. If you do not see a fine mist, try a second time.

- *To use the inhaler:*

    —Using your thumb and one or two fingers, hold the inhaler upright with the mouthpiece end down and pointing toward you.

    —Take the cover off the mouthpiece. Check the mouthpiece and remove any foreign objects. Then gently shake the inhaler three or four times.

    —Hold the mouthpiece away from your mouth and breathe out slowly and completely.

—Use the inhalation method recommended by your doctor.

- Open-mouth method—Place the mouthpiece about 1 or 2 inches (2 fingerwidths) in front of your widely opened mouth. Make sure the inhaler is aimed into your mouth so that the spray does not hit the roof of your mouth or your tongue.

- Closed-mouth method—Place the mouthpiece in your mouth between your teeth and over your tongue with your lips closed tightly around it. Do not block the mouthpiece with your teeth or tongue.

—Tilt your head back a little. Start to breathe in slowly and deeply through your mouth and, at the same time, press the top of the canister one time to get one puff of medicine. Continue to breathe in slowly for 5 to 10 seconds. Count the seconds while inhaling. It is important to press the top of the canister and breathe in slowly at the same time so the medicine is pulled into your lungs. This step may be difficult at first. If you are using the closed-mouth method and you see a fine mist coming from your mouth or nose, the inhaler is not being used correctly.

—Hold your breath as long as you can up to 10 seconds. This gives the medicine time to settle in your airways and lungs.

—Take the mouthpiece away from your mouth and breathe out slowly.

—If your doctor has told you to inhale more than one puff of medicine at each dose, gently shake the inhaler again, and take the second puff following exactly the same steps you used for the first puff.

—When you are finished, wipe off the mouthpiece and replace the cover to keep the mouthpiece clean and free of foreign objects.

- Your doctor may want you to use a spacer device with the inhaler. A spacer makes the inhaler easier to use. With a spacer, more of the medicine is able to reach your lungs, and less of it stays in the mouth and throat.

—*To use a spacer device with the inhaler:*

- Attach the spacer to the inhaler according to the manufacturer's directions. There are different types of spacers available, but the method of breathing remains the same with most spacers.

- Gently shake the inhaler and spacer three or four times.

- Hold the mouthpiece of the spacer away from your mouth and breathe out slowly to the end of a normal breath.

- Place the mouthpiece into your mouth between your teeth and over your tongue with your lips closed around it.

- Press down on the canister top once to release one puff of medicine into the spacer. Within one or two seconds, start to breathe in slowly and deeply through your mouth for 5 to 10 seconds. Count the seconds while inhaling. Do not breathe in through your nose.

- Then hold your breath as long as you can up to 10 seconds.

- Breathe out slowly. Do not remove the mouthpiece from your mouth. Breathe in and out slowly two or three times to make sure the spacer device is emptied.

- If your doctor has told you to take more than one puff of medicine at each dose, gently shake the inhaler and spacer again and take the second puff, following exactly the same steps you used for the first puff. Do not spray more than one puff at a time into the spacer.

- When you are finished, remove the spacer device from the inhaler and replace the cover of the mouthpiece.

- Clean the inhaler, mouthpiece, and spacer at least twice a week to prevent build-up of medicine and blockage of the mouthpiece.

  —*To clean the inhaler:*

  - Remove the metal canister from the inhaler and set it aside.

  - Wash the mouthpiece and cover, the plastic case, and spacer with soap and warm water. Rinse well with warm, running water.

  - Shake off the excess water and let the inhaler parts air dry completely before replacing the metal canister and cover.

- Check with your pharmacist to see if you should save the inhaler piece that comes with this medicine after the medicine is used up. Refill units may be available at a lower cost. However, remember that the inhaler is meant to be used only for the medicine that comes with it. Do not use the inhaler for any other inhalation aerosol medicine, even if the cartridge fits.

For patients using *beclomethasone capsules for inhalation:*

- *Do not swallow the capsules. The medicine will not work if you swallow it.*

- *To load the inhaler:*

  —Make sure your hands are clean and dry.

  —Do not insert the capsule into the inhaler until just before you are ready to use this medicine.

  —Take the inhaler from its container. Hold the inhaler by the mouthpiece and twist the barrel in either direction until it stops.

  —Take a capsule from its container. Hold the inhaler upright with the mouthpiece pointing downward.

Press the capsule, with the clear end first, firmly into the raised small hole.

—Make sure the top of the capsule is even with the top of the hole. This will push the old used capsule shell, if there is one, into the inhaler.

—Hold the inhaler on its side with the white dot facing up. Twist the barrel quickly until it stops. This will break the capsule into two halves so the powder can be inhaled.

* *To use the inhaler:*

—Hold the inhaler away from your mouth and breathe out slowly to the end of a normal breath.

—Keep the inhaler on its side and place the mouthpiece in your mouth. Close your lips around it, and tilt your head slightly back. Do not block the mouthpiece with your teeth or tongue.

—Breathe in slowly through your mouth until you have taken a full deep breath.

—Take the inhaler from your mouth and hold your breath as long as you can up to 10 seconds. This gives the medicine time to settle in your airways and lungs.

—Hold the inhaler well away from your mouth and breathe out to the end of a normal breath.

—If your doctor has told you to use a second capsule, follow the same steps you used for the first capsule.

—When you have finished using the inhaler, pull the two halves of the inhaler apart and throw away the empty capsule shells. There is no need to remove the shell left in the small hole, except before cleaning.

—Put the two halves of the inhaler back together again and place it into its container to keep it clean.

* *To clean the inhaler:*

—Every two weeks, take the inhaler apart and wash

the two halves of the inhaler in clean, warm water. Make sure the empty capsule shell is removed from the small raised hole.

—Shake out the excess water.

—Allow all parts of the inhaler to dry before you put it back together.

• The inhaler should be replaced every 6 months.

For patients using *beclomethasone powder for inhalation:*

• *To load the inhaler:*

—Make sure your hands are clean and dry.

—Do not insert the cartridge until just before you are ready to use this medicine.

—Take off the dark brown mouthpiece cover and make sure the mouthpiece is clean.

—Hold the white cartridge by the exposed corners and gently pull it out until you see the ribbed sides of the cartridge.

—Squeeze the ribbed sides and take out the cartridge unit from the body of the inhaler.

—Place the disk containing the medicine onto the white wheel with the numbers facing up. Allow the underside of the disk to fit into the holes of the wheel.

—Slide the cartridge unit with wheel and disk back into the body of the inhaler. Gently push the cartridge in and pull it out again. The disk will turn.

—Continue to turn the disk in this way until the number 8 appears in the side indicator window. Each disk has eight blisters containing the medicine. The window will display how many doses you have left after you use it each time, by counting down from 8. For example, when you see the number 1, you have one dose left.

—To replace the empty disk with a full disk, follow

the same steps you used to load the inhaler. Do not throw away the wheel when you discard the empty disk.

• *To use the inhaler:*

—Hold the inhaler flat in your hand. Lift the rear edge of the lid until it is fully upright.

—The plastic needle on the front of the lid will break the blister containing one inhalation of medicine. When the lid is raised as far as it will go, both the upper and the lower surfaces of the blister will be pierced. Do not lift the lid if the cartridge is not in the inhaler. Doing this will break the needle and you will need a new inhaler.

—After the blister is broken open, close the lid. Keeping the inhaler flat and well away from your mouth, breathe out to the end of a normal breath.

—Raise the inhaler to your mouth, and place the mouthpiece in your mouth.

—Close your lips around the mouthpiece and tilt your head slightly back. Do not block the mouthpiece with your teeth or tongue. Do not cover the air holes on the side of the mouthpiece.

—Breathe in through your mouth as fast as you can until you have taken a full deep breath.

—Hold your breath and remove the mouthpiece from your mouth. Continue holding your breath as long as you can up to 10 seconds before breathing out. This gives the medicine time to settle in your airways and lungs.

—Hold the inhaler well away from your mouth and breathe out to the end of a normal breath.

—Prepare the cartridge for your next inhalation. Pull the cartridge out once and push it in once. The disk will turn to the next numbered dose as seen in the indicator window. Do not pierce the blister until just before the inhalation.

- *To clean the inhaler:* Brush away the loose powder each day with the brush provided.

- The inhaler should be replaced every 6 months.

For patients using *budesonide powder for inhalation:*

- *To load the inhaler:*

   —Unscrew the cover of the inhaler and lift it off.

   —Hold the inhaler upright with the brown piece pointing downward. Turn the brown piece of the inhaler in one direction as far as it will go. Then twist it back until it clicks.

- *To use the inhaler:*

   —Hold the inhaler away from your mouth and breathe out slowly to the end of a normal breath.

   —Place the mouthpiece in your mouth and close your lips around it. Tilt your head slightly back. Do not block the mouthpiece with your teeth or tongue.

   —Breathe in quickly and evenly through your mouth until you have taken a full deep breath.

   —Hold your breath and remove the inhaler from your mouth. Continue holding your breath as long as you can up to 10 seconds before breathing out. This gives the medicine time to settle in your airways and lungs.

   —Hold the inhaler well away from your mouth and breathe out to the end of a normal breath.

   —Replace the cover on the mouthpiece to keep it clean.

- When the indicator window begins to show a red mark, there are about 20 doses left. When the red mark covers the window, the inhaler is empty.

For patients using *budesonide suspension for inhalation:*

- This medicine is to be used in a power-operated nebulizer equipped with a face mask or mouthpiece. Your doctor will advise you on which nebulizer to use.

Make sure you understand how to use the nebulizer. If you have any questions about this, check with your doctor.

- Any opened ampul should be protected from light. The medicine in an open ampul must be used within 12 hours after the ampul is opened. Ampuls should be used within 3 months after the envelope containing them is opened.

- *To prepare the medicine for use in the nebulizer:*

  —Remove one ampul from the sheet of five units and shake it gently.

  —Hold the ampul upright. Open it by twisting off the wing.

  —Squeeze the contents of the ampul into the cup of the nebulizer. If you use only half of the contents of an ampul, add enough of the sodium chloride solution provided to dilute the solution.

  —Gently shake the nebulizer. Then attach the face mask to the nebulizer and connect the nebulizer to the air pump.

- *To use the medicine in the nebulizer:*

  —This medicine should be inhaled over a period of 10 to 15 minutes.

  —Breathe slowly and evenly, in and out, until no more mist is left in the nebulizer cup.

  —Rinse your mouth when you are finished with the treatment. Wash your face if you used a face mask.

- *To clean the nebulizer:*

  —After each treatment, wash the cup of the nebulizer and the mask or mouthpiece in warm water with a mild detergent.

  —Allow the nebulizer parts to dry before putting them back together again.

Dosing—The dose of these medicines will be different for different patients. *Follow your doctor's orders or the* *directions on the label.* The following information includes only the average doses of these medicines. *If your dose is different, do not change it* unless your doctor tells you to do so.

For beclomethasone

- For inhalation *aerosol:*

  —For bronchial asthma:

    - Adults and children 12 years of age and older— 84 to 100 micrograms (mcg) (2 puffs) three or four times a day, or 168 to 200 mcg (4 puffs) two times a day. In severe asthma, your doctor may want you to take a higher dose.

    - Children 6 to 12 years of age—42 to 100 mcg (1 or 2 puffs) three or four times a day, or 168 to 200 mcg (4 puffs) two times a day.

    - Children up to 6 years of age—Use and dose must be determined by the doctor.

- For *capsules* for inhalation or *powder* for inhalation:

  —For bronchial asthma:

    - Adults and teenagers 14 years of age and older—At first, 200 mcg three or four times a day. Then your doctor may reduce the dose, based on your condition.

    - Children 6 to 14 years of age—At first, 100 mcg two to four times a day. Then your doctor may reduce the dose, based on your condition.

    - Children up to 6 years of age—Use and dose must be determined by the doctor.

For budesonide

- For *powder* for inhalation:

  —For bronchial asthma:

    - Adults and children 12 years of age and older— At first, 400 to 2400 micrograms (mcg) a day, divided into two to four doses. The higher dose is usually used for treatment of severe asthma or when the dose of corticosteroids taken by mouth is being reduced or stopped. Later, your doctor may reduce the dose to 200 to 400 mcg two times a day.

• Children 6 to 12 years of age—At first, 100 to 200 mcg two times a day. The higher dose is usually used for treatment of severe asthma or when the dose of corticosteroids taken by mouth is being reduced or stopped.

• Children up to 6 years of age—Use and dose must be determined by the doctor.

• For *suspension* for inhalation:

—For bronchial asthma:

• Adults and children 12 years of age and older— 500 to 2000 micrograms (mcg) mixed with enough sterile sodium chloride solution for inhalation, if necessary, to make 2 to 4 milliliters (mL). This solution is used in a nebulizer for a period of ten to fifteen minutes. The medicine should be used two times a day.

• Children 3 months to 12 years of age—250 to 1000 mcg mixed with enough sterile sodium chloride solution for inhalation, if necessary, to make 2 to 4 mL. This solution is used in a nebulizer for a period of ten to fifteen minutes. The medicine should be used two times a day.

• Children up to 3 months of age—Use and dose must be determined by the doctor.

For flunisolide

• For inhalation *aerosol:*

—For bronchial asthma:

• Adults and children 4 years of age and older— 500 micrograms (mcg) (2 puffs) two times a day, morning and evening.

• Children up to 4 years of age—Use and dose must be determined by the doctor.

For triamcinolone

- For inhalation *aerosol:*

  —For bronchial asthma:

  • Adults and children 12 years of age and older—At first, 200 micrograms (mcg) (2 puffs) two to four times a day. Then your doctor may reduce the dose, based on your condition. In severe asthma, your doctor may want you to take a higher dose.

  • Children 6 to 12 years of age—At first, 100 to 200 mcg (1 or 2 puffs) three or four times a day. Then your doctor may adjust your dose, based on your condition.

  • Children up to 6 years of age—Use and dose must be determined by the doctor.

Missed dose—If you miss a dose of this medicine, use it as soon as possible. Then use any remaining doses for that day at regularly spaced times.

Storage—To store this medicine:

- Keep out of the reach of children.
- Store away from heat and direct light.
- Do not store the capsule form of this medicine in the bathroom, near the kitchen sink, or in other damp places. Heat or moisture may cause the medicine to break down.
- Keep the aerosol or suspension form of this medicine from getting too cold or freezing. This medicine may be less effective if the container is cold when you use it.
- Do not puncture, break, or burn the aerosol container, even after it is empty.
- Do not keep outdated medicine or medicine no longer needed. Be sure that any discarded medicine is out of the reach of children.

Precautions While Using This Medicine

Check with your doctor if:

- *You go through a period of unusual stress to your body, such as surgery, injury, or infection.*
- *You have an asthma attack that does not improve after you take a bronchodilator medicine.*
- *Signs of mouth, throat, or lung infection occur.*
- *Your symptoms do not improve or if your condition gets worse.*

Your doctor may want you to carry a medical identification card stating that you are using this medicine and that you may need additional medicine during times of emergency, a severe asthma attack or other illness, or unusual stress.

Before you have any kind of surgery (including dental surgery) or emergency treatment, tell the medical doctor or dentist in charge that you are using this medicine.

For patients who are also regularly taking a corticosteroid by mouth in tablet or liquid form:

- *Do not stop taking the corticosteroid taken by mouth without your doctor's advice, even if your asthma seems better.* Your doctor may want you to reduce gradually the amount you are taking before stopping completely to lessen the chance of unwanted effects.
- When your doctor tells you to reduce the dose, or to stop taking the corticosteroid taken by mouth, follow the directions carefully. Your body may need time to adjust to the change. The length of time this takes may depend on the amount of medicine you were taking and how long you took it. *It is especially important that your doctor check your progress at regular visits during this time.* Ask your doctor if there are special directions you should follow if you have a severe asthma attack, if you need any other medical or surgical treatment, or if certain side effects occur. Be certain that you understand these directions, and follow them carefully.

Side Effects of This Medicine

Along with its needed effects, a medicine may cause some unwanted effects. Although not all of these side effects may occur, if they do occur they may need medical attention.

Check with your doctor immediately if any of the following side effects occur just after you use this medicine:

   Rare

   Troubled breathing, tightness in chest, or wheezing

Also, check with your doctor as soon as possible if any of the following side effects occur:

   Less common

   Creamy white, curd-like patches in the mouth or throat and/or pain when eating or swallowing

   Rare

   Behavior changes; mental depression; nervousness; restlessness; pain or burning in the chest

Other side effects may occur that usually do not need medical attention. These side effects may go away during treatment as your body adjusts to the medicine. However, check with your doctor if any of the following side effects continue or are bothersome:

   More common

   Cough; dry mouth; hoarseness or other voice changes; sore throat

   Less common or rare

   Dry throat; headache; nausea; skin bruising or thinning; unpleasant taste

Other side effects not listed above may also occur in some patients. If you notice any other effects, check with your doctor.

CORTICOSTEROIDS   Nasal

Some commonly used brand names are:

In the U.S.—
Beconase[1]
Beconase AQ[1]
Decadron Turbinaire[3]
Nasacort[5]

Nasalide[4]
Vancenase[1]
Vancenase AQ[1]

In Canada—
Beconase[1]
Beconase AQ[1]
Nasacort[5]
Rhinalar[4]

Rhinocort Aqua[2]
Rhinocort Turbuhaler[2]
Vancenase[1]

Another commonly used name for beclomethasone is beclometasone.

Note: For quick reference, the following corticosteroids are numbered to match the corresponding brand names.

This information applies to the following medicines:

1. Beclomethasone (be-kloe-METH-a-sone)§
2. Budesonide (byoo-DES-oh-nide)*
3. Dexamethasone (dex-a-METH-a-sone)†
4. Flunisolide (floo-NISS-oh-lide)
5. Triamcinolone (trye-am-SIN-oh-lone)

---

*Not commercially available in the U.S.
†Not commercially available in Canada.
§Generic name product may also be available in Canada.

Description

Nasal corticosteroids (kor-ti-ko-STER-oids) are cortisone-like medicines. They belong to the family of medicines called steroids. These medicines are sprayed or inhaled into the nose to help relieve the stuffy nose, irritation, and discomfort of hay fever, other allergies, and other nasal problems. These medicines are also used to prevent nasal polyps from growing back after they have been removed by surgery.

These medicines are available only with your doctor's prescription, in the following dosage forms:

Nasal

Beclomethasone
- Aerosol (U.S. and Canada)
- Solution (U.S. and Canada)

Budesonide
- Powder (Canada)
- Solution (Canada)

Dexamethasone
- Aerosol (U.S.)

Flunisolide
- Solution (U.S. and Canada)

Triamcinolone
- Aerosol (U.S. and Canada)

Before Using This Medicine

In deciding to use a medicine, the risks of taking the medicine must be weighed against the good it will do. This is a decision you and your doctor will make. For corticosteroids, the following should be considered:

Allergies—Tell your doctor if you have ever had any unusual or allergic reaction to corticosteroids. Also tell your health care professional if you are allergic to any other substances, such as foods, preservatives, or dyes.

Pregnancy—In one human study, use of beclomethasone oral inhalation by pregnant women did not cause birth defects or other problems. Studies on birth defects with budesonide, dexamethasone, flunisolide, or triamcinolone have not been done in humans.

In animal studies, corticosteroids taken by mouth or injection during pregnancy were shown to cause birth defects. Also, too much use of corticosteroids during pregnancy may cause other unwanted effects in the infant, such as slower growth and reduced adrenal gland function.

If corticosteroids are medically necessary during pregnancy to control nasal problems, nasal corticosteroids are generally considered safer than corticosteroids taken by mouth or injection. Also, use of nasal corticosteroids may allow some patients to stop using or decrease the amount of corticosteroids taken by mouth or injection.

Breast-feeding—Use of dexamethasone is not recommended in nursing mothers, since dexamethasone passes into breast milk and may affect the infant's growth.

It is not known whether beclomethasone, budesonide, flunisolide, or triamcinolone passes into breast milk. Although most medicines pass into breast milk in small amounts, many of them may be used safely while breast-feeding. Mothers who are taking this medicine and who wish to breast-feed should discuss this with their doctor.

Children—Corticosteroids taken by mouth or injection have been shown to slow or stop growth in children and cause reduced adrenal gland function. If corticosteroids are medically necessary to control nasal problems in a child, nasal corticosteroids are generally considered to be safer than corticosteroids taken by mouth or injection. Most nasal corticosteroids have not been shown to affect growth. Also, use of most nasal corticosteroids may allow some children to stop using or decrease the amount of corticosteroids taken by mouth or injection.

Before this medicine is given to a child, you and your child's doctor should talk about the good this medicine will do as well as the risks of using it. Follow the doctor's directions very carefully to lessen the chance of unwanted effects.

Older adults—Although there is no specific information comparing use of nasal corticosteroids in the elderly with use in other age groups, they are not expected to cause different side effects or problems in older people than they do in younger adults.

Other medicines—Although certain medicines should not be used together at all, in other cases two different medi-

cines may be used together even if an interaction might occur. In these cases, your doctor may want to change the dose, or other precautions may be necessary. Tell your health care professional if you are taking any prescription or nonprescription (over-the-counter [OTC]) medicines.

Other medical problems—The presence of other medical problems may affect the use of corticosteroids. Make sure you tell your doctor if you have any other medical problems, especially:

- Amebiasis—Nasal corticosteroids may make this condition worse
- Glaucoma—Long-term use of nasal corticosteroids may worsen glaucoma by increasing the pressure within the eye
- Herpes simplex (virus) infection of the eye or
- Infections (virus, bacteria, or fungus)—Nasal corticosteroids may cover up the signs of these conditions
- Injury to the nose (recent) or
- Nose surgery (recent) or
- Sores in the nose—Nasal corticosteroids may prevent proper healing of these conditions
- Liver disease
- Tuberculosis (active or history of)
- Underactive thyroid

Proper Use of This Medicine

This medicine usually comes with patient directions. *Read them carefully before using the medicine.* Beclomethasone, budesonide, dexamethasone, and triamcinolone are used with a special inhaler. If you do not understand the directions, or if you are not sure how to use the inhaler, check with your health care professional.

Before using this medicine, clear the nasal passages by blowing your nose. Then, with the nosepiece inserted into the nostril, aim the spray towards the inner corner of the eye.

In order for this medicine to help you, it must be used regularly as ordered by your doctor. This medicine usually begins to work in about 1 week, but up to 3 weeks may pass before you feel its full effects.

Use this medicine only as directed. Do not use more of it and do not use it more often than your doctor ordered. To do so may increase the chance of absorption through the lining of the nose and the chance of unwanted effects.

Check with your doctor before using this medicine for nasal problems other than the one for which it was prescribed, since it should not be used on many bacterial, virus, or fungus nasal infections.

Save the inhaler that comes with beclomethasone or dexamethasone, since refill units may be available at lower cost.

Dosing—The dose of nasal corticosteroids will be different for different patients. *Follow your doctor's orders or the directions on the label.* The following information includes only the average doses of nasal corticosteroids. *If your dose is different, do not change it* unless your doctor tells you to do so.

For beclomethasone

- For allergies or other nasal conditions:
  - —For *nasal aerosol* dosage form:
    - Adults and children 6 years of age and older—One spray in each nostril two to four times a day.
    - Children up to 6 years of age—Use and dose must be determined by your doctor.
  - —For *nasal solution* dosage form:
    - Adults and children 6 years of age and older—One or two sprays in each nostril two times a day.
    - Children up to 6 years of age—Use and dose must be determined by your doctor.

For budesonide
- For allergies or other nasal conditions:
    - —For *nasal powder* dosage form:
        - Adults and children 6 years of age and older—Two inhalations in each nostril once a day in the morning.
        - Children up to 6 years of age—Use and dose must be determined by your doctor.
    - —For *nasal solution* dosage form:
        - Adults and children 6 years of age and older—One or two sprays in each nostril one or two times a day.
        - Children up to 6 years of age—Use and dose must be determined by your doctor.

For dexamethasone
- For allergies or other nasal conditions:
    - —For *nasal aerosol* dosage form:
        - Adults and children 6 years of age and older—One or two sprays in each nostril two or three times a day for up to two weeks.
        - Children up to 6 years of age—Use and dose must be determined by your doctor.

For flunisolide
- For allergies or other nasal conditions:
    - —For *nasal solution* dosage form:
        - Adults and children 6 years of age and older—One or two sprays in each nostril one to three times a day.
        - Children up to 6 years of age—Use and dose must be determined by your doctor.

For triamcinolone
- For allergies or other nasal conditions:
    - —For *nasal aerosol* dosage form:

- Adults and children 12 years of age and older—
Two sprays in each nostril once a day.

- Children up to 12 years of age—Use and dose
must be determined by your doctor.

Missed dose—If you miss a dose of this medicine and
remember within an hour or so, use it right away. However, if you do not remember until later, skip the missed
dose and go back to your regular dosing schedule. Do not
double doses.

Storage—To store this medicine:

- Keep out of the reach of children.

- Store away from heat and direct light.

- Do not store budesonide powder in the bathroom,
near the kitchen sink, or in other damp places, especially if the cap has not been tightly screwed back
on. Moisture may cause the medicine to break down.

- Keep the medicine from getting too cold or freezing.
This medicine may be less effective if it is too cold
when you use it.

- Do not puncture, break, or burn the beclomethasone,
dexamethasone, or triamcinolone aerosol container,
even after it is empty.

- Do not keep outdated medicine or medicine no longer
needed. Also, discard any unused flunisolide or beclomethasone solution 3 months after you open the package. Be sure that any discarded medicine is out of
the reach of children.

Precautions While Using This Medicine

If you will be using this medicine for more than a few
weeks, your doctor should check your progress at regular visits.

Check with your doctor:
- *if signs of a nose, sinus, or throat infection occur.*
- *if your symptoms do not improve within 7 days (for dexamethasone) or within 3 weeks (for beclomethasone, budesonide, flunisolide, or triamcinolone).*
- *if your condition gets worse.*

Side Effects of This Medicine

Along with its needed effects, a medicine may cause some unwanted effects. Although not all of these side effects may occur, if they do occur they may need medical attention.

Check with your doctor as soon as possible if any of the following side effects occur:

Less common or rare

Bad smell; bloody mucus or unexplained nosebleeds; burning or stinging after use of spray or irritation inside nose (continuing); crusting, white patches, or sores inside nose; eye pain; gradual loss of vision; headache; hives; lightheadedness or dizziness; loss of sense of taste or smell; nausea or vomiting; shortness of breath, troubled breathing, tightness in chest, or wheezing; skin rash; sore throat, cough, or hoarseness; stomach pains; stuffy, dry, or runny nose or watery eyes (continuing); swelling of eyelids, face, or lips; unusual tiredness or weakness; white patches in throat

Symptoms of overdose

Acne; fullness or rounding of the face; menstrual changes

Other side effects may occur that usually do not need medical attention. These side effects may go away during treatment as your body adjusts to the medicine. However, check with your doctor if any of the following side effects continue or are bothersome:

More common

Burning, dryness, or other irritation inside the nose (mild, lasting only a short time); increase in sneezing; irritation of throat ·

Less common

Throat discomfort or itching

Not all of the side effects listed above have been reported for each of these medicines, but they have been reported for at least one of them. All of the nasal corticosteroids are very similar, so any of the above side effects may occur with any of these medicines.

Other side effects not listed above may also occur in some patients. If you notice any other effects, check with your doctor.

CORTICOSTEROIDS/ CORTICOTROPIN— Glucocorticoid Effects   Systemic

Some commonly used brand names are:

In the U.S.—

Acthar[2]

A-hydroCort[5]

AK-Dex[4]

Amcort[9]

A-methaPred[6]

Aristocort[9]

Aristocort Forte[9]

Aristocort Intralesional[9]

Aristospan Intra-articular[9]

Aristospan Intralesional[9]

Articulose-50[7]

Articulose-L.A.[9]

Celestone[1]

Celestone Phosphate[1]

Celestone Soluspan[1]

Cenocort A-40[9]

Cenocort Forte[9]

Cinalone 40[9]

Cinonide 40[9]

Cortef[5]

Cortenema[5]

Cortifoam[5]

Cortone Acetate[3]

Cortrophin-Zinc[2]

Dalalone[4]

Dalalone D.P.[4]

Dalalone L.A.[4]

Decadrol[4]

Decadron[4]

Decadron-LA[4]

Decadron Phosphate[4]

Decaject[4]

In the U.S. (cont'd)—

Decaject-L.A.[4]
Delta-Cortef[7]
Deltasone[8]
depMedalone 40[6]
depMedalone 80[6]
Depoject-40[6]
Depoject-80[6]
Depo-Medrol[6]
Depopred-40[6]
Depopred-80[6]
Depo-Predate 40[6]
Depo-Predate 80[6]
Deronil[4]
Dexacen-4[4]
Dexacen LA-8[4]
Dexamethasone Intensol[4]
Dexasone[4]
Dexasone-LA[4]
Dexone[4]
Dexone 0.5[4]
Dexone 0.75[4]
Dexone 1.5[4]
Dexone 4[4]
Dexone LA[4]
Duralone-40[6]
Duralone-80[6]
Hexadrol[4]
Hexadrol Phosphate[4]
H.P. Acthar Gel[2]
Hydeltrasol[7]
Hydeltra-T.B.A.[7]
Hydrocortone[5]
Hydrocortone Acetate[5]
Hydrocortone Phosphate[5]
Kenacort[9]
Kenacort Diacetate[9]
Kenaject-40[9]
Kenalog-10[9]
Kenalog-40[9]
Key-Pred 25[7]
Key-Pred 50[7]
Key-Pred SP[7]
Liquid Pred[8]
Medralone-40[6]

Medralone-80[6]
Medrol[6]
Medrol Enpak[6]
Meprolone[6]
Meticorten[8]
Mymethasone[4]
Orasone 1[8]
Orasone 5[8]
Orasone 10[8]
Orasone 20[8]
Orasone 50[8]
Pediapred[7]
Predaject-50[7]
Predalone 50[7]
Predalone T.B.A.[7]
Predate 50[7]
Predate S[7]
Predate TBA[7]
Predcor-25[7]
Predcor-50[7]
Predcor-TBA[7]
Predicort-50[7]
Predicort-RP[7]
Prednicen-M[8]
Prednisone Intensol[8]
Prelone[7]
Rep-Pred 40[6]
Rep-Pred 80[6]
Selestoject[1]
Solu-Cortef[5]
Solu-Medrol[6]
Solurex[4]
Solurex-LA[4]
Sterapred[8]
Sterapred DS[8]
Tac-3[9]
Triam-A[9]
Triam-Forte[9]
Triamolone 40[9]
Triamonide 40[9]
Tri-Kort[9]
Trilog[9]
Trilone[9]
Tristoject[9]

In Canada—

Acthar[2]	Decadron[4]
Acthar Gel (H.P.)[2]	Decadron Phosphate[4]
Apo-Prednisone[8]	Deltasone[8]
Aristocort[9]	Depo-Medrol[6]
Aristocort Forte[9]	Deronil[4]
Aristocort Intralesional[9]	Dexasone[4]
Aristospan Intra-articular[9]	Hexadrol[4]
Betnelan[1]	Kenacort[9]
Betnesol[1]	Kenalog-10[9]
Celestone[1]	Kenalog-40[9]
Celestone Soluspan[1]	Medrol[6]
Cortef[5]	Oradexon[4]
Cortenema[5]	Solu-Cortef[5]
Cortifoam[5]	Solu-Medrol[6]
Cortone[3]	Winpred[8]

Other commonly used names are:
   ACTH[2]
   Cortisol[5]

Note: For quick reference, the following corticosteroids/corticotropins are numbered to match the corresponding brand names.

This information applies to the following medicines:

1. Betamethasone (bay-ta-METH-a-sone)‡
2. Corticotropin (kor-ti-koe-TROE-pin)‡
3. Cortisone (KOR-ti-sone)‡§
4. Dexamethasone (dex-a-METH-a-sone)‡§
5. Hydrocortisone (hye-droe-KOR-ti-sone)
6. Methylprednisolone (meth-ill-pred-NISS-oh-lone)‡
7. Prednisolone (pred-NISS-oh-lone)‡
8. Prednisone (PRED-ni-sone)‡§
9. Triamcinolone (trye-am-SIN-oh-lone)‡§

The following information does *not* apply to desoxycorticosterone or fludrocortisone.

---

‡Generic name product may also be available in the U.S.
§Generic name product may also be available in Canada.

Description

Corticosteroids (kor-ti-koe-STER-oyds) (cortisone-like medicines) are used to provide relief for inflamed areas of the body. They lessen swelling, redness, itching, and allergic reactions. They are often used as part of the treatment for a number of different diseases, such as severe allergies or skin problems, asthma, or arthritis. Corticosteroids may also be used for other conditions as determined by your doctor.

Your body naturally produces certain cortisone-like hormones that are necessary to maintain good health. If your body does not produce enough, your doctor may have prescribed this medicine to help make up the difference.

Corticotropin is not a corticosteroid. It is a hormone that occurs naturally in the body. Corticotropin is known as an adrenocorticotropic hormone, which means it causes the adrenal glands to produce cortisone-like hormones. Corticotropin is used as a test to determine whether your adrenal glands are producing enough hormones. Also, it is sometimes used instead of corticosteroids to treat many of the same medical problems.

Corticosteroids and corticotropin are very strong medicines. In addition to their helpful effects in treating your medical problem, they have side effects that can be very serious. If your adrenal glands are not producing enough cortisone-like hormones, taking this medicine is not likely to cause problems unless you take too much of it. If you are taking this medicine to treat another medical problem, be sure that you discuss the risks and benefits of this medicine with your doctor.

These medicines are available only with your doctor's prescription, in the following dosage forms:

Oral

Betamethasone
- Syrup (U.S.)
- Tablets (U.S. and Canada)
- Effervescent tablets (Canada)
- Extended-release tablets (Canada)

Cortisone
- Tablets (U.S. and Canada)

Dexamethasone
- Elixir (U.S.)
- Oral solution (U.S.)
- Tablets (U.S. and Canada)

Hydrocortisone
- Oral suspension (U.S.)
- Tablets (U.S. and Canada)

Methylprednisolone
- Tablets (U.S. and Canada)

Prednisolone
- Oral solution (U.S.)
- Syrup (U.S.)
- Tablets (U.S.)

Prednisone
- Oral solution (U.S.)
- Syrup (U.S.)
- Tablets (U.S. and Canada)

Triamcinolone
- Syrup (U.S. and Canada)
- Tablets (U.S. and Canada)

Parenteral

Betamethasone
- Injection (U.S. and Canada)

Corticotropin
- Injection (U.S. and Canada)

Cortisone
- Injection (U.S. and Canada)

Dexamethasone
- Injection (U.S. and Canada)

Hydrocortisone
- Injection (U.S. and Canada)

Methylprednisolone
- Injection (U.S. and Canada)

Prednisolone
- Injection (U.S.)

Triamcinolone
- Injection (U.S. and Canada)

Rectal

Betamethasone
- Enema (Canada)

Hydrocortisone
- Aerosol foam (U.S. and Canada)
- Enema (U.S. and Canada)

Methylprednisolone
- Enema (U.S.)

Before Using This Medicine

In deciding to use a medicine, the risks of taking the medicine must be weighed against the good it will do. This is a decision you and your doctor will make. For corticosteroids and corticotropin, the following should be considered:

Allergies—Tell your doctor if you have ever had any unusual or allergic reaction to corticosteroids or corticotropin. Also tell your health care professional if you are allergic to any other substances, such as foods, preservatives, or dyes.

Diet—If you will be using this medicine for a long time, your doctor may want you to:

- Follow a low-salt diet and/or a potassium-rich diet.
- Watch your calories to prevent weight gain.
- Add extra protein to your diet. Make certain your health care professional knows if you are already on any special diet, such as a low-sodium or low-sugar diet.

Pregnancy—Studies on birth defects with corticosteroids or with corticotropin have not been done in humans. However, too much use of corticosteroids during pregnancy may cause the baby to have problems after birth, such as slower growth. Also, studies in animals have shown that corticosteroids cause birth defects and that corticotropin may cause other unwanted effects in the fetus.

Breast-feeding—Corticosteroids pass into breast milk and may cause problems with growth or other unwanted effects in nursing babies. Depending on the amount of medicine you are taking every day, it may be necessary for you to take another medicine or to stop breast-feeding during treatment. Corticotropin has not been shown to cause problems in nursing babies.

Children—Corticosteroids or corticotropin may cause infections such as chickenpox or measles to be more serious in children who catch them. These medicines can also slow or stop growth in children and in growing teenagers, especially when they are used for a long time. Before this medicine is given to children or teenagers, you should discuss its use with your child's doctor and then carefully follow the doctor's instructions.

Older adults—Older patients may be more likely to develop high blood pressure or bone disease from corticosteroids. Women are especially at risk of developing bone disease.

Other medicines—Although certain medicines should not be used together at all, in other cases two different medicines may be used together even if an interaction might occur. In these cases, your doctor may want to change the dose, or other precautions may be necessary. When you are taking corticosteroids or corticotropin, it is especially important that your health care professional know if you are taking any of the following:

- Aminoglutethimide or
- Antacids (in large amounts) or
- Barbiturates, except butalbital, or
- Carbamazepine (e.g., Tegretol) or
- Griseofulvin (e.g., Fulvicin) or
- Mitotane (e.g., Lysodren) or
- Phenylbutazone (e.g., Butazolidin) or
- Phenytoin (e.g., Dilantin) or
- Primidone (e.g., Mysoline) or
- Rifampin (e.g., Rifadin)—Use of these medicines may make corticotropin or certain corticosteroids less effective

- Amphotericin B by injection (e.g., Fungizone)—Corticosteroids and this medicine decrease the amount of potassium in the blood. Serious side effects could occur if the level of potassium gets too low

- Antidiabetics, oral (diabetes medicine taken by mouth) or
- Insulin—Corticosteroids may increase blood glucose (sugar) levels

- Digitalis glycosides (heart medicine)—Corticosteroids decrease the amount of potassium in the blood. Digitalis can cause an irregular heartbeat or other problems more commonly if the blood potassium gets too low

- Diuretics (water pills) or
- Medicine containing potassium—Using corticosteroids with diuretics may cause the diuretic to be less effective. Also, corticosteroids may increase the risk of low blood potassium, which is also a problem with certain diuretics. Potassium supplements or a different type of diuretic is used in treating high blood pressure in those people who have problems keeping their blood potassium at a normal level. Corticosteroids may make these medicines less able to do this

- Immunizations (vaccinations)—While you are being treated with this medicine, and even after you stop taking it, do not have any immunizations without your doctor's approval. Also, other people living in your home should not receive oral polio vaccine, since there is a chance they could pass the polio virus on to you. In addition, you should avoid close contact with other people at school or work who have recently taken oral polio vaccine

- Skin test injections—Corticosteroids may cause false results in skin tests

- Sodium-containing medicine—Corticosteroids and corticotropin cause the body to retain (keep) more salt and water. Too much sodium may cause high blood sodium, high blood pressure, and excess body water

Other medical problems—The presence of other medical problems may affect the use of corticosteroids and corticotropin. Make sure you tell your doctor if you have any other medical problems, especially:

- Bone disease—These medicines may worsen bone disease because they cause the body to lose more calcium

- Chickenpox (including recent exposure) or
- Measles (including recent exposure)—Risk of severe disease affecting other parts of the body

- Colitis or
- Diverticulitis or
- Stomach ulcer or other stomach or intestine problems— These medicines may cover up symptoms of a worsening stomach or intestinal condition. A patient would not know if his/her condition was getting worse and would not get medical help when needed

- Diabetes mellitus (sugar diabetes)—Corticosteroids may cause a loss of control of diabetes by increasing blood glucose (sugar)

- Fungus infection or any other infection or
- Herpes simplex infection of the eye or
- Infection at the place of treatment or
- Recent surgery or serious injury or
- Tuberculosis (active TB, nonactive TB, or past history of)—These medicines can cause slower healing, worsen existing infections, or cause new infections

- Glaucoma—Corticosteroids may cause the pressure within the eye to increase

- Heart disease or
- High blood pressure or
- Kidney disease (especially if you are receiving dialysis) or
- Kidney stones—These medicines cause the body to retain (keep) more salt and water. These conditions may be made worse by this extra body water

- High cholesterol levels—Corticosteroids may increase blood cholesterol levels

- Liver disease or
- Overactive thyroid or
- Underactive thyroid—With these conditions, the body may not eliminate the corticosteroid at the usual rate, which may change the medicine's effect

- Myasthenia gravis—When these medicines are first started, muscle weakness may occur. Your doctor may want to take special precautions because this could cause problems with breathing

• Systemic lupus erythematosus (SLE)—This condition may cause certain side effects of corticosteroids to occur more easily

---

Proper Use of This Medicine

For patients taking this medicine by mouth:

• *Take this medicine with food* to help prevent stomach upset. If stomach upset, burning, or pain continues, check with your doctor.

• Stomach problems may be more likely to occur if you drink alcoholic beverages while being treated with this medicine. You should not drink alcoholic beverages while taking this medicine, unless you have first checked with your doctor.

For patients using this medicine rectally:

• This medicine usually comes with patient directions. Read them carefully before using this medicine.

• For patients using hydrocortisone enema:

—Each bottle contains a single dose. Use it all, unless otherwise directed by your doctor.

—For best results, use this medicine right after a bowel movement. Lie down on your left side when giving the enema.

—Insert the rectal tip of the enema applicator gently to prevent damage to the rectal wall.

—Stay on your left side for at least 30 minutes after the enema is given so the medicine can work. If you can, keep the medicine inside the rectum all night.

• For patients using hydrocortisone acetate rectal aerosol foam:

—This medicine is used with a special applicator.

Do not insert any part of the aerosol container into the rectum.

- For patients using methylprednisolone acetate for enema:

    —Each bottle contains a single dose. Use it all, unless otherwise directed by your doctor.

    —Insert the rectal tip of the enema applicator gently to prevent damage to the rectal wall.

    —If you have been directed to use this enema slowly (not all at once), shake the bottle once in a while while you are giving the enema.

    —Save your applicator. Refill units of this medicine may be available at a lower cost.

Use this medicine only as directed by your doctor. Do not use more or less of it, do not use it more often, and do not use it for a longer time than your doctor ordered. To do so may increase the chance of side effects.

Dosing—The dose of these medicines will be different for different patients. *Follow your doctor's orders or the directions on the label.* The following information gives the range of doses of these medicines for all uses, which can vary widely. The dose that you are receiving may be very different. *If your dose is different, do not change it* unless your doctor tells you to do so.

The number of capsules, tablets, teaspoonfuls of liquid or amount of injection that you use depends on the strength of the medicine. Also, *the number of doses you take each day, the time allowed between doses, and the length of time you take the medicine depend on the medical problem for which you are taking the corticosteroid. In addition, your doctor may need to change the dose from time to time.*

For betamethasone

- For *oral* dosage forms:

    —Syrup, tablets, effervescent tablets:

- Adults and teenagers—Dose may range from 0.6 milligrams (mg) to 7.2 mg a day.

- Children—Dose is based on body weight or size and must be determined by your doctor.

—Extended-release tablets:

- Adults and teenagers—2 to 6 mg a day.

- Children—Dose is based on body weight or size and must be determined by your doctor.

• For *injection* dosage form:

—Adults and teenagers: Up to 9 mg (betamethasone) a day, injected into a muscle, vein, joint, or lesion.

—Children: Dose is based on body weight or size and must be determined by your doctor.

• For *rectal* dosage form (enema):

—Adults and teenagers: 5 mg (betamethasone), given as directed, each night.

—Children: Dose must be determined by your doctor.

For corticotropin

• For *injection* dosage forms:

—Regular:

- Adults and teenagers—10 to 80 Units every twelve to twenty-four hours, injected into a vein or muscle or under the skin.

- Children—Dose is based on body weight or size and must be determined by your doctor.

—Long-acting:

- Adults and teenagers—40 to 80 Units every one to three days, injected into a muscle or under the skin.

- Children—Dose is based on body weight or size and must be determined by your doctor.

For cortisone

- For *oral* dosage form (tablets):

  —Adults and teenagers: 25 to 300 milligrams (mg) a day, as a single dose or divided into several doses.

  —Children: Dose is based on body weight or size and must be determined by your doctor.

- For *injection* dosage form:

  —Adults and teenagers: 20 to 300 mg a day, injected into a muscle.

  —Children: Dose is based on body weight or size and must be determined by your doctor.

For dexamethasone

- For *oral* dosage forms (elixir, solution, tablets):

  —Adults and teenagers: 0.5 to 9 milligrams (mg) a day, as a single dose or divided into several doses.

  —Children: Dose is based on body weight or size and must be determined by your doctor.

- For *injection* dosage form:

  —Adults and teenagers: 0.2 to 16 mg (dexamethasone or dexamethasone phosphate) every three days to three weeks as needed. It is injected into a muscle, joint, or lesion.

  —Children: Dose is based on body weight or size and must be determined by your doctor.

For hydrocortisone

- For *oral* dosage forms (tablets, suspension):

  —Adults and teenagers: 20 to 240 milligrams (mg) (hydrocortisone) a day, as a single dose or divided into several doses.

  —Children: Dose is based on body weight or size and must be determined by your doctor.

- For *injection* dosage form:

  —Adults and teenagers:

    - 15 to 240 mg a day, injected into a muscle; or

• 5 to 75 mg every two to three weeks, injected into a joint or lesion; or

• 100 to 500 mg (hydrocortisone) every two to six hours as needed, injected into a muscle or vein or under the skin.

—Children: Dose is based on body weight or size and must be determined by your doctor.

• For *rectal* dosage forms (enema, aerosol foam):

—Enema:

• Adults and teenagers—100 mg, given as directed, every night.

• Children—Dose must be determined by your doctor.

—Aerosol foam:

• Adults and teenagers—90 mg (one applicatorful) one or two times a day.

• Children—Dose must be determined by your doctor.

For methylprednisolone

• For *oral* dosage form (tablets):

—Adults and teenagers: 4 to 160 milligrams (mg) a day, as a single dose or divided into several doses.

—Children: Dose is based on body weight or size and must be determined by your doctor.

• For *injection* dosage form:

—Adults and teenagers:

• 4 to 120 mg every one day to five weeks as needed, injected into a muscle, joint, or lesion; or

• 10 to 160 mg (methylprednisolone) repeated as needed, injected into a muscle or vein.

—Children: Dose is based on body weight or size and must be determined by your doctor.

• For *rectal* dosage form (enema):

—Adults and teenagers: 40 mg, given as directed, three to seven times a week.

—Children: Dose is based on body weight or size and must be determined by your doctor.

For prednisolone

• For *oral* dosage forms (solution, syrup, tablets):

—Adults and teenagers: 5 to 200 milligrams (mg) (prednisolone) a day, as needed, as a single dose or divided into several doses.

—Children: Dose is based on body weight or size and must be determined by your doctor.

• For *injection* dosage form:

—Adults and teenagers: 2 to 100 mg (prednisolone or prednisolone phosphate) a day as needed, injected into a muscle, vein, joint, or lesion.

—Children: Dose is based on body weight or size and must be determined by your doctor.

For prednisone

• For *oral* dosage forms (solution, syrup, tablets):

—Adults and teenagers: 5 to 200 milligrams (mg) a day, as needed, as a single dose or divided into several doses.

—Children: Dose is usually based on body weight or size and must be determined by your doctor.

For triamcinolone

• For *oral* dosage forms (syrup, tablets):

—Adults and teenagers: 4 to 60 milligrams (mg) (triamcinolone) a day, as needed, as a single dose or divided into several doses.

—Children: Dose is based on body weight or size and must be determined by your doctor.

• For *injection* dosage form:

—Adults and teenagers: 0.5 to 80 mg repeated as

needed, injected into a muscle, joint, or lesion, or under the skin.

—Children: Dose is usually based on body weight or size and must be determined by your doctor.

Missed dose—If you miss a dose of this medicine and your dosing schedule is:

- One dose every other day—Take the missed dose as soon as possible if you remember it the same morning, then go back to your regular dosing schedule. If you do not remember the missed dose until later, wait and take it the following morning. Then skip a day and start your regular dosing schedule again.

- One dose a day—Take the missed dose as soon as possible, then go back to your regular dosing schedule. If you do not remember until the next day, skip the missed dose and do not double the next one.

- Several doses a day—Take the missed dose as soon as possible, then go back to your regular dosing schedule. If you do not remember until your next dose is due, double the next dose.

If you have any questions about this, check with your health care professional.

Storage—To store this medicine:

- Keep out of the reach of children.

- Store away from heat and direct light.

- Do not store tablets in the bathroom, near the kitchen sink, or in other damp places. Heat or moisture may cause the medicine to break down.

- Keep the liquid dosage forms of this medicine, including enemas, and hydrocortisone rectal aerosol foam from freezing.

- Do not puncture, break, or burn the hydrocortisone rectal aerosol foam container, even when it is empty.

- Do not keep outdated medicine or medicine no longer

needed. Be sure that any discarded medicine is out of the reach of children.

Precautions While Using This Medicine

Your doctor should check your progress at regular visits. Also, your progress may have to be checked after you have stopped using this medicine, since some of the effects may continue.

Do not stop using this medicine without first checking with your doctor. Your doctor may want you to reduce gradually the amount you are using before stopping completely.

Check with your doctor if your condition reappears or worsens after the dose has been reduced or treatment with this medicine is stopped.

If you will be using corticosteroids or corticotropin for a long time:

- *Your doctor may want you to follow a low-salt diet and/or a potassium-rich diet.*
- Your doctor may want you to watch your calories to prevent weight gain.
- Your doctor may want you to add extra protein to your diet.
- Your doctor may want you to have your eyes examined by an ophthalmologist (eye doctor) before and also sometime later during treatment.
- Your doctor may want you to carry a medical identification card stating that you are using this medicine.

Tell the doctor in charge that you are using this medicine:

- *Before having skin tests.*
- *Before having any kind of surgery (including dental surgery) or emergency treatment.*
- *If you get a serious infection or injury.*

Avoid close contact with anyone who has chickenpox or measles. This is especially important for children. *Tell your doctor right away if you think you have been exposed to chickenpox or measles.*

While you are being treated with this medicine, and after you stop taking it, *do not have any immunizations without your doctor's approval.* Also, other people living in your home should not receive oral polio vaccine, since there is a chance they could pass the polio virus on to you. In addition, you should avoid close contact with other people at school or work who have recently taken oral polio vaccine.

For *diabetic patients:*
- This medicine may affect blood sugar levels. If you notice a change in the results of your blood or urine sugar tests or if you have any questions, check with your doctor.

For patients having this medicine *injected into their joints:*
- If this medicine is injected into one of your joints, you should be careful not to put too much stress or strain on that joint for a while, even if it begins to feel better. Make sure your doctor has told you how much you are allowed to move this joint while it is healing.
- If redness or swelling occurs at the place of injection, and continues or gets worse, check with your doctor.

For patients using this medicine *rectally:*
- Check with your doctor if you notice rectal bleeding, pain, burning, itching, blistering, or any other sign of irritation not present before you started using this medicine, or if signs of infection occur.

Side Effects of This Medicine

Corticosteroids or corticotropin may lower your resistance to infections. Also, any infection you get may be harder to treat. Always check with your doctor as soon as possible if you notice any signs of a possible infection, such as sore throat, fever, sneezing, or coughing.

Along with its needed effects, a medicine may cause some unwanted effects. Although not all of these side effects may occur, if they do occur they may need medical attention. When this medicine is used for short periods of time, side effects usually are rare. However, check with your doctor as soon as possible if any of the following side effects occur:

Less common

> Decreased or blurred vision; frequent urination; increased thirst; rectal bleeding, blistering, burning, itching, or pain not present before use of this medicine (when used rectally)

Rare

> Blindness (sudden, when injected in the head or neck area); confusion; excitement; false sense of well-being; hallucinations (seeing, hearing, or feeling things that are not there); mental depression; mood swings (sudden and wide); mistaken feelings of self-importance or being mistreated; redness, swelling, pain, or other sign of allergy or infection at place of injection; restlessness

Additional side effects may occur if you take this medicine for a long time. Check with your doctor if any of the following side effects occur:

> Abdominal or stomach pain or burning (continuing); acne or other skin problems; bloody or black, tarry stools; filling or rounding out of the face; irregular heartbeat; menstrual problems; muscle cramps or pain; muscle weakness; nausea; pain in back, hips, ribs, arms, shoulders, or legs; pitting, scarring, or depression of skin at place of injection; reddish purple lines on arms, face, legs, trunk, or groin; swelling of feet or lower legs; thin, shiny skin; unusual bruising; unusual tiredness or weakness; vomiting; weight gain (rapid); wounds that will not heal

Other side effects may occur that usually do not need medical attention. These side effects may go away during

treatment as your body adjusts to the medicine. However, check with your doctor if any of the following side effects continue or are bothersome:

More common

Increased appetite; indigestion; loss of appetite (for triamcinolone only); nervousness or restlessness; trouble in sleeping

Less common or rare

Darkening or lightening of skin color; dizziness; flushing of face or cheeks (after injection into the nose); headache; increased joint pain (after injection into a joint); increased sweating; lightheadedness; nosebleeds (after injection into the nose); unusual increase in hair growth on body or face

After you stop using this medicine, your body may need time to adjust. The length of time this takes depends on the amount of medicine you were using and how long you used it. If you have taken large doses of this medicine for a long time, your body may need one year to adjust. During this time, *check with your doctor immediately if any of the following side effects occur:*

Abdominal, stomach, or back pain; dizziness; fainting; fever; loss of appetite (continuing); muscle or joint pain; nausea; reappearance of disease symptoms; shortness of breath; unexplained headaches (frequent or continuing); unusual tiredness or weakness; vomiting; weight loss (rapid)

Other side effects not listed above may also occur in some patients. If you notice any other effects, check with your doctor.

COUGH/COLD COMBINATIONS Systemic

Some commonly used brand names are:

In the U.S.—

Actagen-C Cough[41]
Actifed with Codeine Cough[41]
Adatuss D.C. Expectorant[97]
Alamine-C Liquid[28]
Alamine Expectorant[113]
Alka-Seltzer Plus Cold and Cough[49]
Alka-Seltzer Plus Night-Time Cold[42a]
Allerfrin with Codeine[41]
All-Nite Cold Formula[51]
Ambay Cough[1]
Ambenyl Cough[1]
Ambenyl-D Decongestant Cough Formula[114]
Ambophen Expectorant[9]
Amgenal Cough[1]
Ami-Tex LA[121]
Anamine HD[23]
Anaplex HD[23]
Anatuss[74]
Anatuss with Codeine[75]
Anatuss DM[114]
Anatuss LA[122]
Anti-Tuss DM Expectorant[94]
Aprodine with Codeine[41]
Banex[120]
Banex-LA[121]
Banex Liquid[120]
Bayaminic Expectorant[121]
Bayaminicol[27]
Baycodan[89]
Baycomine[103]
Baycomine Pediatric[103]
BayCotussend Liquid[106]
Baydec DM Drops[20]
Bayer Select Chest Cold Caplets[88a]
Bayer Select Flu Relief Caplets[50]
Bayer Select Head and Chest Cold Caplets[117]
Bayer Select Night Time Cold Caplets[54b]
Bayhistine DH[28]
Bayhistine Expectorant[113]
Baytussin AC[91]
Baytussin DM[94]
Benylin Expectorant Cough Formula[94]
Biphetane DC Cough[19]
Brexin[81]
Bromanate DC Cough[19]
Bromanyl[1]
Bromarest DX Cough[19b]
Bromatane DX Cough[19b]
Bromfed-DM[19b]
Bromotuss with Codeine[1]
Bromphen DC with Codeine Cough[19]
Bromphen DX Cough[19b]
Broncholate[118]
Bronkotuss Expectorant[82]
Brotane DX Cough[19b]
Calcidrine[90]
Carbinoxamine Compound[20]
Carbinoxamine Compound-Drops[20]
Carbodec DM Drops[20]
Cardec DM[20]
Cardec DM Drops[20]
Cardec DM Pediatric[20]
Cerose-DM[22]
Cheracol[91]
Cheracol D Cough[94]
Cheracol Plus[27]

In the U.S. (cont'd)—

Children's Formula Cough[94]
Children's Tylenol Cold Multi
  Symptom Plus Cough[50]
Children's Vicks NyQuil Cold/
  Cough Relief [29]
Chlorgest-HD[23]
Citra Forte[15] [44]
Co-Apap[50]
Codamine[103]
Codamine Pediatric[103]
Codan[89]
Codegest Expectorant[111]
Codehist DH[28]
Codiclear DH[97]
Codimal DH[40]
Codimal DM[39]
Codimal Expectorant[121]
Codimal PH[38]
Codistan No. 1[94]
Comtrex Cough Formula[117]
Comtrex Daytime Caplets[108]
Comtrex Daytime Maximum
  Strength Cold, Cough, and
  Flu Relief[108]
Comtrex Daytime Maximum
  Strength Cold and Flu
  Relief[108]
Comtrex Hot Flu Relief[50]
Comtrex Maximum Strength
  Liqui-Gels[48]
Comtrex Multi-Symptom Cold
  Reliever[48]
Comtrex Multi-Symptom Non-
  Drowsy Caplets[108]
Comtrex Nighttime[50]
Comtrex Nighttime Maximum
  Strength Cold, Cough, and
  Flu Relief[50]
Comtrex Nighttime Maximum
  Strength Cold and Flu
  Relief[50]
Concentrin[114]
Conex[121]
Conex with Codeine Liquid[111]
Congess JR[122]

Congess SR[122]
Congestac Caplets[122]
Contac Cough & Chest Cold[117]
Contac Cough and Sore
  Throat[88a]
Contac Day Caplets[108]
Contac Jr. Children's Cold
  Medicine[107]
Contac Night Caplets[50b]
Contac Severe Cold and Flu
  Formula Caplets[48]
Contac Severe Cold Formula[50]
Contac Severe Cold Formula
  Night Strength[51]
Contuss[120]
Cophene-S[26]
Cophene-X[109a]
Cophene XP[115]
Cophene-XP[64]
Co-Tuss V[97]
CoTylenol Cold Medication[50]
C-Tussin Expectorant[113]
DayQuil Multi-Symptom Cold/
  Flu LiquiCaps[117]
DayQuil Non-Drowsy Cold/
  Flu[117]
DayQuil Sinus Pressure and
  Congestion Relief
  Caplets[121]
Decohistine DH[28]
Deconsal II[122]
Deconsal Pediatric[113]
Deconsal Sprinkle[120a]
Deproist Expectorant with
  Codeine[113]
Despec[120]
De-Tuss[106]
Detussin Expectorant[115]
Detussin Liquid[106]
Dexafed Cough[109]
Diabetic Tussin DM[94]
Dihistine DH[28]
Dihistine Expectorant[113]
Dilaudid Cough[99]
Dimacol Caplets[114]

In the U.S. (cont'd)—

Dimetane-DC Cough[19]
Dimetane-DX Cough[19b]
Dimetapp DM[19a]
Dimetapp DM Cold and Cough[19a]
Donatussin[62]
Donatussin DC[110]
Donatussin Drops[83]
Dondril[22]
Dorcol Children's Cough[114]
Dristan Cold and Flu[50]
Dristan Juice Mix-in Cold, Flu, and Cough[108]
Dura-Gest[120]
Duratuss[122]
Duratuss HD[115]
Dura-Vent[121]
ED-TLC[23]
ED Tuss HC[23]
Effective Strength Cough Formula[3]
Effective Strength Cough Formula with Decongestant[105]
Efficol Cough Whip (Cough Suppressant/ Decongestant)[102]
Efficol Cough Whip (Cough Suppressant/Decongestant/ Antihistamine)[27]
Efficol Cough Whip (Cough Suppressant/Expectorant)[94]
Endagen-HD[23]
Endal[120a]
Endal Expectorant[111]
Endal-HD[23]
Endal-HD Plus[23]
Enomine[120]
Entex[120]
Entex LA[121]
Entex Liquid[120]
Entex PSE[122]
Entuss-D[106 115]
Entuss Expectorant[97 98]
Entuss Pediatric Expectorant[115]

Eudal-SR[122]
Exgest LA[121]
Extra Action Cough[94]
Father John's Medicine Plus[63]
Fendol[123]
2/G-DM Cough[94]
Genatuss DM[94]
Genite[51]
Glycofed[122]
Glycotuss-dM[94]
Glydeine Cough[91]
GP-500[122]
Guaifed[122]
Guaifed-PD[122]
GuaiMAX-D[122]
Guaipax[121]
Guaitab[122]
GuiaCough CF[112]
GuiaCough PE[122]
Guiamid D.M. Liquid[94]
Guiatuss A.C.[91]
Guiatuss CF[112]
Guiatuss DAC[113]
Guiatuss-DM[94]
Guiatussin with Codeine Liquid [91]
Guiatussin DAC[113]
Guiatussin w/ Dextromethorphan[94]
Guiatuss PE[122]
Halotussin-DM Expectorant[94]
Histafed C[41]
Histalet X[122]
Histatuss Pediatric[21]
Histine DM[19a]
Histussin HC[23]
Humibid DM[94]
Humibid DM Sprinkle[94]
Hycodan[89]
Hycomine[103]
Hycomine Compound[47]
Hycomine Pediatric[103]
Hycotuss Expectorant[97]
Hydromet[89]
Hydromine[103]

In the U.S. (cont'd)—

Hydromine Pediatric[103]
Hydropane[89]
Hydrophen[103]
Improved Sino-Tuss[46]
Iophen-C Liquid[92]
Iophen DM[95]
Ipsatol Cough Formula for Children[112]
Kiddy Koff[112]
KIE[119]
Kolephrin/DM Caplets[49,50a]
Kolephrin GG/DM[94]
Kolephrin NN Liquid[54]
Kophane[65]
Kophane Cough and Cold Formula[27]
Kwelcof Liquid[97]
Lanatuss Expectorant[85]
Mapap Cold Formula[50]
Marcof Expectorant[98]
Meda Syrup Forte[62]
Medi-Flu[50]
Medi-Flu Caplets[50]
Mediquell Decongestant Formula[105]
Midahist DH[28]
Mycotussin[106]
Myhistine DH[28]
Myhistine Expectorant[113]
Myhydromine[103]
Myhydromine Pediatric[103]
Myminic Expectorant[121]
Myminicol[27]
Myphetane DC Cough[19]
Myphetane DX Cough[19b]
Mytussin AC[91]
Mytussin DAC[113]
Mytussin DM[94]
Naldecon-CX Adult Liquid[111]
Naldecon-DX Adult Liquid[112]
Naldecon-DX Children's Syrup[112]
Naldecon-DX Pediatric Drops[112]
Naldecon-EX[121]

Naldecon-EX Pediatric Drops[121]
Naldecon Senior DX[94]
Naldelate DX Adult[112]
Nasatab LA[122]
Nolex LA[121]
Noratuss II Liquid[114]
Normatane DC[19]
Nortussin with Codeine[91]
Novagest Expectorant w/ Codeine[113]
Novahistine DH Liquid[28]
Novahistine DMX Liquid[114]
Novahistine Expectorant[113]
Nucochem[104]
Nucochem Expectorant[113]
Nucochem Pediatric Expectorant[113]
Nucofed[104]
Nucofed Expectorant[113]
Nucofed Pediatric Expectorant[113]
Nucotuss Expectorant[113]
Nucotuss Pediatric Expectorant[113]
Nytcold Medicine[51]
Nytime Cold Medicine Liquid[51]
Omnicol[43]
Ordrine AT[101]
Ornex Severe Cold No Drowsiness Caplets[108]
Orthoxicol Cough[27]
Para-Hist HD[23]
Partuss LA[121]
PediaCare Children's Cough-Cold[29]
PediaCare Cough-Cold[29]
PediaCare Night Rest Cough-Cold Liquid[29]
Pediacof Cough[61]
Pedituss Cough[61]
Pentazine VC w/Codeine[5]
Pertussin All Night CS[94]
Pertussin All Night PM[51]
Phanadex[72a]

In the U.S. (cont'd)—

Phanatuss[94]
Phenameth DM[6]
Phenameth VC with Codeine[37]
Phenergan with Codeine[5]
Phenergan with Dextromethorphan[6]
Phenergan VC with Codeine[37]
Phenhist DH w/Codeine[28]
Phenhist Expectorant[113]
Phenylfenesin L.A.[121]
Pherazine w/Codeine[5]
Pherazine DM[6]
Pherazine VC with Codeine[37]
Pneumotussin HC[97]
Polaramine Expectorant[87]
Poly-Histine-CS[19]
Poly-Histine-DM[19a]
Primatuss Cough Mixture 4[3]
Primatuss Cough Mixture 4D[114]
Promethazine DM[6]
Promethazine VC w/Codeine[37]
Prometh w/Dextromethorphan[6]
Prometh VC with Codeine[37]
Promethist w/Codeine[37]
Prominic Expectorant[121]
Prominicol Cough[69]
Promist HD Liquid[30]
Pseudo-Car DM[20]
Pseudodine C Cough[41]
P-V-Tussin[13 30]
Quelidrine Cough[57]
Remcol-C[8]
Rentamine Pediatric[21]
Rescaps-D S.R.[101]
Rescon-DM[29]
Rescon-GG[120a]
Respaire-60 SR[122]
Respaire-120 SR[122]
Rhinosyn-DM[29]
Rhinosyn-DMX Expectorant[94]
Rhinosyn-X[114]
Robafen AC Cough[91]
Robafen CF[112]
Robafen DAC[113]

Robafen DM[94]
Robitussin A-C[91]
Robitussin-CF[112]
Robitussin Cold and Cough Liqui-Gels[114]
Robitussin-DAC[113]
Robitussin-DM[94]
Robitussin Maximum Strength Cough and Cold[105]
Robitussin Night Relief[54a]
Robitussin Night Relief Colds Formula Liquid[53]
Robitussin-PE[122]
Robitussin Pediatric Cough & Cold[105]
Robitussin Severe Congestion Liqui-Gels[122]
Rolatuss Expectorant[60]
Rolatuss w/Hydrocodone[34]
Rondamine-DM Drops[20]
Rondec-DM[20]
Rondec-DM Drops[20]
Ru-Tuss DE[122]
Ru-Tuss Expectorant[114]
Ru-Tuss with Hydrocodone Liquid[34]
Rymed[122]
Rymed Liquid[122]
Rymed-TR Caplets[122]
Ryna-C Liquid[28]
Ryna-CX Liquid[113]
Rynatuss[21]
Rynatuss Pediatric[21]
Safe Tussin 30[94]
Saleto-CF[107]
Scot-Tussin DM[3]
Silexin Cough[94]
Sinufed Timecelles[122]
Sinupan[120a]
SINUvent[121]
Snaplets-DM[102]
Snaplets-EX[121]
Snaplets-Multi[27]
SRC Expectorant[115]
Stamoist E[122]

In the U.S. (cont'd)—

Stamoist LA[121]

Statuss Green[34]

S-T Forte[71a]

S-T Forte 2[3a]

Sudafed Cold & Cough Liquid Caps[117]

Sudafed Cough[114]

Sudafed Severe Cold Formula Caplets[108]

Syracol Liquid[102]

TheraFlu/Flu, Cold and Cough Medicine[50]

TheraFlu Maximum Strength Non-Drowsy Formula Flu, Cold and Cough Medicine[108]

TheraFlu Nighttime Maximum Strength[50]

Threamine DM[27]

Threamine Expectorant[121]

T-Koff[24]

Tolu-Sed Cough[91]

Tolu-Sed DM[94]

Touro LA Caplets[122]

Triacin C Cough[41]

Triafed w/Codeine[41]

Triaminic-DM Cough Formula[102]

Triaminic Expectorant[121]

Triaminic Expectorant with Codeine[111]

Triaminic Expectorant DH[71]

Triaminic Nite Light[29]

Triaminic Sore Throat Formula[108]

Triaminicol Multi-Symptom Relief[27]

Triaminicol Multi-Symptom Relief Colds with Coughs[27]

Tricodene Cough & Cold[7]

Tricodene Forte[27]

Tricodene NN[27]

Tricodene Pediatric[102]

Tricodene Sugar Free[3]

Trifed-C Cough[41]

Triminol Cough[27]

Trinex[86]

Triphenyl Expectorant[121]

Tri-Tannate Plus Pediatric[21]

Tusquelin[25]

Tuss-Ade[101]

Tussafed[20]

Tussafed Drops[20]

Tussafin Expectorant[115]

Tuss Allergine Modified T.D.[101]

Tussanil DH[23 116]

Tussar-2[113]

Tussar DM[29]

Tussar SF[113]

Tuss-DM[94]

Tussex Cough[109]

Tussgen[106]

Tuss-Genade Modified[101]

Tussigon[89]

Tussionex[3a 4]

Tussi-Organidin DM Liquid[95]

Tussi-Organidin Liquid[92]

Tussirex with Codeine Liquid[78]

Tuss-LA[122]

Tusso-DM[95]

Tussogest[101]

Ty-Cold Cold Formula[50]

Tylenol Cold and Flu[50]

Tylenol Cold and Flu No Drowsiness Powder[108]

Tylenol Cold Medication[50]

Tylenol Cold Medication, Non-Drowsy[108]

Tylenol Cold Night Time[50a]

Tylenol Cough with Decongestant Maximum Strength[108]

Tylenol Maximum Strength Cough[88a]

Tylenol Maximum Strength Flu Gelcaps[108]

Tyrodone[106]

ULR-LA[121]

Uni-tussin DM[94]

Unproco[94]

Utex-S.R.[121]

In the U.S. (cont'd)—

Vanex Expectorant[115]
Vanex-HD[23]
Vanex-LA[121]
V-Dec-M[122]
Versacaps[122]
Vicks 44 Cough and Cold Relief LiquiCaps[105]
Vicks 44D Dry Hacking Cough and Head Congestion[105]
Vicks 44M Cough, Cold and Flu Relief[50]
Vicks 44M Cough, Cold and Flu Relief LiquiCaps[50]
Vicks NyQuil Multi-Symptom Cold/Flu Relief[51]
Vicks NyQuil Multi-Symptom LiquiCaps[51]
Vicks Pediatric Formula 44D Cough & Decongestant[105]
Vicks Pediatric Formula 44E[94]
Vicks Pediatric Formula 44M Multi-Symptom Cough & Cold[29]
Vicodin Tuss[97]
Viro-Med[50]
Zephrex[122]
Zephrex-LA[122]

In Canada—

Actifed DM[42]
Benylin with Codeine[113]
Caldomine-DH Forte[36]
Caldomine-DH Pediatric[36]
Calmylin with Codeine[11]
CoActifed[41]
CoActifed Expectorant[73]
Coristex-DH[100a]
Coristine-DH[100a]
Dimetane Expectorant[80]
Dimetane Expectorant-C[55]
Dimetane Expectorant-DC[56]
Dimetapp-DM[18]
Dorcol DM[112]
Entex LA[121]
Hycomine[72]
Hycomine-S Pediatric[72]
Novahistex C[100]
Novahistex DH[100a]
Novahistex DH Expectorant[110]
Novahistex DM[32]
Novahistine DH[33]
Novahistine DH Expectorant[68]
Omni-Tuss[67]
Ornade-DM 10[27]
Ornade-DM 15[27]
Ornade-DM 30[27]
Ornade Expectorant[84]
Robitussin A-C[14]
Robitussin-CF[112]
Robitussin with Codeine[14]
Robitussin-DM[94]
Sudafed DM[105]
Sudafed Expectorant[122]
Triaminic-DM Expectorant[70]
Triaminic Expectorant[88]
Triaminic Expectorant DH[71]
Triaminicin with Codeine[52]
Triaminicol DM[35]
Tussaminic C [34a]
Tussaminic C Pediatric[34a]
Tussaminic DH[36]
Tussaminic DH Pediatric[36]
Tussionex[4]
Tuss-Ornade Spansules[26a]
Tylenol Cold Medication[50]
Tylenol Cold Medication, Non-Drowsy[108]

Note: For quick reference the following cough/cold combinations are numbered to match the preceding corresponding brand names.

Antihistamine and antitussive combinations—

1. Bromodiphenhydramine (broe-moe-dye-fen-HYE-dra-meen) and Codeine (KOE-deen)

2. No product available
3. Chlorpheniramine (klor-fen-EER-a-meen) and Dextromethorphan (dex-troe-meth-OR-fan)
3a. Chlorpheniramine and Hydrocodone (hye-droe-KOE-done)
4. Phenyltoloxamine (fen-ill-tole-OX-a-meen) and Hydrocodone
5. Promethazine (proe-METH-a-zeen) and Codeine†
6. Promethazine and Dextromethorphan
7. Pyrilamine and Codeine

Antihistamine, antitussive, and analgesic combinations—
8. Chlorpheniramine, Dextromethorphan (dex-troe-meth-OR-fan), and Acetaminophen (a-seat-a-MIN-oh-fen)

Antihistamine, antitussive, and expectorant combinations—
9. Bromodiphenhydramine (broe-moe-dye-fen-HYE-dra-meen), Diphenhydramine (dye-fen-HYE-dra-meen), Codeine (KOE-deen), Ammonium Chloride (a-MOE-nee-um KLOR-ide), and Potassium Guaiacolsulfonate (poe-TAS-ee-um gwye-a-kol-SUL-fon-ate)
10. No product available
11. Diphenhydramine, Codeine, and Ammonium Chloride
12. No product available
13. Phenindamine (fen-IN-da-meen), Hydrocodone (hye-droe-KOE-done), and Guaifenesin
14. Pheniramine (fen-EER-a-meen), Codeine, and Guaifenesin
15. Pheniramine, Pyrilamine (peer-ILL-a-meen), Hydrocodone, Potassium Citrate (poe-TAS-ee-um SI-trate), and Ascorbic Acid
16. No product available

Antihistamine, decongestant, and antitussive combinations—
17. No product available
18. Brompheniramine, Phenylephrine, Phenylpropanolamine, and Dextromethorphan (dex-troe-meth-OR-fan)
19. Brompheniramine, Phenylpropanolamine, and Codeine
19a. Brompheniramine, Phenylpropanolamine, and Dextromethorphan
19b. Brompheniramine, Pseudoephedrine (soo-doe-e-FED-rin), and Dextromethorphan
20. Carbinoxamine (kar-bi-NOX-a-meen), Pseudoephedrine, and Dextromethorphan

21. Chlorpheniramine (klor-fen-EER-a-meen), Ephedrine (e-FED-rin), Phenylephrine, and Carbetapentane (kar-bay-ta-PEN-tane)
22. Chlorpheniramine, Phenylephrine, and Dextromethorphan
23. Chlorpheniramine, Phenylephrine, and Hydrocodone (hye-droe-KOE-done)
24. Chlorpheniramine, Phenylephrine, Phenylpropanolamine, and Codeine
25. Chlorpheniramine, Phenylephrine, Phenylpropanolamine, and Dextromethorphan
26. Chlorpheniramine, Phenylephrine, Phenylpropanolamine, and Dihydrocodeine (dye-hye-droe-KOE-deen)
26a. Chlorpheniramine, Phenylpropanolamine, and Caramiphen (kar-AM-i-fen)
27. Chlorpheniramine, Phenylpropanolamine, and Dextromethorphan
28. Chlorpheniramine, Pseudoephedrine, and Codeine
29. Chlorpheniramine, Pseudoephedrine, and Dextromethorphan
30. Chlorpheniramine, Pseudoephedrine, and Hydrocodone
31. No product available
32. Diphenylpyraline, Phenylephrine, and Dextromethorphan
33. Diphenylpyraline, Phenylephrine, and Hydrocodone
34. Pheniramine (fen-EER-a-meen), Pyrilamine (peer-ILL-a-meen), Phenylephrine, Phenylpropanolamine, and Hydrocodone
34a. Pheniramine, Pyrilamine, Phenylpropanolamine, and Codeine
35. Pheniramine, Pyrilamine, Phenylpropanolamine, and Dextromethorphan
36. Pheniramine, Pyrilamine, Phenylpropanolamine, and Hydrocodone
37. Promethazine (proe-METH-a-zeen), Phenylephrine, and Codeine
38. Pyrilamine, Phenylephrine, and Codeine
39. Pyrilamine, Phenylephrine, and Dextromethorphan
40. Pyrilamine, Phenylephrine, and Hydrocodone
41. Triprolidine (trye-PROE-li-deen), Pseudoephedrine, and Codeine

42. Triprolidine, Pseudoephedrine, and Dextromethorphan

Antihistamine, decongestant, antitussive, and analgesic combinations—

42a. Brompheniramine (brome-fen-EER-a-meen), Phenylpropanolamine (fen-ill-proe-pa-NOLE-a-meen), Dextromethorphan (dex-troe-meth-OR-fan), and Aspirin

43. Chlorpheniramine (klor-fen-EER-a-meen), Phenindamine (fen-IN-da-meen), Phenylephrine (fen-ill-EF-rin), Dextromethorphan, Acetaminophen (a-seat-a-MIN-oh-fen), Salicylamide (sal-i-SILL-a-mide), Caffeine (kaf-EEN), and Ascorbic (a-SKOR-bik) Acid

44. Chlorpheniramine, Pheniramine (fen-EER-a-meen), Pyrilamine (peer-ILL-a-meen), Phenylephrine, Hydrocodone (hye-droe-KOE-done), Salicylamide, Caffeine, and Ascorbic Acid

45. No product available

46. Chlorpheniramine, Phenylephrine, Dextromethorphan, Acetaminophen, and Salicylamide

47. Chlorpheniramine, Phenylephrine, Hydrocodone (hye-droe-KOE-done), Acetaminophen, and Caffeine

48. Chlorpheniramine, Phenylpropanolamine (fen-ill-proe-pa-NOLE-a-meen), Dextromethorphan, and Acetaminophen

49. Chlorpheniramine, Phenylpropanolamine, Dextromethorphan, and Aspirin

50. Chlorpheniramine, Pseudoephedrine (soo-doe-e-FED-rin), Dextromethorphan, and Acetaminophen

50a. Chlorpheniramine, Pseudoephedrine, Dextromethorphan, Acetaminophen, and Caffeine

50b. Diphenhydramine (dye-fen-HYE-dra-meen), Pseudoephedrine, Dextromethorphan, and Acetaminophen

51. Doxylamine (dox-ILL-a-meen), Pseudoephedrine, Dextromethorphan, and Acetaminophen

52. Pheniramine, Pyrilamine, Phenylpropanolamine, Codeine, Acetaminophen, and Caffeine

53. Pyrilamine, Phenylephrine, Dextromethorphan, and Acetaminophen

54. Pyrilamine, Phenylpropanolamine, Dextromethorphan, and Sodium Salicylate (sa-LI-si-late)

54a. Pyrilamine, Pseudoephedrine, Dextromethorphan, and Acetaminophen

54b. Triprolidine, Pseudoephedrine, Dextromethorphan, and Acetaminophen

Antihistamine, decongestant, antitussive, and expectorant combinations—

55. Brompheniramine (brome-fen-EER-a-meen), Phenylephrine (fen-ill-EF-rin), Phenylpropanolamine (fen-ill-proe-pa-NOLE-a-meen), Codeine (KOE-deen), and Guaifenesin (gwye-FEN-e-sin)

56. Brompheniramine, Phenylephrine, Phenylpropanolamine, Hydrocodone (hye-droe-KOE-done), and Guaifenesin

57. Chlorpheniramine, Ephedrine, Phenylephrine, Dextromethorphan (dex-troe-meth-OR-fan), Ammonium Chloride, and Ipecac (IP-e-kak)

58. No product available

59. No product available

60. Chlorpheniramine, Phenylephrine, Codeine and Ammonium Chloride

61. Chlorpheniramine, Phenylephrine, Codeine, and Potassium Iodide (EYE-oh-dyed)

62. Chlorpheniramine, Phenylephrine, Dextromethorphan, and Guaifenesin

63. Chlorpheniramine, Phenylephrine, Dextromethorphan, Guaifenesin, and Ammonium Chloride

64. Chlorpheniramine, Phenylephrine, Phenylpropanolamine, Carbetapentane (kar-bay-ta-PEN-tane), and Potassium (poe-TAS-see-um) Guaiacolsulfonate (gwye-a-kol-SUL-fon-ate)

65. Chlorpheniramine, Phenylpropanolamine, Dextromethorphan, and Ammonium Chloride

66. No product available

67. Chlorpheniramine, Phenyltoloxamine (fen-ill-tole-OX-a-meen), Ephedrine, Codeine, and Guaiacol Carbonate (GYWE-a-kole KAR-bone-ate)

68. Diphenylpyraline (dye-fen-il-PEER-a-leen), Phenylephrine, Hydrocodone, and Guaifenesin

69. Pheniramine (fen-EER-a-meen), Pyrilamine, Phenylpropanolamine, Dextromethorphan, and Ammonium Chloride

70. Pheniramine, Pyrilamine, Phenylpropanolamine, Dextromethorphan, and Guaifenesin

71. Pheniramine, Pyrilamine, Phenylpropanolamine, Hydrocodone, and Guaifenesin
71a. Pheniramine, Phenylephrine, Phenylpropanolamine, Hydrocodone, and Guaifenesin
72. Pyrilamine, Phenylephrine, Hydrocodone, and Ammonium Chloride
72a. Pyrilamine, Phenylpropanolamine, Dextromethorphan, Guaifenesin, Potassium Citrate, and Citric Acid
73. Triprolidine (trye-PROE-li-deen), Pseudoephedrine (soo-doe-e-FED-rin), Codeine, and Guaifenesin

Antihistamine, decongestant, antitussive, expectorant, and analgesic combinations—

74. Chlorpheniramine (klor-fen-EER-a-meen), Phenylephrine (fen-ill-EF-rin), Phenylpropanolamine (fen-ill-proe-pa-NOLE-a-meen), Dextromethorphan (dex-troe-meth-OR-fan), Guaifenesin (gwye-FEN-e-sin), and Acetaminophen (a-seat-a-MIN-oh-fen)
75. Chlorpheniramine, Phenylpropanolamine, Codeine (KOE-deen), Guaifenesin, and Acetaminophen
76. No product available
77. No product available
78. Pheniramine (fen-EER-a-meen), Phenylephrine, Codeine, Sodium Citrate (SOE-dee-um SI-trate), Sodium Salicylate (sa-LI-sill-ate), and Caffeine (kaf-EEN)
79. No product available

Antihistamine, decongestant, and expectorant combinations—

80. Brompheniramine (brome-fen-EER-a-meen), Phenylephrine (fen-ill-EF-rin), Phenylpropanolamine (fen-ill-proe-pa-NOLE-a-meen), and Guaifenesin (gwye-FEN-e-sin)
81. Carbinoxamine (kar-bi-NOX-a-meen), Pseudoephedrine (soo-doe-e-FED-rin), and Guaifenesin
82. Chlorpheniramine (klor-fen-EER-a-meen), Ephedrine (e-FED-rin), and Guaifenesin
83. Chlorpheniramine, Phenylephrine, and Guaifenesin
84. Chlorpheniramine, Phenylpropanolamine, and Guaifenesin
85. Chlorpheniramine, Phenylpropanolamine, Guaifenesin, Sodium Citrate (SOE-dee-um SI-trate), and Citric (SI-trik) Acid
86. Chlorpheniramine, Pseudoephedrine, and Guaifenesin

87. Dexchlorpheniramine (dex-klor-fen-EER-a-meen), Pseudoephedrine, and Guaifenesin
88. Pheniramine (fen-EER-a-meen), Pyrilamine (peer-ILL-a-meen), Phenylpropanolamine, and Guaifenesin

Antitussive and analgesic combination—

88a. Dextromethorphan (dex-troe-meth-OR-fan) and Acetaminophen (a-seat-a-MIN-oh-fen)

Antitussive and anticholinergic combination—

89. Hydrocodone (hye-droe-KOE-done) and Homatropine (hoe-MA-troe-peen)†

Antitussive and expectorant combinations—

90. Codeine (KOE-deen) and Calcium Iodide (KAL-see-um EYE-oh-dyed)
91. Codeine and Guaifenesin (gwye-FEN-e-sin)
92. Codeine and Iodinated Glycerol (EYE-oh-di-nay-ted GLI-ser-ole)
93. No product available
94. Dextromethorphan and Guaifenesin
95. Dextromethorphan and Iodinated Glycerol
96. No product available
97. Hydrocodone (hye-droe-KOE-done) and Guaifenesin
98. Hydrocodone and Potassium Guaiacolsulfonate
99. Hydromorphone (hye-droe-MOR-fone) and Guaifenesin

Decongestant and antitussive combinations—

100. Phenylephrine (fen-ill-EF-rin) and Codeine (KOE-deen)
100a. Phenylephrine and Hydrocodone (hye-droe-KOE-done)
101. Phenylpropanolamine (fen-ill-proe-pa-NOLE-a-meen) and Caramiphen (kar-AM-i-fen)
102. Phenylpropanolamine and Dextromethorphan
103. Phenylpropanolamine and Hydrocodone (hye-droe-KOE-done)
104. Pseudoephedrine (soo-doe-e-FED-rin) and Codeine
105. Pseudoephedrine and Dextromethorphan
106. Pseudoephedrine and Hydrocodone

Decongestant, antitussive, and analgesic combinations—

107. Phenylpropanolamine (fen-ill-proe-pa-NOLE-a-meen), Dextromethorphan (dex-troe-meth-OR-fan), and Acetaminophen (a-seat-a-MIN-oh-fen)

108. Pseudoephedrine (soo-doe-e-FED-rin), Dextromethorphan, and Acetaminophen

Decongestant, antitussive, and expectorant combinations—

109. Phenylephrine (fen-ill-EF-rin), Dextromethorphan (dextroe-meth-OR-fan), and Guaifenesin (gwye-FEN-e-sin)

109a. Phenylephrine, Phenylpropanolamine, Carbetapentane (kar-bay-ta-PEN-tane), and Potassium Guaiacolsulfonate (poe-TAS-see-um gwye-a-kol-SUL-fon-ate)

110. Phenylephrine, Hydrocodone (hye-droe-KOE-done), and Guaifenesin

111. Phenylpropanolamine (fen-ill-proe-pa-NOLE-a-meen), Codeine (KOE-deen), and Guaifenesin

112. Phenylpropanolamine, Dextromethorphan, and Guaifenesin

113. Pseudoephedrine (soo-doe-e-FED-rin), Codeine, and Guaifenesin

114. Pseudoephedrine, Dextromethorphan, and Guaifenesin

115. Pseudoephedrine, Hydrocodone, and Guaifenesin

Decongestant, antitussive, expectorant, and analgesic combinations—

116. Phenylpropanolamine (fen-ill-proe-pa-NOLE-a-meen), Hydrocodone (hye-droe-KOE-done), Guaifenesin (gwye-FEN-e-sin), and Salicylamide (sal-i-SILL-amide)

117. Pseudoephedrine (soo-doe-e-FED-rin), Dextromethorphan, Guaifenesin, and Acetaminophen

Decongestant and expectorant combinations—

118. Ephedrine (e-FED-rin) and Guaifenesin (gwye-FEN-e-sin)

119. Ephedrine and Potassium Iodide (poe-TAS-ee-um EYE-oh-dyed)

120. Phenylephrine (fen-ill-EF-rin), Phenylpropanolamine (fen-ill-proe-pa-NOLE-a-meen), and Guaifenesin

120a. Phenylephrine and Guaifenesin

121. Phenylpropanolamine and Guaifenesin

122. Pseudoephedrine (soo-doe-e-FED-rin) and Guaifenesin

Decongestant, expectorant, and analgesic combination—

123. Phenylephrine (fen-ill-EF-rin), Guaifenesin (gwye-FEN-e-sin), Acetaminophen (a-seat-a-MIN-oh-fen), Salicylamide and Caffeine

---

†Generic name product available in the U.S.

Description

Cough/cold combinations are used mainly to relieve the cough due to colds, influenza, or hay fever. They are not to be used for the chronic cough that occurs with smoking, asthma, or emphysema or when there is an unusually large amount of mucus or phlegm (pronounced flem) with the cough.

Cough/cold combination products contain more than one ingredient. For example, some products may contain an antihistamine, a decongestant, and an analgesic, in addition to a medicine for coughing. If you are treating yourself, it is important to select a product that is best for your symptoms. Also, in general, it is best to buy a product that includes only those medicines you really need. If you have questions about which product to buy, check with your pharmacist.

Since different products contain ingredients that will have different precautions and side effects, it is important that you know the ingredients of the medicine you are taking. The different kinds of ingredients that may be found in cough/cold combinations include:

Antihistamines—Antihistamines are used to relieve or prevent the symptoms of hay fever and other types of allergy. They also help relieve some symptoms of the common cold, such as sneezing and runny nose. They work by preventing the effects of a substance called histamine, which is produced by the body. Some examples of antihistamines contained in these combinations are: chlorpheniramine, diphenhydramine, pheniramine, promethazine, and triprolidine.

Decongestants—Decongestants, such as ephedrine, phenylephrine, phenylpropanolamine (also known as PPA), and pseudoephedrine, produce a narrowing of blood vessels. This leads to clearing of nasal congestion. However, this effect may also increase blood pressure in patients who have high blood pressure.

Antitussives—To help relieve coughing, these combinations contain either a narcotic (codeine, dihydrocodeine, hydrocodone or hydromorphone) or a non-narcotic (carbetapentane, dextromethorphan, or noscapine) antitussive. These antitussives act directly on the cough center in the brain. Narcotics may become habit-forming, causing mental or physical dependence, if used for a long time. Physical dependence may lead to withdrawal side effects when you stop taking the medicine.

Expectorants—Guaifenesin works by loosening the mucus or phlegm in the lungs. Other ingredients added as expectorants (for example, ammonium chloride, calcium iodide, iodinated glycerol, ipecac, potassium guaiacolsulfonate, potassium iodide, and sodium citrate) have not been proven to be effective. In general, the best thing you can do to loosen mucus or phlegm is to drink plenty of water.

Analgesics—Analgesics, such as acetaminophen, aspirin, and other salicylates (such as salicylamide and sodium salicylate), are used in these combination medicines to help relieve the aches and pain that may occur with the common cold.

The use of too much acetaminophen and salicylates at the same time may cause kidney damage or cancer of the kidney or urinary bladder. This may occur if large amounts of both medicines are taken together for a long time. However, taking the recommended amounts of combination medicines that contain both acetaminophen and a salicylate for short periods of time has not been shown to cause these unwanted effects.

Anticholinergics—Anticholinergics such as homatropine may help produce a drying effect in the nose and chest.

Some of these combinations are available only with your doctor's prescription. Others are available without a prescription; however, your doctor or pharmacist may have special instructions on the proper dose of the medicine for your medical condition.

Cough/cold combinations are available in the following dosage forms:

Antihistamine and antitussive combinations—
Oral

 Bromodiphenhydramine and Codeine
 • Syrup (U.S.)
 Chlorpheniramine and Dextromethorphan
 • Oral solution (U.S.)
 Chlorpheniramine and Hydrocodone
 • Oral suspension (U.S.)
 Phenyltoloxamine and Hydrocodone
 • Capsules (Canada)
 • Oral suspension (U.S. and Canada)
 Promethazine and Codeine
 • Syrup (U.S.)
 Promethazine and Dextromethorphan
 • Syrup (U.S.)
 Pyrilamine and Codeine
 • Oral solution (U.S.)

Antihistamine, antitussive, and analgesic combinations—
Oral

 Chlorpheniramine, Dextromethorphan, and Acetaminophen
 • Capsules (U.S.)

Antihistamine, antitussive, and expectorant combinations—
Oral

 Bromodiphenhydramine, Diphenhydramine, Codeine, Ammonium Chloride, and Potassium Guaiacolsulfonate
 • Oral solution (U.S.)
 Diphenhydramine, Codeine, and Ammonium Chloride
 • Syrup (Canada)
 Phenindamine, Hydrocodone, and Guaifenesin
 • Tablets (U.S.)

Pheniramine, Codeine, and Guaifenesin
  • Syrup (Canada)
Pheniramine, Pyrilamine, Hydrocodone, and Potassium Citrate
  • Syrup (U.S.)

Antihistamine, decongestant, and antitussive combinations—

Oral

Brompheniramine, Phenylephrine, Phenylpropanolamine, and Dextromethorphan
  • Elixir (Canada)
  • Tablets (Canada)
Brompheniramine, Phenylpropanolamine, and Codeine
  • Syrup (U.S.)
Brompheniramine, Phenylpropanolamine, and Dextromethorphan
  • Syrup (U.S.)
Brompheniramine, Pseudoephedrine, and Dextromethorphan
  • Syrup (U.S.)
Carbinoxamine, Pseudoephedrine, and Dextromethorphan
  • Oral solution (U.S.)
  • Syrup (U.S.)
Chlorpheniramine, Ephedrine, Phenylephrine, and Carbetapentane
  • Oral suspension (U.S.)
  • Tablets (U.S.)
Chlorpheniramine, Phenylephrine, and Dextromethorphan
  • Oral solution (U.S.)
  • Tablets (U.S.)
Chlorpheniramine, Phenylephrine, and Hydrocodone
  • Syrup (U.S.)
Chlorpheniramine, Phenylephrine, Phenylpropanolamine, and Codeine
  • Syrup (U.S.)
Chlorpheniramine, Phenylephrine, Phenylpropanolamine, and Dextromethorphan
  • Syrup (U.S.)
Chlorpheniramine, Phenylephrine, Phenylpropanolamine, and Dihydrocodeine
  • Syrup (U.S.)

Chlorpheniramine, Phenylpropanolamine, and Caramiphen
- Extended-release capsules (Canada)

Chlorpheniramine, Phenylpropanolamine, and Dextromethorphan
- Granules (U.S.)
- Oral gel (U.S.)
- Oral solution (U.S. and Canada)
- Syrup (U.S.)
- Tablets (U.S.)

Chlorpheniramine, Pseudoephedrine, and Codeine
- Elixir (U.S.)
- Oral solution (U.S.)
- Syrup (U.S.)

Chlorpheniramine, Pseudoephedrine, and Dextromethorphan
- Oral solution (U.S.)
- Syrup (U.S.)

Chlorpheniramine, Pseudoephedrine, and Hydrocodone
- Oral solution (U.S.)

Diphenylpyraline, Phenylephrine, and Dextromethorphan
- Syrup (Canada)

Diphenylpyraline, Phenylephrine, and Hydrocodone
- Oral solution (Canada)
- Syrup (Canada)

Pheniramine, Pyrilamine, Phenylephrine, Phenylpropanolamine, and Hydrocodone
- Oral solution (U.S.)

Pheniramine, Pyrilamine, Phenylpropanolamine, and Codeine
- Syrup (Canada)

Pheniramine, Pyrilamine, Phenylpropanolamine, and Dextromethorphan
- Syrup (Canada)

Pheniramine, Pyrilamine, Phenylpropanolamine, and Hydrocodone
- Oral solution (Canada)

Promethazine, Phenylephrine, and Codeine
- Syrup (U.S.)

Pyrilamine, Phenylephrine, and Codeine
- Syrup (U.S.)

Pyrilamine, Phenylephrine, and Dextromethorphan

• Oral solution (U.S.)

Pyrilamine, Phenylephrine, and Hydrocodone
  • Syrup (U.S.)

Triprolidine, Pseudoephedrine, and Codeine
  • Syrup (U.S. and Canada)
  • Tablets (Canada)

Triprolidine, Pseudoephedrine, and Dextromethorphan
  • Oral solution (Canada)

Antihistamine, decongestant, antitussive, and analgesic combinations—

Oral

Brompheniramine, Phenylpropanolamine, Dextromethorphan, and Aspirin
  • Tablets (U.S.)

Chlorpheniramine, Phenindamine, Phenylephrine, Dextromethorphan, Acetaminophen, Salicylamide, Caffeine, and Ascorbic Acid
  • Tablets (U.S.)

Chlorpheniramine, Pheniramine, Pyrilamine, Phenylephrine, Hydrocodone, Salicylamide, Caffeine, and Ascorbic Acid
  • Capsules (U.S.)

Chlorpheniramine, Phenylephrine, Dextromethorphan, Acetaminophen, and Salicylamide
  • Tablets (U.S.)

Chlorpheniramine, Phenylephrine, Hydrocodone, Acetaminophen, and Caffeine
  • Tablets (U.S.)

Chlorpheniramine, Phenylpropanolamine, Dextromethorphan, and Acetaminophen
  • Capsules (U.S.)
  • Oral solution (U.S.)
  • Tablets (U.S.)

Chlorpheniramine, Phenylpropanolamine, Dextromethorphan, and Aspirin
  • Tablets (U.S.)

Chlorpheniramine, Pseudoephedrine, Dextromethorphan, and Acetaminophen
  • Capsules (U.S.)
  • Oral solution (U.S.)
  • Tablets (U.S./Canada)

Chlorpheniramine, Pseudoephedrine, Dextromethorphan, Acetaminophen, and Caffeine
- Tablets (U.S.)

Diphenhydramine, Pseudoephedrine, Dextromethorphan, and Acetaminophen
- Capsules (U.S.)
- Oral solution (U.S.)

Doxylamine, Pseudoephedrine, Dextromethorphan, and Acetaminophen
- Oral solution (U.S.)

Pheniramine, Pyrilamine, Phenylpropanolamine, Codeine, Acetaminophen, and Caffeine
- Tablets (Canada)

Pyrilamine, Phenylephrine, Dextromethorphan, and Acetaminophen
- Oral solution (U.S.)

Pyrilamine, Phenylpropanolamine, Dextromethorphan, and Sodium Salicylate
- Oral solution (U.S.)

Pyrilamine, Pseudoephedrine, Dextromethorphan, and Acetaminophen
- Oral solution (U.S.)

Triprolidine, Pseudoephedrine, Dextromethorphan, and Acetaminophen
- Tablets (U.S.)

Antihistamine, decongestant, antitussive, and expectorant combinations—
Oral

Brompheniramine, Phenylephrine, Phenylpropanolamine, Codeine, and Guaifenesin
- Syrup (Canada)

Brompheniramine, Phenylephrine, Phenylpropanolamine, Hydrocodone, and Guaifenesin
- Oral solution (Canada)

Chlorpheniramine, Ephedrine, Phenylephrine, Dextromethorphan, Ammonium Chloride, and Ipecac
- Syrup (U.S.)

Chlorpheniramine, Phenylephrine, Codeine, and Ammonium Chloride
- Oral solution (U.S.)

Chlorpheniramine, Phenylephrine, Codeine, and Potassium Iodide
- Syrup (U.S.)

Chlorpheniramine, Phenylephrine, Dextromethorphan, and Guaifenesin
- Syrup (U.S.)

Chlorpheniramine, Phenylephrine, Dextromethorphan, Guaifenesin, and Ammonium Chloride
- Oral solution (U.S.)

Chlorpheniramine, Phenylephrine, Phenylpropanolamine, Carbetapentane, and Potassium Guaiacolsulfonate
- Capsules (U.S.)
- Syrup (U.S.)

Chlorpheniramine, Phenylpropanolamine, Dextromethorphan, and Ammonium Chloride
- Syrup (U.S.)

Chlorpheniramine, Phenyltoloxamine, Ephedrine, Codeine, and Guaiacol Carbonate
- Oral suspension (Canada)

Diphenylpyraline, Phenylephrine, Hydrocodone, and Guaifenesin
- Oral solution (Canada)

Pheniramine, Pyrilamine, Phenylpropanolamine, Dextromethorphan, and Ammonium Chloride
- Syrup (U.S.)

Pheniramine, Pyrilamine, Phenylpropanolamine, Dextromethorphan, and Guaifenesin
- Oral solution (Canada)

Pheniramine, Pyrilamine, Phenylpropanolamine, Hydrocodone, and Guaifenesin
- Oral solution (U.S.)

Pheniramine, Phenylephrine, Phenylpropanolamine, Hydrocodone, and Guaifenesin
- Oral solution (U.S.)

Pyrilamine, Phenylephrine, Hydrocodone, and Ammonium Chloride
- Syrup (Canada)

Pyrilamine, Phenylpropanolamine, Dextromethorphan, Guaifenesin, Potassium Citrate, and Citric Acid
- Syrup (U.S.)

Triprolidine, Pseudoephedrine, Codeine, and Guaifenesin
- Oral solution (Canada)

Antihistamine, decongestant, antitussive, expectorant, and analgesic combinations—

Oral

Chlorpheniramine, Phenylephrine, Phenylpropanolamine, Dextromethorphan, Guaifenesin, and Acetaminophen
- Syrup (U.S.)
- Tablets (U.S.)

Chlorpheniramine, Phenylpropanolamine, Codeine, Guaifenesin, and Acetaminophen
- Syrup (U.S.)
- Tablets (U.S.)

Pheniramine, Phenylephrine, Codeine, Sodium Citrate, Sodium Salicylate, and Caffeine
- Syrup (U.S.)

Antihistamine, decongestant, and expectorant combinations—

Oral

Brompheniramine, Phenylephrine, Phenylpropanolamine, and Guaifenesin
- Syrup (Canada)

Carbinoxamine, Pseudoephedrine, and Guaifenesin
- Capsules (U.S.)
- Oral solution (U.S.)

Chlorpheniramine, Ephedrine, and Guaifenesin
- Oral solution (U.S.)

Chlorpheniramine, Phenylephrine, and Guaifenesin
- Oral solution (U.S.)

Chlorpheniramine, Phenylpropanolamine, and Guaifenesin
- Oral solution (Canada)

Chlorpheniramine, Phenylpropanolamine, Guaifenesin, Sodium Citrate, and Citric Acid
- Oral solution (U.S.)

Chlorpheniramine, Pseudoephedrine, and Guaifenesin
- Extended-release tablets (U.S.)

Dexchlorpheniramine, Pseudoephedrine, and Guaifenesin
- Oral solution (U.S.)

Pheniramine, Pyrilamine, Phenylpropanolamine, and Guaifenesin
- Oral solution (Canada)

Antitussive and anticholinergic combination—
Oral

    Hydrocodone and Homatropine
- Syrup (U.S.)
- Tablets (U.S.)

Antitussive and expectorant combinations—
Oral

    Codeine and Calcium Iodide
- Syrup (U.S.)

    Codeine and Guaifenesin
- Oral solution (U.S.)
- Syrup (U.S.)

    Codeine and Iodinated Glycerol
- Oral solution (U.S.)

    Dextromethorphan and Guaifenesin
- Capsules (U.S.)
- Extended-release capsules (U.S.)
- Oral gel (U.S.)
- Lozenges (U.S.)
- Oral solution (U.S.)
- Syrup (U.S.)
- Tablets (U.S.)
- Extended-release tablets (U.S.)

    Dextromethorphan and Iodinated Glycerol
- Oral solution (U.S.)

    Hydrocodone and Guaifenesin
- Oral solution (U.S.)
- Syrup (U.S.)
- Tablets (U.S.)

    Hydrocodone and Potassium Guaiacolsulfonate
- Syrup (U.S.)

    Hydromorphone and Guaifenesin
- Syrup (U.S.)

Decongestant and antitussive combinations—
Oral

    Phenylephrine and Codeine
- Oral solution (Canada)

    Phenylephrine and Hydrocodone
- Oral solution (Canada)

Phenylpropanolamine and Caramiphen
- Extended-release capsules (U.S.)
- Oral solution (U.S.)

Phenylpropanolamine and Dextromethorphan
- Oral gel (U.S.)
- Granules (U.S.)
- Lozenges (U.S.)
- Oral solution (U.S.)
- Syrup (U.S.)

Phenylpropanolamine and Hydrocodone
- Oral solution (U.S.)
- Syrup (U.S.)

Pseudoephedrine and Codeine
- Capsules (U.S.)
- Syrup (U.S.)

Pseudoephedrine and Dextromethorphan
- Oral solution (Canada)
- Chewable tablets (U.S.)

Pseudoephedrine and Hydrocodone
- Oral solution (U.S.)
- Syrup (U.S.)

Decongestant, antitussive, and analgesic combinations—
Oral

Phenylpropanolamine, Dextromethorphan, and Acetaminophen
- Oral solution (U.S.)
- Tablets (U.S.)

Pseudoephedrine, Dextromethorphan, and Acetaminophen
- Oral solution (U.S.)
- Tablets (U.S./Canada)

Decongestant, antitussive, and expectorant combinations—
Oral

Phenylephrine, Dextromethorphan, and Guaifenesin
- Syrup (U.S.)

Phenylephrine, Phenylpropanolamine, Carbetapentane and Potassium Guaiacolsulfonate
- Capsules (U.S.)

Phenylephrine, Hydrocodone, and Guaifenesin
- Syrup (U.S.)

Phenylpropanolamine, Codeine, and Guaifenesin
- Oral solution (U.S.)
- Oral suspension (U.S.)
- Syrup (U.S.)

Phenylpropanolamine, Dextromethorphan, and Guaifenesin
- Oral solution (U.S.)
- Syrup (U.S.)

Pseudoephedrine, Codeine, and Guaifenesin
- Oral solution (U.S.)
- Syrup (U.S.)

Pseudoephedrine, Dextromethorphan, and Guaifenesin
- Capsules (U.S.)
- Oral solution (U.S.)
- Syrup (U.S.)

Pseudoephedrine, Hydrocodone, and Guaifenesin
- Oral solution (U.S.)
- Tablets (U.S.)

Decongestant, antitussive, expectorant, and analgesic combinations—
Oral

Phenylpropanolamine, Hydrocodone, Guaifenesin, and Salicylamide
- Tablets (U.S.)

Pseudoephedrine, Dextromethorphan, Guaifenesin, and Acetaminophen
- Oral solution (U.S.)
- Tablets (U.S.)

Decongestant and expectorant combinations—
Oral

Ephedrine and Guaifenesin
- Capsules (U.S.)
- Syrup (U.S.)

Ephedrine and Potassium Iodide
- Syrup (U.S.)

Phenylephrine, Phenylpropanolamine, and Guaifenesin
- Capsules (U.S.)
- Oral solution (U.S.)
- Tablets (U.S.)

Phenylephrine and Guaifenesin
- Extended-release capsules (U.S.)

Phenylpropanolamine and Guaifenesin
- Oral solution (U.S.)
- Syrup (U.S.)
- Extended-release tablets (U.S. and Canada)

Pseudoephedrine and Guaifenesin
- Extended-release capsules (U.S.)
- Oral solution (U.S.)
- Syrup (U.S.)
- Tablets (U.S.)
- Extended-release tablets (U.S.)

Decongestant, expectorant, and analgesic combination—
Oral

Phenylephrine, Guaifenesin, Acetaminophen, Salicylamide and Caffeine
- Tablets (U.S.)

Before Using This Medicine

If you are taking this medicine without a prescription, carefully read and follow any precautions on the label. For cough/cold combinations, the following should be considered:

Allergies—Tell your doctor if you have ever had any unusual or allergic reaction to any of the ingredients contained in this medicine. Also tell your health care professional if you are allergic to any other substances, such as foods, preservatives, or dyes. In addition, if this medicine contains *aspirin or other salicylates*, before taking it, check with your doctor if you have ever had any unusual or allergic reaction to any of the following medicines:

Aspirin or other salicylates
Diclofenac (e.g., Voltaren)
Diflunisal (e.g., Dolobid)

Fenoprofen (e.g., Nalfon)
Floctafenine
Flurbiprofen, by mouth (e.g., Ansaid)
Ibuprofen (e.g., Motrin)
Indomethacin (e.g., Indocin)
Ketoprofen (e.g., Orudis)
Ketorolac (e.g., Toradol)
Meclofenamate (e.g., Meclomen)
Mefenamic acid (e.g., Ponstel)
Methyl salicylate (oil of wintergreen)
Naproxen (e.g., Naprosyn)
Oxyphenbutazone (e.g., Tandearil)
Phenylbutazone (e.g., Butazolidin)
Piroxicam (e.g., Feldene)
Sulindac (e.g., Clinoril)
Suprofen (e.g., Suprol)
Tiaprofenic acid (e.g., Surgam)
Tolmetin (e.g., Tolectin)
Zomepirac (e.g., Zomax)

Diet—Make certain your health care professional knows if you are on any special diet, such as a low-sodium or low-sugar diet.

Pregnancy—The occasional use of a cough/cold combination is not likely to cause problems in the fetus or in the newborn baby. However, when these medicines are used at higher doses and/or for a long time, the chance that problems might occur may increase. For the individual ingredients of these combinations, the following information should be considered before you decide to use a particular cough/cold combination:

- *Acetaminophen*—Studies on birth defects have not been done in humans. However, acetaminophen has not been shown to cause birth defects or other problems in humans.

- *Alcohol*—Some of these combination medicines contain a large amount of alcohol. Too much use of alcohol during pregnancy may cause birth defects.

- *Antihistamines*—Antihistamines have not been shown to cause problems in humans.
- *Caffeine*—Studies in humans have not shown that caffeine causes birth defects. However, studies in animals have shown that caffeine causes birth defects when given in very large doses (amounts equal to the amount of caffeine contained in 12 to 24 cups of coffee a day).
- *Codeine*—Although studies on birth defects with codeine have not been done in humans, it has not been reported to cause birth defects in humans. Codeine has not been shown to cause birth defects in animal studies, but it caused other unwanted effects. Also, regular use of narcotics during pregnancy may cause the baby to become dependent on the medicine. This may lead to withdrawal side effects after birth. In addition, narcotics may cause breathing problems in the newborn baby if taken by the mother just before delivery.
- *Hydrocodone*—Although studies on birth defects with hydrocodone have not been done in humans, it has not been reported to cause birth defects in humans. However, hydrocodone has been shown to cause birth defects in animals when given in very large doses. Also, regular use of narcotics during pregnancy may cause the baby to become dependent on the medicine. This may lead to withdrawal side effects after birth. In addition, narcotics may cause breathing problems in the newborn baby if taken by the mother just before delivery.
- *Iodides (e.g., calcium iodide and iodinated glycerol)*—Not recommended during pregnancy. Iodides have caused enlargement of the thyroid gland in the fetus and resulted in breathing problems in newborn babies whose mothers took iodides in large doses for a long period of time.
- *Phenylephrine*—Studies on birth defects with phenyl-

ephrine have not been done in either humans or animals.

- *Phenylpropanolamine*—Studies on birth defects with phenylpropanolamine have not been done in either humans or animals. However, it seems that women who take phenylpropanolamine in the weeks following delivery are more likely to suffer mental or mood changes.

- *Pseudoephedrine*—Studies on birth defects with pseudoephedrine have not been done in humans. In animal studies pseudoephedrine did not cause birth defects but did cause a decrease in average weight, length, and rate of bone formation in the animal fetus when given in high doses.

- *Salicylates (e.g., aspirin)*—Studies on birth defects in humans have been done with aspirin, but not with salicylamide or sodium salicylate. Salicylates have not been shown to cause birth defects in humans. However, salicylates have been shown to cause birth defects in animals.

Some reports have suggested that too much use of aspirin late in pregnancy may cause a decrease in the newborn's weight and possible death of the fetus or newborn infant. However, the mothers in these reports had been taking much larger amounts of aspirin than are usually recommended. Studies of mothers taking aspirin in the doses that are usually recommended did not show these unwanted effects. However, there is a chance that regular use of salicylates late in pregnancy may cause unwanted effects on the heart or blood flow in the fetus or newborn baby.

Use of salicylates, especially aspirin, during the last 2 weeks of pregnancy may cause bleeding problems in the fetus before or during delivery, or in the newborn baby. Also, too much use of salicylates during the last 3 months of pregnancy may increase the length of pregnancy, prolong labor, cause other problems during delivery, or cause severe bleeding in the mother before, during, or after delivery. *Do not take aspirin during the last 3 months of pregnancy unless it has been ordered by your doctor.*

Breast-feeding—If you are breast-feeding, the chance that problems might occur depends on the ingredients of the combination. For the individual ingredients of these combinations, the following apply:

- *Acetaminophen*—Acetaminophen passes into the breast milk. However, it has not been reported to cause problems in nursing babies.

- *Alcohol*—Alcohol passes into the breast milk. However, the amount of alcohol in recommended doses of this medicine does not usually cause problems in nursing babies.

- *Antihistamines*—Small amounts of antihistamines pass into the breast milk. Antihistamine-containing medicine is not recommended for use while breast-feeding since most antihistamines are especially likely to cause side effects, such as unusual excitement or irritability, in the baby. Also, since antihistamines tend to decrease the secretions of the body, the flow of breast milk may be reduced in some patients.

- *Caffeine*—Small amounts of caffeine pass into the breast milk and may build up in the nursing baby. However, the amount of caffeine in recommended doses of this medicine does not usually cause problems in nursing babies.

- *Decongestants (e.g., ephedrine, phenylephrine, phenylpropanolamine, pseudoephedrine)*—Phenylephrine and phenylpropanolamine have not been reported to cause problems in nursing babies. Ephedrine and pseudoephedrine pass into the breast milk and may cause unwanted effects in nursing babies (especially newborn and premature babies).

- *Iodides (e.g., calcium iodide and iodinated gly-*

cerol)—These medicines pass into the breast milk and may cause unwanted effects, such as underactive thyroid, in the baby.

- *Narcotic antitussives (e.g., codeine, dihydrocodeine, hydrocodone, and hydromorphone)*—Small amounts of codeine have been shown to pass into the breast milk. However, the amount of codeine or other narcotic antitussives in recommended doses of this medicine has not been reported to cause problems in nursing babies.

- *Salicylates (e.g., aspirin)*—Salicylates pass into the breast milk. Although salicylates have not been reported to cause problems in nursing babies, it is possible that problems may occur if large amounts are taken regularly.

Children—Very young children are usually more sensitive to the effects of this medicine. *Before giving any of these combination medicines to a child, check the package label very carefully. Some of these medicines are too strong for use in children.* If you are not certain whether a specific product can be given to a child, or if you have any questions about the amount to give, check with your health care professional, especially if it contains:

- *Antihistamines*—Nightmares, unusual excitement, nervousness, restlessness, or irritability may be more likely to occur in children taking antihistamines.

- *Decongestants (e.g., ephedrine, phenylephrine, phenylpropanolamine, pseudoephedrine)*—Increases in blood pressure may be more likely to occur in children taking decongestants. Also, mental changes may be more likely to occur in young children taking phenylpropanolamine-containing combinations.

- *Narcotic antitussives (e.g., codeine, hydrocodeine, hydrocodone, and hydromorphone)*—Breathing problems may be especially likely to occur in children younger than 2 years of age taking narcotic antitussives. Also, unusual excitement or restlessness may be more likely to occur in children receiving these medicines.

- *Salicylates (e.g., aspirin)—Do not give medicines containing aspirin or other salicylates to a child with a fever or other symptoms of a virus infection, especially flu or chickenpox, without first discussing its use with your child's doctor.* This is very important because salicylates may cause a serious illness called Reye's syndrome in children with fever caused by a virus infection, especially flu or chickenpox. Also, children may be more sensitive to the aspirin or other salicylates contained in some of these medicines, especially if they have a fever or have lost large amounts of body fluid because of vomiting, diarrhea, or sweating.

Teenagers—*Do not give medicines containing aspirin or other salicylates to a teenager with a fever or other symptoms of a virus infection, especially flu or chickenpox, without first discussing its use with your child's doctor.* This is very important because salicylates may cause a serious illness called Reye's syndrome in teenagers with fever caused by a virus infection, especially flu or chickenpox.

Older adults—The elderly are usually more sensitive to the effects of this medicine, especially if it contains:

- *Antihistamines*—Confusion, difficult or painful urination, dizziness, drowsiness, feeling faint, or dryness of mouth, nose, or throat may be more likely to occur in elderly patients. Also, nightmares or unusual excitement, nervousness, restlessness, or irritability may be more likely to occur in the elderly taking antihistamines.
- *Decongestants (e.g., ephedrine, phenylephrine, phenylpropanolamine, pseudoephedrine)*—Confusion, hallucinations, drowsiness, or convulsions (seizures) may

be more likely to occur in the elderly, who are usually more sensitive to the effects of this medicine. Also, increases in blood pressure may be more likely to occur in elderly persons taking decongestants.

Other medicines—Although certain medicines should not be used together at all, in other cases two different medicines may be used together even if an interaction might occur. In these cases, your doctor may want to change the dose, or other precautions may be necessary. Tell your health care professional if you are taking *any* other prescription or nonprescription (over-the-counter [OTC]) medicine, for example, aspirin or other medicine for allergies. Some medicines may change the way this medicine affects your body. Also, the effect of other medicines may be increased or reduced by some of the ingredients in this medicine. Check with your health care professional about which medicines you should not take with this medicine.

Other medical problems—The presence of other medical problems may affect the use of the cough/cold combination medicine. Make sure you tell your doctor if you have any other medical problems, especially:

- Alcohol abuse (or history of)—Acetaminophen-containing medicines increase the chance of liver damage; also, some of the liquid medicines contain a large amount of alcohol
- Anemia or
- Gout or
- Hemophilia or other bleeding problems or
- Stomach ulcer or other stomach problems—These conditions may become worse if you are taking a combination medicine containing aspirin or another salicylate
- Brain disease or injury or
- Colitis or
- Convulsions (seizures) (history of) or
- Diarrhea or
- Gallbladder disease or gallstones—These conditions may become worse if you are taking a combination medicine containing codeine, dihydrocodeine, hydrocodone, or hydromorphone

- Cystic fibrosis (in children)—Side effects of iodinated glycerol may be more likely in children with cystic fibrosis
- Diabetes mellitus (sugar diabetes)—Decongestants may put diabetic patients at greater risk of having heart or blood vessel disease
- Emphysema, asthma, or chronic lung disease (especially in children)—Salicylate-containing medicine may cause an allergic reaction in which breathing becomes difficult
- Enlarged prostate or
- Urinary tract blockage or difficult urination—Some of the effects of anticholinergics (e.g., homatropine) or antihistamines may make urinary problems worse
- Glaucoma—A slight increase in inner eye pressure may occur with the use of anticholinergics (e.g., homatropine) or antihistamines, which may make the condition worse
- Heart or blood vessel disease or
- High blood pressure—Decongestant-containing medicine may increase the blood pressure and speed up the heart rate; also, caffeine-containing medicine, if taken in large amounts, may speed up the heart rate
- Kidney disease—This condition may increase the chance of side effects of this medicine because the medicine may build up in the body
- Liver disease—Liver disease increases the chance of side effects because the medicine may build up in the body; also, if liver disease is severe, there is a greater chance that aspirin-containing medicine may cause bleeding
- Thyroid disease—If an overactive thyroid has caused a fast heart rate, the decongestant in this medicine may cause the heart rate to speed up further; also, if the medicine contains narcotic antitussives (e.g., codeine), iodides (e.g., iodinated glycerol), or salicylates, the thyroid problem may become worse

---

Proper Use of This Medicine

To help loosen mucus or phlegm in the lungs, *drink a glass of water after each dose of this medicine*, unless otherwise directed by your doctor.

Take this medicine only as directed. Do not take more of it and do not take it more often than recommended on the label, unless otherwise directed by your doctor. To do so may increase the chance of side effects.

For patients *taking the extended-release capsule or tablet form of this medicine:*
- Swallow the capsule or tablet whole.
- Do not crush, break, or chew before swallowing.
- If the capsule is too large to swallow, you may mix the contents of the capsule with applesauce, jelly, honey, or syrup and swallow without chewing.

For patients *taking a combination medicine containing an antihistamine and/or aspirin or other salicylate:*
- Take with food or a glass of water or milk to lessen stomach irritation, if necessary.

If a combination medicine containing aspirin has a strong vinegar-like odor, do not use it. This odor means the medicine is breaking down. If you have any questions about this, check with your pharmacist.

Missed dose—If you must take this medicine regularly and you miss a dose, take it as soon as possible. However, if it is almost time for your next dose, skip the missed dose and go back to your regular dosing schedule. Do not double doses.

Storage—To store this medicine:
- Keep this medicine out of the reach of children. Overdose is very dangerous in young children.
- Store away from heat and direct light.
- Do not store the capsule or tablet form of this medicine in the bathroom, near the kitchen sink, or in other damp places. Heat or moisture may cause the medicine to break down.
- Keep the liquid form of this medicine from freezing. Do not refrigerate the syrup.

- Do not keep outdated medicine or medicine no longer needed. Be sure that any discarded medicine is out of the reach of children.

Precautions While Using This Medicine

If your cough has not improved after 7 days or if you have a high fever, skin rash, continuing headache, or sore throat with the cough, check with your doctor. These signs may mean that you have other medical problems.

For patients *taking antihistamine-containing medicine:*

- Before you have any skin tests for allergies, tell the doctor in charge that you are taking this medicine. The results of the test may be affected by the antihistamine in this medicine.

- This medicine will add to the effects of alcohol and other CNS depressants (medicines that slow down the nervous system, possibly causing drowsiness). Some examples of CNS depressants are antihistamines or medicine for hay fever, other allergies, or colds; sedatives, tranquilizers, or sleeping medicine; prescription pain medicine or narcotics; barbiturates; medicine for seizures; muscle relaxants; or anesthetics, including some dental anesthetics. *Check with your doctor before taking any of the above while you are taking this medicine.*

- This medicine may cause some people to become drowsy, dizzy, or less alert than they are normally. *Make sure you know how you react to this medicine before you drive, use machines, or do anything else that could be dangerous if you are dizzy or are not alert.*

- When taking antihistamines on a regular basis, make sure your doctor knows if you are taking large amounts of aspirin at the same time (as in arthritis or rheumatism). Effects of too much aspirin, such as ringing in the ears, may be covered up by the antihistamine.

- Antihistamines may cause dryness of the mouth. For temporary relief, use sugarless candy or gum, melt bits of ice in your mouth, or use a saliva substitute. However, if your mouth continues to feel dry for more than 2 weeks, check with your medical doctor or dentist. Continuing dryness of the mouth may increase the chance of dental disease, including tooth decay, gum disease, and fungus infections.

For patients *taking decongestant-containing medicine:*

- This medicine may add to the central nervous system (CNS) stimulant and other effects of phenylpropanolamine (PPA)-containing diet aids. *Do not use medicines for diet or appetite control while taking this medicine unless you have checked with your doctor.*

- This medicine may cause some people to be nervous or restless or to have trouble in sleeping. If you have trouble in sleeping, *take the last dose of this medicine for each day a few hours before bedtime.* If you have any questions about this, check with your doctor.

- Before having any kind of surgery (including dental surgery) or emergency treatment, tell the medical doctor or dentist in charge that you are taking this medicine.

For patients *taking narcotic antitussive (codeine, dihydrocodeine, hydrocodone, or hydromorphone)–containing medicine:*

- This medicine will add to the effects of alcohol and other CNS depressants (medicines that slow down the nervous system, possibly causing drowsiness). Some examples of CNS depressants are antihistamines or medicine for hay fever, other allergies, or colds; sedatives, tranquilizers, or sleeping medicine; prescription pain medicine or narcotics; barbiturates; medicine for seizures; muscle relaxants; or anesthetics, including some dental anesthetics. *Check with your doctor before taking any of the above while you are taking this medicine.*

- This medicine may cause some people to become drowsy, dizzy, less alert than they are normally, or to feel a false sense of well-being. *Make sure you know how you react to this medicine before you drive, use machines, or do anything else that could be dangerous if you are dizzy or are not alert and clearheaded.*

- Nausea or vomiting may occur after taking a narcotic antitussive. This effect may go away if you lie down for a while. However, if nausea or vomiting continues, check with your doctor.

- Dizziness, lightheadedness, or fainting may be especially likely to occur when you get up suddenly from a lying or sitting position. Getting up slowly may help lessen this problem.

- Before having any kind of surgery (including dental surgery) or emergency treatment, tell the medical doctor or dentist in charge that you are taking this medicine.

For patients *taking iodide (calcium iodide, iodinated glycerol, or potassium iodide)-containing medicine:*

- Make sure your doctor knows if you are planning to have any future thyroid tests. The results of the thyroid test may be affected by the iodine in this medicine.

For patients *taking analgesic-containing medicine:*

- *Check the label of all nonprescription (over-the-counter [OTC]), and prescription medicines you now take.* If any contain acetaminophen or aspirin or other salicylates, including diflunisal or bismuth subsalicylate, be especially careful. Taking them while taking

a cough/cold combination medicine that already contains them may lead to overdose. If you have any
questions about this, check with your health care
professional.

- Do not take aspirin-containing medicine for 5 days
before any surgery, including dental surgery, unless
otherwise directed by your medical doctor or dentist.
Taking aspirin during this time may cause bleeding
problems.

For *diabetic patients taking aspirin- or sodium salicylate–
containing medicine:*

- False urine sugar test results may occur:

  —If you take 8 or more 325-mg (5-grain) doses of
  aspirin every day for several days in a row.

  —If you take 8 or more 325-mg (5-grain), or 4 or
  more 500-mg (10-grain) doses of sodium salicylate.

- Smaller doses or occasional use of aspirin or sodium
salicylate usually will not affect urine sugar tests. If
you have any questions about this, check with your
health care professional, especially if your diabetes is
not well controlled.

For patients *taking homatropine-containing medicine:*

- This medicine may make you sweat less, causing
your body temperature to increase. *Use extra care
not to become overheated during exercise or hot
weather while you are taking this medicine,* since
overheating may result in heat stroke. Also, hot baths
or saunas may make you feel dizzy or faint while
you are taking this medicine.

Side Effects of This Medicine

Along with its needed effects, a medicine may cause some
unwanted effects. Although serious side effects occur

rarely when this medicine is taken as recommended, they may be more likely to occur if:

- too much medicine is taken.
- it is taken in large doses.
- it is taken for a long period of time.

Get emergency help immediately if any of the following symptoms of overdose occur:

For narcotic antitussive (codeine, dihydrocodeine, hydrocodone, or hydromorphone)–containing

> Cold, clammy skin; confusion (severe); convulsions (seizures); drowsiness or dizziness (severe); nervousness or restlessness (severe); pinpoint pupils of eyes; slow heartbeat; slow or troubled breathing; weakness (severe)

For acetaminophen-containing

> Diarrhea; increased sweating; loss of appetite; nausea or vomiting; stomach cramps or pain; swelling or tenderness in the upper abdomen or stomach area

For salicylate-containing

> Any loss of hearing; bloody urine; confusion; convulsions (seizures); diarrhea (severe or continuing); dizziness or lightheadedness; drowsiness (severe); excitement or nervousness (severe); fast or deep breathing; fever; hallucinations (seeing, hearing, or feeling things that are not there); increased sweating; nausea or vomiting (severe or continuing); shortness of breath or troubled breathing (for salicylamide only); stomach pain (severe or continuing); uncontrollable flapping movements of the hands, especially in elderly patients; unusual thirst; vision problems

For decongestant-containing

> Fast, pounding, or irregular heartbeat; headache (continuing and severe); nausea or vomiting (severe); nervousness or restlessness (severe); shortness of breath or troubled breathing (severe or continuing)

Also, check with your doctor as soon as possible if any of the following side effects occur:

For all combinations

Skin rash, hives, and/or itching

For antihistamine- or anticholinergic-containing

Clumsiness or unsteadiness; convulsions (seizures); drowsiness (severe); dryness of mouth, nose, or throat (severe); flushing or redness of face; hallucinations (seeing, hearing, or feeling things that are not there); restlessness (severe); shortness of breath or troubled breathing; slow or fast heartbeat

For iodine-containing

Headache (continuing); increased watering of mouth; loss of appetite; metallic taste; skin rash, hives, or redness; sore throat; swelling of face, lips, or eyelids

For acetaminophen-containing

Unexplained sore throat and fever; unusual tiredness or weakness; yellow eyes or skin

Other side effects may occur that usually do not need medical attention. These side effects may go away during treatment as your body adjusts to the medicine. However, check with your doctor if any of the following side effects continue or are bothersome:

Constipation; decreased sweating; difficult or painful urination; dizziness or lightheadedness; drowsiness; dryness of mouth, nose, or throat; false sense of well-being; increased sensitivity of skin to sun; nausea or vomiting; nightmares; stomach pain; thickening of mucus; trouble in sleeping; unusual excitement, nervousness, restlessness, or irritability; unusual tiredness or weakness

Not all of the side effects listed above have been reported for each of these medicines, but they have been reported for at least one of them. There are some similarities among these combination medicines, so many of the above side effects may occur with any of these medicines.

Other side effects not listed above may also occur in some patients. If you notice any other effects, check with your doctor.

CROMOLYN Inhalation

A commonly used brand name in the U.S. and Canada is Intal.
Another commonly used name is sodium cromoglycate.

Description

Cromolyn (KROE-moe-lin) is used to prevent the symptoms of asthma. When it is used regularly, cromolyn lessens the number and severity of asthma attacks by reducing inflammation in the lungs. Cromolyn is also used just before exposure to conditions or substances (for example, allergens, chemicals, cold air, or air pollutants) that cause bronchospasm (wheezing or difficulty in breathing). In addition, this medicine is used to prevent bronchospasm following exercise. Cromolyn will not help an asthma or bronchospasm attack that has already started.

Cromolyn may be used alone or with other asthma medicines, such as bronchodilators (medicines that open up narrowed breathing passages) or corticosteroids (cortisone-like medicines).

Cromolyn inhalation works by acting on certain inflammatory cells in the lungs to prevent them from releasing substances that cause asthma symptoms or bronchospasm.

This medicine is available only with your doctor's prescription, in the following dosage forms:

Inhalation
- Capsules for inhalation (U.S. and Canada)
- Inhalation aerosol (U.S. and Canada)
- Inhalation solution (U.S. and Canada)

Before Using This Medicine

In deciding to use a medicine, the risks of using the medicine must be weighed against the good it will do. This is

a decision you and your doctor will make. For cromolyn inhalation, the following should be considered:

Allergies—Tell your doctor if you have ever had any unusual or allergic reaction to cromolyn or to any other inhalation aerosol medicine.

Pregnancy—Cromolyn has not been studied in pregnant women. However, when taken during pregnancy to control the mother's asthma, cromolyn has not been shown to cause problems in the baby. Studies in animals have shown that cromolyn causes a decrease in successful pregnancies and a decrease in the weight of the animal fetus only when given by injection in very large amounts.

Breast-feeding—It is not known whether cromolyn passes into the breast milk. However, this medicine has not been reported to cause problems in nursing babies. Although most medicines pass into breast milk in small amounts, many of them may be used safely while breast-feeding. Mothers who are using this medicine and who wish to breast-feed should discuss this with their doctor.

Children—Although there is no specific information comparing use of cromolyn inhalation in children 2 years of age and older with use in other age groups, this medicine is not expected to cause different side effects or problems in children than it does in adults.

Older adults—Many medicines have not been studied specifically in older people. Therefore, it may not be known whether they work exactly the same way they do in younger adults. Although there is no specific information comparing the use of cromolyn inhalation in the elderly with use in other age groups, this medicine is not expected to cause different side effects or problems in older people than it does in younger adults.

Proper Use of This Medicine

Cromolyn oral inhalation is used to help prevent symptoms of asthma or bronchospasm (wheezing or difficulty in breathing). Cromolyn will not relieve an asthma or a bronchospasm attack that has already started.

Use cromolyn inhalation only as directed. Do not use more of it and do not use it more often than your doctor ordered. To do so may increase the chance of side effects.

Cromolyn inhalation usually comes with patient directions. Read them carefully before using this medicine. If you do not understand the directions that come with the inhaler or if you are not sure how to use the inhaler, ask your health care professional to show you how to use it. Also, ask your health care professional to check regularly how you use the inhaler to make sure you are using it properly.

For patients using *cromolyn inhalation aerosol:*

- The cromolyn aerosol canister provides about 112 or 200 inhalations, depending on the size of the canister your doctor ordered. You should try to keep a record of the number of inhalations you use so you will know when the canister is almost empty. This canister, unlike some other aerosol canisters, cannot be floated in water to test its fullness.

- When you use the inhaler for the first time, or if you have not used it for several days, the inhaler may not deliver the right amount of medicine with the first puff. Therefore, before using the inhaler, test it to make sure it works properly.

- *To test the inhaler:*

  —Insert the metal canister firmly into the clean mouthpiece according to the manufacturer's instructions. Check to make sure the canister is placed properly into the mouthpiece.

—Take the cover off the mouthpiece and shake the inhaler well.

—Hold the canister well away from you against a light background and press the top of the canister, spraying the medicine one time into the air. If you see a fine mist, you will know the inhaler is working properly to provide the right amount of medicine when you use it. If you do not see a fine mist, try a second time.

• *To use the inhaler:*

—Using your thumb and one or two fingers, hold the inhaler upright with the mouthpiece end down and pointing toward you.

—Take the cover off the mouthpiece. Check the mouthpiece for any foreign objects. Do not use the inhaler with any other mouthpieces.

—Gently shake the inhaler three or four times.

—Hold the mouthpiece away from your mouth and breathe out slowly and completely to the end of a normal breath.

—Use the inhalation method recommended by your doctor.

> • Open-mouth method: Place the mouthpiece about 1 to 2 inches (2 fingerwidths) in front of your widely opened mouth. Make sure the inhaler is aimed into your mouth so the spray does not hit the roof of your mouth or your tongue.
>
> • Closed-mouth method: Place the mouthpiece in your mouth between your teeth and over your tongue with your lips closed tightly around it. Make sure your tongue or teeth are not blocking the opening.

—Tilt your head back a little. Start to breathe in slowly and deeply through your mouth and, at the same time, press the top of the canister once to get one puff of medicine. Continue to breathe in slowly for 3 to 4 seconds until you have taken a full deep breath. It is important to press down on the canister and breathe in slowly at the same time so the medicine is pulled into your lungs. This step may be difficult at first. If you are using the closed-mouth method and you see a fine mist coming from your mouth or nose, the inhaler is not being used correctly.

—Hold your breath as long as you can up to 10 seconds (count slowly to ten). This gives the medicine time to get into your airways and lungs.

—Take the mouthpiece away from your mouth and breathe out slowly.

—Wait 1 minute between puffs. Then, gently shake the inhaler again, and take the second puff following exactly the same steps you used for the first puff. Breathe in only one puff at a time.

—If your doctor has told you to use an inhaled bronchodilator before using cromolyn, you should wait at least 2 minutes after using the bronchodilator before using cromolyn. This allows the cromolyn to get deeper into your lungs.

—When you are finished using the inhaler, wipe off the mouthpiece and replace the cover to keep the mouthpiece clean and free of foreign objects.

Your doctor may want you to use a spacer device with the inhaler. A spacer makes the inhaler easier to use. It allows more of the medicine to reach your lungs, rather than staying in your mouth and throat.

• *To use a spacer device with the inhaler:*

—Attach the spacer to the inhaler according to the manufacturer's directions. There are different types of spacers available, but the method of breathing remains the same with most spacers.

—Gently shake the inhaler and spacer well.

—Hold the mouthpiece of the spacer away from your mouth and breathe out slowly and completely.

—Place the mouthpiece of the spacer into your mouth between your teeth and over your tongue with your lips closed around it.

—Press down on the canister top once to release one puff of medicine into the spacer. Then, within one or two seconds, begin to breathe in slowly and deeply through your mouth for 5 to 10 seconds. Count the seconds while inhaling.

—Hold your breath as long as you can up to 10 seconds (count slowly to 10).

—Breathe out slowly. Do not remove the mouthpiece from your mouth. Breathe in and out slowly two or three times to make sure the spacer is emptied.

—Wait a minute between puffs. Then, gently shake the inhaler and spacer again and take the second puff, following exactly the same steps you used for the first puff. Do not spray more than one puff at a time into the spacer.

—When you are finished using the inhaler, remove the spacer device from the inhaler and replace the cover of the mouthpiece.

Clean the inhaler, mouthpiece, and spacer at least two times a week to prevent build-up of medicine and blockage of the mouthpiece.

• *To clean the inhaler:*

—Remove the metal canister from the inhaler and set the canister aside. Do not get the canister wet.

—Wash the mouthpiece and cover, the plastic case, and the spacer in warm soapy water. Rinse well with warm, running water.

—Shake off the excess water and let the inhaler parts air dry completely before putting the inhaler back together.

For patients using *cromolyn capsules for inhalation:*

- *Do not swallow the capsules. The medicine will not work if you swallow it.*
- This medicine is used with a special inhaler, either the *Spinhaler* or the *Halermatic*. If you do not understand the directions that come with the inhaler or if you are not sure how to use the inhaler, ask your health care professional to show you how to use it. Also, ask your health care professional to check regularly how you use the inhaler to make sure you are using it properly.
- If you are using *cromolyn capsules for inhalation* with the *Spinhaler:*

  —*To load the Spinhaler:*
  - Make sure your hands are clean and dry.
  - Insert the capsule into the inhaler just before using this medicine.
  - Hold the inhaler upright with the mouthpiece pointing downward. Unscrew the body of the inhaler from the mouthpiece.
  - Keep the mouthpiece pointing downward and the propeller on the spindle. Remove the foil from the capsule and insert the colored end of the cromolyn capsule firmly into the cup of the propeller. Avoid too much handling of the capsule, because moisture from your hands may make the capsule soft.
  - Make sure the propeller moves freely.
  - Screw the body of the inhaler back into the mouthpiece and make certain that it is fastened well.
  - While keeping the inhaler upright with the mouthpiece pointing downward, slide the grey outer sleeve down firmly until it stops. This will puncture the capsule. Then slide the sleeve up as far as it will go. This step may be repeated

a second time to make sure the capsule is punctured.

—*To use the Spinhaler:*

- Check to make sure the mouthpiece is properly attached to the body of the inhaler.
- Hold the inhaler away from your mouth and breathe out slowly to the end of a normal breath.
- Place the mouthpiece in your mouth, close your lips around it, and tilt your head back. Do not block the mouthpiece with your teeth or tongue.
- Take a deep and rapid breath. You should hear and feel the vibrations of the rotating propeller as you breathe in.
- Take the inhaler from your mouth and hold your breath for a few seconds or as long as possible.
- Hold the inhaler away from your mouth and breathe out slowly and completely to the end of a normal breath. Do not breathe out through the inhaler because this may prevent the inhaler from working properly.
- Keep taking inhalations of this medicine until all the powder from the capsule is inhaled. A light dusting of powder remaining in the capsule is normal and is not a sign that the inhaler is not working properly.
- Throw away the empty capsule. Then return the inhaler to the container and replace the lid on the container.

—*To clean the Spinhaler:*

- At least once a week, brush off any powder left sticking to the propeller.
- Take the inhaler apart and wash the parts of the inhaler with clean, warm water.

- Wash the inside of the propeller shaft by moving the propeller on and off the steel spindle under water.
- Shake out the excess water.
- Allow all parts of the inhaler to dry completely before putting it back together.
- The Spinhaler should be replaced after 6 months.

• If you are using *cromolyn capsules for inhalation* with the *Halermatic:*

  —*To load the Halermatic:*
  - Make sure your hands are clean and dry.
  - Insert the capsule cartridge into the inhaler just before using this medicine.
  - Remove the mouthpiece cover. Then pull off the mouthpiece.
  - Push a cromolyn capsule cartridge firmly down to the bottom of the slot.
  - Slide the mouthpiece back on the body of the inhaler. Push down slowly as far as the mouthpiece will go. This punctures the capsule cartridge and lifts it into the rotation chamber. Do not repeat this step because the capsule cartridge needs to be punctured only once.

  —*To use the Halermatic:*
  - Hold the inhaler away from your mouth and breathe out slowly to the end of a normal breath.
  - Place the mouthpiece in your mouth, close your lips around it, and tilt your head back. Do not block the flow of medicine into the lungs with your teeth or tongue.
  - Breathe in quickly and steadily through the mouthpiece.

- Hold your breath for a few seconds to keep the medicine in the lungs as long as possible. Then take the inhaler away from your mouth.

- Hold the inhaler well away from your mouth and breathe out to the end of a normal breath. Do not breathe out through the inhaler because this may prevent the inhaler from working properly.

- Keep taking inhalations of this medicine until all the powder from the capsule is inhaled. A light dusting of powder remaining in the capsule is normal and is not a sign that the inhaler is not working properly.

- Throw away the empty capsule cartridge.

—*To clean the Halermatic:*

- Brush away powder deposits each day with a brush.

- When powder deposits build up, wipe them away with a slightly damp cloth.

- The mouthpiece may be washed separately if necessary. However, do not wet the blue-based body of the inhaler. Be sure the mouthpiece grid is dry before putting the inhaler back together.

- The Halermatic should be replaced every 6 months.

For patients using *cromolyn inhalation solution:*

- Cromolyn inhalation solution comes in a small glass container called an ampul. The ampul must be broken gently to empty the contents. If you do not understand the manufacturer's directions, ask your health care professional to show you what to do.

- Do not use the solution in the ampul if it is cloudy or contains particles.

- *To break and empty the ampul:*

    —The glass ampul is weak at each end so the ends can be broken easily by hand.

    —Hold the ampul away from the nebulizer and your face when you break it. Hold the ampul at an angle and carefully break off the lower end. No solution will come out.

    —Turn the ampul over so the open end faces upward. Place a forefinger carefully over the open end.

    —Keep your finger firmly in place and break off the lower end of the ampul.

    —To empty the ampul, hold it over the bowl of the nebulizer unit and remove your finger to let the solution flow out.

    —Throw away any solution left in the nebulizer after you have taken your treatment.

- Use this medicine only in a power-operated nebulizer that has an adequate flow rate and is equipped with a face mask or mouthpiece. Your doctor will advise you on which nebulizer to use. Make sure you understand exactly how to use it. Hand-squeezed bulb nebulizers cannot be used with this medicine. If you have any questions about this, check with your doctor.

For patients using *cromolyn oral inhalation* regularly (for example, every day):

- *In order for cromolyn to work properly, it must be inhaled every day in regularly spaced doses as ordered by your doctor.* Up to 4 weeks may pass before you feel the full effects of the medicine.

Dosing—The dose of cromolyn will be different for different patients. *Follow your doctor's orders or the directions on the label.* The following information includes only the average doses of cromolyn inhalation. *If your dose is different, do not change it* unless your doctor tells you to do so.

The number of doses you take each day, the time allowed between doses, and the length of time you take the medicine depend on the medical problem for which you are taking cromolyn inhalation.

- For *inhalation aerosol* dosage form:

  —For prevention of asthma symptoms:

    • Adults and children 5 years of age or older— 1.6 or 2 milligrams (mg) (2 puffs) taken four times a day with doses spaced four to six hours apart.

    • Children up to 5 years of age—Use and dose must be determined by your doctor.

  —For prevention of bronchospasm caused by exercise or a condition or substance:

    • Adults and children 5 years of age or older— 1.6 or 2 milligrams (mg) (2 puffs) taken at least ten to fifteen (but not more than sixty) minutes before exercise or exposure to any condition or substance that may cause an attack.

    • Children up to 5 years of age—Use and dose must be determined by your doctor.

- For *capsule for inhalation* dosage form:

  —For prevention of asthma symptoms:

    • Adults and children 2 years of age or older— 20 mg (contents of 1 capsule) taken four times a day with doses spaced four to six hours apart.

    • Children up to 2 years of age—Use and dose must be determined by your doctor.

  —For prevention of bronchospasm caused by exercise or a condition or substance:

    • Adults and children 2 years of age or older— 20 mg (contents of 1 capsule) taken at least ten to fifteen (but not more than sixty) minutes before exercise or exposure to any condition or substance that may cause an attack.

• Children up to 2 years of age—Use and dose must be determined by your doctor.

• For *inhalation solution* dosage form:

—For prevention of asthma symptoms:

• Adults and children 2 years of age or older—20 mg (contents of 1 ampul) used in a nebulizer. This medicine should be used four times a day with doses spaced four to six hours apart. Use a new ampul of solution for each dose.

• Children up to 2 years of age—Use and dose must be determined by your doctor.

—For prevention of bronchospasm caused by exercise or a condition or substance:

• Adults and children 2 years of age or older—20 mg (contents of 1 ampul) used in a nebulizer. This medicine should be used at least ten to fifteen (but not more than sixty) minutes before exercise or exposure to any condition or substance that may cause an attack. Use a new ampul of solution for each dose.

• Children up to 2 years of age—Use and dose must be determined by your doctor.

Missed dose—If you are using cromolyn regularly and you miss a dose, use it as soon as possible. Then use any remaining doses for that day at regularly spaced times.

Storage—To store this medicine:

• Keep out of the reach of children.

• Store the aerosol or solution form of this medicine at room temperature away from heat or cold. Keep this medicine from freezing.

• Store the capsule or solution form of this medicine away from direct light. Store the aerosol form of this medicine away from direct sunlight.

• Do not store the capsule form of this medicine in the

bathroom, near the kitchen sink, or in other damp places. Heat or moisture may cause the medicine to break down.

- Do not puncture, break, or burn the aerosol container, even if it is empty.

- Do not keep outdated medicine or medicine no longer needed. Be sure that any discarded medicine is out of the reach of children.

Precautions While Using This Medicine

If your symptoms do not improve within 4 weeks or if your condition becomes worse after you begin using cromolyn, check with your doctor.

If you are also taking a corticosteroid or a bronchodilator for your asthma along with this medicine, do not stop taking the corticosteroid or bronchodilator even if your asthma seems better, unless you are told to do so by your doctor.

Dryness of the mouth or throat, throat irritation, and hoarseness may occur after you use this medicine. Gargling and rinsing your mouth or taking a drink of water after each dose may help prevent these effects.

Side Effects of This Medicine

Along with its needed effects, a medicine may cause some unwanted effects. Although not all of these side effects may occur, if they do occur they may need medical attention.

Check with your doctor as soon as possible if any of the following side effects occur:

Less common
>   Increased wheezing, tightness in chest, or difficulty in breathing

Rare
>   Chest pain; chills; difficult or painful urination; difficulty in swallowing; dizziness; frequent urge to urinate; headache (severe or continuing); joint pain or swelling; muscle pain or weakness; skin rash, hives, or itching; sweating; swelling of the face, lips, eyelids, hands, feet, or inside of mouth

Other side effects may occur that usually do not need medical attention. These side effects may go away during treatment as your body adjusts to the medicine. However, check with your doctor if any of the following side effects continue or are bothersome:

More common
>   Cough; dryness of the mouth or throat; nausea; stuffy nose; throat irritation

Less common
>   Hoarseness; watering of the eyes

If you are using the cromolyn inhalation aerosol, you may notice an unpleasant taste. This may be expected and will go away when you stop using the medicine.

Other side effects not listed above may also occur in some patients. If you notice any other effects, check with your doctor.

CYCLOBENZAPRINE Systemic

Some commonly used brand names are:

In the U.S.—
Cycoflex   Flexeril
Generic name product may also be available.
In Canada—
Flexeril

Description

Cyclobenzaprine (sye-kloe-BEN-za-preen) is used to help relax certain muscles in your body. It helps relieve the pain, stiffness, and discomfort caused by strains, sprains, or injuries to your muscles. However, this medicine does not take the place of rest, exercise or physical therapy, or other treatment that your doctor may recommend for your medical problem. Cyclobenzaprine acts on the central nervous system (CNS) to produce its muscle relaxant effects. Its actions on the CNS may also cause some of this medicine's side effects.

Cyclobenzaprine may also be used for other conditions as determined by your doctor.

Cyclobenzaprine is available only with your doctor's prescription, in the following dosage form:

Oral
- Tablets (U.S. and Canada)

Before Using This Medicine

In deciding to use a medicine, the risks of taking the medicine must be weighed against the good it will do. This is a decision you and your doctor will make. For cyclobenzaprine, the following should be considered:

Allergies—Tell your doctor if you have ever had any unusual or allergic reaction to cyclobenzaprine. Also tell your health care professional if you are allergic to any other substances, such as foods, preservatives, or dyes.

Pregnancy—Studies on birth defects with cyclobenzaprine have not been done in humans. However, cyclobenzaprine has not been shown to cause birth defects or other problems in animal studies.

Breast-feeding—It is not known whether cyclobenzaprine passes into breast milk. Although most medicines pass into the breast milk in small amounts, many of them may be used safely while breast-feeding. Mothers who are taking this medicine and who wish to breast-feed should discuss this with their doctor.

Children—Studies on this medicine have been done only in adult patients, and there is no specific information comparing use of cyclobenzaprine in children with use in other age groups.

Teenagers—Studies on this medicine have been done only in adult patients, and there is no specific information comparing use of cyclobenzaprine in teenagers up to 15 years of age with use in other age groups.

Older adults—Many medicines have not been studied specifically in older people. Therefore, it may not be known whether they work exactly the same way they do in younger adults or if they cause different side effects or problems in older people. There is no specific information comparing use of cyclobenzaprine in the elderly with use in other age groups.

Other medicines—Although certain medicines should not be used together at all, in other cases two different medicines may be used together even if an interaction might occur. In these cases, your doctor may want to change the dose, or other precautions may be necessary. When you are taking cyclobenzaprine, it is especially important that your health care professional know if you are taking any of the following:

- Alcohol or
- Central nervous system (CNS) depressants or
- Tricyclic antidepressants (amitriptyline [e.g., Elavil], amoxapine [e.g., Asendin], clomipramine [e.g., Anafranil], desipramine [e.g., Pertofrane], doxepin [e.g., Sinequan], imipramine [e.g., Tofranil], nortriptyline [e.g., Aventyl], protriptyline [e.g., Vivactil], trimipramine [e.g., Surmontil])—The chance of side effects may be increased
- Monoamine oxidase (MAO) inhibitors (furazolidone [e.g.,

Furoxone], isocarboxazid [e.g., Marplan], phenelzine [e.g., Nardil], procarbazine [e.g., Matulane], selegiline (e.g., Eldepryl), tranylcypromine [e.g., Parnate])—Taking cyclobenzaprine while you are taking or within 2 weeks of taking monoamine oxidase (MAO) inhibitors may increase the chance of side effects

Other medical problems—The presence of other medical problems may affect the use of cyclobenzaprine. Make sure you tell your doctor if you have any other medical problems, especially:

- Glaucoma or
- Problems with urination—Cyclobenzaprine can make your condition worse

- Heart or blood vessel disease or
- Overactive thyroid—The chance of side effects may be increased

---

Proper Use of This Medicine

Take this medicine only as directed by your doctor. Do not take more of it and do not take it more often than your doctor ordered. To do so may increase the chance of serious side effects.

Dosing—The dose of cyclobenzaprine will be different for different people. *Follow your doctor's orders or the directions on the label.* The following information includes only the average doses of cyclobenzaprine. *If your dose is different, do not change it* unless your doctor tells you to do so.

- For the *oral* dosage form (tablets):

    —For relaxing stiff muscles:

        • Adults and teenagers 15 years of age and older—The usual dose is 10 milligrams (mg) three times a day. The largest amount should be no more than 60 mg (six 10-mg tablets) a day.

- Children and teenagers up to 15 years of age—Dose must be determined by your doctor.

Missed dose—If you miss a dose of this medicine and remember within an hour or so of the missed dose, take it right away. Then go back to your regular dosing schedule. But if you do not remember until later, skip the missed dose and go back to your regular dosing schedule. Do not double doses.

Storage—To store this medicine:

- Keep out of the reach of children.
- Store away from heat and direct light.
- Do not store this medicine in the bathroom, near the kitchen sink, or in other damp places. Heat or moisture may cause the medicine to break down.
- Do not keep outdated medicine or medicine no longer needed. Be sure that any discarded medicine is out of the reach of children.

Precautions While Using This Medicine

This medicine will add to the effects of alcohol and other CNS depressants (medicines that slow down the nervous system, possibly causing drowsiness). Some examples of CNS depressants are antihistamines or medicine for hay fever, other allergies, or colds; sedatives, tranquilizers, or sleeping medicine; prescription pain medicine or narcotics; barbiturates; medicine for seizures; other muscle relaxants; or anesthetics, including some dental anesthetics. *Check with your doctor before taking any of the above while you are using this medicine.*

This medicine may cause some people to have blurred vision or to become drowsy, dizzy, or less alert than they are normally. *Make sure you know how you react to this medicine before you drive, use machines, or do anything else that could be dangerous if you are dizzy or are not alert and able to see well.*

Cyclobenzaprine may cause dryness of the mouth. For temporary relief, use sugarless candy or gum, melt bits of ice in your mouth, or use a saliva substitute. However, if your mouth continues to feel dry for more than 2 weeks, check with your medical doctor or dentist. Continuing dryness of the mouth may increase the chance of dental disease, including tooth decay, gum disease, and fungus infections.

Side Effects of This Medicine

Along with its needed effects, a medicine may cause some unwanted effects. Although not all of these side effects may occur, if they do occur they may need medical attention.

The following side effects may mean that you are having a serious allergic reaction to the medicine. *Get emergency help right away if any of them occurs:*

> *Rare*
>> Changes in the skin color of the face; fast or irregular breathing; large swellings that look like hives on the face, eyelids, mouth, lips, and/or tongue; puffiness or swelling of the eyelids or the area around the eyes; shortness of breath, troubled breathing, tightness in chest, and/or wheezing; skin rash, hives, or itching

Also, check with your doctor immediately if any of the following side effects occur:

> *Rare*
>> Fainting
>
> *Symptoms of overdose*
>> Convulsions (seizures); drowsiness (severe); dry, hot, flushed skin; fast or irregular heartbeat; hallucinations (seeing, hearing, or feeling things that are not there); increase or decrease in body temperature; troubled

breathing; unexplained muscle stiffness; unusual nervousness or restlessness (severe); vomiting (occurring together with other symptoms of overdose)

Also, check with your doctor as soon as possible if any of the following side effects occur:

Rare

Clumsiness or unsteadiness; confusion; mental depression or other mood or mental changes; problems in urinating; ringing or buzzing in the ears; skin rash, hives, or itching occurring without other symptoms of an allergic reaction listed above; unusual thoughts or dreams; yellow eyes or skin

Other side effects may occur that usually do not need medical attention. These side effects may go away during treatment as your body adjusts to the medicine. However, check with your doctor if any of the following side effects continue or are bothersome:

More common

Dizziness or lightheadedness; drowsiness; dryness of mouth

Less common or rare

Bloated feeling or gas, indigestion, nausea or vomiting, or stomach cramps or pain; blurred vision; constipation; decrease in blood pressure; diarrhea; excitement or nervousness; frequent urination; general feeling of discomfort or illness; headache; muscle twitching; numbness, tingling, pain, or weakness in hands or feet; pounding heartbeat; problems in speaking; trembling; trouble in sleeping; unpleasant taste or other taste changes; unusual muscle weakness; unusual tiredness

Other side effects not listed above may also occur in some patients. If you notice any other effects, check with your doctor.

Additional Information

Once a medicine has been approved for marketing for a certain use, experience may show that it is also useful for

other medical problems. Although this use is not included in product labeling, cyclobenzaprine is used in certain patients with fibromyalgia syndrome (also called fibrositis or fibrositis syndrome).

There is no additional information relating to proper use, precautions, or side effects for this use of cyclobenzaprine.

DIDANOSINE   Systemic

A commonly used brand name in the U.S. and Canada is Videx.
Another commonly used name is ddI.

Description

Didanosine (di-DAN-oe-seen) (also known as ddI) is used in the treatment of the infection caused by the human immunodeficiency virus (HIV). HIV is the virus responsible for acquired immune deficiency syndrome (AIDS).

Didanosine (ddI) will not cure or prevent HIV infection or AIDS; however, it helps keep HIV from reproducing and appears to slow down the destruction of the immune system. This may help delay the development of problems usually related to AIDS or HIV disease. Didanosine will not keep you from spreading HIV to other people. People who receive this medicine may continue to have the problems usually related to AIDS or HIV disease.

Didanosine may cause some serious side effects, including pancreatitis (inflammation of the pancreas). Symptoms of pancreatitis include stomach pain, and nausea and vomiting. Didanosine may also cause peripheral neuropathy. Symptoms of peripheral neuropathy include tingling, burning, numbness, and pain in the hands or feet. *Check with your doctor if any new health problems or symptoms occur while you are taking didanosine.*

Didanosine is available only with your doctor's prescription, in the following dosage forms:

Oral

- Oral solution (U.S.)
- Oral suspension (U.S. and Canada)
- Tablets (U.S. and Canada)

Before Using This Medicine

In deciding to use a medicine, the risks of taking the medicine must be weighed against the good it will do. This is a decision you and your doctor will make. For didanosine, the following should be considered:

Allergies—Tell your doctor if you have ever had any unusual or allergic reaction to didanosine. Also tell your health care professional if you are allergic to any other substances, such as foods, preservatives, or dyes.

Diet—Make certain your health care professional knows if you are on any special diet, such as a low-sodium (low-salt) diet. Didanosine chewable tablets and the oral solution packets contain a large amount of sodium. Also, didanosine tablets contain phenylalanine, which must be restricted in patients with phenylketonuria.

Pregnancy—Didanosine crosses the placenta. Studies in pregnant women have not been done. However, didanosine has not been shown to cause birth defects or other problems in animal studies. Also, it is not known whether didanosine reduces the chances that a baby born to an HIV-infected mother will also be infected.

Breast-feeding—It is not known whether didanosine passes into the breast milk. However, if your baby does not already have the AIDS virus, there is a chance that you could pass it to your baby by breast-feeding. Talk to your doctor first if you are thinking about breast-feeding your baby.

Children—Didanosine can cause serious side effects in any patient. Therefore, it is especially important that you discuss with your child's doctor the good that this medicine may do as well as the risks of using it. Your child must be carefully followed, and frequently seen, by the doctor while taking didanosine.

Older adults—Many medicines have not been studied specifically in older people. Therefore, it may not be known whether they work exactly the same way they do in younger adults or if they cause different side effects or problems in older people. There is no specific information comparing use of didanosine in the elderly with use in other age groups.

Other medicines—Although certain medicines should not be used together at all, in other cases two different medicines may be used together even if an interaction might occur. In these cases, your doctor may want to change the dose, or other precautions may be necessary. When you are taking didanosine, it is especially important that your health care professional know if you are taking any of the following:

- Alcohol or
- Asparaginase (e.g., Elspar) or
- Azathioprine (e.g., Imuran) or
- Estrogens (female hormones) or
- Furosemide (e.g., Lasix) or
- Methyldopa (e.g., Aldomet) or
- Pentamidine (e.g., Pentam, Pentacarinat) or
- Sulfonamides (e.g., Bactrim, Septra) or
- Sulindac (e.g., Clinoril) or
- Thiazide diuretics (e.g., Diuril, Hydrodiuril) or
- Valproic acid (e.g., Depakote)—Use of these medicines with didanosine may increase the chance of pancreatitis (inflammation of the pancreas)
- Chloramphenicol (e.g., Chloromycetin) or

- Cisplatin (e.g., Platinol) or
- Ethambutol (e.g., Myambutol) or
- Ethionamide (e.g., Trecator-SC) or
- Hydralazine (e.g., Apresoline) or
- Isoniazid (e.g., Nydrazid) or
- Lithium (e.g., Eskalith, Lithobid) or
- Metronidazole (e.g., Flagyl) or
- Nitrous oxide or
- Phenytoin (e.g., Dilantin) or
- Stavudine (e.g., D4T) or
- Vincristine (e.g., Oncovin) or
- Zalcitabine (e.g., HIVID)—Use of these medicines with didanosine may increase the chance of peripheral neuropathy (tingling, burning, numbness, or pain in your hands or feet)
- Ciprofloxacin (e.g., Cipro) or
- Enoxacin (e.g., Penetrex) or
- Itraconazole (e.g., Sporanox) or
- Ketoconazole (e.g., Nizoral) or
- Lomefloxacin (e.g., Maxaquin) or
- Norfloxacin (e.g., Noroxin) or
- Ofloxacin (e.g., Floxin) or
- Trimethoprim (e.g., Proloprim, Trimpex)—Use of these medicines with didanosine may keep these medicines from working properly; these medicines should be taken at least 2 hours before or 2 hours after taking didanosine
- Dapsone (e.g., Avlosulfon)—Use of dapsone with didanosine may increase the chance of peripheral neuropathy (tingling, burning, numbness, or pain in your hands or feet); it may also keep dapsone from working properly; dapsone should be taken at least 2 hours before or 2 hours after taking didanosine
- Nitrofurantoin (e.g., Macrodantin)—Use of nitrofurantoin with didanosine may increase the chance of pancreatitis (inflammation of the pancreas) and peripheral neuropathy (tingling, burning, numbness, or pain in your hands or feet)
- Tetracyclines (e.g., Achromycin, Minocin)—Use of tetracyclines with didanosine may increase the chance of pancreatitis (inflammation of the pancreas); it may also keep the tetracycline from working properly; tetracyclines should be taken at least 2 hours before or 2 hours after taking didanosine

Other medical problems—The presence of other medical problems may affect the use of didanosine. Make sure you tell your doctor if you have any other medical problems, especially:

- Alcoholism, active, or
- Increased blood triglycerides (substance formed in the body from fats in foods) or
- Pancreatitis (or a history of)—Patients with these medical problems may be at increased risk of pancreatitis (inflammation of the pancreas)

- Edema or
- Heart disease or
- High blood pressure or
- Kidney disease or
- Liver disease or
- Toxemia of pregnancy—The salt contained in the didanosine tablets and the oral solution packets may make these conditions worse

- Gouty arthritis—Didanosine may cause an attack or worsen gout

- Peripheral neuropathy—Didanosine may make this condition worse

- Phenylketonuria (PKU)—Didanosine tablets contain phenylalanine, which must be restricted in patients with PKU

Proper Use of This Medicine

Take this medicine exactly as directed by your doctor. Do not take more of it, do not take it more often, and do not take it for a longer time than your doctor ordered. Also, do not stop taking this medicine without checking with your doctor first. However, stop taking didanosine and call your doctor right away if you get severe nausea, vomiting, and stomach pain.

Otherwise, keep taking didanosine for the full time of treatment, even if you begin to feel better.

For patients taking *didanosine pediatric oral suspension:*

- Use a specially marked measuring spoon or other device to measure each dose accurately. The average household teaspoon may not hold the right amount of liquid.

For patients taking *didanosine for oral solution:*

- Open the foil packet and pour its contents into approximately 1/2 glass (4 ounces) of water. *Do not mix with fruit juice* or other acid-containing drinks.
- Stir for approximately 2 to 3 minutes until the powder is dissolved.
- Drink at once.

For patients taking *didanosine tablets:*

- Tablets should be thoroughly chewed or crushed or mixed in at least 1 ounce of water before swallowing. The tablets are hard and some people may find them difficult to chew. If the tablets are mixed in water, stir well until a uniform suspension is formed and take at once.
- *Two tablets must be taken together by patients over 1 year of age.* These tablets contain a special buffer to keep didanosine from being destroyed in the stomach. In order to get the correct amount of buffer, 2 tablets always need to be taken together. Infants from 6 to 12 months of age will get enough buffer from just 1 tablet.

Didanosine should be taken on an empty stomach since food may decrease the absorption in the stomach and keep it from working properly. Didanosine should be taken at least 2 hours before or 2 hours after you eat.

This medicine works best when there is a constant amount in the blood. *To help keep the amount constant, do not miss any doses.* If you need help in planning the best times to take your medicine, check with your health care professional.

Dosing—The dose of didanosine will be different for different patients. *Follow your doctor's orders or the directions on the label.* The following information includes only the average doses of didanosine. *If your dose is different, do not change it* unless your doctor tells you to do so.

The number of tablets or teaspoonfuls of solution or suspension that you take depends on the strength of the medicine.

• For the treatment of advanced HIV infection or AIDS:

—For *oral* dosage form (solution):

• Adults and teenagers—Dose is based on body weight.

—For patients weighing less than 60 kilograms (kg) (132 pounds): 167 milligrams (mg) every twelve hours.

—For patients weighing 60 kg (132 pounds) or more: 250 mg every twelve hours.

• Children—The oral solution is usually not used for small children.

—For *oral* dosage form (pediatric suspension):

• Adults and teenagers—The pediatric oral suspension is usually not used in adults and teenagers.

• Children—Dose is based on body size and must be determined by your doctor. The dose usually ranges from 31 to 125 mg every eight to twelve hours.

—For *oral* dosage form (tablets):

• Adults and teenagers—Dose is based on body weight.

—For patients weighing less than 60 kg (132 pounds): 125 mg every twelve hours.

—For patients weighing 60 kg (132 pounds) or more: 200 mg every twelve hours.

• Children—Dose is based on body size and must be determined by your doctor. The dose usually ranges from 25 to 100 mg every eight to twelve hours.

Missed dose—If you do miss a dose of this medicine, take it as soon as possible. However, if it is almost time for your next dose, skip the missed dose and go back to your regular dosing schedule. Do not double doses.

Only take medicine that your doctor has prescribed specifically for you. Do not share your medicine with others.

Storage—To store this medicine:

• Keep out of the reach of children.

• Store away from heat and direct light.

• Do not store in the bathroom, near the kitchen sink, or in other damp places. Heat or moisture may cause the medicine to break down.

• Do not keep outdated medicine or medicine no longer needed. Be sure that any discarded medicine is out of the reach of children.

Precautions While Using This Medicine

It is very important that your doctor check your progress at regular visits.

Do not take any other medicines without checking with your doctor first. To do so may increase the chance of side effects from didanosine.

HIV may be acquired from or spread to other people through infected body fluids, including blood, vaginal fluid, or semen. *If you are infected, it is best to avoid any sexual activity involving an exchange of body fluids with other people. If you do have sex, always wear (or have your partner wear) a condom ("rubber").* Only use condoms made of latex, and *use them every time you have vaginal, anal, or oral sex.* The use of a spermicide (such as nonoxynol-9) may also help prevent transmission of HIV if it is not irritating to the vagina, rectum, or mouth. Spermicides have been shown to kill HIV in lab tests. Do not use oil-based jelly, cold cream, baby oil, or shortening as a lubricant—these products can cause the condom to break. Lubricants without oil, such as *K-Y jelly*, are recommended. Women may wish to carry their own condoms. Birth control pills and diaphragms will help protect against pregnancy, but they will not prevent someone from giving or getting the AIDS virus. *If you inject drugs,* get help to stop. *Do not share needles or equipment with anyone.* In some cities, more than half of the drug users are infected and sharing even one needle or syringe can spread the virus. If you have any questions about this, check with your health care professional.

Side Effects of This Medicine

Along with its needed effects, a medicine may cause some unwanted effects. Although not all of these side effects may occur, if they do occur they may need medical attention.

Check with your doctor immediately if any of the following side effects occur:

Less common

Nausea and vomiting; stomach pain; tingling, burning, numbness, and pain in the hands or feet

Rare

Convulsions (seizures); fever and chills; shortness of breath; skin rash and itching; sore throat; swelling of feet or lower legs; unusual bleeding and bruising; unusual tiredness and weakness; yellow skin and eyes

Other side effects may occur that usually do not need medical attention. These side effects may go away during treatment as your body adjusts to the medicine. However, check with your doctor if any of the following side effects continue or are bothersome:

More common

Anxiety; diarrhea; difficulty in sleeping; dryness of mouth; headache; irritability; restlessness

Other side effects not listed above may also occur in some patients. If you notice any other effects, check with your doctor.

DIGITALIS MEDICINES Systemic

Some commonly used brand names are:

In the U.S.—

Crystodigin[1]   Lanoxin[2]
Lanoxicaps[2]

In Canada—

Digitaline[1]   Novodigoxin[2]
Lanoxin[2]

Note: For quick reference, the following digitalis medicines are numbered to match the corresponding brand names.

This information applies to the following medicines:

1. Digitoxin (di-ji-TOX-in)§
2. Digoxin (di-JOX-in)‡§

‡Generic name product may also be available in U.S.
§Generic name product may also be available in Canada

Description

Digitalis medicines are used to improve the strength and efficiency of the heart, or to control the rate and rhythm of the heartbeat. This leads to better blood circulation and reduced swelling of hands and ankles in patients with heart problems.

Although digitalis has been prescribed to help some patients lose weight, it should *never* be used in this way. When used improperly, digitalis can cause serious problems.

Digitalis medicines are available only with your doctor's prescription, in the following dosage forms:

  Oral
    Digitoxin
      • Tablets (U.S. and Canada)
    Digoxin
      • Capsules (U.S.)
      • Elixir (U.S. and Canada)
      • Tablets (U.S. and Canada)

  Parenteral
    Digoxin
      • Injection (U.S. and Canada)

Before Using This Medicine

In deciding to use a medicine, the risks of taking the medicine must be weighed against the good it will do. This is a decision you and your doctor will make. For digitalis medicines, the following should be considered:

Allergies—Tell your doctor if you have ever had any unusual or allergic reaction to digitalis medicines. Also tell your health care professional if you are allergic to any other substances, such as foods, preservatives, or dyes.

Pregnancy—Digitalis medicines pass from the mother to the fetus. However, studies on effects in pregnancy have not been done in either humans or animals. Make sure your doctor knows if you are pregnant or if you may become pregnant before taking digitalis medicines.

Breast-feeding—Although small amounts of digitalis medicines pass into breast milk, they have not been reported to cause problems in nursing babies.

Children—This medicine has been tested in children and, in effective doses, has not been shown to cause different side effects or problems than it does in adults. However, the dose is very different for babies and children, and it is important to follow your doctor's instructions exactly.

Older adults—Signs and symptoms of overdose may be especially likely to occur in elderly patients, who are usually more sensitive than younger adults to the effects of digitalis medicines.

Other medicines—Although certain medicines should not be used together at all, in other cases two different medicines may be used together even if an interaction might occur. In these cases, your doctor may want to change the dose, or other precautions may be necessary. When you are taking or receiving digitalis medicines it is especially important that your health care professional know if you are taking any of the following:

- Amiodarone (e.g., Cordarone)—May cause levels of digitalis medicines in the body to be higher than usual, which could lead to signs or symptoms of overdose

- Amphetamines or
- Appetite suppressants (diet pills) or
- Digitalis medicines (other) or other heart medicine or
- Medicine for asthma or other breathing problems or
- Medicine for colds, sinus problems, or hay fever or other allergies (including nose drops or sprays)—May increase the risk of heart rhythm problems

- Calcium channel blocking agents (bepridil [e.g., Bepadin, Vascor], diltiazem [e.g., Cardizem, Cardizem CD, Cardizem SR], felodipine [e.g., Plendil], flunarizine [e.g., Sibelium], isradipine [e.g., DynaCirc], nicardipine [e.g., Cardene], nifedipine [e.g., Adalat, Procardia, Procardia XL], nimodipine [e.g., Nimotop], verapamil [e.g., Calan, Calan SR, Isoptin, Isoptin SR, Verelan] or

- Propafenone—May cause levels of digitalis medicines in the body to be higher than usual, which could lead to signs or symptoms of overdose

- Cholestyramine (e.g., Questran) or

- Colestipol (e.g., Colestid) or
- Diarrhea medicine or
- Sucralfate or
- If your diet contains large amounts of fiber, such as bran—
  May decrease effects of digitalis medicines by keeping
  them from being absorbed into the body; digitalis medi-
  cines should be taken several hours apart from these

- Diuretics (water pills) or
- Other medicines that decrease the amount of potassium in
  the body (corticosteroids [cortisone-like medicines], alcohol, capreomycin, corticotropin, insulin, laxatives, salicylates [aspirin], vitamin B_{12}, vitamin D [high doses])—
  These medicines can cause hypokalemia (low levels of
  potassium in the body), which can increase the unwanted
  effects of digitalis medicines

- Potassium-containing medicines or supplements—If levels
  of potassium in the body become too high, there is a serious risk of heart rhythm problems being caused by digitalis medicines

- Quinidine (e.g., Quinidex)—May cause levels of digitalis
  medicines in the body to be higher than usual, which could
  lead to signs or symptoms of overdose

Other medical problems—The presence of other medical
problems may affect the use of digitalis medicines. Make
sure you tell your doctor if you have any other medical
problems, especially:

- Heart disease or
- Lung disease (severe)—The heart may be more sensitive to
  the effects of digitalis medicines
- Heart rhythm problems—Digitalis glycosides may make
  certain heart rhythm problems worse
- Kidney disease or
- Liver disease—Effects may be increased because of slower
  removal of digitalis medicines from the body
- Thyroid disease—Patients with low or high thyroid gland
  activity may be more or less sensitive to the effects of
  digitalis glycosides

Proper Use of This Medicine

To keep your heart working properly, *take this medicine exactly as directed even though you may feel well.* Do not take more of it than your doctor ordered and do not miss any doses.

For patients taking the *liquid form of digoxin:*

• This medicine is to be taken by mouth even if it comes in a dropper bottle. The amount you should take is to be measured only with the specially marked dropper.

To help you remember to take your dose of medicine, try to take it at the same time every day.

Ask your doctor about checking your pulse rate. Then, while you are taking this medicine, check your pulse regularly. If it is much slower, or faster, than your usual rate (or less than 60 beats per minute), or if it changes in rhythm or force, check with your doctor. Such changes may mean that side effects are developing.

Dosing—When you are taking digitalis medicines, it is very important that you get the exact amount of medicine that you need. The dose of digitalis medicine will be different for different patients. Your doctor will determine the proper dose of digitalis medicine for you. *Follow your doctor's orders or the directions on the label.*

After you begin taking digitalis medicines, your doctor may sometimes check your blood level of digitalis medicine to find out if your dose needs to be changed. *Do not change your dose of digitalis medicine* unless your doctor tells you to do so.

The number of capsules or tablets or teaspoonfuls of solution that you take depends on the strength of the medicine.

Missed dose—If you do miss a dose of this medicine, and you remember it within 12 hours, take it as soon as you remember. However, if you do not remember until later, do not take the missed dose at all and do not double the next one. Instead, go back to your regular dosing schedule. If you have any questions about this or if you miss doses for 2 or more days in a row, check with your doctor.

Storage—To store this medicine:

- Keep out of the reach of children.
- Store away from heat and direct light.
- Do not store in the bathroom, near the kitchen sink, or in other damp places. Heat or moisture may cause the medicine to break down.
- Keep the oral liquid form of this medicine from freezing.
- Do not keep outdated medicine or medicine no longer needed. Be sure that any discarded medicine is out of the reach of children.

Precautions While Using This Medicine

It is important that your doctor check your progress at regular visits to make sure the medicine is working properly. This will allow your doctor to make any changes in directions for taking it, if necessary.

Do not stop taking this medicine without first checking with your doctor. Stopping suddenly may cause a serious change in heart function.

Keep this medicine out of the reach of children. Digitalis medicines are a major cause of accidental poisoning in children.

Watch for signs and symptoms of overdose while you are taking digitalis medicine. Follow your doctor's directions carefully. The amount of this medicine needed to help most people is very close to the amount that could cause serious problems from overdose. Some early warning signs of overdose are loss of appetite, nausea, vomiting, diarrhea, or extremely slow heartbeat. In infants and small children, the earliest signs of overdose are changes in the rate and rhythm of the heartbeat. Children may not show the other symptoms as soon as adults.

Before having any kind of surgery (including dental surgery) or emergency treatment, tell the medical doctor or dentist in charge that you are using this medicine.

Your doctor may want you to carry a medical identification card or bracelet stating that you are taking this medicine.

Do not take any other medicine unless ordered by your doctor. Many over-the-counter (OTC) or nonprescription medicines contain ingredients that interfere with digitalis medicines or that may make your condition worse. These medicines include antacids; laxatives; asthma remedies; cold, cough, or sinus preparations; medicine for diarrhea; and reducing or diet medicines.

For patients taking the *tablet or capsule* form of this medicine:

- This medicine may look like other tablets or capsules you now take. It is very important that you do not get the medicines mixed up since this may have serious results. Ask your pharmacist for ways to avoid mix-ups with medicines that look alike.

Side Effects of This Medicine

Along with its needed effects, a medicine may cause some unwanted effects. Although not all of these side effects may occur, if they do occur they may need medical attention.

Check with your doctor as soon as possible if any of the following side effects or symptoms of overdose occur:

Rare

Skin rash or hives

Signs and symptoms of overdose (in the order in which they may occur)

Loss of appetite; nausea or vomiting; lower stomach pain; diarrhea;. unusual tiredness or weakness (extreme); slow or irregular heartbeat (may be fast heartbeat in children); blurred vision or "yellow, green, or white vision" (yellow, green, or white halo seen around objects); drowsiness; confusion or mental depression; headache; fainting

Note: Overdose symptoms in infants and small children may occur at first only as changes in the heartbeat rate or rhythm, while in adults and older children the first symptoms may be mostly stomach upset, stomach pain, loss of appetite, or unusually slow heartbeat.

Other side effects not listed above may also occur in some patients. If you notice any other effects, check with your doctor.

DISOPYRAMIDE   Systemic

Some commonly used brand names are:

In the U.S.—
Norpace
Norpace CR

Generic name product may also be available.

In Canada—

Norpace	Rythmodan
Norpace CR	Rythmodan-LA

Description

Disopyramide (dye-soe-PEER-a-mide) is used to correct irregular heartbeats to a normal rhythm and to slow an overactive heart. This allows the heart to work more efficiently.

Disopyramide is available only with your doctor's prescription, in the following dosage forms:

Oral
- Capsules (U.S. and Canada)
- Extended-release capsules (U.S.)
- Extended-release tablets (Canada)

Parenteral
- Injection (Canada)

Before Using This Medicine

In deciding to use a medicine, the risks of taking the medicine must be weighed against the good it will do. This is a decision you and your doctor will make. For disopyramide, the following should be considered:

Allergies—Tell your doctor if you have ever had any unusual or allergic reaction to disopyramide. Also tell your health care professional if you are allergic to any other substance, such as foods, preservatives, or dyes.

Pregnancy—Disopyramide has not been studied in pregnant women. However, use of disopyramide in a small number of pregnant women seems to show that this medicine may cause contractions of the uterus. Studies in animals have shown that disopyramide increases the risk of miscarriages. Before taking this medicine, make sure your doctor knows if you are pregnant or if you may become pregnant.

Breast-feeding—Disopyramide passes into breast milk.

Children—This medicine has been tested in children and has not been shown to cause different side effects or problems than it does in adults.

Older adults—Some side effects, such as difficult urination and dry mouth, may be especially likely to occur in elderly patients, who are usually more sensitive than younger adults to the effects of disopyramide.

Other medicines—Although certain medicines should not be used together at all, in other cases two different medicines may be used together even if an interaction might occur. In these cases, your doctor may want to change the dose, or other precautions may be necessary. When you are taking disopyramide, it is especially important that your health care professional know if you are taking any of the following:

- Other heart medicine—Effects on the heart may be increased
- Pimozide (e.g., Orap)—Risk of heart rhythm problems may be increased

Other medical problems—The presence of other medical problems may affect the use of disopyramide. Make sure you tell your doctor if you have any other medical problems, especially:

- Diabetes mellitus (sugar diabetes)—Disopyramide may cause low blood sugar
- Difficult urination or
- Enlarged prostate—Disopyramide may cause difficult urination
- Glaucoma (history of) or
- Myasthenia gravis—Disopyramide may make these conditions worse
- Kidney disease or
- Liver disease—Effects may be increased because of slower removal of disopyramide from the body

Proper Use of This Medicine

Take disopyramide exactly as directed by your doctor even though you may feel well. Do not take more medicine than ordered.

For patients taking the *extended-release capsules:*

- Swallow the capsule whole without breaking, crushing, or chewing.

For patients taking the *extended-release tablets:*

• Do not crush or chew the tablet.

This medicine works best when there is a constant amount in the blood. *To help keep the amount constant, do not miss any doses. Also, it is best to take the doses at evenly spaced times day and night.* For example, if you are to take 4 doses a day, the doses should be spaced about 6 hours apart. If this interferes with your sleep or other daily activities, or if you need help in planning the best times to take your medicine, check with your health care professional.

Dosing—The dose of disopyramide will be different for different patients. *Follow your doctor's orders or the directions on the label.* The following information includes only the average doses of disopyramide. *If your dose is different, do not change it* unless your doctor tells you to do so:

The number of tablets or capsules that you take depends on the strength of the medicine.

• For *treatment* of arrhythmias:

—For *short-acting oral* dosage forms (capsules):

• Adults—300 milligrams (mg) for the first dose. Then 100 to 150 mg taken every six to eight hours.

• Children—Dose is based on body weight and age. It must be determined by your doctor. The dose is usually 6 to 30 mg per kilogram (kg) of body weight (2.73 to 13.64 mg per pound) per day. This dose is evenly divided and taken every six hours.

—For *long-acting oral* dosage forms (extended-release capsules or tablets):

• Adults—200 or 300 mg every twelve hours.

• Children—Use is not recommended.

—For *injection* dosage form:
- Adults—
  —*First few doses:* Dose is based on body weight and must be determined by your doctor. It is usually 2 mg per kg of body weight (0.91 mg per pound) injected in three divided doses, or, 2 mg per kg of body weight (0.91 mg per pound) infused over fifteen minutes.

  —*Dose following first few doses:* Dose is based on body weight and must be determined by your doctor. It is usually 0.4 mg per kg of body weight (0.18 mg per pound) per hour given for up to twenty-four hours.
- Children—Use is not recommended.

Missed dose—*If you do miss a dose of this medicine, take it as soon as possible unless the next scheduled dose is in less than 4 hours.* If you do not remember until later, skip the missed dose and go back to your regular dosing schedule. Do not double doses.

Storage—To store this medicine:
- Keep out of the reach of children.
- Store away from heat and direct light.
- Do not store in the bathroom, near the kitchen sink, or in other damp places. Heat or moisture may cause the medicine to break down.
- Do not keep outdated medicine or medicine no longer needed. Be sure that any discarded medicine is out of the reach of children.

Precautions While Using This Medicine

Your doctor should check your progress at regular visits to make sure the medicine is working properly.

Do not stop taking this medicine without first checking with your doctor. Stopping suddenly may cause a serious change in heart function.

Dizziness, lightheadedness, or fainting may occur, especially when you get up from a lying or sitting position. This is due to lowered blood pressure. Getting up slowly may help. This effect does not occur often at doses of disopyramide usually used; however, *make sure you know how you react to this medicine before you drive, use machines, or do anything else that could be dangerous if you are not alert.* If the problem continues or gets worse, check with your doctor.

Avoid alcoholic beverages until you have discussed their use with your doctor. Alcohol may make the low blood sugar effect worse and/or increase the possibility of dizziness or fainting.

Disopyramide may cause hypoglycemia (low blood sugar) in some people. Patients with congestive heart disease or diabetes especially should be aware of the signs of hypoglycemia. (See *Side Effects of This Medicine.*) *If these signs appear, eat or drink a food containing sugar and call your doctor right away.*

This medicine may cause blurred vision or other vision problems. If any of these occur, *do not drive, use machines, or do anything else that could be dangerous if you are not able to see well.*

Disopyramide may cause dryness of the mouth, nose, and throat. For temporary relief of mouth dryness, use sugarless candy or gum, melt bits of ice in your mouth, or use a saliva substitute. However, if dry mouth continues for more than 2 weeks, check with your medical doctor or dentist. Continuing dryness of the mouth may increase the chance of dental disease, including tooth decay, gum disease, and fungus infections.

This medicine will often make you sweat less, allowing your body temperature to increase. *Use extra care not to become overheated during exercise or hot weather while you are taking this medicine*, since overheating could possibly result in heat stroke.

Side Effects of This Medicine

Along with its needed effects, a medicine may cause some unwanted effects. Although not all of these side effects may occur, if they do occur they may need medical attention.

Check with your doctor as soon as possible if any of the following side effects occur:

More common
    Difficult urination

Less common
    Chest pains; dizziness, lightheadedness, or fainting; fast or slow heartbeat; muscle weakness; shortness of breath (unexplained); swelling of feet or lower legs; weight gain (rapid)

Rare
    Eye pain; mental depression; sore throat and fever; yellow eyes or skin

Signs and symptoms of hypoglycemia (low blood sugar)
    Anxious feeling; chills; cold sweats; confusion; cool, pale skin; drowsiness; fast heartbeat; headache; hunger (excessive); nausea; nervousness; shakiness; unsteady walk; unusual tiredness or weakness

Other side effects may occur that usually do not need medical attention. These side effects may go away during treatment as your body adjusts to the medicine. However, check with your health care professional if any of the following side effects continue or are bothersome:

More common
    Dryness of mouth and throat

Less common

Bloating or stomach pain; blurred vision; constipation; decreased sexual ability; dry eyes and nose; frequent urge to urinate; loss of appetite

Other side effects not listed above may also occur in some patients. If you notice any other effects, check with your doctor.

DIURETICS, LOOP   Systemic

Some commonly used brand names are:

In the U.S.—

Bumex[1]   Lasix[3]
Edecrin[2]   Myrosemide[3]

In Canada—

Apo-Furosemide[3]   Lasix Special[3]
Edecrin[2]   Novosemide[3]
Furoside[3]   Uritol[3]
Lasix[3]

Note: For quick reference, the following loop diuretics are numbered to match the corresponding brand names.

This information applies to the following medicines:

1. Bumetanide (byoo-MET-a-nide)†
2. Ethacrynic Acid (eth-a-KRIN-ik AS-id)
3. Furosemide (fur-OH-se-mide)‡§

---

†Not commercially available in Canada.
‡Generic name product may also be available in the U.S.
§Generic name product may also be available in Canada.

Description

Loop diuretics are given to help reduce the amount of water in the body. They work by acting on the kidneys to increase the flow of urine.

Furosemide is also used to treat high blood pressure (hypertension) in those patients who are not helped by other medicines or in those patients who have kidney problems.

High blood pressure adds to the work load of the heart and arteries. If it continues for a long time, the heart and arteries may not function properly. This can damage the blood vessels of the brain, heart, and kidneys, resulting in a stroke, heart failure, or kidney failure. High blood pressure may also increase the risk of heart attacks. These problems may be less likely to occur if blood pressure is controlled.

Loop diuretics may also be used for other conditions as determined by your doctor.

This medicine is available only with your doctor's prescription, in the following dosage forms:

Oral

Bumetanide
   • Tablets (U.S.)
Ethacrynic Acid
   • Oral solution (U.S. and Canada)
   • Tablets (U.S. and Canada)
Furosemide
   • Oral solution (U.S. and Canada)
   • Tablets (U.S. and Canada)

Parenteral

Bumetanide
   • Injection (U.S.)
Ethacrynic Acid
   • Injection (U.S. and Canada)
Furosemide
   • Injection (U.S. and Canada)

Before Using This Medicine

In deciding to use a medicine, the risks of taking the medicine must be weighed against the good it will do. This is a decision you and your doctor will make. For loop diuretics, the following should be considered:

Allergies—Tell your doctor if you have ever had any unusual or allergic reaction to bumetanide, ethacrynic acid, furosemide, sulfonamides (sulfa drugs), or thiazide diuretics (water pills). Also tell your health care professional if you are allergic to any other substances, such as foods, preservatives, or dyes.

Pregnancy—Studies have not been done in pregnant women. However, studies in animals have shown this medicine to cause harmful effects.

In general, diuretics are not useful for normal swelling of feet and hands that occurs during pregnancy. Diuretics should not be taken during pregnancy unless recommended by your doctor.

Breast-feeding—These medicines have not been reported to cause problems in nursing babies. Furosemide passes into breast milk; it is not known whether bumetanide or ethacrynic acid passes into breast milk.

Children—Although there is no specific information comparing the use of loop diuretics in children with use in any other age group, these medicines are not expected to cause different side effects in children than they do in adults.

Older adults—Dizziness, lightheadedness, or signs of too much potassium loss may be more likely to occur in the elderly, who are more sensitive to the effects of this medicine. Elderly patients may also be more likely to develop blood clots.

Other medicines—Although certain medicines should not be used together at all, in other cases two different medicines may be used together even if an interaction might occur. In these cases, your doctor may want to change the dose, or other precautions may be necessary. When you are taking loop diuretics, it is especially important that your health care professional know if you are taking *any* other medicines.

Other medical problems—The presence of other medical problems may affect the use of loop diuretics. Make sure you tell your doctor if you have any other medical problems, especially:

- Diabetes mellitus (sugar diabetes)—Loop diuretics may increase the amount of sugar in the blood
- Gout or
- Hearing problems or
- Pancreatitis (inflammation of the pancreas)—Loop diuretics may make these conditions worse
- Heart attack, recent—Use of loop diuretics after a recent heart attack may increase the chance of side effects
- Kidney disease (severe) or
- Liver disease—Higher blood levels of the loop diuretic may occur, which may increase the chance of side effects
- Lupus erythematosus (history of)—Ethacrynic acid and furosemide may make this condition worse

---

Proper Use of This Medicine

This medicine may cause you to have an unusual feeling of tiredness when you begin to take it. You may also notice an increase in the amount of urine or in your frequency of urination. After you have taken the medicine for a while, these effects should lessen. In general, to keep the increase in urine from affecting your sleep:

- If you are to take a single dose a day, take it in the morning after breakfast.
- If you are to take more than one dose a day, take the last dose no later than 6 p.m., unless otherwise directed by your doctor.

However, it is best to plan your dose or doses according to a schedule that will least affect your personal activities and sleep. Ask your health care professional to help you plan the best time to take this medicine.

To help you remember to take your medicine, try to get into the habit of taking it at the same time each day.

For patients taking the *oral liquid form* of furosemide:

- This medicine is to be taken by mouth even if it comes in a dropper bottle. If this medicine does not come in a dropper bottle, use a specially marked measuring spoon or other device to measure each dose accurately, since the average household teaspoon may not hold the right amount of liquid.

For patients taking this medicine for *high blood pressure:*

- In addition to the use of the medicine your doctor has prescribed, appropriate treatment for your high blood pressure may include weight control and care in the types of foods you eat, especially foods high in sodium. Your doctor will tell you which factors are most important for you. You should check with your doctor before changing your diet.

- Many patients who have high blood pressure will not notice any signs of the problem. In fact, many may feel normal. It is very important that you *take your medicine exactly as directed* and that you keep your appointments with your doctor even if you feel well.

- Remember that this medicine will not cure your high blood pressure but it does help control it. Therefore, you must continue to take it as directed if you expect to lower your blood pressure and keep it down. *You may have to take high blood pressure medicine for the rest of your life.* If high blood pressure is not treated, it can cause serious problems such as heart failure, blood vessel disease, stroke, or kidney disease.

If this medicine upsets your stomach, it may be taken with meals or milk. If stomach upset (nausea, vomiting, or stomach pain) continues or gets worse, or if you suddenly get severe diarrhea, check with your doctor.

Dosing—The dose of loop diuretics will be different for different patients. *Follow your doctor's orders or the directions on the label.* The following information includes only the average doses of loop diuretics. *If your dose is different, do not change it* unless your doctor tells you to do so.

The number of tablets or teaspoonfuls of solution that you take depends on the strength of the medicine. Also, *the number of doses you take each day, the time allowed between doses, and the length of time you take the medicine depend on the medical problem for which you are taking loop diuretics.*

For bumetanide

- For *oral* dosage form (tablets):

  —To lower the amount of water in the body:

    • Adults—0.5 to 2 milligrams (mg) once a day. Your doctor may increase your dose if needed.

    • Children—Dose must be determined by your doctor.

- For *injection* dosage form:

  —To lower the amount of water in the body:

    • Adults—0.5 to 1 mg injected into a muscle or a vein every two to three hours as needed.

    • Children—Dose must be determined by your doctor.

For ethacrynic acid

- For *oral* dosage form (oral solution or tablets):

  —To lower the amount of water in the body:

    • Adults—50 to 200 milligrams (mg) a day. This may be taken as a single dose or divided into smaller doses.

• Children—At first, 25 mg a day. Your doctor may increase your dose as needed.

• For *injection* dosage form:

—To lower the amount of water in the body:

• Adults—50 mg injected into a vein every two to six hours as needed.

• Children—Dose is based on body weight and must be determined by your doctor. The usual dose is 1 mg per kilogram (kg) (0.45 mg per pound) of body weight injected into a vein.

For furosemide

• For *oral* dosage form (oral solution or tablets):

—To lower the amount of water in the body:

• Adults—At first, 20 to 80 milligrams (mg) once a day. Then, your doctor may increase your dose as needed. Your doctor may tell you to take a dose once a day, two or three times a day, or every other day.

• Children—Dose is based on body weight and must be determined by your doctor. The usual dose is 2 mg per kilogram (kg) (0.91 mg per pound) of body weight for one dose. Then, your doctor may increase your dose every six to eight hours as needed.

—For high blood pressure:

• Adults—40 mg two times a day. Your doctor may increase your dose.

• For *injection* dosage form:

—To lower the amount of water in the body:

• Adults—At first, 20 to 40 mg injected into a muscle or a vein for one dose. Then, your doctor may increase your dose every two hours as needed. Once the medicine is working, the dose is injected into a muscle or a vein one or two times a day.

• Children—Dose is based on body weight and must be determined by your doctor. The usual dose is 1 mg per kg (0.45 mg per pound) of body weight injected into a muscle or a vein for one dose. Your doctor may increase your dose every two hours as needed.

—For very high blood pressure:

• Adults—40 to 200 mg injected into a vein.

Missed dose—If you miss a dose of this medicine, take it as soon as possible. However, if it is almost time for your next dose, skip the missed dose and go back to your regular dosing schedule. Do not double doses.

Storage—To store this medicine:

• Keep out of the reach of children.

• Store away from heat and direct light.

• Do not store in the bathroom, near the kitchen sink, or in other damp places. Heat or moisture may cause the medicine to break down.

• Keep the oral liquid form of this medicine from freezing.

• Do not keep outdated medicine or medicine no longer needed. Be sure that any discarded medicine is out of the reach of children.

Precautions While Using This Medicine

It is important that your doctor check your progress at regular visits to make sure that this medicine is working properly.

This medicine may cause a loss of potassium from your body:

• To help prevent this, your doctor may want you to:

—eat or drink foods that have a high potassium content (for example, orange or other citrus fruit juices), or

—take a potassium supplement, or

—take another medicine to help prevent the loss of the potassium in the first place.

- It is very important to follow these directions. Also, it is important not to change your diet on your own. This is more important if you are already on a special diet (as for diabetes), or if you are taking a potassium supplement or a medicine to reduce potassium loss. Extra potassium may not be necessary and, in some cases, too much potassium could be harmful.

To prevent the loss of too much water and potassium, tell your doctor if you become sick, especially with severe or continuing nausea and vomiting or diarrhea.

Before having any kind of surgery (including dental surgery) or emergency treatment, make sure the medical doctor or dentist in charge knows that you are taking this medicine.

Dizziness, lightheadedness, or fainting may occur, especially when you get up from a lying or sitting position. This is more likely to occur in the morning. *Getting up slowly may help.* When you get up from lying down, sit on the edge of the bed with your feet dangling for 1 or 2 minutes. Then stand up slowly. If the problem continues or gets worse, check with your doctor.

The dizziness, lightheadedness, or fainting is also more likely to occur if you drink alcohol, stand for long periods of time, exercise, or if the weather is hot. *While you are taking this medicine, be careful to limit the amount of alcohol you drink. Also, use extra care during exercise or hot weather or if you must stand for long periods of time.*

For *diabetic patients:*

- This medicine may affect blood sugar levels. While

you are using this medicine, be especially careful in testing for sugar in your blood or urine.

For patients taking this medicine for *high blood pressure:*

• *Do not take other medicines unless they have been discussed with your doctor.* This especially includes over-the-counter (nonprescription) medicines for appetite control, asthma, colds, cough, hay fever, or sinus problems, since they may tend to increase your blood pressure.

For patients taking *furosemide:*

• Furosemide may cause your skin to be more sensitive to sunlight than it is normally. Exposure to sunlight, even for brief periods of time, may cause a skin rash, itching, redness or other discoloration of the skin, or a severe sunburn. When you begin taking this medicine:

—Stay out of direct sunlight, especially between the hours of 10:00 a.m. and 3:00 p.m., if possible.

—Wear protective clothing, including a hat. Also, wear sunglasses.

—Apply a sun block product that has a skin protection factor (SPF) of at least 15. Some patients may require a product with a higher SPF number, especially if they have a fair complexion. If you have any questions about this, check with your health care professional.

—Apply a sun block lipstick that has an SPF of at least 15 to protect your lips.

—Do not use a sunlamp or tanning bed or booth.

If you have a severe reaction from the sun, check with your doctor.

Side Effects of This Medicine

Along with its needed effects, a medicine may cause some unwanted effects. Although not all of these side effects

may occur, if they do occur they may need medical attention.

Check with your doctor as soon as possible if any of the following side effects occur:

Rare

Black, tarry stools; blood in urine or stools; cough or hoarseness; fever or chills; joint pain; lower back or side pain; painful or difficult urination; pinpoint red spots on skin; ringing or buzzing in ears or any loss of hearing—more common with ethacrynic acid; skin rash or hives; stomach pain (severe) with nausea and vomiting; unusual bleeding or bruising; yellow eyes or skin; yellow vision—for furosemide only

Signs and symptoms of too much potassium loss

Dryness of mouth; increased thirst; irregular heartbeat; mood or mental changes; muscle cramps or pain; nausea or vomiting; unusual tiredness or weakness; weak pulse

Other side effects may occur that usually do not need medical attention. These side effects may go away during treatment as your body adjusts to the medicine. However, check with your doctor if any of the following side effects continue or are bothersome:

More common

Dizziness or lightheadedness when getting up from a lying or sitting position

Less common or rare

Blurred vision; chest pain—with bumetanide only; confusion—with ethacrynic acid only; diarrhea—more common with ethacrynic acid; headache; increased sensitivity of skin to sunlight—with furosemide only; loss of appetite—more common with ethacrynic acid; nervousness—with ethacrynic acid only; premature ejaculation or difficulty in keeping an erection—with bumetanide only; redness or pain at place of injection; stomach cramps or pain

Other side effects not listed above may also occur in some patients. If you notice any other effects, check with your doctor.

Additional Information

Once a medicine has been approved for marketing for a certain use, experience may show that it is also useful for other medical problems. Although these uses are not included in product labeling, loop diuretics are used in certain patients with the following medical conditions:

- Hypercalcemia (too much calcium in the blood)
- Diagnostic aid for kidney disease

Other than the above information, there is no additional information relating to proper use, precautions, or side effects for these uses.

DIURETICS, POTASSIUM-SPARING   Systemic

Some commonly used brand names are:

In the U.S.—

Aldactone[2]   Midamor[1]

Dyrenium[3]

In Canada—

Aldactone[2]   Midamor[1]

Dyrenium[3]   Novospiroton[2]

Note: For quick reference, the following potassium-sparing diuretics are numbered to match the corresponding brand names.

This information applies to the following medicines:

1. Amiloride (a-MILL-oh-ride)‡
2. Spironolactone (speer-on-oh-LAK-tone)‡
3. Triamterene (trye-AM-ter-een)

‡Generic name product may also be available in the U.S.

Description

Potassium-sparing diuretics are commonly used to help reduce the amount of water in the body. Unlike some other diuretics, these medicines do not cause your body to lose potassium.

Amiloride and spironolactone are also used to treat high blood pressure (hypertension). High blood pressure adds to the workload of the heart and arteries. If the condition continues for a long time, the heart and arteries may not function properly. This can damage the blood vessels of the brain, heart, and kidneys, resulting in a stroke, heart failure, or kidney failure. High blood pressure may also increase the risk of heart attacks. These problems may be less likely to occur if blood pressure is controlled.

Spironolactone is also used to help increase the amount of potassium in the body when it is getting too low.

Potassium-sparing diuretics help to reduce the amount of water in the body by acting on the kidneys to increase the flow of urine. This also helps to lower blood pressure.

These medicines can also be used for other conditions as determined by your doctor.

Potassium-sparing diuretics are available only with your doctor's prescription, in the following dosage forms:

Oral

Amiloride
• Tablets (U.S. and Canada)
Spironolactone
• Tablets (U.S. and Canada)
Triamterene
• Capsules (U.S.)
• Tablets (Canada)

Before Using This Medicine

In deciding to use a medicine, the risks of taking the medicine must be weighed against the good it will do. This is a decision you and your doctor will make. For potassium-sparing diuretics, the following should be considered:

Allergies—Tell your doctor if you have ever had any unusual or allergic reaction to amiloride, spironolactone, or triamterene. Also tell your health care professional if you are allergic to any other substances, such as foods, preservatives, or dyes.

Pregnancy—Studies have not been done in pregnant women. However, this medicine has not been shown to cause birth defects or other problems in animals.

In general, diuretics are not useful for normal swelling of feet and hands that occurs during pregnancy. Diuretics should not be taken during pregnancy unless recommended by your doctor.

Breast-feeding—Although amiloride, spironolactone, and triamterene may pass into breast milk, these medicines have not been reported to cause problems in nursing babies.

Children—This medicine has been tested in children and, in effective doses, has not been shown to cause different side effects or problems in children than it does in adults.

Older adults—Signs and symptoms of too much potassium are more likely to occur in the elderly, who are more sensitive than younger adults to the effects of this medicine.

Other medicines—Although certain medicines should not be used together at all, in other cases two different medicines may be used together even if an interaction might occur. In these cases, your doctor may want to change the dose, or other precautions may be necessary. When you are taking potassium-sparing diuretics, it is especially important that your health care professional know if you are taking any of the following:

- Angiotensin-converting enzyme (ACE) inhibitors (benazepril [e.g., Lotensin], captopril [e.g., Capoten], enalapril [e.g., Vasotec], fosinopril [e.g., Monopril], lisinopril [e.g., Prinivil, Zestril], quinapril [e.g., Accupril], ramipril [e.g., Altace]) or

- Cyclosporine (e.g., Sandimmune) or
- Potassium-containing medicines or supplements—Use with potassium-sparing diuretics may cause high blood levels of potassium, which may increase the chance of side effects
- Digoxin—Use with spironolactone may cause high blood levels of digoxin, which may increase the chance of side effects
- Lithium (e.g., Lithane)—Use with potassium-sparing diuretics may cause high blood levels of lithium, which may increase the chance of side effects

Other medical problems—The presence of other medical problems may affect the use of potassium-sparing diuretics. Make sure you tell your doctor if you have any other medical problems, especially:

- Diabetes mellitus (sugar diabetes) or
- Kidney disease or
- Liver disease—Higher blood levels of potassium may occur, which may increase the chance of side effects
- Gout or
- Kidney stones (history of)—Triamterene may make these conditions worse
- Menstrual problems or breast enlargement—Spironolactone may make these conditions worse

---

Proper Use of This Medicine

This medicine may cause you to have an unusual feeling of tiredness when you begin to take it. You may also notice an increase in the amount of urine or in your frequency of urination. After you have taken the medicine for a while, these effects should lessen. In general, to keep the increase in urine from affecting your sleep:

- If you are to take a single dose a day, take it in the morning after breakfast.

- If you are to take more than one dose a day, take the last dose no later than 6 p.m., unless otherwise directed by your doctor.

However, it is best to plan your dose or doses according to a schedule that will least affect your personal activities and sleep. Ask your health care professional to help you plan the best time to take this medicine.

To help you remember to take your medicine, try to get into the habit of taking it at the same time each day.

If this medicine upsets your stomach, it may be taken with meals or milk. If stomach upset (nausea, vomiting, stomach pain or cramps) continues, check with your doctor.

For patients taking this medicine for *high blood pressure:*

- In addition to the use of the medicine your doctor has prescribed, treatment for your high blood pressure may include weight control and care in the types of foods you eat, especially foods high in sodium. Your doctor will tell you which of these are most important for you. You should check with your doctor before changing your diet.

- Many patients who have high blood pressure will not notice any signs of the problem. In fact, many may feel normal. It is very important that you *take your medicine exactly as directed* and that you keep your appointments with your doctor even if you feel well.

- Remember that this medicine will not cure your high blood pressure but it does help control it. Therefore, you must continue to take it as directed if you expect to lower your blood pressure and keep it down. *You may have to take high blood pressure medicine for the rest of your life.* If high blood pressure is not treated, it can cause serious problems such as heart failure, blood vessel disease, stroke, or kidney disease.

Dosing—The dose of potassium-sparing diuretics will be different for different patients. *Follow your doctor's orders* *or the directions on the label.* The following information includes only the average doses of potassium-sparing diuretics. *If your dose is different, do not change it* unless your doctor tells you to do so.

The number of capsules or tablets that you take depends on the strength of the medicine. Also, *the number of doses you take each day, the time allowed between doses, and the length of time you take the medicine depend on the medical problem for which you are taking potassium-sparing diuretics.*

For amiloride

• For *oral* dosage form (tablets):

—For high blood pressure or to lower the amount of water in the body:

• Adults—5 to 10 milligrams (mg) once a day.

• Children—Dose must be determined by your doctor.

For spironolactone

• For *oral* dosage form (tablets):

—To lower the amount of water in the body:

• Adults—At first, 25 to 200 milligrams (mg) a day. This is divided into two to four doses. Your doctor may increase your dose to 75 to 400 mg a day.

• Children—Dose is based on body weight and must be determined by your doctor. The usual dose is 1 to 3 mg per kilogram (kg) (0.45 to 1.36 mg per pound) of body weight a day. The dose may be taken as a single dose or divided into two to four doses. Your doctor may increase your dose as needed.

—For high blood pressure:

• Adults—At first, 50 to 100 milligrams (mg) a day. This may be taken as a single dose or divided into two to four doses. Your doctor may gradually increase your dose up to 200 mg a day.

• Children—Dose is based on body weight and must be determined by your doctor. The usual dose is 1 to 3 mg per kg (0.45 to 1.36 mg per pound) of body weight a day. The dose may be taken as a single dose or divided into two to four doses. Your doctor may increase your dose as needed.

—To treat high aldosterone levels in the body:

• Adults—100 to 400 mg a day. This is divided into two to four doses and taken until you have surgery. If you are not having surgery, your doses may be smaller.

—For detecting high aldosterone levels in the body:

• Adults—400 mg a day, taken in two to four divided doses. Your doctor may want you to take this dose for as little as four days or as long as three to four weeks. Follow your doctor's instructions.

—To treat low potassium levels in the blood:

• Adults—25 to 100 mg a day. This may be taken as a single dose or divided into two to four doses.

For triamterene

• For *oral* dosage form (capsules or tablets):

—To lower the amount of water in the body:

• Adults—25 to 100 milligrams (mg) a day. Your doctor may gradually increase your dose.

• Children—Dose is based on body weight and must be determined by your doctor. To start, the usual dose is 2 to 4 mg per kilogram (kg) (0.9 to 1.82 mg per pound) of body weight a day or every other day. This is divided into smaller doses. Your doctor may increase your dose as needed.

Missed dose—If you miss a dose of this medicine, take it as soon as possible. However, if it is almost time for

your next dose, skip the missed dose and go back to your regular dosing schedule. Do not double doses.

Storage—To store this medicine:

- Keep out of the reach of children.
- Store away from heat and direct light.
- Do not store in the bathroom, near the kitchen sink, or in other damp places. Heat or moisture may cause the medicine to break down.
- Do not keep outdated medicine or medicine no longer needed. Be sure that any discarded medicine is out of the reach of children.

Precautions While Using This Medicine

It is important that your doctor check your progress at regular visits to make sure that this medicine is working properly.

This medicine does not cause a loss of potassium from your body as some other diuretics (water pills) do. Therefore, it is not necessary for you to get extra potassium in your diet, and too much potassium could even be harmful. Since salt substitutes and low-sodium milk may contain potassium, do not use them unless told to do so by your doctor.

Check with your doctor if you become sick and have severe or continuing nausea, vomiting, or diarrhea. These problems may cause you to lose additional water, which could be harmful, or to lose potassium, which could lessen the medicine's helpful effects.

Before having any kind of surgery (including dental surgery) or emergency treatment, tell the medical doctor or dentist in charge that you are taking this medicine.

Before you have any medical tests, tell the doctor in charge that you are taking this medicine. The results of some tests may be affected by this medicine.

For patients taking this medicine for *high blood pressure:*

• *Do not take other medicines unless they have been discussed with your doctor.* This especially includes over-the-counter (nonprescription) medicines for appetite control, asthma, colds, cough, hay fever, or sinus problems, since these medicines may tend to increase your blood pressure.

For patients taking *triamterene:*

• This medicine may cause your skin to be more sensitive to sunlight than it is normally. Exposure to sunlight, even for brief periods of time, may cause a skin rash, itching, redness or other discoloration of the skin, or a severe sunburn. When you begin taking this medicine:

—Stay out of direct sunlight, especially between the hours of 10:00 a.m. and 3:00 p.m., if possible.

—Wear protective clothing, including a hat. Also, wear sunglasses.

—Apply a sun block product that has a skin protection factor (SPF) of at least 15. Some patients may require a product with a higher SPF number, especially if they have a fair complexion. If you have any questions about this, check with your health care professional.

—Apply a sun block lipstick that has an SPF of at least 15 to protect your lips.

—Do not use a sunlamp or tanning bed or booth.

—If you have a severe reaction from the sun, check with your doctor.

Side Effects of This Medicine

In rats, spironolactone has been found to increase the risk of tumors. It is not known if spironolactone increases the chance of tumors in humans.

Along with its needed effects, a medicine may cause some unwanted effects. Although not all of these side effects may occur, if they do occur they may need medical attention.

Check with your doctor as soon as possible if any of the following side effects occur:

Rare

For amiloride, spironolactone, and triamterene

Skin rash or itching; shortness of breath

For spironolactone and triamterene only (in addition to effects listed above)

Cough or hoarseness; fever or chills; lower back or side pain; painful or difficult urination

For triamterene only (in addition to effects listed above)

Black, tarry stools; blood in urine or stools; bright red tongue; burning, inflamed feeling in tongue; cracked corners of mouth; lower back pain (severe); pinpoint red spots on skin; unusual bleeding or bruising; weakness

Signs and symptoms of too much potassium

Confusion; irregular heartbeat; nervousness; numbness or tingling in hands, feet, or lips; shortness of breath or difficult breathing; unusual tiredness or weakness; weakness or heaviness of legs

Other side effects may occur that usually do not need medical attention. These side effects may go away during treatment as your body adjusts to the medicine. However, check with your doctor if any of the following side effects continue or are bothersome:

More common (less common with amiloride and triamterene)

Nausea and vomiting; stomach cramps and diarrhea

Less common

For amiloride, spironolactone, and triamterene

Dizziness; headache

For amiloride and spironolactone only (in addition to effects listed above)

Decreased sexual ability

For amiloride only (in addition to effects listed above)

Constipation; muscle cramps

For spironolactone only (in addition to effects listed above for spironolactone)

Breast tenderness in females; clumsiness; deepening of voice in females; enlargement of breasts in males; inability to have or keep an erection; increased hair growth in females; irregular menstrual periods; sweating

For triamterene only (in addition to effects listed above for triamterene)

Increased sensitivity of skin to sunlight

Signs and symptoms of too little sodium

Drowsiness; dryness of mouth; increased thirst; lack of energy

For *male patients:*

• Spironolactone sometimes causes enlarged breasts in males, especially when they take large doses of it for a long time. Breasts usually decrease in size gradually over several months after this medicine is stopped. If you have any questions about this, check with your doctor.

Other side effects not listed above may also occur in some patients. If you notice any other effects, check with your doctor.

Additional Information

Once a medicine has been approved for marketing for a certain use, experience may show that it is also useful for other medical problems. Although these uses are not in-

cluded in product labeling, spironolactone is used in certain patients with the following medical conditions:

- Polycystic ovary syndrome
- Hirsutism, female (increased hair growth)

Other than the above information, there is no additional information relating to proper use, precautions, or side effects for this use.

DIURETICS, THIAZIDE   Systemic

Some commonly used brand names are:

In the U.S.—

Anhydron[5]	Hydromox[11]
Aquatensen[8]	Hygroton[4]
Diucardin[7]	Metahydrin[12]
Diulo[9]	Mykrox[9]
Diuril[3]	Naqua[12]
Enduron[8]	Naturetin[1]
Esidrix[6]	Oretic[6]
Exna[2]	Renese[10]
Hydrex[2]	Saluron[7]
Hydro-chlor[6]	Thalitone[4]
Hydro-D[6]	Trichlorex[12]
HydroDIURIL[6]	Zaroxolyn[9]

In Canada—

Apo-Chlorthalidone[4]	Neo-Codema[6]
Apo-Hydro[6]	Novo-Hydrazide[6]
Diuchlor H[6]	Novo-Thalidone[4]
Duretic[8]	Uridon[4]
HydroDIURIL[6]	Urozide[6]
Hygroton[4]	Zaroxolyn[9]
Naturetin[1]	

Note: For quick reference, the following thiazide diuretics are numbered to match the corresponding brand names.

This information applies to the following medicines:

1. Bendroflumethiazide (ben-droe-floo-meth-EYE-a-zide)
2. Benzthiazide (benz-THYE-a-zide)†‡
3. Chlorothiazide (klor-oh-THYE-a-zide)†‡
4. Chlorthalidone (klor-THAL-i-doan)‡§
5. Cyclothiazide (sye-kloe-THYE-a-zide)†

6. Hydrochlorothiazide (hye-droe-klor-oh-THYE-a-zide)‡§
7. Hydroflumethiazide (hye-droe-floo-meth-EYE-a-zide)†‡
8. Methyclothiazide (meth-ee-kloe-THYE-a-zide)‡
9. Metolazone (me-TOLE-a-zone)
10. Polythiazide (pol-i-THYE-a-zide)†
11. Quinethazone (kwin-ETH-a-zone)†
12. Trichlormethiazide (trye-klor-meth-EYE-a-zide)†‡

†Not commercially available in Canada.
‡Generic name product may also be available in the U.S.
§Generic name product may also be available in Canada.

Description

Thiazide or thiazide-like diuretics are commonly used to treat high blood pressure (hypertension). High blood pressure adds to the workload of the heart and arteries. If it continues for a long time, the heart and arteries may not function properly. This can damage the blood vessels of the brain, heart, and kidneys, resulting in a stroke, heart failure, or kidney failure. High blood pressure may also increase the risk of heart attacks. These problems may be less likely to occur if blood pressure is controlled.

Thiazide diuretics are also used to help reduce the amount of water in the body by increasing the flow of urine. They may also be used for other conditions as determined by your doctor.

Thiazide diuretics are available only with your doctor's prescription, in the following dosage forms:

Oral

Bendroflumethiazide
• Tablets (U.S. and Canada)
Benzthiazide
• Tablets (U.S.)
Chlorothiazide
• Oral suspension (U.S.)
• Tablets (U.S.)
Chlorthalidone
• Tablets (U.S. and Canada)

Cyclothiazide
  • Tablets (U.S.)
Hydrochlorothiazide
  • Oral solution (U.S.)
  • Tablets (U.S. and Canada)
Hydroflumethiazide
  • Tablets (U.S.)
Methyclothiazide
  • Tablets (U.S. and Canada)
Metolazone
  • Tablets (U.S. and Canada)
Polythiazide
  • Tablets (U.S.)
Quinethazone
  • Tablets (U.S.)
Trichlormethiazide
  • Tablets (U.S.)

Parenteral

Chlorothiazide
  • Injection (U.S.)

Before Using This Medicine

In deciding to use a medicine, the risks of taking the medicine must be weighed against the good it will do. This is a decision you and your doctor will make. For thiazide diuretics, the following should be considered:

Allergies—Tell your doctor if you have ever had any unusual or allergic reaction to sulfonamides (sulfa drugs), bumetanide, furosemide, acetazolamide, dichlorphenamide, methazolamide, or to any of the thiazide diuretics. Also tell your health care professional if you are allergic to any other substances, such as foods, preservatives, or dyes.

Pregnancy—When this medicine is used during pregnancy, it may cause side effects including jaundice, blood problems, and low potassium in the newborn infant. In addition, although this medicine has not been shown to cause birth defects or other problems in animals, studies have not been done in humans.

In general, diuretics are not useful for normal swelling of feet and hands that occurs during pregnancy. They should not be taken during pregnancy unless recommended by your doctor.

Breast-feeding—Thiazide diuretics pass into breast milk. These medicines also may decrease the flow of breast milk. Therefore, you should avoid use of thiazide diuretics during the first month of breast-feeding.

Children—Although there is no specific information comparing the use of thiazide diuretics in children with use in other age groups, these medicines are not expected to cause different side effects or problems in children than they do in adults. However, extra caution may be necessary in infants with jaundice, because these medicines can make the condition worse.

Older adults—Dizziness or lightheadedness and signs of too much potassium loss may be more likely to occur in the elderly, who are more sensitive than younger adults to the effects of thiazide diuretics.

Other medicines—Although certain medicines should not be used together at all, in other cases two different medicines may be used together even if an interaction might occur. In these cases, your doctor may want to change the dose, or other precautions may be necessary. When you are taking thiazide diuretics, it is especially important that your health care professional know if you are taking any of the following:

- Cholestyramine or
- Colestipol—Use with thiazide diuretics may prevent the diuretic from working properly; take the diuretic at least 1 hour before or 4 hours after cholestyramine or colestipol
- Digitalis glycosides (heart medicine)—Use with thiazide di-

uretics may cause high blood levels of digoxin, which may increase the chance of side effects
- Lithium (e.g., Lithane)—Use with thiazide diuretics may cause high blood levels of lithium, which may increase the chance of side effects

Other medical problems—The presence of other medical problems may affect the use of thiazide diuretics. Make sure you tell your doctor if you have any other medical problems, especially:
- Diabetes mellitus (sugar diabetes)—Thiazide diuretics may increase the amount of sugar in the blood
- Gout (history of) or
- Lupus erythematosus (history of) or
- Pancreatitis (inflammation of the pancreas)—Thiazide diuretics may make these conditions worse
- Heart or blood vessel disease—Thiazide diuretics may cause high cholesterol levels or high triglyceride levels
- Liver disease or
- Kidney disease (severe)—Higher blood levels of the thiazide diuretic may occur, which may prevent the thiazide diuretic from working properly

---

Proper Use of This Medicine

This medicine may cause you to have an unusual feeling of tiredness when you begin to take it. You may also notice an increase in the amount of urine or in your frequency of urination. After you have taken the medicine for a while, these effects should lessen. In general, to keep the increase in urine from affecting your sleep:
- If you are to take a single dose a day, take it in the morning after breakfast.
- If you are to take more than one dose a day, take the last dose no later than 6 p.m., unless otherwise directed by your doctor.

However, it is best to plan your dose or doses according

to a schedule that will least affect your personal activities and sleep. Ask your health care professional to help you plan the best time to take this medicine.

To help you remember to take your medicine, try to get into the habit of taking it at the same time each day.

For patients taking this medicine for *high blood pressure:*

- In addition to the use of the medicine your doctor has prescribed, appropriate treatment for your high blood pressure may include weight control and care in the types of foods you eat, especially foods high in sodium. Your doctor will tell you which factors are most important for you. You should check with your doctor before changing your diet.

- Many patients who have high blood pressure will not notice any signs of the problem. In fact, many may feel normal. It is very important that you *take your medicine exactly as directed* and that you keep your appointments with your doctor even if you feel well.

- Remember that this medicine will not cure your high blood pressure, but it does help control it. Therefore, you must continue to take it as directed if you expect to lower your blood pressure and keep it down. *You may have to take high blood pressure medicine for the rest of your life*. If high blood pressure is not treated, it can cause serious problems such as heart failure, blood vessel disease, stroke, or kidney disease.

For patients taking the *oral liquid form of hydrochlorothiazide,* which comes in a dropper bottle:

- This medicine is to be taken by mouth. The amount you should take is to be measured only with the specially marked dropper.

Dosing—The dose of these medicines will be different for different patients. *Follow your doctor's orders or the directions on the label.* The following information includes only the average doses of these medicines. *If your dose is different, do not change it* unless your doctor tells you to do so.

The number of tablets or teaspoonfuls of solution or suspension that you take depends on the strength of the medicine. Also, *the number of doses you take each day, the time allowed between doses, and the length of time you take the medicine depend on the medical problem for which you are taking thiazide diuretics.*

For bendroflumethiazide

- For *oral* dosage form (tablets):

    —To lower the amount of water in the body:

    - Adults—At first, 2.5 to 10 milligrams (mg) one or two times a day. Then, your doctor may lower your dose to 2.5 to 5 mg once a day. Or, your doctor may want you to take this dose once every other day or once a day for only three to five days out of the week.

    - Children—Dose is based on body weight and must be determined by your doctor. The usual dose is 50 to 100 micrograms (mcg) per kilogram (kg) (22.7 to 45.4 mcg per pound) of body weight once a day.

    —For high blood pressure:

    - Adults—2.5 to 20 mg a day. This may be taken as a single dose or divided into two doses.

    - Children—Dose is based on body weight and must be determined by your doctor. The usual dose is 50 to 400 mcg per kg (22.7 to 181.8 mcg per pound) of body weight a day. This may be taken as a single dose or divided into two doses.

For benzthiazide

- For *oral* dosage form (tablets):

    —To lower the amount of water in the body:

    - Adults—25 to 100 milligrams (mg) two times

a day. Or, your doctor may want you to take this dose once every other day or once a day for only three to five days out of the week.

• Children—Dose is based on body weight and must be determined by your doctor.

—For high blood pressure:

• Adults—50 to 100 mg a day. This may be taken as a single dose or divided into two doses.

• Children—Dose is based on body weight and must be determined by your doctor.

For chlorothiazide

• For *oral* dosage forms (oral suspension or tablets):

—To lower the amount of water in the body:

• Adults—250 milligrams (mg) every six to twelve hours.

• Children—Dose is based on body weight and must be determined by your doctor.

—For high blood pressure:

• Adults—250 to 1000 mg a day. This may be taken as a single dose or divided into smaller doses.

• Children—Dose is based on body weight and must be determined by your doctor.

• For *injection* dosage form:

—To lower the amount of water in the body:

• Adults—250 mg injected into a vein every six to twelve hours.

• Children—Use and dose must be determined by your doctor.

—For high blood pressure:

• Adults—500 to 1000 mg a day, injected into a vein. This dose may be given as a single dose or divided into two doses.

- Children—Use and dose must be determined by your doctor.

For chlorthalidone
- For *oral* dosage form (tablets):
  —To lower the amount of water in the body:
  - Adults—25 to 100 milligrams (mg) once a day. Or, 100 to 200 mg taken once every other day or once a day for three days out of the week.
  - Children—Dose is based on body weight and must be determined by your doctor.
  —For high blood pressure:
  - Adults—25 to 100 mg once a day.
  - Children—Dose is based on body weight and must be determined by your doctor.

For cyclothiazide
- For *oral* dosage form (tablets):
  —To lower the amount of water in the body:
  - Adults—1 to 2 milligrams (mg) once a day. Or, your doctor may want you to take this dose once every other day or once a day for only two or three days out of the week.
  - Children—Dose is based on body weight and must be determined by your doctor.
  —For high blood pressure:
  - Adults—2 mg once a day.
  - Children—Dose is based on body weight and must be determined by your doctor.

For hydrochlorothiazide
- For *oral* dosage forms (oral solution or tablets):
  —To lower the amount of water in the body:
  - Adults—25 to 100 milligrams (mg) one or two times a day. Or, your doctor may want you to take this dose once every other day or once a day for three to five days out of the week.

• Children—Dose is based on body weight and must be determined by your doctor.

—For high blood pressure:

• Adults—25 to 100 mg a day. This may be taken as a single dose or divided into two doses.

• Children—Dose is based on body weight and must be determined by your doctor.

For hydroflumethiazide

• For *oral* dosage form (tablets):

—To lower the amount of water in the body:

• Adults—25 to 100 milligrams (mg) one or two times a day. Or, your doctor may want you to take this dose once every other day or once a day for three to five days out of the week.

• Children—Dose is based on body weight and must be determined by your doctor.

—For high blood pressure:

• Adults—50 to 100 mg a day. This may be taken as a single dose or divided into two doses.

• Children—Dose is based on body weight and must be determined by your doctor.

For methyclothiazide

• For *oral* dosage form (tablets):

—To lower the amount of water in the body:

• Adults—2.5 to 10 milligrams (mg) once a day. Or, your doctor may want you to take this dose once every other day or once a day for three to five days out of the week.

• Children—Dose is based on body weight and must be determined by your doctor.

—For high blood pressure:

• Adults—2.5 to 5 mg once a day.

• Children—Dose is based on body weight and must be determined by your doctor.

For metolazone

- For *oral* dosage form (*extended* metolazone tablets):

  —To lower the amount of water in the body:

  - Adults—5 to 20 milligrams (mg) once a day.
  - Children—Dose must be determined by your doctor.

  —For high blood pressure:

  - Adults—2.5 to 5 mg once a day.
  - Children—Dose must be determined by your doctor.

- For *oral* dosage form (*prompt* metolazone tablets):

  —For high blood pressure:

  - Adults—At first, 500 micrograms (mcg) once a day. Then, 500 to 1000 mcg once a day.
  - Children—Dose must be determined by your doctor.

For polythiazide

- For *oral* dosage form (tablets):

  —To lower the amount of water in the body:

  - Adults—1 to 4 milligrams (mg) once a day. Or, your doctor may want you to take this dose once every other day or once a day for three to five days out of the week.
  - Children—Dose is based on body weight and must be determined by your doctor.

  —For high blood pressure:

  - Adults—2 to 4 mg once a day.
  - Children—Dose is based on body weight and must be determined by your doctor.

For quinethazone

- For *oral* dosage form (tablets):

  —To lower the amount of water in the body or for high blood pressure:

- Adults—50 to 200 milligrams (mg) a day. This may be taken as a single dose or divided into two doses.

- Children—Dose must be determined by your doctor.

For trichlormethiazide

- For *oral* dosage form (tablets):

   —To lower the amount of water in the body:

   - Adults—1 to 4 milligrams (mg) once a day. Or, your doctor may want you to take this dose once every other day or once a day for three to five days out of the week.

   - Children—Dose is based on body weight and must be determined by your doctor.

   —For high blood pressure:

   - Adults—2 to 4 mg once a day.

   - Children—Dose is based on body weight and must be determined by your doctor.

Missed dose—If you miss a dose of this medicine, take it as soon as possible. However, if it is almost time for your next dose, skip the missed dose and go back to your regular dosing schedule. Do not double doses.

Storage—To store this medicine:

- Keep out of the reach of children.

- Store away from heat and direct light.

- Do not store in the bathroom, near the kitchen sink, or in other damp places. Heat or moisture may cause the medicine to break down.

- Keep the oral liquid form of this medicine from freezing.

- Do not keep outdated medicine or medicine no longer needed. Be sure that any discarded medicine is out of the reach of children.

Precautions While Using This Medicine

It is important that your doctor check your progress at regular visits to make sure that this medicine is working properly.

This medicine may cause a loss of potassium from your body:

- To help prevent this, your doctor may want you to:
    - —eat or drink foods that have a high potassium content (for example, orange or other citrus fruit juices), or
    - —take a potassium supplement, or
    - —take another medicine to help prevent the loss of the potassium in the first place.
- It is very important to follow these directions. Also, it is important not to change your diet on your own. This is more important if you are already on a special diet (as for diabetes), or if you are taking a potassium supplement or a medicine to reduce potassium loss. Extra potassium may not be necessary and, in some cases, too much potassium could be harmful.

Check with your doctor if you become sick and have severe or continuing vomiting or diarrhea. These problems may cause you to lose additional water and potassium.

For *diabetic patients:*

- Thiazide diuretics may raise blood sugar levels. While you are using this medicine, be especially careful in testing for sugar in your blood or urine.

Thiazide diuretics may cause your skin to be more sensitive to sunlight than it is normally. Exposure to sunlight, even for brief periods of time, may cause a skin rash, itching, redness or other discoloration of the skin, or a severe sunburn. When you begin taking this medicine:

- Stay out of direct sunlight, especially between the hours of 10:00 a.m. and 3:00 p.m., if possible.
- Wear protective clothing, including a hat. Also, wear sunglasses.
- Apply a sun block product that has a skin protection factor (SPF) of at least 15. Some patients may require a product with a higher SPF number, especially if they have a fair complexion. If you have any questions about this, check with your health care professional.
- Apply a sun block lipstick that has an SPF of at least 15 to protect your lips.
- Do not use a sunlamp or tanning bed or booth.

If you have a severe reaction from the sun, check with your doctor.

For patients taking this medicine for *high blood pressure:*

- *Do not take other medicines unless they have been discussed with your doctor.* This especially includes over-the-counter (nonprescription) medicines for appetite control, asthma, colds, cough, hay fever, or sinus problems, since they may tend to increase your blood pressure.

Side Effects of This Medicine

Along with its needed effects, a medicine may cause some unwanted effects. Although not all of these side effects may occur, if they do occur they may need medical attention.

Check with your doctor as soon as possible if any of the following side effects occur:

Rare

Black, tarry stools; blood in urine or stools; cough or hoarseness; fever or chills; joint pain; lower back or side pain; painful or difficult urination; pinpoint red spots on skin; skin rash or hives; stomach pain (severe) with nausea and vomiting; unusual bleeding or bruising; yellow eyes or skin

Signs and symptoms of too much potassium loss

Dryness of mouth; increased thirst; irregular heartbeat; mood or mental changes; muscle cramps or pain; nausea or vomiting; unusual tiredness or weakness; weak pulse

Signs and symptoms of too much sodium loss

Confusion; convulsions; decreased mental activity; irritability; muscle cramps; unusual tiredness or weakness

Other side effects may occur that usually do not need medical attention. These side effects may go away during treatment as your body adjusts to the medicine. However, check with your doctor if any of the following side effects continue or are bothersome:

Less common

Decreased sexual ability; diarrhea; dizziness or lightheadedness when getting up from a lying or sitting position; increased sensitivity of skin to sunlight; loss of appetite; upset stomach

Other side effects not listed above may also occur in some patients. If you notice any other effects, check with your doctor.

Additional Information

Once a medicine has been approved for marketing for a certain use, experience may show that it is also useful for other medical problems. Although these uses are not specifically included in product labeling, thiazide diuretics are used in certain patients with the following medical conditions:

- Diabetes insipidus (water diabetes)
- Kidney stones (calcium-containing)

For patients taking this medicine for *diabetes insipidus (water diabetes):*

• Some thiazide diuretics are used in the treatment of diabetes insipidus (water diabetes). In patients with water diabetes, this medicine causes a decrease in the flow of urine and helps the body hold water. Thus, the information given above about increased urine flow will not apply to you.

Other than the above information, there is no additional information relating to proper use, precautions, or side effects for these uses.

DOXAZOSIN   Systemic

A commonly used brand name in the U.S. and Canada is Cardura.

Description

Doxazosin (dox-AY-zoe-sin) belongs to the general class of medicines called antihypertensives. It is used to treat high blood pressure (hypertension).

High blood pressure adds to the workload of the heart and arteries. If it continues for a long time, the heart and arteries may not function properly. This can damage the blood vessels of the brain, heart, and kidneys, resulting in a stroke, heart failure, or kidney failure. High blood pressure may also increase the risk of heart attacks. These problems may be less likely to occur if blood pressure is controlled.

Doxazosin works by relaxing blood vessels so that blood passes through them more easily. This helps to lower blood pressure.

Doxazosin may also be used for other conditions as determined by your doctor.

Doxazosin is available only with your doctor's prescription, in the following dosage form:

Oral
- Tablets (U.S. and Canada)

Before Using This Medicine

In deciding to use a medicine, the risks of taking the medicine must be weighed against the good it will do. This is a decision you and your doctor will make. For doxazosin, the following should be considered:

Allergies—Tell your doctor if you have ever had any unusual or allergic reaction to doxazosin, prazosin, or terazosin. Also tell your health care professional if you are allergic to any other substances, such as foods, preservatives, or dyes.

Pregnancy—Doxazosin has not been studied in pregnant women. However, studies in rabbits have shown that doxazosin given at very high doses may cause death of the fetus. Before taking this medicine, make sure your doctor knows if you are pregnant or if you may become pregnant.

Breast-feeding—It is not known whether doxazosin passes into breast milk. However, doxazosin passes into the milk of rats. Although most medicines pass into breast milk in small amounts, many of them may be used safely while breast-feeding. Mothers who are taking this medicine and who wish to breast-feed should discuss this with their doctor.

Children—Studies on this medicine have been done only in adult patients, and there is no specific information comparing use of doxazosin in children with use in other age groups.

Older adults—Dizziness, lightheadedness, or fainting may be especially likely to occur in elderly patients, who are usually more sensitive than younger adults to the effects of doxazosin.

Other medicines—Although certain medicines should not be used together at all, in other cases two different medicines may be used together even if an interaction might occur. In these cases, your doctor may want to change the dose, or other precautions may be necessary. Tell your health care professional if you are using any other prescription or nonprescription (over-the-counter [OTC]) medicine.

Other medical problems—The presence of other medical problems may affect the use of doxazosin. Make sure you tell your doctor if you have any other medical problems, especially:

- Kidney disease—Possible increased sensitivity to the effects of doxazosin
- Liver disease—The effects of doxazosin may be increased, which may increase the chance of side effects

Proper Use of This Medicine

For patients *taking this medicine for high blood pressure:*

- In addition to the use of the medicine your doctor has prescribed, treatment for your high blood pressure may include weight control and care in the types of foods you eat, especially foods high in sodium. Your doctor will tell you which of these are most important for you. You should check with your doctor before changing your diet.

- Many patients who have high blood pressure will not notice any signs of the problem. In fact, many may feel normal. It is very important that you *take your medicine exactly as directed* and that you keep your appointments with your doctor even if you feel well.

- Remember that doxazosin will not cure your high blood pressure, but it does help control it. Therefore, you must continue to take it as directed if you expect to lower your blood pressure and keep it down. *You may have to take high blood pressure medicine for the rest of your life.* If high blood pressure is not treated, it can cause serious problems such as heart failure, blood vessel disease, stroke, or kidney disease.

To help you remember to take your medicine, try to get into the habit of taking it at the same time each day.

Dosing—The dose of doxazosin will be different for different patients. *Follow your doctor's orders or the directions on the label.* The following information includes only the average doses of doxazosin. *If your dose is different, do not change it* unless your doctor tells you to do so.

The number of tablets that you take depends on the strength of the medicine.

- For *oral* dosage form (tablets):
  —For high blood pressure:
  - Adults—1 milligram (mg) once a day to start. Your doctor may increase your dose slowly to as much as 16 mg once a day.
  - Children—Use and dose must be determined by your doctor.

Missed dose—If you miss a dose of this medicine, take it as soon as possible. However, if it is almost time for your next dose, skip the missed dose and go back to your regular dosing schedule. Do not double doses.

Storage—To store this medicine:

- Keep out of the reach of children.
- Store away from heat and direct light.
- Do not store in the bathroom, near the kitchen sink,

or in other damp places. Heat or moisture may cause
the medicine to break down.

- Do not keep outdated medicine or medicine no longer
  needed. Be sure that any discarded medicine is out
  of the reach of children.

Precautions While Using This Medicine

It is important that your doctor check your progress at
regular visits to make sure that this medicine is working
properly. This is especially important for elderly patients,
who may be more sensitive to the effects of this medicine.

*Do not take other medicines unless they have been dis-
cussed with your doctor.* This especially includes over-the-
counter (nonprescription) medicines for appetite control,
asthma, colds, cough, hay fever, or sinus problems, since
they may tend to increase your blood pressure.

Dizziness, lightheadedness, or sudden fainting may occur
after you take this medicine, especially when you get up
from a lying or sitting position. These effects are more
likely to occur when you take the first dose of this medicine. Taking the first dose at bedtime may prevent problems. However, *be especially careful if you need to get
up during the night.* These effects may also occur with
any doses you take after the first dose. Getting up slowly
may help lessen this problem. *If you feel dizzy, lie down
so that you do not faint.* Then sit for a few moments
before standing to prevent the dizziness from returning.

The dizziness, lightheadedness, or sudden fainting is more
likely to occur if you drink alcohol, stand for a long time,
exercise, or if the weather is hot. *While you are taking
this medicine, be careful to limit the amount of alcohol
you drink. Also, use extra care during exercise or hot
weather or if you must stand for a long time.*

Doxazosin may cause some people to become drowsy or less alert than they are normally. *Make sure you know how you react to this medicine before you drive, use machines, or do anything else that could be dangerous if you are dizzy, drowsy, or are not alert.* After you have taken several doses of this medicine, these effects should lessen.

Side Effects of This Medicine

Along with its needed effects, a medicine may cause some unwanted effects. Although not all of these side effects may occur, if they do occur they may need medical attention.

Check with your doctor as soon as possible if any of the following side effects occur:

More common

Dizziness or lightheadedness

Less common

Dizziness or lightheadedness when getting up from a lying or sitting position; fainting (sudden); fast and pounding heartbeat; irregular heartbeat; shortness of breath; swelling of feet or lower legs

Other side effects may occur that usually do not need medical attention. These side effects may go away during treatment as your body adjusts to the medicine. However, check with your doctor if any of the following side effects continue or are bothersome:

More common

Headache; unusual tiredness

Less common

Nausea; nervousness, restlessness, unusual irritability; runny nose; sleepiness or drowsiness

Other side effects not listed above may also occur in some patients. If you notice any other effects, check with your doctor.

Additional Information

Once a medicine has been approved for marketing for a certain use, experience may show that it is also useful for other medical problems. Although this use is not included in product labeling, doxazosin is used in certain patients with the following medical condition:

- Benign enlargement of the prostate

For patients taking this medicine for *benign enlargement of the prostate*:

- Doxazosin will not shrink the size of your prostate, but it does help to relieve the symptoms.

Other than the above information, there is no additional information relating to proper use, precautions, or side effects for this use.

ERYTHROMYCINS   Systemic

Some commonly used brand names are:

In the U.S.—

E-Base[1]	Erythrocin[5, 6]
E-Mycin[1]	Erythrocot[6]
ERYC[1]	Ilotycin[1, 4]
Ery-Tab	Ilosone[2]
E.E.S.[3]	My-E[6]
EryPed[3]	PCE[1]
Erythro[3]	Wintrocin[6]

In Canada—

Apo-Erythro[1]	ERYC-333[1]
Apo-Erythro E-C[1]	Erythrocin[5, 6]
Apo-Erythro-ES[3]	Erythromid[1]
Apo-Erythro-S[6]	Ilosone[2]
E-Mycin[1]	Ilotycin[4]
E.E.S.[3]	Novo-rythro[2, 6]
Erybid[1]	Novo-rythro Encap[1]
EryPed[3]	PCE[1]
ERYC-250[1]	

Note: For quick reference, the following erythromycins are numbered to match the corresponding brand names.

This information applies to the following medicines:

1. Erythromycin Base (er-ith-roe-MYE-sin)‡§
2. Erythromycin Estolate (ESS-toe-layt)‡
3. Erythromycin Ethylsuccinate (eth-ill-SUK-sin-ayt)‡
4. Erythromycin Gluceptate (gloo-SEP-tayt)
5. Erythromycin Lactobionate (lak-toe-BYE-oh-nayt)‡
6. Erythromycin Stearate (STEER-ate)‡

---

‡Generic name product may also be available in the U.S.
§Generic name product may also be available in Canada.

Description

Erythromycins (eh-rith-roe-MYE-sins) are used to treat many kinds of infections. Erythromycins are also used to prevent "strep" infections in patients with a history of rheumatic heart disease who may be allergic to penicillin.

These medicines may also be used to treat Legionnaires' disease and for other problems as determined by your doctor. They will not work for colds, flu, or other virus infections.

Erythromycins are available only with your doctor's prescription, in the following dosage forms:

Oral

Erythromycin Base
- Delayed-release capsules (U.S. and Canada)
- Delayed-release tablets (U.S. and Canada)
- Tablets (U.S. and Canada)

Erythromycin Estolate
- Capsules (U.S. and Canada)
- Oral suspension (U.S. and Canada)
- Tablets (U.S. and Canada)

Erythromycin Ethylsuccinate
- Chewable tablets (U.S. and Canada)
- Oral suspension (U.S. and Canada)
- Tablets (U.S. and Canada)

Erythromycin Stearate
- Oral suspension (Canada)
- Tablets (U.S. and Canada)

Parenteral

Erythromycin Gluceptate
- Injection (U.S. and Canada)

Erythromycin Lactobionate
- Injection (U.S. and Canada)

Before Using This Medicine

In deciding to use a medicine, the risks of taking the medicine must be weighed against the good it will do. This is a decision you and your doctor will make. For erythromycins, the following should be considered:

Allergies—Tell your doctor if you have ever had any unusual or allergic reaction to erythromycins, or any related medicines, such as azithromycin or clarithromycin. Also tell your health care professional if you are allergic to any other substances, such as foods, preservatives, or dyes.

Pregnancy—Erythromycin estolate has caused side effects involving the liver in some pregnant women. However, none of the erythromycins has been shown to cause birth defects or other problems in human babies.

Breast-feeding—Erythromycins pass into the breast milk. However, erythromycins have not been shown to cause problems in nursing babies.

Children—This medicine has been tested in children and, in effective doses, has not been shown to cause different side effects or problems in children than it does in adults.

Older adults—This medicine has been tested and has not been shown to cause different side effects or problems in older people than it does in younger adults. However, older adults may be at increased risk of hearing loss, especially if they are taking high doses of erythromycin and/or have kidney or liver disease.

Other medicines—Although certain medicines should not be used together at all, in other cases two different medicines may be used together even if an interaction might occur. In these cases, your doctor may want to change the dose, or other precautions may be necessary. When you are taking or receiving erythromycins, it is especially important that your health care professional know if you are taking any of the following:

- Acetaminophen (e.g., Tylenol) (with long-term, high-dose use) or
- Amiodarone (e.g., Cordarone) or
- Anabolic steroids (nandrolone [e.g., Anabolin], oxandrolone [e.g., Anavar], oxymetholone [e.g., Anadrol], stanozolol [e.g., Winstrol]) or
- Androgens (male hormones) or
- Antithyroid agents (medicine for overactive thyroid) or
- Carmustine (e.g., BiCNU) or
- Chloroquine (e.g., Aralen) or
- Dantrolene (e.g., Dantrium) or
- Daunorubicin (e.g., Cerubidine) or
- Disulfiram (e.g., Antabuse) or
- Divalproex (e.g., Depakote) or
- Estrogens (female hormones) or
- Etretinate (e.g., Tegison) or
- Gold salts (medicine for arthritis) or
- Hydroxychloroquine (e.g., Plaquenil) or
- Mercaptopurine (e.g., Purinethol) or
- Methotrexate (e.g., Mexate) or
- Methyldopa (e.g., Aldomet) or
- Naltrexone (e.g., Trexan) (with long-term, high-dose use) or
- Oral contraceptives (birth control pills) containing estrogen or
- Other anti-infectives by mouth or by injection (medicine for infection) or
- Phenothiazines (acetophenazine [e.g., Tindal], chlorpromazine [e.g., Thorazine], fluphenazine [e.g., Prolixin], mesoridazine [e.g., Serentil], perphenazine [e.g., Trilafon], prochlorperazine [e.g., Compazine], promazine [e.g.,

Sparine], promethazine [e.g., Phenergan], thioridazine [e.g., Mellaril], trifluoperazine [e.g., Stelazine], triflupromazine [e.g., Vesprin], trimeprazine [e.g., Temaril]) or

- Phenytoin (e.g., Dilantin) or
- Plicamycin (e.g., Mithracin) or
- Valproic acid (e.g., Depakene)—Use of these medicines with erythromycins, especially erythromycin estolate, may increase the chance of liver problems
- Aminophylline (e.g., Somophyllin) or
- Caffeine (e.g., NoDoz) or
- Oxtriphylline (e.g., Choledyl) or
- Theophylline (e.g., Somophyllin-T, Theo-Dur)—Use of these medicines with erythromycins may increase the chance of side effects from aminophylline, caffeine, oxtriphylline, or theophylline
- Astemizole (e.g., Hismanal) or
- Terfenadine (e.g., Seldane)—Use of astemizole or terfenadine with erythromycins may cause heart problems, such as an irregular heartbeat; these medicines should not be used together
- Carbamazepine (e.g., Tegretol)—Use of carbamazepine with erythromycin may increase the side effects of carbamazepine or increase the chance of liver problems
- Chloramphenicol (e.g., Chloromycetin) or
- Clindamycin (e.g., Cleocin) or
- Lincomycin (e.g., Lincocin)—Use of these medicines with erythromycins may decrease the effectiveness of these other antibiotics
- Cyclosporine (e.g., Sandimmune) or
- Warfarin (e.g., Coumadin)—Use of any of these medicines with erythromycins may increase the side effects of these medicines

Other medical problems—The presence of other medical problems may affect the use of erythromycins. Make sure you tell your doctor if you have any other medical problems, especially:

- Heart disease—High doses of erythromycin may increase the chance of side effects in patients with a history of an irregular heartbeat

- Liver disease—Erythromycins, especially erythromycin estolate, may increase the chance of side effects involving the liver
- Loss of hearing—High doses of erythromycins may, on rare occasion, cause hearing loss, especially if you have kidney or liver disease

---

Proper Use of This Medicine

Generally, erythromycins are best taken with a full glass (8 ounces) of water on an empty stomach (at least 1 hour before or 2 hours after meals). If stomach upset occurs, these medicines may be taken with food. If you have questions about the erythromycin medicine you are taking, check with your health care professional.

For patients taking the *oral liquid form* of this medicine:

- This medicine is to be taken by mouth even if it comes in a dropper bottle. If this medicine does not come in a dropper bottle, use a specially marked measuring spoon or other device to measure each dose accurately. The average household teaspoon may not hold the right amount of liquid.
- Do not use after the expiration date on the label. The medicine may not work properly after that date. Check with your pharmacist if you have any questions about this.

For patients taking the *chewable tablet form* of this medicine:

- Tablets must be chewed or crushed before they are swallowed.

For patients taking the *delayed-release capsule form (with enteric-coated pellets) or the delayed-release tablet form* of this medicine:

- Swallow capsules or tablets whole. Do not break or

crush. If you are not sure about which type of capsule or tablet you are taking, check with your pharmacist.

To help clear up your infection completely, *keep taking this medicine for the full time of treatment,* even if you begin to feel better after a few days. *If you have a "strep" infection, you should keep taking this medicine for at least 10 days. This is especially important in "strep" infections. Serious heart problems could develop later* if your infection is not cleared up completely. Also, if you stop taking this medicine too soon, your symptoms may return.

This medicine works best when there is a constant amount in the blood. *To help keep the amount constant, do not miss any doses. Also, it is best to take the doses at evenly spaced times day and night.* For example, if you are to take 4 doses a day, the doses should be spaced about 6 hours apart. If this interferes with your sleep or other daily activities, or if you need help in planning the best times to take your medicine, check with your health care professional.

Dosing—The dose of erythromycin will be different for different patients. *Follow your doctor's orders or the directions on the label.* The following information includes only the average doses of erythromycin. *If your dose is different, do not change it* unless your doctor tells you to do so.

The number of capsules or tablets or teaspoonfuls of suspension that you take depends on the strength of the medicine. Also, *the number of doses you take each day, the time allowed between doses, and the length of time you take the medicine depend on the medical problem for which you are taking erythromycin.*

For erythromycin base

- For *oral* dosage forms (capsules, tablets):
    - —For treatment of infections:

• Adults and teenagers—250 to 500 milligrams (mg) two to four times a day.

• Children—Dose is based on body weight. The usual dose is 7.5 to 12.5 mg per kilogram (kg) (3.4 to 5.6 mg per pound) of body weight four times a day, or 15 to 25 mg per kg (6.8 to 11.4 mg per pound) of body weight two times a day.

—For prevention of heart infections:

• Adults and teenagers—Take 1 gram two hours before your dental appointment or surgery, then 500 mg six hours after taking the first dose.

• Children—Dose is based on body weight. The usual dose is 20 mg per kg (9.1 mg per pound) of body weight two hours before the dental appointment or surgery, then 10 mg per kg (4.5 mg per pound) of body weight six hours after taking the first dose.

For erythromycin estolate

• For *oral* dosage forms (capsules, oral suspension, tablets):

—For treatment of infections:

• Adults and teenagers—250 to 500 milligrams (mg) two to four times a day.

• Children—Dose is based on body weight. The usual dose is 7.5 to 12.5 mg per kilogram (kg) (3.4 to 5.6 mg per pound) of body weight four times a day, or 15 to 25 mg per kg (6.8 to 11.4 mg per pound) of body weight two times a day.

—For prevention of heart infections:

• Adults and teenagers—Take 1 gram two hours before your dental appointment or surgery, then 500 mg six hours after taking the first dose.

• Children—Dose is based on body weight. The usual dose is 20 mg per kg (9.1 mg per pound) of body weight two hours before the dental appointment or surgery, then 10 mg per kg (4.5 mg per pound) of body weight six hours after taking the first dose.

For erythromycin ethylsuccinate

- For *oral* dosage forms (oral suspension, tablets):

    —For treatment of infections:

    - Adults and teenagers—400 to 800 milligrams (mg) two to four times a day.

    - Children—Dose is based on body weight. The usual dose is 7.5 to 12.5 mg per kilogram (kg) (3.4 to 5.6 mg per pound) of body weight four times a day, or 15 to 25 mg per kg.(6.8 to 11.4 mg per pound) of body weight two times a day.

    —For prevention of heart infections:

    - Adults and teenagers—Take 1.6 grams two hours before your dental appointment or surgery, then 800 mg six hours after taking the first dose.

    - Children—Dose is based on body weight. The usual dose is 20 mg per kg (9.1 mg per pound) of body weight two hours before the dental appointment or surgery, then 10 mg per kg (4.5 mg per pound) of body weight six hours after taking the first dose.

For erythromycin gluceptate

- For *injection* dosage forms:

    —For treatment of infections:

    - Adults and teenagers—250 to 500 milligrams (mg) injected into a vein every six hours; or 3.75 to 5 mg per kilogram (kg) (1.7 to 2.3 mg per pound) of body weight injected into a vein every six hours.

    - Children—Dose is based on body weight. The usual dose is 3.75 to 5 mg per kg (1.7 to 2.3 mg per pound) of body weight injected into a vein every six hours.

For erythromycin lactobionate

• For *injection* dosage forms:

—For treatment of infections:

• Adults and teenagers—250 to 500 milligrams (mg) injected into a vein every six hours; or 3.75 to 5 mg per kilogram (kg) (1.7 to 2.3 mg per pound) of body weight injected into a vein every six hours.

• Children—Dose is based on body weight. The usual dose is 3.75 to 5 mg per kg (1.7 to 2.3 mg per pound) of body weight injected into a vein every six hours.

For erythromycin stearate

• For *oral* dosage forms (oral suspension, tablets):

—For treatment of infections:

• Adults and teenagers—250 to 500 milligrams (mg) two to four times a day.

• Children—Dose is based on body weight. The usual dose is 7.5 to 12.5 mg per kilogram (kg) (3.4 to 5.6 mg per pound) of body weight four times a day; or 15 to 25 mg per kg (6.8 to 11.4 mg per pound) of body weight two times a day.

—For prevention of heart infections:

• Adults and teenagers—Take 1 gram two hours before your dental appointment or surgery, then 500 mg six hours after taking the first dose.

• Children—Dose is based on body weight. The usual dose is 20 mg per kg (9.1 mg per pound) of body weight two hours before the dental appointment or surgery, then 10 mg per kg (4.5 mg per pound) of body weight six hours after taking the first dose.

Missed dose—If you miss a dose of this medicine, take it as soon as possible. This will help to keep a constant amount of medicine in the blood. However, if it is almost time for your next dose, skip the missed dose and go back to your regular dosing schedule. Do not double doses.

Storage—To store this medicine:
- Keep out of the reach of children.
- Store away from heat and direct light.
- Do not store the capsule or tablet form of erythromycins in the bathroom, near the kitchen sink, or in other damp places. Heat or moisture may cause the medicine to break down.
- Store the oral liquid form of some erythromycins in the refrigerator because heat will cause this medicine to break down. However, keep the medicine from freezing. Follow the directions on the label.
- Do not keep outdated medicine or medicine no longer needed. Be sure that any discarded medicine is out of the reach of children.

Precautions While Using This Medicine

If your symptoms do not improve within a few days, or if they become worse, check with your doctor.

Side Effects of This Medicine

Along with its needed effects, a medicine may cause some unwanted effects. Although not all of these side effects may occur, if they do occur they may need medical attention.

Check with your doctor immediately if any of the following side effects occur:

Less common

> Fever; nausea; skin rash, redness, or itching; stomach pain (severe); unusual tiredness or weakness; vomiting; yellow eyes or skin—with erythromycin estolate (rare with other erythromycins)

Less common—with erythromycin injection only

> Pain, swelling, or redness at place of injection

Rare

> Fainting (repeated); irregular or slow heartbeat; loss of hearing (temporary)

Other side effects may occur that usually do not need medical attention. These side effects may go away during treatment as your body adjusts to the medicine. However, check with your doctor if any of the following side effects continue or are bothersome:

More common

> Abdominal or stomach cramping and discomfort; diarrhea; nausea or vomiting

Less common

> Sore mouth or tongue; vaginal itching and discharge

Other side effects not listed above may also occur in some patients. If you notice any other effects, check with your doctor.

Additional Information

Once a medicine has been approved for marketing for a certain use, experience may show that it is also useful for other medical problems. Although these uses are not included in product labeling, erythromycins are used in certain patients with the following medical conditions:

- Acne
- Actinomycosis
- Anthrax
- Chancroid

- Gastroparesis
- Lyme disease
- Lymphogranuloma venereum
- Relapsing fever

Other than the above information, there is no additional information relating to proper use, precautions, or side effects for these uses.

ESTROGENS   Systemic

Some commonly used brand names are:

In the U.S.—

Aquest[6]	Estroject-LA[3]
Clinagen LA 40[3]	Estro-L.A.[3]
Deladiol-40[3]	Estrone '5'[6]
Delestrogen[3]	Estro-Span[3]
depGynogen[3]	Estrovis[9]
Depo-Estradiol[3]	Gynogen L.A. 20[3]
Depogen[3]	Gynogen L.A. 40[3]
Dioval 40[3]	Kestrone-5[6]
Dioval XX[3]	Menaval-20[3]
Dura-Estrin[3]	Menest[5]
Duragen-20[3]	Ogen .625[7]
Duragen-40[3]	Ogen 1.25[7]
E-Cypionate[3]	Ogen 2.5[7]
Estinyl[8]	Ortho-Est[7]
Estrace[3]	Premarin[4]
Estraderm[3]	Premarin Intravenous[4]
Estragyn 5[6]	Stilphostrol[2]
Estragyn LA 5[3]	TACE[1]
Estra-L 40[3]	Valergen-10[3]
Estratab[5]	Valergen-20[3]
Estro-A[6]	Valergen-40[3]
Estro-Cyp[3]	Wehgen[6]
Estrofem[3]	

In Canada—

C.E.S.[4]	Femogex[3]
Congest[4]	Honvol[2]
Delestrogen[3]	Neo-Estrone[5]
Estinyl[8]	Ogen[7]
Estrace[3]	Premarin[4]
Estraderm[3]	Premarin Intravenous[4]

Other commonly used names are:

DES[2]   Piperazine Estrone Sulfate[7]

Note: For quick reference, the following estrogens are numbered to match the corresponding brand names.

This information applies to the following medicines:

1. Chlorotrianisene (klor-oh-trye-AN-i-seen)†
2. Diethylstilbestrol (dye-eth-il-stil-BESS-trole)‡
3. Estradiol (ess-tra-DYE-ole)‡
4. Estrogens, Conjugated (ESS-troe-jenz, CON-ju-gate-ed)§
5. Estrogens, Esterified (ess-TAIR-i-fyed)
6. Estrone (ESS-trone)†‡
7. Estropipate (ess-troe-PI-pate)‡
8. Ethinyl Estradiol (ETH-in-il ess-tra-DYE-ole)
9. Quinestrol (quin-ESS-trole)†

---

†Not commercially available in Canada.
‡Generic name product may also be available in the U.S.
§Generic name product may also be available in Canada.

Description

Estrogens (ESS-troe-jenz) are female hormones. They are produced by the body and are necessary for the normal sexual development of the female and for the regulation of the menstrual cycle during the childbearing years.

The ovaries begin to produce less estrogen after menopause (the change of life). This medicine is prescribed to make up for the lower amount of estrogen. This should relieve signs of menopause, such as hot flashes and unusual sweating, chills, faintness, or dizziness.

Estrogens are prescribed for several reasons:

- to provide additional hormone when the body does not produce enough of its own, as during the menopause or following certain kinds of surgery.

- in the treatment of selected cases of breast cancer in men and women.

- in the treatment of men with certain kinds of cancer of the prostate.

• to help prevent weakening of bones (osteoporosis) in women past menopause.

Estrogens may also be used for other conditions as determined by your doctor.

There is *no* medical evidence to support the belief that the use of estrogens will keep the patient feeling young, keep the skin soft, or delay the appearance of wrinkles. Nor has it been proven that the use of estrogens during the menopause will relieve emotional and nervous symptoms, unless these symptoms are caused by other menopausal symptoms, such as hot flashes or hot flushes.

Estrogens are very useful medicines. However, in addition to their helpful effects in treating your medical problem, they sometimes have side effects that could be very serious. *A paper called "Information for the Patient" should be given to you with your prescription. Read this carefully.* Also, before you use an estrogen, you and your doctor should discuss the good that it will do as well as the risks of using it.

Estrogens are available only with your doctor's prescription, in the following dosage forms:

Oral

Chlorotrianisene
• Capsules (U.S.)
Diethylstilbestrol
• Tablets (U.S. and Canada)
Estradiol
• Tablets (U.S. and Canada)
Estrogens, Conjugated
• Tablets (U.S. and Canada)
Estrogens, Esterified
• Tablets (U.S. and Canada)
Estropipate
• Tablets (U.S. and Canada)
Ethinyl Estradiol
• Tablets (U.S. and Canada)

Quinestrol
- Tablets (U.S.)

Parenteral

Diethylstilbestrol
- Injection (U.S. and Canada)

Estradiol
- Injection (U.S. and Canada)

Estrogens, Conjugated
- Injection (U.S. and Canada)

Estrone
- Injection (U.S.)

Topical

Estradiol
- Transdermal system (stick-on patch) (U.S. and Canada)

Before Using This Medicine

In deciding to use a medicine, the risks of taking the medicine must be weighed against the good it will do. This is a decision you and your doctor will make. For estrogens, the following should be considered:

Allergies—Tell your doctor if you have ever had any unusual or allergic reaction to estrogens. Also tell your health care professional if you are allergic to any other substances, such as foods, preservatives, or dyes.

Pregnancy—Estrogens are not recommended for use during pregnancy, since some have been shown to cause serious birth defects in humans and animals. Some daughters of women who took diethylstilbestrol (DES) during pregnancy have developed reproductive (genital) tract problems and, rarely, cancer of the vagina or cervix (opening to the uterus) when they reached childbearing age. Some sons of women who took DES during pregnancy have developed urinary-genital tract problems.

Breast-feeding—Use of this medicine is not recommended in nursing mothers. Estrogens pass into the breast milk and their possible effect on the baby is not known.

Older adults—This medicine has been tested and has not been shown to cause different side effects or problems in older women than it does in younger women.

Other medicines—Although certain medicines should not be used together at all, in other cases two different medicines may be used together even if an interaction might occur. In these cases, your doctor may want to change the dose, or other precautions may be necessary. When you are taking estrogens, it is especially important that your health care professional know if you are taking any of the following:

- Acetaminophen (e.g., Tylenol) (with long-term, high-dose use) or
- Amiodarone (e.g., Cordarone) or
- Anabolic steroids (nandrolone [e.g., Anabolin], oxandrolone [e.g., Anavar], oxymetholone [e.g., Anadrol], stanozolol [e.g., Winstrol]) or
- Androgens (male hormones) or
- Anti-infectives by mouth or by injection (medicine for infection) or
- Antithyroid agents (medicine for overactive thyroid) or
- Carbamazepine (e.g., Tegretol) or
- Carmustine (e.g., BiCNU) or
- Chloroquine (e.g., Aralen) or
- Dantrolene (e.g., Dantrium) or
- Daunorubicin (e.g., Cerubidine) or
- Disulfiram (e.g., Antabuse) or
- Divalproex (e.g., Depakote) or
- Etretinate (e.g., Tegison) or
- Gold salts (medicine for arthritis) or
- Hydroxychloroquine (e.g., Plaquenil) or
- Mercaptopurine (e.g., Purinethol) or
- Methotrexate (e.g., Mexate) or
- Methyldopa (e.g., Aldomet) or
- Naltrexone (e.g., Trexan) (with long-term, high-dose use) or

- Oral contraceptives (birth control pills) containing estrogen or
- Phenothiazines (acetophenazine [e.g., Tindal], chlorpromazine [e.g., Thorazine], fluphenazine [e.g., Prolixin], mesoridazine [e.g., Serentil], perphenazine [e.g., Trilafon], prochlorperazine [e.g., Compazine], promazine [e.g., Sparine], promethazine [e.g., Phenergan], thioridazine [e.g., Mellaril], trifluoperazine [e.g., Stelazine], triflupromazine [e.g., Vesprin], trimeprazine [e.g., Temaril]) or
- Phenytoin (e.g., Dilantin) or
- Plicamycin (e.g., Mithracin) or
- Valproic acid (e.g., Depakene)—Estrogens and all of these medicines can cause liver damage. Your doctor may want you to have extra blood tests that tell about your liver, if you must take any of these medicines with estrogens
- Bromocriptine (e.g., Parlodel)—Estrogens may interfere with the effects of bromocriptine
- Cyclosporine (e.g., Sandimmune)—Estrogens can increase the chance of toxic effects to the kidney or liver from cyclosporine because estrogens can interfere with the body's ability to get the cyclosporine out of the bloodstream as it normally would

Other medical problems—The presence of other medical problems may affect the use of estrogens. Make sure you tell your doctor if you have any other medical problems, especially:

For all patients

- Blood clots (or history of during previous estrogen therapy)—Estrogens may worsen blood clots or cause new clots to form
- Breast cancer (active or suspected)—Estrogens may cause growth of the tumor in some cases
- Changes in vaginal bleeding of unknown causes—Some irregular vaginal bleeding is a sign that the lining of the uterus is growing too much or is a sign of cancer of the uterus lining; estrogens may make these conditions worse
- Endometriosis—Estrogens may worsen endometriosis by causing growth of endometriosis implants

- Fibroid tumors of the uterus—Estrogens may cause fibroid tumors to increase in size
- Gallbladder disease or gallstones (or history of)—Estrogens may possibly increase the risk of gallbladder disease or gallstones
- Jaundice (or history of during pregnancy)—Estrogens may worsen or cause jaundice in these patients
- Liver disease—Toxic drug effects may occur in patients with liver disease because the body is not able to get this medicine out of the bloodstream as it normally would
- Porphyria—Estrogens can make porphyria worse

For males treated for breast or prostate cancer

- Blood clots or
- Heart or circulation disease or
- Stroke—Males with these medical problems may be more likely to have clotting problems while taking estrogens; the doses of estrogens used to treat male breast or prostate cancer have been shown to increase the chances of heart attack, phlebitis (inflamed veins) caused by a blood clot, or blood clots in the lungs

Proper Use of This Medicine

For patients taking any of the estrogens by mouth:

- *Take this medicine only as directed by your doctor. Do not take more of it and do not take it for a longer time than your doctor ordered.* Try to take the medicine at the same time each day to reduce the possibility of side effects and to allow it to work better.
- Nausea may occur during the first few weeks after you start taking estrogens. This effect usually disappears with continued use. If the nausea is bothersome, it can usually be prevented or reduced by taking each dose with food or immediately after food.

For patients using the transdermal (stick-on patch) form of estradiol:

- This medicine comes with patient directions. Read them carefully before using this medicine.
- Wash and dry your hands thoroughly before and after handling.
- Apply the patch to a clean, dry, non-oily skin area of your abdomen (stomach) or buttocks that has little or no hair and is free of cuts or irritation.
- *Do not apply to the breasts.* Also, do not apply to the waistline or anywhere else where tight clothes may rub the patch loose.
- Press the patch firmly in place with the palm of your hand for about 10 seconds. Make sure there is good contact, especially around the edges.
- If a patch becomes loose or falls off, you may reapply it or discard it and apply a new patch.
- Each dose is best applied to a different area of skin on your abdomen so that at least 1 week goes by before the same area is used again. This will help prevent skin irritation.

Dosing—The dose of these medicines will be different for different patients. *Follow your doctor's orders or the directions on the label.* The following information includes only the average doses of these medicines. *If your dose is different, do not change it* unless your doctor tells you to do so.

The number of capsules or tablets that you take or the amount of injection you use depends on the strength of the medicine. Also, *the number of doses you take or use each day, the time allowed between doses, and the length of time you take or use the medicine depend on the medical problem for which you are taking or using estrogen.*

For chlorotrianisene

- For *oral* dosage form (capsules):

  —For treating a genital skin condition (vulvar squamous hyperplasia), inflammation of the vagina

(atrophic vaginitis), ovary disorders (female hypogonadism), or symptoms of menopause:

• Adults—12 to 25 milligrams (mg) a day. Your
doctor may want you to take this medicine every
day or only on certain days each month.

—For treating prostate cancer:

• Adults—12 to 25 mg a day.

For conjugated estrogens

• For *oral* dosage form (tablets):

—For treating a genital skin condition (vulvar squamous hyperplasia), inflammation of the vagina
(atrophic vaginitis), or to prevent loss of bone
(osteoporosis):

• Adults—0.3 to 1.25 milligrams (mg) a day.
Your doctor may want you to take the medicine
each day or only on certain days of the month.

—For treating ovary problems (female hypogonadism):

• Adults—2.5 to 7.5 mg a day. This dose is divided up and taken in smaller doses. Your doctor
may want you to take the medicine only on certain days of the month.

—For treating symptoms of menopause:

• Adults—0.625 to 1.25 mg a day. Your doctor
may want you to take the medicine each day or
only on certain days of the month.

—For treating ovary problems (failure or removal of
the ovary):

• Adults—1.25 mg a day. Your doctor may want
you to take the medicine each day or only on
certain days of the month.

—For treating breast cancer in women after menopause and in men:

• Adults—10 mg three times a day for at least
three months.

—For treating prostate cancer:

- Adults—1.25 to 2.5 mg three times a day.

• For *injection* dosage form:

—For controlling abnormal bleeding of the uterus:

- Adults—25 mg injected into a muscle or vein. This may be repeated in six to twelve hours if needed.

For diethylstilbestrol

• For *oral* dosage forms (tablets and enteric-coated tablets):

—For treating breast cancer in women after menopause and in men:

- Adults—15 milligrams (mg) a day.

—For treating prostate cancer:

- Adults—At first, 1 to 3 mg a day. Later, your doctor may decrease your dose to 1 mg a day.

For diethylstilbestrol diphosphate

• For *oral* dosage form (tablets):

—For treating prostate cancer:

- Adults—50 to 200 milligrams (mg) three times a day.

• For *injection* dosage form:

—For treating prostate cancer:

- Adults—At first, 500 mg mixed in solution with sodium chloride or dextrose injection and injected slowly into a vein. Your doctor may increase your dose to 1 gram a day for five or more straight days as needed. Then, your doctor may lower your dose to 250 to 500 mg one or two times a week.

For esterified estrogens

• For *oral* dosage form (tablets):

—For treating a genital skin condition (vulvar squamous hyperplasia) or inflammation of the vagina (atrophic vaginitis):

- • Adults—0.3 to 1.25 milligrams (mg) a day. Your doctor may want you to take the medicine each day or only on certain days of the month.

—For treating ovary problems (female hypogonadism):

- • Adults—2.5 to 7.5 mg a day. This dose may be divided up and taken in smaller doses. Your doctor may want you to take the medicine each day or only on certain days of the month.

—For treating symptoms of menopause:

- • Adults—0.625 to 1.25 mg a day. Your doctor may want you to take the medicine each day or only on certain days of the month.

—For treating ovary problems (failure or removal of the ovary):

- • Adults—1.25 mg a day. Your doctor may want you to take the medicine each day or only on certain days of the month.

—For treating breast cancer in women after menopause and in men:

- • Adults—10 mg three times a day for at least three months.

—For treating prostate cancer:

- • Adults—1.25 to 2.5 mg three times a day.

For estradiol

- • For *oral* dosage form (tablets):

—For treating a genital skin condition (vulvar squamous hyperplasia), inflammation of the vagina (atrophic vaginitis), ovary problems (female hypogonadism or failure or removal of the ovary), or symptoms of menopause:

- • Adults—0.5 to 2 milligrams (mg) a day. Your

doctor may want you to take the medicine each day or only on certain days of the month.

—For treating breast cancer in women after menopause and in men:

- Adults—10 mg three times a day for at least three months.

—For treating prostate cancer:

- Adults—1 to 2 mg three times a day.

—For preventing bone loss (osteoporosis):

- Adults—0.5 mg a day. Your doctor may want you to take the medicine each day or only on certain days of the month.

- For *transdermal* dosage form (patches):

—For treating a genital skin condition (vulvar squamous hyperplasia), inflammation of the vagina (atrophic vaginitis), symptoms of menopause, ovary problems (female hypogonadism or failure or removal of the ovary), or to prevent bone loss (osteoporosis):

- Adults—0.05 or 0.1 milligram (mg) (one patch) applied to the skin and worn for one-half of a week. Then, remove that patch and apply a new patch. A new patch should be applied two times a week.

For estradiol cypionate

- For *injectable* dosage form:

—For treating ovary problems (female hypogonadism):

- Adults—1.5 to 2 milligrams (mg) injected into a muscle once a month.

—For treating symptoms of menopause:

- Adults—1 to 5 mg injected into a muscle every three to four weeks.

For estradiol valerate

• For *injection* dosage form:

—For treating a genital skin condition (vulvar squamous hyperplasia), inflammation of the vagina (atrophic vaginitis), symptoms of menopause, or ovary problems (female hypogonadism or failure or removal of the ovary):

• Adults—10 to 20 milligrams (mg) injected into a muscle every four weeks as needed.

—For treating prostate cancer:

• Adults—30 mg injected into a muscle every one or two weeks.

For estrone

• For *injection* dosage form:

—For controlling abnormal bleeding of the uterus:

• Adults—2 to 5 milligrams (mg) a day, injected into a muscle for several days.

—For treating ovary problems (female hypogonadism, failure or removal of the ovary):

• Adults—0.1 to 2 mg a week. This is injected into a muscle as a single dose or divided into more than one dose. Your doctor may want you to receive the medicine each week or only during certain weeks of the month.

—For treating a genital skin condition (vulvar squamous hyperplasia), inflammation of the vagina (atrophic vaginitis), or symptoms of menopause:

• Adults—0.1 to 0.5 mg injected into a muscle two or three times a week. Your doctor may want you to receive the medicine each week or only during certain weeks of the month.

—For treating prostate cancer:

• Adults—2 to 4 mg injected into a muscle two or three times a week.

For estropipate

- For oral dosage form (tablets):

  —For treating a genital skin condition (vulvar squamous hyperplasia), inflammation of the vagina (atrophic vaginitis), or symptoms of menopause:

  • Adults—0.75 to 6 milligrams (mg) a day. Your doctor may want you to take the medicine each day or only on certain days of the month.

  —For treating ovary problems (female hypogonadism, failure or removal of the ovary):

  • Adults—1.5 to 9 mg a day. Your doctor may want you to take the medicine each day or only on certain days of the month.

For ethinyl estradiol

- For *oral* dosage form (tablets):

  —For treating ovary problems (female hypogonadism):

  • Adults—0.05 milligrams (mg) one to three times a day for three to six months. Your doctor may want you to take the medicine each day or only on certain days of the month.

  —For treating symptoms of menopause:

  • Adults—0.02 to 0.05 mg a day. Your doctor may want you to take the medicine each day or only on certain days of the month.

  —For treating breast cancer in women after menopause:

  • Adults—1 mg three times a day.

  —For treating prostate cancer:

  • Adults—0.15 to 3 mg a day.

For quinestrol

- For *oral* dosage form (tablets):

  —For treating a genital skin condition (vulvar squamous hyperplasia), inflammation of the vagina (atrophic vaginitis), symptoms of menopause, or ovary problems (female hypogonadism, failure or removal of the ovary):

• Adults—At first, 100 micrograms (mcg) a day for seven days. Then, no medicine is taken for seven days. After that, your doctor will lower your dose to 100 to 200 mcg taken once a week.

Missed dose—

• For patients taking any of the estrogens by mouth: If you miss a dose of this medicine, take it as soon as possible. However, if it is almost time for your next dose, skip the missed dose and go back to your regular dosing schedule. Do not double doses.

• For patients using the transdermal (stick-on patch) form of estradiol: If you forget to apply a new patch when you are supposed to, apply it as soon as possible. However, if it is almost time for the next patch, skip the missed one and go back to your regular schedule. Do not apply more than one patch at a time.

Storage—To store this medicine:

• Keep out of the reach of children.

• Store away from heat and direct light.

• Do not store in the bathroom medicine cabinet because the heat or moisture may cause the medicine to break down.

• Keep the injectable form of this medicine from freezing.

• Do not keep outdated medicine or medicine no longer needed. Be sure that any discarded medicine is out of the reach of children.

Precautions While Using This Medicine

It is very important that your doctor check your progress at regular visits to make sure this medicine does not cause unwanted effects. These visits will usually be every year, but some doctors require them more often.

It is not yet known whether the use of estrogens increases the risk of breast cancer in women. Therefore, it is very important that you regularly check your breasts for any unusual lumps or discharge. You should also have a mammogram (x-ray pictures of the breasts) done if your doctor recommends it. Because breast cancer has occurred in men taking estrogens, regular self-breast exams and exams by your doctor for any unusual lumps or discharge should be done.

In some patients using estrogens, tenderness, swelling, or bleeding of the gums may occur. Brushing and flossing your teeth carefully and regularly and massaging your gums may help prevent this. See your dentist regularly to have your teeth cleaned. Check with your medical doctor or dentist if you have any questions about how to take care of your teeth and gums, or if you notice any tenderness, swelling, or bleeding of your gums.

If you think that you may be pregnant, stop using the medicine immediately and check with your doctor. Continued use of some estrogens during pregnancy may cause birth defects in the child. DES may also increase the risk of vaginal cancer developing in daughters when they reach childbearing age.

Do not give this medicine to anyone else. Your doctor has prescribed it only for you after studying your health record and the results of your physical examination. Estrogens may be dangerous for other people because of differences in their health and body make-up.

Side Effects of This Medicine

Discuss these possible effects with your doctor:

- The prolonged use of estrogens has been reported to

increase the risk of endometrial cancer (cancer of the lining of the uterus) in women after the menopause. This risk seems to increase as the dose and the length of use increase. When estrogens are used in low doses for less than 1 year, there is less risk. The risk is also reduced if a progestin (another female hormone) is added to, or replaces part of, your estrogen dose. If the uterus has been removed by surgery (total hysterectomy), there is no risk of endometrial cancer.

- It is not yet known whether the use of estrogens increases the risk of breast cancer in women. Although some large studies show an increased risk, most studies and information gathered to date do not support this idea. Breast cancer has been reported in men taking estrogens.

- In studies with oral contraceptives (birth control pills) containing estrogens, cigarette smoking was shown to cause an increased risk of serious side effects affecting the heart or blood circulation, such as dangerous blood clots, heart attack, or stroke. The risk increased as the amount of smoking and the age of the smoker increased. Women aged 35 and over were at greatest risk when they smoked while using oral contraceptives containing estrogens. It is not known if this risk exists with the use of estrogens for symptoms of menopause. However, smoking may make estrogens less effective.

The following side effects may be caused by blood clots, which could lead to stroke, heart attack, or death. These side effects rarely occur, and, when they do occur, they occur in men treated for cancer using high doses of estrogens. *Get emergency help immediately* if any of the following side effects occur:

Rare—For males being treated for breast or prostate cancer only

Headache (sudden or severe); loss of coordination (sudden); loss of vision or change of vision (sudden); pains

in chest, groin, or leg, especially in calf of leg; shortness of breath (sudden and unexplained); slurring of
speech (sudden); weakness or numbness in arm or leg

Also, check with your doctor as soon as possible if any
of the following side effects occur:

More common

Breast pain (in females and males); increased breast size
(in females and males); swelling of feet and lower legs;
weight gain (rapid)

Less common or rare

Changes in vaginal bleeding (spotting, breakthrough bleeding, prolonged or heavier bleeding, or complete stoppage of bleeding); lumps in, or discharge from, breast
(in females and males); pains in stomach, side, or abdomen; uncontrolled jerky muscle movements; yellow
eyes or skin

Other side effects may occur that usually do not need
medical attention. These side effects may go away during
treatment as your body adjusts to the medicine. However,
check with your doctor if any of the following side effects
continue or are bothersome:

More common

Bloating of stomach; cramps of lower stomach; loss of
appetite; nausea; skin irritation or redness where skin
patch was worn

Less common

Diarrhea (mild); dizziness (mild); headaches (mild); migraine headaches; problems in wearing contact lenses;
unusual decrease in sexual desire (in males); unusual
increase in sexual desire (in females); vomiting (usually
with high doses)

Also, many women who are taking estrogens with a progestin (another female hormone) will start having monthly
vaginal bleeding, similar to menstrual periods again. This
effect will continue for as long as the medicine is taken.
However, monthly bleeding will not occur in women who

have had the uterus removed by surgery (total hysterectomy).

Other side effects not listed above may also occur in some patients. If you notice any other effects, check with your doctor.

ESTROGENS AND PROGESTINS—
Oral Contraceptives   Systemic

Some commonly used brand names are:

In the U.S.—

Brevicon[5]	Nelova 1/50M[6]
Demulen 1/35[2]	Nelulen 1/35E[2]
Demulen 1/50[2]	Nelulen 1/50E[2]
Desogen[1]	Nordette[3]
GenCept 0.5/35[5]	Norethin 1/35E[5]
GenCept 1/35[5]	Norethin 1/50M[6]
GenCept 10/11[5]	Norinyl 1+50[6]
Genora 0.5/35[5]	Norinyl 1+35[5]
Genora 1/35[5]	Ortho-Cept[1]
Genora 1/50[6]	Ortho-Cyclen[7]
Jenest[5]	Ortho-Novum 1/35[5]
Levlen[3]	Ortho-Novum 7/7/7[5]
Loestrin 1/20[4]	Ortho-Novum 10/11[5]
Loestrin 1.5/30[4]	Ortho-Novum 1/50[6]
Lo/Ovral[8]	Ortho Tri-Cyclen[7]
ModiCon[5]	Ovcon-35[5]
N.E.E. 1/35[5]	Ovcon-50[5]
N.E.E. 1/50[5]	Ovral[8]
Nelova 0.5/35E[5]	Tri-Levlen[3]
Nelova 1/35E[5]	Tri-Norinyl[5]
Nelova 10/11[5]	Triphasil[3]

In Canada—

Brevicon 0.5/35[5]	Minestrin 1/20[4]
Brevicon 1/35[5]	Min-Ovral[3]
Cyclen[7]	Norinyl 1/50[6]
Demulen 30[2]	Ortho 0.5/35[5]
Demulen 50[2]	Ortho 1/35[5]
Loestrin 1.5/30[4]	Ortho 7/7/7[5]
Marvelon[1]	Ortho 10/11[5]

In Canada—

Ortho-Cept[1]

Ortho-Novum 0.5[6]

Ortho-Novum 1/50[6]

Ortho-Novum 1/80[6]

Ortho-Novum 2[6]

Ovral[8]

Synphasic[5]

Tri-Cyclen[7]

Triphasil[3]

Triquilar[3]

Note: For quick reference, the following estrogens and progestins are numbered to match the corresponding brand names.

This information applies to the following medicines:

1. Desogestrel (des-oh-JES-trel) and Ethinyl Estradiol (ETH-in-il ess-tra-DYE-ole)
2. Ethynodiol (e-thye-noe-DYE-ole) Diacetate and Ethinyl Estradiol
3. Levonorgestrel (LEE-voe-nor-jess-trel) and Ethinyl Estradiol
4. Norethindrone (nor-eth-IN-drone) Acetate and Ethinyl Estradiol
5. Norethindrone and Ethinyl Estradiol
6. Norethindrone and Mestranol
7. Norgestimate (nor-JES-ti-mate) and Ethinyl Estradiol
8. Norgestrel (nor-JESS-trel) and Ethinyl Estradiol

For information about Norethindrone (e.g., Micronor) or Norgestrel (e.g., Ovrette) when used as single-ingredient oral contraceptives, see *Progestins (Systemic)*.

Description

Oral contraceptives are known also as the Pill, OC's, BC's, BC tablets, or birth control pills. They usually contain two types of female hormones, estrogens (ESS-troe-jenz) and progestins (proe-JESS-tins). When taken by mouth on a regular schedule, they change the hormone balance of the body, which prevents pregnancy.

Sometimes these preparations can be used in the treatment of conditions that are helped by added hormones. Oral contraceptives do not prevent or cure venereal diseases (VD), however.

Before you take an oral contraceptive, you and your doctor should discuss the benefits and risks of using these medicines. Besides surgery or not having intercourse, these medicines are the most effective method of preventing pregnancy. However, oral contraceptives sometimes have side effects that could be very serious.

To make the use of oral contraceptives as safe and reliable as possible, you should understand how and when to take them and what effects may be expected. *A paper with information for the patient will be given to you with your filled prescription, and will provide many details concerning the use of oral contraceptives. Read this paper carefully* and ask your health care professional if you need additional information or explanation.

Oral contraceptives are available only with your doctor's prescription, in the following dosage forms:

Oral

    Desogestrel and Ethinyl Estradiol
      • Tablets (U.S. and Canada)
    Ethynodiol Diacetate and Ethinyl Estradiol
      • Tablets (U.S. and Canada)
    Levonorgestrel and Ethinyl Estradiol
      • Tablets (U.S. and Canada)
    Norethindrone Acetate and Ethinyl Estradiol
      • Tablets (U.S. and Canada)
    Norethindrone and Ethinyl Estradiol
      • Tablets (U.S. and Canada)
    Norethindrone and Mestranol
      • Tablets (U.S. and Canada)
    Norgestimate and Ethinyl Estradiol
      • Tablets (U.S. and Canada)
    Norgestrel and Ethinyl Estradiol
      • Tablets (U.S. and Canada)

Before Using This Medicine

In deciding to use a medicine, the risks of taking the medicine must be weighed against the good it will do. This is a decision you and your doctor will make. For estrogen and progestin birth control pills, the following should be considered:

Allergies—Tell your doctor if you have ever had any unusual or allergic reaction to estrogens or progestins. Also tell your health care professional if you are allergic to any other substances, such as foods, preservatives, or dyes.

Pregnancy—Oral contraceptives are not recommended for use during pregnancy.

Breast-feeding—The estrogens in oral contraceptives pass into the breast milk. It is not known what effect oral contraceptives may have on the infant. Studies have shown oral contraceptives to cause tumors in humans and animals. Use of "high-dose" birth control medicines is not recommended during breast-feeding. It may be necessary for you to use another method of birth control or to stop breast-feeding while taking oral contraceptives. However, your doctor may allow you to begin using one of the "low-dose" oral contraceptives after you have been breast-feeding for a while.

Children—This medicine is frequently used for birth control in teenage females and has not been shown to cause different side effects or problems than it does in adults. However, some teenagers may need extra information on the importance of taking this medication exactly as prescribed in order for it to work.

Other medicines—Although certain medicines should not be used together at all, in other cases two different medicines may be used together even if an interaction might occur. In these cases, your doctor may want to change the dose, or other precautions may be necessary. When you are taking estrogen and progestin birth control pills, it is especially important that your health care professional know if you are taking any of the following:

- Acetaminophen (e.g., Tylenol) (with long-term, high-dose use)
- Adrenocorticoids (cortisone-like medicine)
- Amiodarone (e.g., Cordarone)
- Anabolic steroids (nandrolone [e.g., Anabolin], oxandrolone [e.g., Anavar], oxymetholone [e.g., Anadrol], stanozolol [e.g., Winstrol])

- Androgens (male hormones)
- Anticoagulants (blood thinners)
- Anti-infectives by mouth or by injection (medicine for infection)
- Antithyroid agents (medicine for overactive thyroid)
- Barbiturates
- Bromocriptine (e.g., Parlodel)
- Carbamazepine (e.g., Tegretol)
- Carmustine (e.g., BiCNU)
- Chloroquine (e.g., Aralen)
- Dantrolene (e.g., Dantrium)
- Daunorubicin (e.g., Cerubidine)
- Disulfiram (e.g., Antabuse)
- Divalproex (e.g., Depakote)
- Estrogens (female hormones)
- Etretinate (e.g., Tegison)
- Gold salts (medicine for arthritis)
- Griseofulvin (e.g., Fulvicin)
- Hydroxychloroquine (e.g., Plaquenil)
- Mercaptopurine (e.g., Purinethol)
- Methotrexate (e.g., Mexate)
- Methyldopa (e.g., Aldomet)
- Naltrexone (e.g., Trexan) (with long-term, high-dose use)
- Phenothiazines (acetophenazine [e.g., Tindal], chlorproma-zine [e.g., Thorazine], fluphenazine [e.g., Prolixin], mesori-dazine [e.g., Serentil], perphenazine [e.g., Trilafon], prochlorperazine [e.g., Compazine], promazine [e.g., Sparine], promethazine [e.g., Phenergan], thioridazine [e.g., Mellaril], trifluoperazine [e.g., Stelazine], triflupro-mazine [e.g., Vesprin], trimeprazine [e.g., Temaril])
- Phenylbutazone (e.g., Butazolidin)
- Phenytoin (e.g., Dilantin)
- Plicamycin (e.g., Mithracin)
- Primidone (e.g., Mysoline)
- Rifampin (e.g., Rifadin)
- Tricyclic antidepressants (amitriptyline [e.g., Elavil], amox-

apine [e.g., Asendin], clomipramine [e.g., Anafranil], desipramine [e.g., Pertofrane], doxepin [e.g., Sinequan], imipramine [e.g., Tofranil], nortriptyline [e.g., Aventyl], protriptyline [e.g., Vivactil], trimipramine [e.g., Surmontil])

• Valproic acid (e.g., Depakene)

Other medical problems—The presence of other medical problems may affect the use of estrogen and progestin birth control pills. Make sure you tell your doctor if you have any other medical problems, especially:

• Angina pectoris (chest pains on exertion)
• Asthma
• Blood clots (or history of)
• Bone disease
• Breast disease (not cancerous, such as fibrocystic disease [breast cysts], breast lumps, or abnormal mammograms [x-ray pictures of the breast])
• Cancer (or history of or family history of breast cancer)
• Changes in vaginal bleeding
• Diabetes mellitus (sugar diabetes)
• Endometriosis
• Epilepsy
• Fibroid tumors of the uterus
• Gallbladder disease or gallstones (or history of)
• Heart or circulation disease
• High blood cholesterol
• High blood pressure (hypertension)
• Jaundice (or history of, including jaundice during pregnancy)
• Kidney disease
• Liver disease (such as jaundice or porphyria)
• Lumps in breasts
• Mental depression (or history of)
• Migraine headaches
• Scanty or irregular menstrual periods
• Stroke (history of)

- Too much calcium in the blood
- Tuberculosis
- Varicose veins

Proper Use of This Medicine

Take this medicine only as directed by your doctor. This medicine must be taken exactly on schedule to prevent pregnancy. Try to take the medicine at the same time each day, not more than 24 hours apart, to reduce the possibility of side effects and to provide the best protection.

Nausea may occur during the first few weeks after you start taking this medicine. This effect usually disappears with continued use. If the nausea is bothersome, it can usually be prevented or reduced by taking each dose with food or immediately after food.

Since one of the most important factors in the proper use of oral contraceptives is taking every dose exactly on schedule, you should never let your tablet supply run out. Always keep 1 extra month's supply of tablets on hand. To keep the extra month's supply from becoming too old, use it next, after the pills now being used, and replace the extra supply each month on a regular schedule. The tablets will keep well when kept dry and at room temperature (light will fade some tablet colors but will not change the medicine's effect).

Keep the tablets in the container in which you received them. Most containers aid you in keeping track of your dosage schedule.

It is very important that you take the tablets in the same order that they appear in the container. Tablets of different colors in the same package are also different in strength. *Taking the tablets out of order may reduce the effectiveness of the medicine.*

- *Monophasic (one-phase) cycle* dosing schedule: Most available dosing schedules are of the monophasic type. If you are taking tablets of one strength (color) for 20 or 21 days, you are using a monophasic schedule. For the 28-day monophasic cycle you will also take an additional 7 inactive tablets, which are of another color.

- *Biphasic (two-phase) cycle* dosing schedule:

  —If you are using a biphasic 21-day schedule, you are taking tablets of one strength (color) for 7 to 10 days (the 1st phase). You then take tablets of a second strength (color) for the next 11 to 14 days (the 2nd phase). For the 28-day biphasic cycle you will also take an additional 7 inactive tablets, which are of a third color.

  —If you are using a biphasic 24-day schedule, you are taking tablets of one strength (color) for 17 days (the 1st phase). You then take tablets of a second strength (color) for the next 7 days (the 2nd phase).

- *Triphasic (three-phase) cycle* dosing schedule: If you are using a triphasic 21-day schedule, you are taking tablets of one strength (color) for 6 or 7 days depending on the medicine prescribed (the 1st phase). You then take tablets of a second strength (color) for the next 5 to 9 days depending on the medicine prescribed (the 2nd phase). After that, you take tablets of a third strength (color) for the next 5 to 10 days depending on the medicine prescribed (the 3rd phase). At this point, you will have taken a total of 21 tablets. For the 28-day triphasic cycle you will also take an additional 7 inactive tablets, which are of a fourth color.

Dosing—Your health care professional may begin your dose on the first day of your menstrual period (called day-1 start), on the fifth day of your menstrual period (called day-5 start), or on Sunday (called Sunday start). *When you* *begin on a certain day it is important that you follow that schedule, even when you miss a dose. Do not change your schedule on your own.* If the schedule that you have been put on is not convenient, check with your health care professional about changing schedules.

- For *oral* dosage forms (monophasic, biphasic, or triphasic tablets):
  —For contraception:
    - Adults and teenagers—

      For 21-day cycle: Take one tablet a day for twenty-one days. Skip seven days. Then repeat the cycle.

      For 28-day cycle: Take one tablet a day for twenty-eight days. Then repeat the cycle.

Missed dose—*Follow your doctor's orders or the directions on the label* if you miss a dose of this medicine. The following information includes only some of the ways to handle missed doses. Your health care professional may want you to stop taking the medicine and use other birth control methods for the rest of the month until you have your menstrual period. Then your health care professional can help you begin your medicine again.

For monophasic, biphasic, or triphasic cycles:

- If you miss the first tablet of a new cycle—Take the missed tablet as soon as you remember and take the next tablet at the usual time. You may take 2 tablets in one day. Then continue your regular dosing schedule. Also, use another birth control method until you have taken seven days of your tablets after the last missed dose.

- If you miss 1 tablet during the cycle—Take the missed tablet as soon as you remember. Take the next tablet at the usual time. You may take 2 tablets in one day. Then continue your regular dosing schedule.

- If you miss 2 tablets in a row in the first or second

week—Take 2 tablets on the day that you remember and 2 tablets the next day. Continue taking 1 tablet a day. Also, use another birth control method until you begin a new cycle.

- If you miss 2 tablets in a row in the third week; or
- If you miss 3 or more tablets in a row at any time during the cycle—

Using a day-1 start: Throw out your current cycle and begin taking a new cycle. Also, use another birth control method until you have taken seven days of your tablets after the last missed dose. You may not have a menstrual period this month. But if you miss two menstrual periods in a row, call your health care professional.

Using a day-5 start: Keep taking one tablet a day from your current pack until the end of the cycle. Use another birth control method until you begin a new cycle. You should have a menstrual period this month. If you do not, call your health care professional.

Using a Sunday start: Keep taking one tablet a day from your current pack until Sunday. Then, on Sunday, throw out your old pack and begin a new pack. Also, use another birth control method until you have taken seven days of your tablets after the last missed dose. You may not have a menstrual period this month. But if you miss two menstrual periods in a row, call your health care professional.

If you miss any of the last 7 (inactive) tablets of a 28-day cycle, there is no danger of pregnancy. However, the first tablet (active) of the next month's cycle must be taken on the regularly scheduled day, in spite of any missed doses, if pregnancy is to be avoided. The active and inactive tablets are colored differently for your convenience.

Storage—To store this medicine:

- Keep out of the reach of children.

- Store away from heat and direct light.
- Do not store in the bathroom, near the kitchen sink, or in other damp places. Heat and moisture may cause the medicine to break down.
- Do not keep outdated medicine or medicine no longer needed. Be sure that any discarded medicine is out of the reach of children.

Precautions While Using This Medicine

It is very important that your doctor check your progress at regular visits to make sure this medicine does not cause unwanted effects. These visits will usually be every 6 to 12 months, but some doctors require them more often.

When you begin to use oral contraceptives, your body will require at least 7 days to adjust before pregnancy will be prevented; therefore, you should *use a second method of birth control for the first cycle (or 3 weeks)* to ensure full protection.

Tell the medical doctor or dentist in charge that you are taking this medicine before any kind of surgery (including dental surgery) or emergency treatment, since this medicine may cause serious blood clots, heart attack, or stroke.

The following medicines may reduce the effectiveness of oral contraceptives. *You should use a second method of birth control during each cycle in which any of the following medicines are used:*

Ampicillin
Adrenocorticoids (cortisone-like medicine)
Bacampicillin
Barbiturates
Carbamazepine (e.g., Tegretol)
Chloramphenicol (e.g., Chloromycetin)
Dihydroergotamine (e.g., D.H.E. 45)
Griseofulvin (e.g., Fulvicin)

Mineral oil
Neomycin, oral
Penicillin V
Phenylbutazone (e.g., Butazolidin)
Phenytoin (e.g., Dilantin)
Primidone (e.g., Mysoline)
Rifampin (e.g., Rifadin)
Sulfonamides (sulfa medicine)
Tetracyclines (medicine for infection)
Tranquilizers
Valproic acid (e.g., Depakene)

Check with your doctor if you have any questions about this.

Vaginal bleeding of various amounts may occur between your regular menstrual periods during the first 3 months of use. This is sometimes called spotting when slight, or breakthrough bleeding when heavier. If this should occur:

- Continue on your regular dosing schedule.
- The bleeding usually stops within 1 week.
- Check with your doctor if the bleeding continues for more than 1 week.
- After you have been taking oral contraceptives on schedule and for more than 3 months, check with your doctor.

Missed menstrual periods may occur:

- if you have not taken the medicine exactly as scheduled. Pregnancy must be considered a possibility.
- if the medicine is not properly adjusted for your needs.
- if you have taken oral contraceptives for a long time, usually 2 or more years, and stop their use.

Check with your doctor if you miss any menstrual periods so that the cause may be determined.

In some patients using estrogen-containing oral contraceptives, tenderness, swelling, or bleeding of the gums may occur. Brushing and flossing your teeth carefully and regularly and massaging your gums may help prevent this. See your dentist regularly to have your teeth cleaned. Check with your medical doctor or dentist if you have any questions about how to take care of your teeth and gums, or if you notice any tenderness, swelling, or bleeding of your gums. Also, it has been shown that estrogen-containing oral contraceptives may cause a healing problem called dry socket after a tooth has been removed. If you are going to have a tooth removed, tell your dentist or oral surgeon that you are taking oral contraceptives.

Some people who take oral contraceptives may become more sensitive to sunlight than they are normally. When you begin taking this medicine, avoid too much sun and do not use a sunlamp until you see how you react to the sun, especially if you tend to burn easily. If you have a severe reaction, check with your doctor. Some people may develop brown, blotchy spots on exposed areas. These spots usually disappear gradually when the medicine is stopped.

If you wear contact lenses and notice a change in vision or are not able to wear them, check with your doctor.

If you suspect that you may have become pregnant, stop taking this medicine immediately and check with your doctor.

If you are scheduled for any laboratory tests, tell your doctor that you are taking birth control pills.

Do not give this medicine to anyone else. Your doctor has prescribed it only for you after studying your health record and the results of your physical examination. Oral contraceptives may be dangerous for other people because of differences in their health and body make-up.

Check with your doctor before taking any leftover oral contraceptives from an old prescription, especially after a pregnancy. Your old prescription may be dangerous to you now or may allow you to become pregnant if your health has changed since your last physical examination.

Side Effects of This Medicine

Discuss these possible effects with your doctor:

- Along with their needed effects, birth control tablets sometimes cause some unwanted effects such as benign (not cancerous) liver tumors, liver cancer, blood clots, heart attack, and stroke, and problems of the gallbladder, liver, and uterus. Although these effects are rare, they can be very serious and may cause death.

- *Cigarette smoking* during the use of oral contraceptives has been found to increase the risk of serious side effects affecting the heart and/or blood circulation, such as dangerous blood clots, heart attack, or stroke. The risk increases as the age of the patient and the amount of smoking increase. This risk is greater in women age 35 and over. *To reduce the risk of serious side effects, do not smoke cigarettes while using oral contraceptives.*

The following side effects may be caused by blood clots, which could lead to stroke, heart attack, or death. Although these side effects rarely occur, they require immediate medical attention. *Get emergency help immediately* if any of the following side effects occur:

Abdominal or stomach pain (sudden, severe, or continuing); coughing up blood; headache (severe or sudden); loss of coordination (sudden); loss of vision or change in vision (sudden); pains in chest, groin, or leg (especially in calf of leg); shortness of breath (sudden or unexplained); slurring of speech (sudden); weakness, numbness, or pain in arm or leg (unexplained)

Check with your doctor as soon as possible if any of the following side effects occur:

Less common or rare

Bulging eyes; changes in vaginal bleeding (spotting, break-through bleeding, prolonged bleeding, or complete stoppage of bleeding); double vision; fainting; frequent urge to urinate or painful urination; increased blood pressure; loss of vision (gradual, partial, or complete); lumps in, or discharge from, breast; mental depression; pains in stomach, side, or abdomen; skin rash, redness, or other skin irritation; swelling, pain, or tenderness in upper abdomen (stomach) area; unusual or dark-colored mole; vaginal discharge (thick, white, or curd-like); vaginal itching or irritation; yellow eyes or skin

Other side effects may occur that usually do not need medical attention. These side effects may go away during treatment as your body adjusts to the medicine. However, check with your doctor if any of the following side effects continue or are bothersome:

More common

Acne (usually less common after first 3 months); bloating of stomach; cramps of lower stomach; increase or decrease in appetite; nausea; swelling of ankles and feet; swelling and increased tenderness of breasts; unusual tiredness or weakness; unusual weight gain

Less common or rare

Brown, blotchy spots on exposed skin;. diarrhea (mild); dizziness; headaches or migraine headaches; increased body and facial hair; increased sensitivity to contact lenses; increased skin sensitivity to sun; irritability; some loss of scalp hair; unusual decrease or increase in sexual desire; vomiting; weight loss

Other side effects not listed above may also occur in some patients. If you notice any other effects, check with your doctor.

FAMCICLOVIR   Systemic†

A commonly used brand name in the U.S. is Famvir.

†Not commercially available in Canada.

Description

Famciclovir (fam-SYE-kloe-veer) is used to treat the symptoms of herpes zoster (also known as shingles), a herpes virus infection of the skin. Although famciclovir will not cure herpes zoster, it does help relieve the pain and discomfort and helps the sores heal faster.

Famciclovir is available only with your doctor's prescription, in the following dosage form:

Oral
- Tablets (U.S.)

Before Using This Medicine

In deciding to use a medicine, the risks of taking the medicine must be weighed against the good it will do. This is a decision you and your doctor will make. For famciclovir, the following should be considered:

Allergies—Tell your doctor if you have ever had any unusual or allergic reaction to famciclovir. Also tell your health care professional if you are allergic to any other substances, such as foods, sulfites or other preservatives, or dyes.

Pregnancy—Famciclovir has not been studied in pregnant women. However, famciclovir has not been shown to cause birth defects or other problems in animal studies.

Breast-feeding—It is not known whether famciclovir

passes into the breast milk of humans; however, it does pass into the milk of rats. Famciclovir is not recommended during breast-feeding because it may cause unwanted effects in nursing babies.

Children—Studies on this medicine have been done only in adult patients, and there is no specific information comparing use of famciclovir in children with use in other age groups.

Older adults—Famciclovir has been used in the elderly and has not been shown to cause different side effects or problems in older people than it does in younger adults.

Other medicines—Although certain medicines should not be used together at all, in other cases two different medicines may be used together even if an interaction might occur. In these cases, your doctor may want to change your dose or other precautions may be necessary. Tell your health care professional if you are taking any other prescription or nonprescription (over-the-counter [OTC]) medicine.

Other medical problems—The presence of other medical problems may affect the use of famciclovir. Make sure you tell your doctor if you have any other medical problems, especially:

• Kidney disease—Kidney disease may increase blood levels of this medicine, increasing the chance of side effects

Proper Use of This Medicine

Famciclovir is best used within 48 hours after the symptoms of shingles (for example, pain, burning, blisters) begin to appear.

Famciclovir may be taken with meals.

To help clear up your herpes infection, *keep taking famciclovir for the full time of treatment,* even if your symptoms begin to clear up after a few days. *Do not miss any doses*. However, *do not use this medicine more often or for a longer time than your doctor ordered*.

Dosing—The dose of famciclovir will be different for different patients. *Follow your doctor's orders or the directions on the label*. The following information includes only the average doses of famciclovir. Your dose may be different if you have kidney disease. *If your dose is different, do not change it* unless your doctor tells you to do so.

- For *oral* dosage form (tablets):

    —For treatment of shingles:

    - Adults—500 milligrams (mg) every eight hours for seven days.
    - Children—Use and dose must be determined by your doctor.

Missed dose—If you miss a dose of this medicine, take it as soon as possible. However, if it is almost time for your next dose, skip the missed dose and go back to your regular dosing schedule. Do not double doses.

Storage—To store this medicine:

- Keep out of the reach of children.
- Store away from heat and direct light.
- Do not store the tablets in the bathroom, near the kitchen sink, or in other damp places. Heat or moisture may cause the medicine to break down.
- Do not keep outdated medicine or medicine no longer needed. Be sure that any discarded medicine is out of the reach of children.

Precautions While Using This Medicine

If your symptoms do not improve within a few days, or if they become worse, check with your doctor.

The areas affected by herpes should be kept as clean and dry as possible. Also, wear loose-fitting clothing to avoid irritating the sores (blisters).

Side Effects of This Medicine

Along with its needed effects, a medicine may cause some unwanted effects. Although not all of these side effects may occur, if they do occur they may need medical attention.

Side effects may occur that usually do not need medical attention. These side effects may go away during treatment as your body adjusts to the medicine. However, check with your doctor if any of the following side effects continue or are bothersome:

More common
   Headache
Less common
   Diarrhea; dizziness; nausea; unusual tiredness or weakness; vomiting

Other side effects not listed above may also occur in some patients. If you notice any other effects, check with your doctor.

FINASTERIDE   Systemic

A commonly used brand name in the in the U.S. and Canada is Proscar.

Description

Finasteride (fi-NAS-teer-ide) belongs to the group of medicines called enzyme inhibitors. It is used to treat enlargement of the prostate (benign prostatic hyperplasia or BPH), a condition that causes urinary problems in men.

Finasteride blocks an enzyme called 5-alpha-reductase, which is necessary to change testosterone to another hormone that causes the prostate to grow. As a result, the size of the prostate is decreased. The effect of finasteride on the prostate lasts only as long as the medicine is taken. If it is stopped, the prostate begins to grow again.

Oral

• Tablets (U.S. and Canada)

Before Using This Medicine

In deciding to use a medicine, the risks of taking the medicine must be weighed against the good it will do. This is a decision you and your doctor will make. For finasteride, the following should be considered:

Allergies—Tell your doctor if you have ever had any unusual or allergic reaction to finasteride. Also tell your health care professional if you are allergic to any other substances, such as foods, preservatives, or dyes.

Pregnancy—Women who are or may become pregnant should not be exposed to finasteride, because it can cause changes in the genitals (sex organs) of male infants. Therefore, you should use a condom to prevent contact of your semen with your sexual partner while you are taking finasteride. Discuss with your doctor the need to stop taking finasteride if your partner wishes to become pregnant.

While you are taking finasteride, you may notice a decrease in the amount of semen when you ejaculate. This should not affect your sexual performance and is not a sign of any change in fertility.

Older adults—This medicine has been tested and has not been shown to cause different side effects or problems in older people than it does in younger adults.

Other medicines—Although certain medicines should not be used together at all, in other cases two different medi-

cines may be used together even if an interaction might occur. In these cases, your doctor may want to change the dose, or other precautions may be necessary. When you are taking finasteride, it is especially important that your health care professional know if you are taking any of the following:

- Amantadine (e.g., Symmetrel) or
- Amphetamines or
- Anticholinergics (medicine for abdominal or stomach spasms or cramps) or
- Antidepressants (medicine for depression) or
- Antidyskinetics (medicine for Parkinson's disease or other conditions affecting control of muscles) or
- Antihistamines or
- Antipsychotics (medicine for mental illness) or
- Appetite suppressants (diet pills) or
- Buclizine (e.g., Bucladin) or
- Carbamazepine (e.g., Tegretol) or
- Cyclizine (e.g., Marezine) or
- Cyclobenzaprine (e.g., Flexerel) or
- Disopyramide (e.g., Norpace) or
- Flavoxate (e.g., Urispas) or
- Ipratropium (e.g., Atrovent) or
- Meclizine (e.g., Antivert) or
- Medicine for asthma or other breathing problems or
- Medicine for colds, sinus problems, or hay fever or other allergies (including nose drops or sprays) or
- Methylphenidate (e.g., Ritalin) or
- Orphenadrine (e.g., Norflex) or
- Oxybutynin (e.g., Ditropan) .
- Procainamide (e.g., Pronestyl) or
- Promethazine (e.g., Phenergan) or
- Quinidine (e.g., Quinidex) or
- Trimeprazine (e.g., Temaril)—These medicines can cause problems with urination, which could reduce the effects of finasteride

Other medical problems—The presence of other medical problems may affect the use of finasteride. Make sure you tell your doctor if you have any other medical problems, especially:

- Liver disease—Effects of finasteride may be increased because of slower removal from the body

---

Proper Use of This Medicine

To help you remember to take your medicine, try to get into the habit of taking it at the same time each day.

Remember that this medicine does not cure BPH, but it does help reduce the size of the prostate. Therefore, you must continue to take it if you expect to keep the size of your prostate down. *You may have to take medicine for the rest of your life.* Do not stop taking this medicine without first discussing it with your doctor.

Finasteride tablets may be crushed to make them easier to swallow.

This medicine helps to reduce urinary problems in men with BPH. In general, it is best to avoid drinking fluids, especially coffee or alcohol, in the evening. Then your sleep will not be disturbed by your needing to urinate during the night.

Dosing—The dose of finasteride will be different for different patients. *Follow your doctor's orders or the directions on the label.* The following information includes only the average dose of finasteride. *If your dose is different, do not change it* unless your doctor tells you to do so:

- Adults: 5 mg (one tablet) once a day.

Missed dose—If you miss a dose of this medicine, take it as soon as possible. However, if it is almost time for your next dose, skip the missed dose and go back to your regular dosing schedule. Do not double doses.

Storage—To store this medicine:

- Keep out of the reach of children.
- Store away from heat and direct light.

- Do not store in the bathroom, near the kitchen sink, or in other damp places. Heat or moisture may cause the medicine to break down.
- Do not keep outdated medicine or medicine no longer needed. Be sure that any discarded medicine is out of the reach of children.

Precautions While Using This Medicine

Do not take other medicines unless they have been discussed with your doctor. This especially includes over-the-counter (nonprescription) medicines for appetite control, asthma, colds, cough, hay fever, or sinus problems. These medicines may cause problems with urination and could reduce the effects of finasteride.

Women who are or who may become pregnant should not handle crushed finasteride tablets because of the risk that it could be absorbed into the body and harm the infant.

Side Effects of This Medicine

Along with its needed effects, a medicine may cause some unwanted effects. The following side effects may go away during treatment as your body adjusts to the medicine. However, check with your doctor if any of the following side effects continue or are bothersome:

Less common or rare

Decreased libido (decreased interest in sex); decreased volume of ejaculate (amount of semen); impotence (inability to have or keep an erection)

Other side effects not listed above may also occur in some patients. If you notice any other effects, check with your doctor.

FLUOROQUINOLONES   Systemic

Some commonly used brand names are:

In the U.S.—

Cipro[1]

Cipro IV[1]

Floxin[5]

Floxin IV[5]

Maxaquin[3]

Noroxin[4]

Penetrex[2]

In Canada—

Cipro[1]

Floxin[5]

Maxaquin[3]

Penetrex[2]

Note: For quick reference, the following fluoroquinolones are numbered to match the corresponding brand names.

This information applies to the following medicines:

1. Ciprofloxacin (sip-roe-FLOX-a-sin)
2. Enoxacin (en-OX-a-sin)
3. Lomefloxacin (loe-me-FLOX-a-sin)
4. Norfloxacin (nor-FLOX-a-sin)
5. Ofloxacin (oe-FLOX-a-sin)

Description

Fluoroquinolones (flu-roe-KWIN-a-lones) are used to treat bacterial infections in many different parts of the body. They work by killing bacteria or preventing their growth. However, these medicines will not work for colds, flu, or other virus infections. Fluoroquinolones may be used for other problems as determined by your doctor.

Fluoroquinolones are available only with your doctor's prescription, in the following dosage forms:

Oral

Ciprofloxacin
  • Tablets (U.S. and Canada)
Enoxacin
  • Tablets (U.S. and Canada)
Lomefloxacin
  • Tablets (U.S. and Canada)
Norfloxacin
  • Tablets (U.S. and Canada)

Ofloxacin
- Tablets (U.S. and Canada)

Parenteral

Ciprofloxacin
- Injection (U.S. and Canada)

Ofloxacin
- Injection (U.S.)

Before Using This Medicine

In deciding to use a medicine, the risks of taking the medicine must be weighed against the good it will do. This is a decision you and your doctor will make. For the fluoroquinolones, the following should be considered:

Allergies—Tell your doctor if you have ever had any unusual or allergic reaction to any of the fluoroquinolones or to any related medicines such as cinoxacin (e.g., Cinobac) or nalidixic acid (e.g., NegGram). Also tell your health care professional if you are allergic to any other substances, such as foods, preservatives, or dyes.

Pregnancy—Studies have not been done in humans. However, use is not recommended during pregnancy since fluoroquinolones have been reported to cause bone development problems in young animals.

Breast-feeding—Some of the fluoroquinolones are known to pass into human breast milk. Since fluoroquinolones have been reported to cause bone development problems in young animals, breast-feeding is not recommended during treatment with these medicines.

Children—Use is not recommended for infants or children since fluoroquinolones have been shown to cause bone development problems in young animals. However, your doctor may choose to use one of these medicines if other medicines cannot be used.

Teenagers—Use is not recommended for teenagers up to 18 years of age since fluoroquinolones have been shown to cause bone development problems in young animals. However, your doctor may choose to use one of these medicines if other medicines cannot be used.

Older adults—These medicines have been tested and, in effective doses, have not been shown to cause different side effects or problems in older people than they do in younger adults.

Other medicines—Although certain medicines should not be used together at all, in other cases two different medicines may be used together even if an interaction might occur. In these cases, your doctor may want to change the dose, or other precautions may be necessary. When you are taking a fluoroquinolone, it is especially important that your health care professional know if you are taking any of the following:

- Aminophylline or
- Oxtriphylline (e.g., Choledyl) or
- Theophylline (e.g., Somophyllin-T, Theodur, Elixophyllin)—Enoxacin, ciprofloxacin, and norfloxacin may increase the chance of side effects of aminophylline, oxtriphylline, or theophylline
- Antacids, aluminum-, calcium-, or magnesium-containing, or
- Iron supplements or
- Sucralfate—Antacids, iron, or sucralfate may keep any of the fluoroquinolones from working properly
- Caffeine—Enoxacin, ciprofloxacin, and norfloxacin may increase the chance of side effects of caffeine
- Didanosine (e.g., Videx, ddI)—Didanosine may keep any of the fluoroquinolones from working properly
- Warfarin (e.g., Coumadin)—Enoxacin, ciprofloxacin, and norfloxacin may increase the effect of warfarin, increasing the chance of bleeding

Other medical problems—The presence of other medical problems may affect the use of fluoroquinolones. Make sure you tell your doctor if you have any other medical problems, especially:

- Brain or spinal cord disease, including hardening of the arteries in the brain or epilepsy or other seizures—Fluoroquinolones may cause nervous system side effects
- Kidney disease or
- Kidney disease and liver disease—Patients with kidney disease (alone) or kidney disease and liver disease (together) may have an increased chance of side effects

---

Proper Use of This Medicine

Do not take fluoroquinolones if you are pregnant. Do not give fluoroquinolones to infants, children, or teenagers unless otherwise directed by your doctor. These medicines have been shown to cause bone development problems in young animals.

Fluoroquinolones are best taken with a full glass (8 ounces) of water. Several additional glasses of water should be taken every day, unless you are otherwise directed by your doctor. Drinking extra water will help to prevent some unwanted effects of ciprofloxacin and norfloxacin.

Ciprofloxacin and lomefloxacin may be taken with meals or on an empty stomach.

Enoxacin, norfloxacin, and ofloxacin should be taken on an empty stomach.

To help clear up your infection completely, *keep taking your medicine for the full time of treatment,* even if you begin to feel better after a few days. If you stop taking this medicine too soon, your symptoms may return.

This medicine works best when there is a constant amount in the blood or urine. *To help keep the amount constant, do not miss any doses. Also, it is best to take the doses*

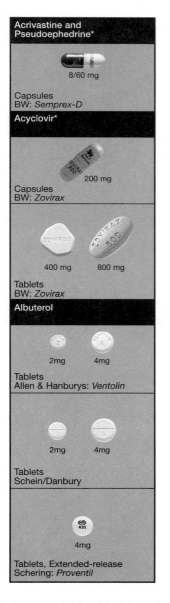

Acrivastine and Pseudoephedrine*

8/60 mg
Capsules
BW: *Semprex-D*

Acyclovir*

200 mg
Capsules
BW: *Zovirax*

400 mg   800 mg
Tablets
BW: *Zovirax*

Albuterol

2mg   4mg
Tablets
Allen & Hanburys: *Ventolin*

2mg   4mg
Tablets
Schein/Danbury

4mg
Tablets, Extended-release
Schering: *Proventil*

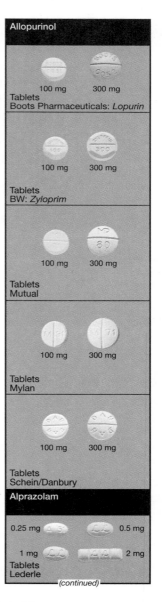

Allopurinol

100 mg   300 mg
Tablets
Boots Pharmaceuticals: *Lopurin*

100 mg   300 mg
Tablets
BW: *Zyloprim*

100 mg   300 mg
Tablets
Mutual

100 mg   300 mg
Tablets
Mylan

100 mg   300 mg
Tablets
Schein/Danbury

Alprazolam

0.25 mg   0.5 mg
1 mg   2 mg
Tablets
Lederle

(continued)

*Single source product for solid oral dosage forms in the U.S.

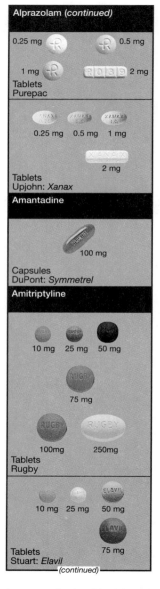

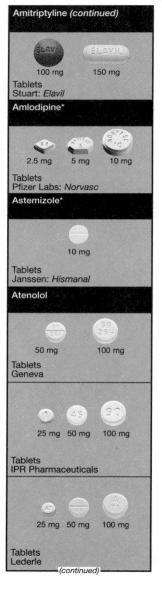

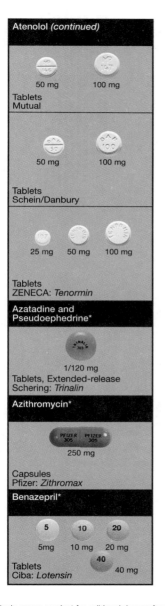

Atenolol *(continued)*

50 mg   100 mg

Tablets
Mutual

50 mg   100 mg

Tablets
Schein/Danbury

25 mg   50 mg   100 mg

Tablets
ZENECA: *Tenormin*

Azatadine and Pseudoephedrine*

1/120 mg

Tablets, Extended-release
Schering: *Trinalin*

Azithromycin*

250 mg

Capsules
Pfizer: *Zithromax*

Benazepril*

5mg   10 mg   20 mg

40 mg

Tablets
Ciba: *Lotensin*

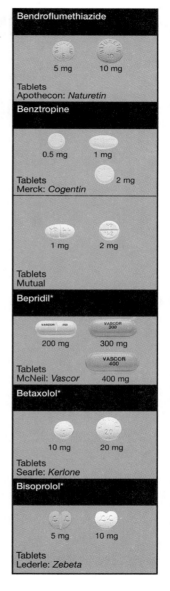

Bendroflumethiazide

5 mg   10 mg

Tablets
Apothecon: *Naturetin*

Benztropine

0.5 mg   1 mg

2 mg

Tablets
Merck: *Cogentin*

1 mg   2 mg

Tablets
Mutual

Bepridil*

200 mg   300 mg

400 mg

Tablets
McNeil: *Vascor*

Betaxolol*

10 mg   20 mg

Tablets
Searle: *Kerlone*

Bisoprolol*

5 mg   10 mg

Tablets
Lederle: *Zebeta*

*Single source product for solid oral dosage forms in the U.S.

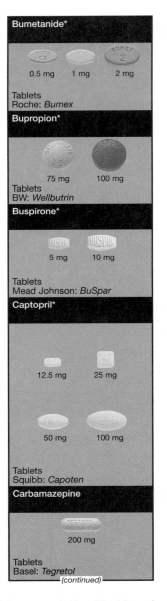

Bumetanide*

0.5 mg   1 mg   2 mg

Tablets
Roche: *Bumex*

Bupropion*

75 mg   100 mg

Tablets
BW: *Wellbutrin*

Buspirone*

5 mg   10 mg

Tablets
Mead Johnson: *BuSpar*

Captopril*

12.5 mg   25 mg

50 mg   100 mg

Tablets
Squibb: *Capoten*

Carbamazepine

200 mg

Tablets
Basel: *Tegretol*
(continued)

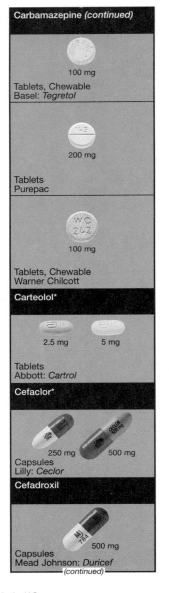

Carbamazepine *(continued)*

100 mg

Tablets, Chewable
Basel: *Tegretol*

200 mg

Tablets
Purepac

100 mg

Tablets, Chewable
Warner Chilcott

Carteolol*

2.5 mg   5 mg

Tablets
Abbott: *Cartrol*

Cefaclor*

250 mg   500 mg

Capsules
Lilly: *Ceclor*

Cefadroxil

500 mg

Capsules
Mead Johnson: *Duricef*
(continued)

*Single source product for solid oral dosage forms in the U.S.

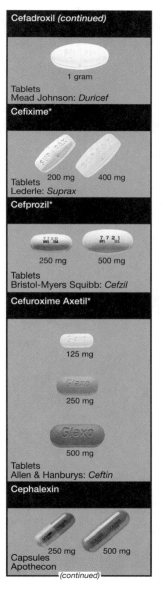

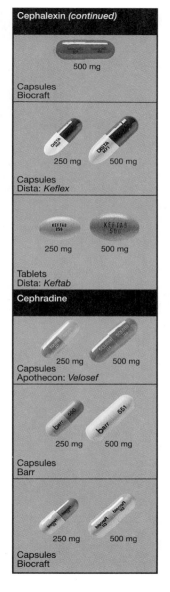

Cefadroxil *(continued)*

1 gram

Tablets
Mead Johnson: *Duricef*

Cefixime*

200 mg   400 mg

Tablets
Lederle: *Suprax*

Cefprozil*

250 mg   500 mg

Tablets
Bristol-Myers Squibb: *Cefzil*

Cefuroxime Axetil*

125 mg

250 mg

500 mg

Tablets
Allen & Hanburys: *Ceftin*

Cephalexin

250 mg   500 mg

Capsules
Apothecon

(continued)

Cephalexin *(continued)*

500 mg

Capsules
Biocraft

250 mg   500 mg

Capsules
Dista: *Keflex*

250 mg   500 mg

Tablets
Dista: *Keftab*

Cephradine

250 mg   500 mg

Capsules
Apothecon: *Velosef*

250 mg   500 mg

Capsules
Barr

250 mg   500 mg

Capsules
Biocraft

*Single source product for solid oral dosage forms in the U.S.

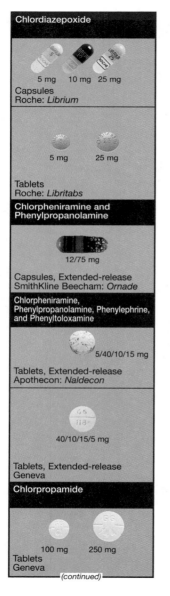

Chlordiazepoxide

5 mg   10 mg   25 mg

Capsules
Roche: *Librium*

5 mg   25 mg

Tablets
Roche: *Libritabs*

Chlorpheniramine and Phenylpropanolamine

12/75 mg

Capsules, Extended-release
SmithKline Beecham: *Ornade*

Chlorpheniramine, Phenylpropanolamine, Phenylephrine, and Phenyltoloxamine

5/40/10/15 mg

Tablets, Extended-release
Apothecon: *Naldecon*

40/10/15/5 mg

Tablets, Extended-release
Geneva

Chlorpropamide

100 mg   250 mg

Tablets
Geneva

(continued)

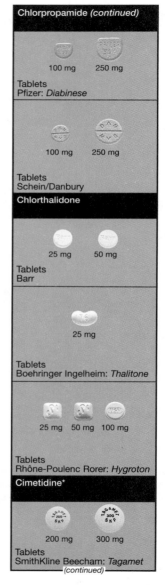

Chlorpropamide *(continued)*

100 mg   250 mg

Tablets
Pfizer: *Diabinese*

100 mg   250 mg

Tablets
Schein/Danbury

Chlorthalidone

25 mg   50 mg

Tablets
Barr

25 mg

Tablets
Boehringer Ingelheim: *Thalitone*

25 mg   50 mg   100 mg

Tablets
Rhône-Poulenc Rorer: *Hygroton*

Cimetidine*

200 mg   300 mg

Tablets
SmithKline Beecham: *Tagamet*

(continued)

*Single source product for solid oral dosage forms in the U.S.

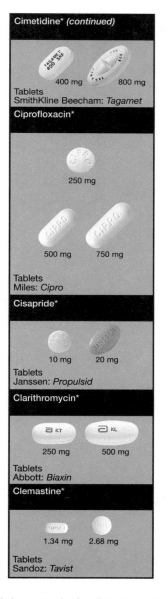

Cimetidine* *(continued)*

400 mg   800 mg

Tablets
SmithKline Beecham: *Tagamet*

Ciprofloxacin*

250 mg

500 mg   750 mg

Tablets
Miles: *Cipro*

Cisapride*

10 mg   20 mg

Tablets
Janssen: *Propulsid*

Clarithromycin*

250 mg   500 mg

Tablets
Abbott: *Biaxin*

Clemastine*

1.34 mg   2.68 mg

Tablets
Sandoz: *Tavist*

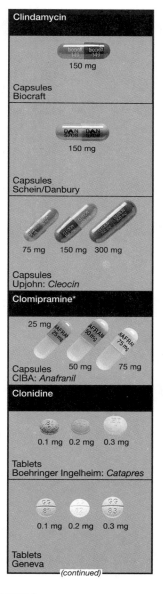

Clindamycin

150 mg

Capsules
Biocraft

150 mg

Capsules
Schein/Danbury

75 mg   150 mg   300 mg

Capsules
Upjohn: *Cleocin*

Clomipramine*

25 mg

50 mg   75 mg

Capsules
CIBA: *Anafranil*

Clonidine

0.1 mg 0.2 mg 0.3 mg

Tablets
Boehringer Ingelheim: *Catapres*

0.1 mg 0.2 mg 0.3 mg

Tablets
Geneva

(continued)

*Single source product for solid oral dosage forms in the U.S.

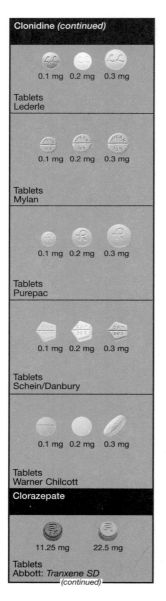

Clonidine *(continued)*

0.1 mg 0.2 mg 0.3 mg

Tablets
Lederle

0.1 mg 0.2 mg 0.3 mg

Tablets
Mylan

0.1 mg 0.2 mg 0.3 mg

Tablets
Purepac

0.1 mg 0.2 mg 0.3 mg

Tablets
Schein/Danbury

0.1 mg 0.2 mg 0.3 mg

Tablets
Warner Chilcott

Clorazepate

11.25 mg 22.5 mg

Tablets
Abbott: *Tranxene SD*
(continued)

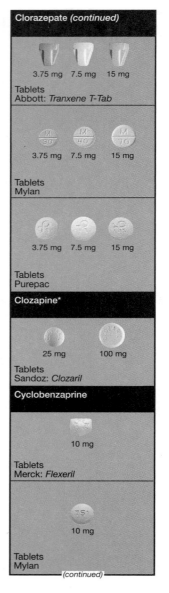

Clorazepate *(continued)*

3.75 mg 7.5 mg 15 mg

Tablets
Abbott: *Tranxene T-Tab*

3.75 mg 7.5 mg 15 mg

Tablets
Mylan

3.75 mg 7.5 mg 15 mg

Tablets
Purepac

Clozapine*

25 mg 100 mg

Tablets
Sandoz: *Clozaril*

Cyclobenzaprine

10 mg

Tablets
Merck: *Flexeril*

10 mg

Tablets
Mylan
(continued)

*Single source product for solid oral dosage forms in the U.S.

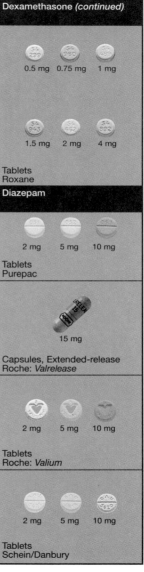

Cyclobenzaprine *(continued)*

DAN
10 mg

Tablets
Schein/Danbury

Desipramine

GG
64
100 mg

GG
160
150 mg

Tablets†   †Also available:
Geneva   10, 25, 50, and 75 mg

10 mg   25 mg   50 mg

75 mg   100 mg   150 mg

Tablets
Marion Merrell Dow: *Norpramin*

Dexamethasone

0.25 mg   0.5 mg   0.75 mg

1.5 mg   4 mg   6 mg

Tablets
Merck: *Decadron*
(continued)

Dexamethasone *(continued)*

54
299
0.5 mg

54
280
0.75 mg

54
339
1 mg

54
943
1.5 mg

54
612
2 mg

54
892
4 mg

Tablets
Roxane

Diazepam

2 mg   5 mg   10 mg

Tablets
Purepac

15 mg

Capsules, Extended-release
Roche: *Valrelease*

2 mg   5 mg   10 mg

Tablets
Roche: *Valium*

2 mg   5 mg   10 mg

Tablets
Schein/Danbury

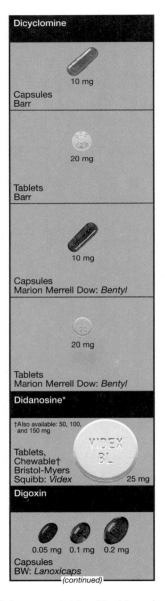

Dicyclomine

10 mg

Capsules
Barr

20 mg

Tablets
Barr

10 mg

Capsules
Marion Merrell Dow: *Bentyl*

20 mg

Tablets
Marion Merrell Dow: *Bentyl*

Didanosine*

†Also available: 50, 100, and 150 mg

Tablets, Chewable†
Bristol-Myers Squibb: *Videx*

VIDEX BL   25 mg

Digoxin

0.05 mg   0.1 mg   0.2 mg

Capsules
BW: *Lanoxicaps*
—(continued)—

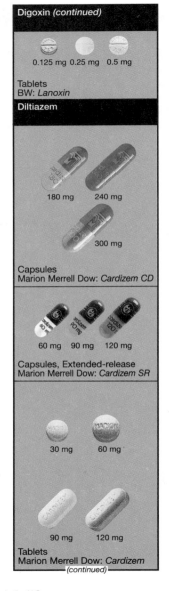

Digoxin *(continued)*

0.125 mg   0.25 mg   0.5 mg

Tablets
BW: *Lanoxin*

Diltiazem

180 mg   240 mg

300 mg

Capsules
Marion Merrell Dow: *Cardizem CD*

60 mg   90 mg   120 mg

Capsules, Extended-release
Marion Merrell Dow: *Cardizem SR*

30 mg   60 mg

90 mg   120 mg

Tablets
Marion Merrell Dow: *Cardizem*
—(continued)—

*Single source product for solid oral dosage forms in the U.S.

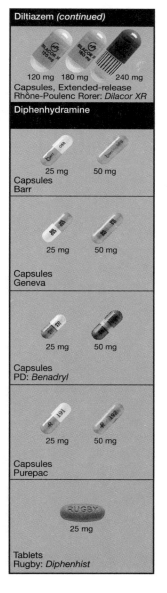

Diltiazem (continued)

120 mg   180 mg   240 mg
Capsules, Extended-release
Rhône-Poulenc Rorer: *Dilacor XR*

Diphenhydramine

25 mg   50 mg
Capsules
Barr

25 mg   50 mg
Capsules
Geneva

25 mg   50 mg
Capsules
PD: *Benadryl*

25 mg   50 mg
Capsules
Purepac

25 mg
Tablets
Rugby: *Diphenhist*

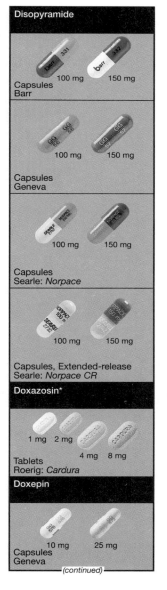

Disopyramide

100 mg   150 mg
Capsules
Barr

100 mg   150 mg
Capsules
Geneva

100 mg   150 mg
Capsules
Searle: *Norpace*

100 mg   150 mg
Capsules, Extended-release
Searle: *Norpace CR*

Doxazosin*

1 mg   2 mg   4 mg   8 mg
Tablets
Roerig: *Cardura*

Doxepin

10 mg   25 mg
Capsules
Geneva

(continued)

*Single source product for solid oral dosage forms in the U.S.

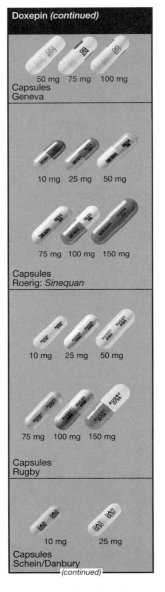

Doxepin *(continued)*

50 mg   75 mg   100 mg
Capsules
Geneva

10 mg   25 mg   50 mg

75 mg   100 mg   150 mg
Capsules
Roerig: *Sinequan*

10 mg   25 mg   50 mg

75 mg   100 mg   150 mg
Capsules
Rugby

10 mg   25 mg
Capsules
Schein/Danbury

(continued)

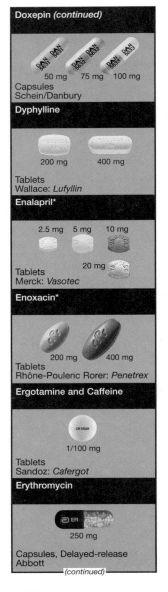

Doxepin *(continued)*

50 mg   75 mg   100 mg
Capsules
Schein/Danbury

Dyphylline

200 mg   400 mg
Tablets
Wallace: *Lufyllin*

Enalapril*

2.5 mg   5 mg   10 mg

20 mg
Tablets
Merck: *Vasotec*

Enoxacin*

200 mg   400 mg
Tablets
Rhône-Poulenc Rorer: *Penetrex*

Ergotamine and Caffeine

1/100 mg
Tablets
Sandoz: *Cafergot*

Erythromycin

250 mg
Capsules, Delayed-release
Abbott

(continued)

*Single source product for solid oral dosage forms in the U.S.

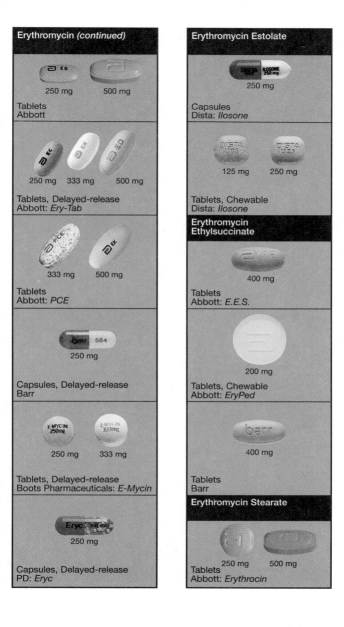

Erythromycin *(continued)*

250 mg   500 mg

Tablets
Abbott

250 mg 333 mg 500 mg

Tablets, Delayed-release
Abbott: *Ery-Tab*

333 mg   500 mg

Tablets
Abbott: *PCE*

250 mg

Capsules, Delayed-release
Barr

250 mg   333 mg

Tablets, Delayed-release
Boots Pharmaceuticals: *E-Mycin*

250 mg

Capsules, Delayed-release
PD: *Eryc*

Erythromycin Estolate

250 mg

Capsules
Dista: *Ilosone*

125 mg   250 mg

Tablets, Chewable
Dista: *Ilosone*

Erythromycin Ethylsuccinate

400 mg

Tablets
Abbott: *E.E.S.*

200 mg

Tablets, Chewable
Abbott: *EryPed*

400 mg

Tablets
Barr

Erythromycin Stearate

250 mg   500 mg
Tablets
Abbott: *Erythrocin*

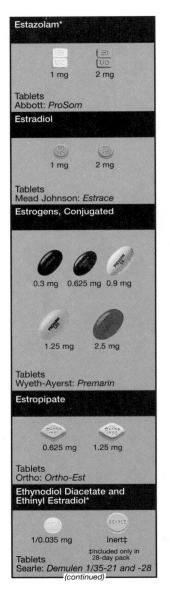

Estazolam*

1 mg   2 mg

Tablets
Abbott: *ProSom*

Estradiol

1 mg   2 mg

Tablets
Mead Johnson: *Estrace*

Estrogens, Conjugated

0.3 mg   0.625 mg   0.9 mg

1.25 mg   2.5 mg

Tablets
Wyeth-Ayerst: *Premarin*

Estropipate

0.625 mg   1.25 mg

Tablets
Ortho: *Ortho-Est*

**Ethynodiol Diacetate and
Ethinyl Estradiol***

1/0.035 mg   Inert‡

‡Included only in
28-day pack

Tablets
Searle: *Demulen 1/35-21 and -28*
(continued)

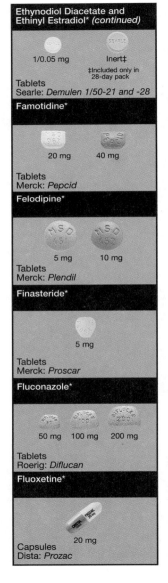

**Ethynodiol Diacetate and
Ethinyl Estradiol*** *(continued)*

1/0.05 mg   Inert‡

‡Included only in
28-day pack

Tablets
Searle: *Demulen 1/50-21 and -28*

Famotidine*

20 mg   40 mg

Tablets
Merck: *Pepcid*

Felodipine*

5 mg   10 mg

Tablets
Merck: *Plendil*

Finasteride*

5 mg

Tablets
Merck: *Proscar*

Fluconazole*

50 mg   100 mg   200 mg

Tablets
Roerig: *Diflucan*

Fluoxetine*

20 mg

Capsules
Dista: *Prozac*

---

*Single source product for solid oral dosage forms in the U.S.

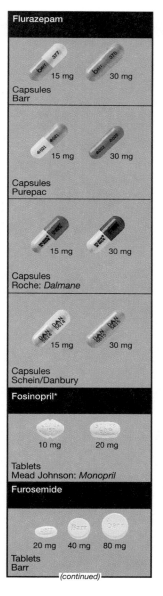

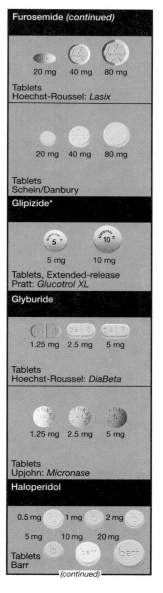

(continued)

*Single source product for solid oral dosage forms in the U.S.

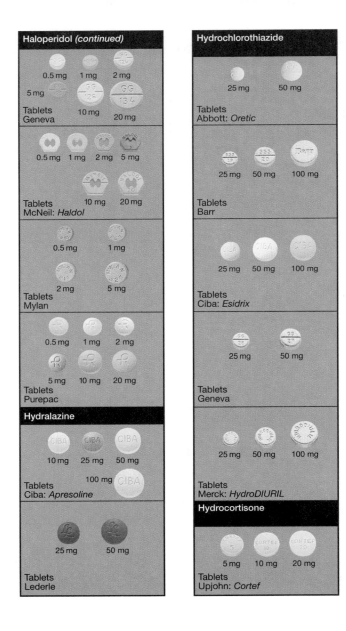

Haloperidol *(continued)*

0.5 mg 1 mg 2 mg
5 mg 10 mg 20 mg
Tablets
Geneva

0.5 mg 1 mg 2 mg 5 mg
10 mg 20 mg
Tablets
McNeil: *Haldol*

0.5 mg 1 mg
2 mg 5 mg
Tablets
Mylan

0.5 mg 1 mg 2 mg
5 mg 10 mg 20 mg
Tablets
Purepac

Hydralazine

10 mg 25 mg 50 mg
100 mg
Tablets
Ciba: *Apresoline*

25 mg 50 mg
Tablets
Lederle

Hydrochlorothiazide

25 mg 50 mg
Tablets
Abbott: *Oretic*

25 mg 50 mg 100 mg
Tablets
Barr

25 mg 50 mg 100 mg
Tablets
Ciba: *Esidrix*

25 mg 50 mg
Tablets
Geneva

25 mg 50 mg 100 mg
Tablets
Merck: *HydroDIURIL*

Hydrocortisone

5 mg 10 mg 20 mg
Tablets
Upjohn: *Cortef*

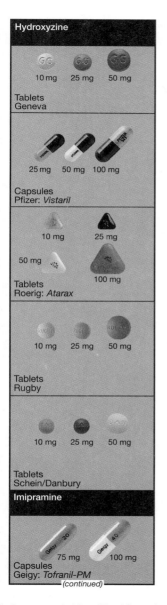

Hydroxyzine

10 mg **25 mg** **50 mg**

Tablets
Geneva

25 mg **50 mg** **100 mg**

Capsules
Pfizer: *Vistaril*

10 mg **25 mg**
50 mg **100 mg**

Tablets
Roerig: *Atarax*

10 mg **25 mg** **50 mg**

Tablets
Rugby

10 mg **25 mg** **50 mg**

Tablets
Schein/Danbury

Imipramine

75 mg **100 mg**

Capsules
Geigy: *Tofranil-PM*
(continued)

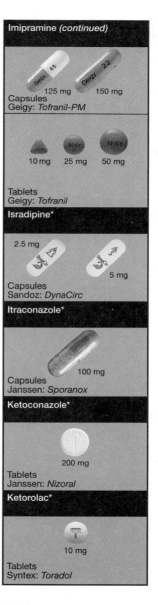

Imipramine *(continued)*

125 mg **150 mg**

Capsules
Geigy: *Tofranil-PM*

10 mg **25 mg** **50 mg**

Tablets
Geigy: *Tofranil*

Isradipine*

2.5 mg **5 mg**

Capsules
Sandoz: *DynaCirc*

Itraconazole*

100 mg

Capsules
Janssen: *Sporanox*

Ketoconazole*

200 mg

Tablets
Janssen: *Nizoral*

Ketorolac*

10 mg

Tablets
Syntex: *Toradol*

*Single source product for solid oral dosage forms in the U.S.

Labetalol

100 mg 200 mg 300 mg

Tablets
Allen & Hanburys: *Trandate*

100 mg 200 mg 300 mg

Tablets
Schering: *Normodyne*

Levonorgestrel and Ethinyl Estradiol

0.15/0.03 mg   Inert‡

‡Included only in 28-day pack

Tablets
Berlex: *Levlen 21 and 28*

0.075/0.04 mg

0.05/0.03 mg   0.125/0.03 mg

‡Included only in 28-day pack

Inert‡

Tablets
Berlex: *Tri-Levlen 21 and 28*

0.15/0.03 mg   Inert‡

‡Included only in 28-day pack

Tablets
Wyeth-Ayerst: *Nordette-21 and -28*

0.05/0.03 mg   0.075/0.04 mg

0.125/0.03 mg   Inert‡

‡Included only in 28-day pack

Tablets
Wyeth-Ayerst: *Triphasil-21 and -28*

Lisinopril

5 mg   10 mg   20 mg

40 mg

Tablets
Merck: *Prinivil*

5 mg   10 mg   20 mg

40 mg

Tablets
Stuart: *Zestril*

Lithium

150 mg

300 mg

Capsules
Roxane   600 mg

300 mg

Tablets
Roxane

300 mg

Capsules
SmithKline Beecham: *Eskalith*

450 mg

Tablets, Extended-release
SmithKline Beecham: *Eskalith CR*
(continued)

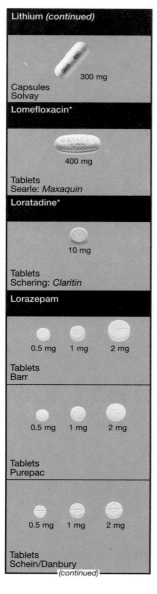

Lithium (continued)

300 mg

Capsules
Solvay

Lomefloxacin*

400 mg

Tablets
Searle: *Maxaquin*

Loratadine*

10 mg

Tablets
Schering: *Claritin*

Lorazepam

0.5 mg   1 mg   2 mg

Tablets
Barr

0.5 mg   1 mg   2 mg

Tablets
Purepac

0.5 mg   1 mg   2 mg

Tablets
Schein/Danbury

(continued)

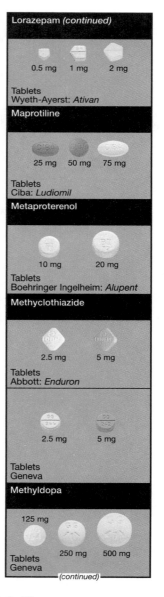

Lorazepam (continued)

0.5 mg   1 mg   2 mg

Tablets
Wyeth-Ayerst: *Ativan*

Maprotiline

25 mg   50 mg   75 mg

Tablets
Ciba: *Ludiomil*

Metaproterenol

10 mg   20 mg

Tablets
Boehringer Ingelheim: *Alupent*

Methyclothiazide

2.5 mg   5 mg

Tablets
Abbott: *Enduron*

2.5 mg   5 mg

Tablets
Geneva

Methyldopa

125 mg

250 mg   500 mg

Tablets
Geneva

(continued)

*Single source product for solid oral dosage forms in the U.S.

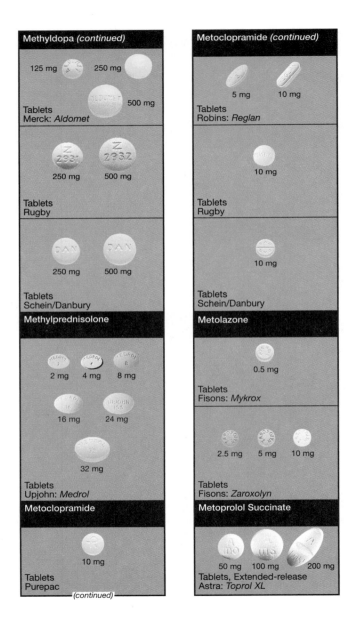

Methyldopa *(continued)*

125 mg 250 mg

500 mg

Tablets
Merck: *Aldomet*

250 mg 500 mg

Tablets
Rugby

250 mg 500 mg

Tablets
Schein/Danbury

Methylprednisolone

2 mg 4 mg 8 mg

16 mg 24 mg

32 mg

Tablets
Upjohn: *Medrol*

Metoclopramide

10 mg

Tablets
Purepac

Metoclopramide *(continued)*

5 mg 10 mg

Tablets
Robins: *Reglan*

10 mg

Tablets
Rugby

10 mg

Tablets
Schein/Danbury

Metolazone

0.5 mg

Tablets
Fisons: *Mykrox*

2.5 mg 5 mg 10 mg

Tablets
Fisons: *Zaroxolyn*

Metoprolol Succinate

50 mg 100 mg 200 mg

Tablets, Extended-release
Astra: *Toprol XL*

(continued)

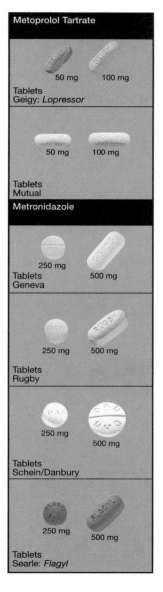

Metoprolol Tartrate

50 mg 100 mg

Tablets
Geigy: *Lopressor*

50 mg 100 mg

Tablets
Mutual

Metronidazole

250 mg 500 mg

Tablets
Geneva

250 mg 500 mg

Tablets
Rugby

250 mg 500 mg

Tablets
Schein/Danbury

250 mg 500 mg

Tablets
Searle: *Flagyl*

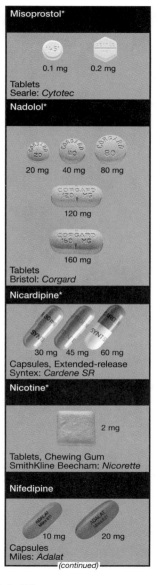

Misoprostol*

0.1 mg 0.2 mg

Tablets
Searle: *Cytotec*

Nadolol*

20 mg 40 mg 80 mg

120 mg

160 mg

Tablets
Bristol: *Corgard*

Nicardipine*

30 mg 45 mg 60 mg

Capsules, Extended-release
Syntex: *Cardene SR*

Nicotine*

2 mg

Tablets, Chewing Gum
SmithKline Beecham: *Nicorette*

Nifedipine

10 mg 20 mg

Capsules
Miles: *Adalat*

(continued)

*Single source product for solid oral dosage forms in the U.S.

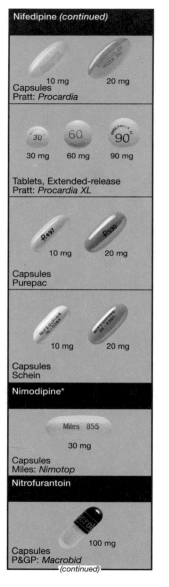

Nifedipine (continued)

10 mg   20 mg
Capsules
Pratt: *Procardia*

30 mg   60 mg   90 mg

Tablets, Extended-release
Pratt: *Procardia XL*

10 mg   20 mg
Capsules
Purepac

10 mg   20 mg
Capsules
Schein

Nimodipine*

30 mg
Capsules
Miles: *Nimotop*

Nitrofurantoin

100 mg
Capsules
P&GP: *Macrobid*
(continued)

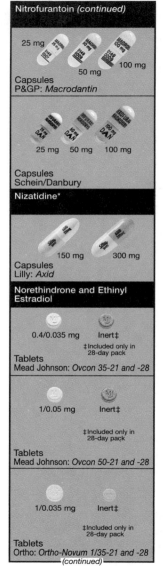

Nitrofurantoin (continued)

25 mg
50 mg   100 mg
Capsules
P&GP: *Macrodantin*

25 mg   50 mg   100 mg
Capsules
Schein/Danbury

Nizatidine*

150 mg   300 mg
Capsules
Lilly: *Axid*

Norethindrone and Ethinyl Estradiol

0.4/0.035 mg   Inert‡
‡Included only in
28-day pack
Tablets
Mead Johnson: *Ovcon 35-21 and -28*

1/0.05 mg   Inert‡
‡Included only in
28-day pack
Tablets
Mead Johnson: *Ovcon 50-21 and -28*

1/0.035 mg   Inert‡
‡Included only in
28-day pack
Tablets
Ortho: *Ortho-Novum 1/35-21 and -28*
(continued)

*Single source product for solid oral dosage forms in the U.S.

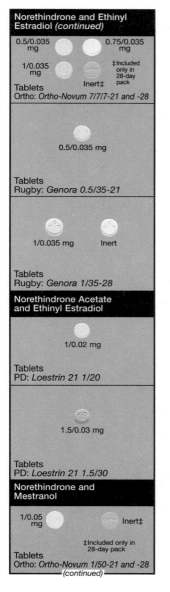

Norethindrone and Ethinyl Estradiol *(continued)*

0.5/0.035 mg   0.75/0.035 mg

1/0.035 mg   ‡Included only in 28-day pack

Inert‡

Tablets
Ortho: *Ortho-Novum 7/7/7-21 and -28*

0.5/0.035 mg

Tablets
Rugby: *Genora 0.5/35-21*

1/0.035 mg   Inert

Tablets
Rugby: *Genora 1/35-28*

Norethindrone Acetate and Ethinyl Estradiol

1/0.02 mg

Tablets
PD: *Loestrin 21 1/20*

1.5/0.03 mg

Tablets
PD: *Loestrin 21 1.5/30*

Norethindrone and Mestranol

1/0.05 mg   Inert‡

‡Included only in 28-day pack

Tablets
Ortho: *Ortho-Novum 1/50-21 and -28*
(continued)

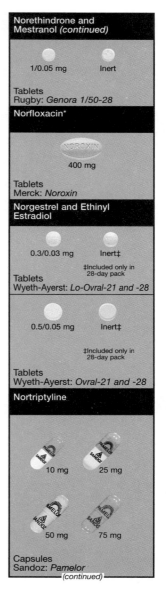

Norethindrone and Mestranol *(continued)*

1/0.05 mg   Inert

Tablets
Rugby: *Genora 1/50-28*

Norfloxacin*

NOROXIN

400 mg

Tablets
Merck: *Noroxin*

Norgestrel and Ethinyl Estradiol

0.3/0.03 mg   Inert‡

‡Included only in 28-day pack

Tablets
Wyeth-Ayerst: *Lo-Ovral-21 and -28*

0.5/0.05 mg   Inert‡

‡Included only in 28-day pack

Tablets
Wyeth-Ayerst: *Ovral-21 and -28*

Nortriptyline

10 mg   25 mg

50 mg   75 mg

Capsules
Sandoz: *Pamelor*
(continued)

*Single source product for solid oral dosage forms in the U.S.

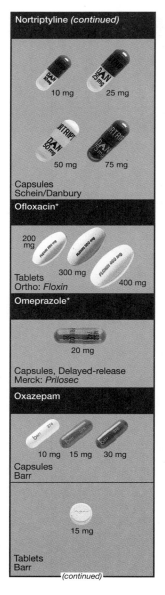

Nortriptyline (continued)

10 mg   25 mg

50 mg   75 mg

Capsules
Schein/Danbury

Ofloxacin*

200 mg   300 mg   400 mg

Tablets
Ortho: *Floxin*

Omeprazole*

20 mg

Capsules, Delayed-release
Merck: *Prilosec*

Oxazepam

10 mg   15 mg   30 mg

Capsules
Barr

15 mg

Tablets
Barr

(continued)

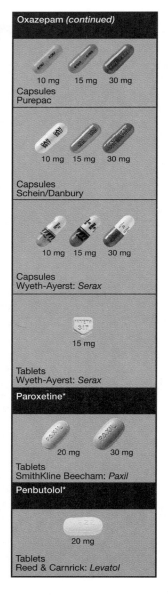

Oxazepam (continued)

10 mg   15 mg   30 mg

Capsules
Purepac

10 mg   15 mg   30 mg

Capsules
Schein/Danbury

10 mg   15 mg   30 mg

Capsules
Wyeth-Ayerst: *Serax*

15 mg

Tablets
Wyeth-Ayerst: *Serax*

Paroxetine*

20 mg   30 mg

Tablets
SmithKline Beecham: *Paxil*

Penbutolol*

20 mg

Tablets
Reed & Carnrick: *Levatol*

*Single source product for solid oral dosage forms in the U.S.

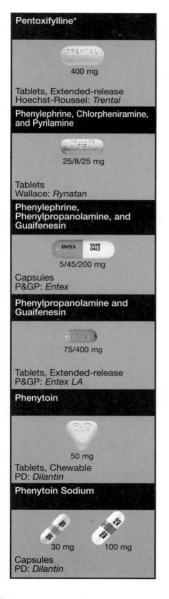

Pentoxifylline*

400 mg

Tablets, Extended-release
Hoechst-Roussel: *Trental*

Phenylephrine, Chlorpheniramine, and Pyrilamine

25/8/25 mg

Tablets
Wallace: *Rynatan*

Phenylephrine, Phenylpropanolamine, and Guaifenesin

5/45/200 mg

Capsules
P&GP: *Entex*

Phenylpropanolamine and Guaifenesin

75/400 mg

Tablets, Extended-release
P&GP: *Entex LA*

Phenytoin

50 mg

Tablets, Chewable
PD: *Dilantin*

Phenytoin Sodium

30 mg   100 mg

Capsules
PD: *Dilantin*

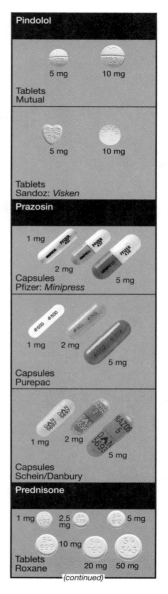

Pindolol

5 mg   10 mg

Tablets
Mutual

5 mg   10 mg

Tablets
Sandoz: *Visken*

Prazosin

1 mg
2 mg
5 mg

Capsules
Pfizer: *Minipress*

1 mg   2 mg
5 mg

Capsules
Purepac

1 mg   2 mg
5 mg

Capsules
Schein/Danbury

Prednisone

1 mg   2.5 mg   5 mg
10 mg
20 mg   50 mg

Tablets
Roxane

(continued)

*Single source product for solid oral dosage forms in the U.S.

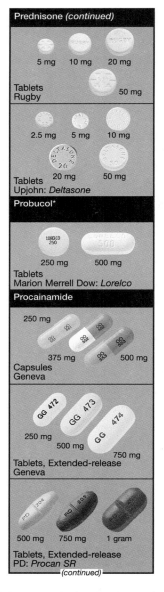

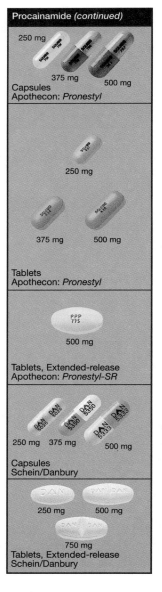

Prednisone *(continued)*

5 mg 10 mg 20 mg
50 mg
Tablets
Rugby

2.5 mg 5 mg 10 mg
20 mg 50 mg
Tablets
Upjohn: *Deltasone*

Probucol*

250 mg 500 mg
Tablets
Marion Merrell Dow: *Lorelco*

Procainamide

250 mg
375 mg 500 mg
Capsules
Geneva

GG 472 GG 473 GG 474
250 mg 500 mg 750 mg
Tablets, Extended-release
Geneva

500 mg 750 mg 1 gram
Tablets, Extended-release
PD: *Procan SR*

Procainamide *(continued)*

250 mg
375 mg 500 mg
Capsules
Apothecon: *Pronestyl*

250 mg
375 mg 500 mg
Tablets
Apothecon: *Pronestyl*

500 mg
Tablets, Extended-release
Apothecon: *Pronestyl-SR*

250 mg 375 mg 500 mg
Capsules
Schein/Danbury

250 mg 500 mg
750 mg
Tablets, Extended-release
Schein/Danbury

(continued)

*Single source product for solid oral dosage forms in the U.S.

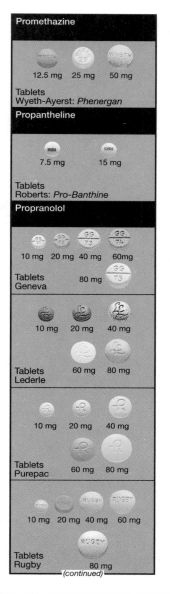

Promethazine

12.5 mg   25 mg   50 mg

Tablets
Wyeth-Ayerst: *Phenergan*

Propantheline

7.5 mg   15 mg

Tablets
Roberts: *Pro-Banthine*

Propranolol

10 mg   20 mg   40 mg   60mg

Tablets
Geneva   80 mg

10 mg   20 mg   40 mg

60 mg   80 mg

Tablets
Lederle

10 mg   20 mg   40 mg

60 mg   80 mg

Tablets
Purepac

10 mg   20 mg   40 mg   60 mg

80 mg

Tablets
Rugby
(continued)

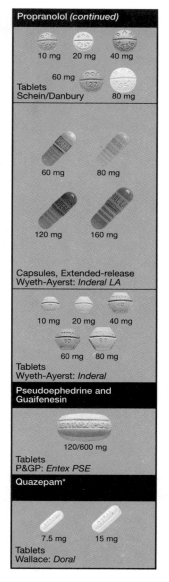

Propranolol *(continued)*

10 mg   20 mg   40 mg

60 mg   80 mg

Tablets
Schein/Danbury

60 mg   80 mg

120 mg   160 mg

Capsules, Extended-release
Wyeth-Ayerst: *Inderal LA*

10 mg   20 mg   40 mg

60 mg   80 mg

Tablets
Wyeth-Ayerst: *Inderal*

Pseudoephedrine and Guaifenesin

120/600 mg

Tablets
P&GP: *Entex PSE*

Quazepam*

7.5 mg   15 mg

Tablets
Wallace: *Doral*

*Single source product for solid oral dosage forms in the U.S.

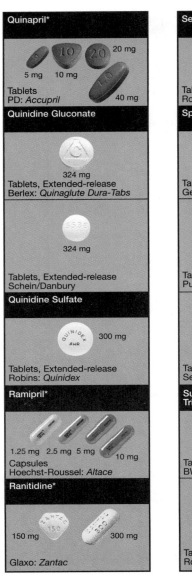

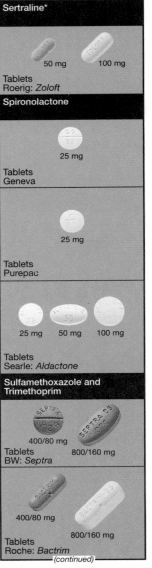

Quinapril*

5 mg 10 mg 20 mg 20 mg 40 mg

Tablets
PD: *Accupril*

Quinidine Gluconate

324 mg

Tablets, Extended-release
Berlex: *Quinaglute Dura-Tabs*

324 mg

Tablets, Extended-release
Schein/Danbury

Quinidine Sulfate

300 mg

Tablets, Extended-release
Robins: *Quinidex*

Ramipril*

1.25 mg 2.5 mg 5 mg 10 mg

Capsules
Hoechst-Roussel: *Altace*

Ranitidine*

150 mg 300 mg

Glaxo: *Zantac*

Sertraline*

50 mg 100 mg

Tablets
Roerig: *Zoloft*

Spironolactone

25 mg

Tablets
Geneva

25 mg

Tablets
Purepac

25 mg 50 mg 100 mg

Tablets
Searle: *Aldactone*

Sulfamethoxazole and Trimethoprim

400/80 mg 800/160 mg

Tablets
BW: *Septra*

400/80 mg 800/160 mg

Tablets
Roche: *Bactrim*

(continued)

*Single source product for solid oral dosage forms in the U.S.

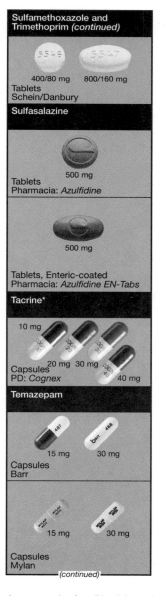

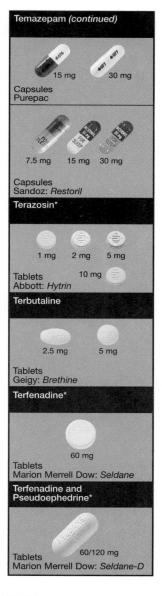

Sulfamethoxazole and Trimethoprim *(continued)*

400/80 mg   800/160 mg

Tablets
Schein/Danbury

Sulfasalazine

500 mg

Tablets
Pharmacia: *Azulfidine*

500 mg

Tablets, Enteric-coated
Pharmacia: *Azulfidine EN-Tabs*

Tacrine*

10 mg
20 mg   30 mg
40 mg

Capsules
PD: *Cognex*

Temazepam

15 mg   30 mg

Capsules
Barr

15 mg   30 mg

Capsules
Mylan

(continued)

Temazepam *(continued)*

15 mg   30 mg

Capsules
Purepac

7.5 mg   15 mg   30 mg

Capsules
Sandoz: *Restoril*

Terazosin*

1 mg   2 mg   5 mg

Tablets   10 mg
Abbott: *Hytrin*

Terbutaline

2.5 mg   5 mg

Tablets
Geigy: *Brethine*

Terfenadine*

60 mg

Tablets
Marion Merrell Dow: *Seldane*

**Terfenadine and
Pseudoephedrine***

60/120 mg

Tablets
Marion Merrell Dow: *Seldane-D*

*Single source product for solid oral dosage forms in the U.S.

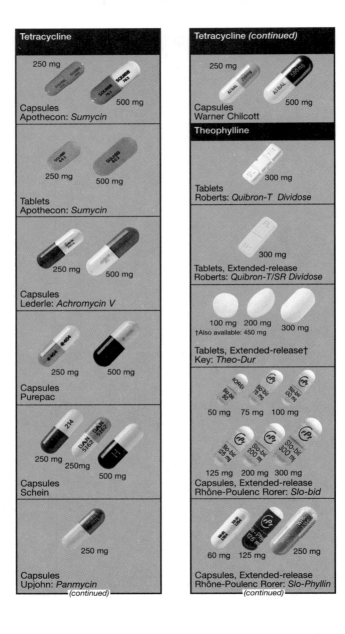

Tetracycline

250 mg
500 mg

Capsules
Apothecon: *Sumycin*

250 mg
500 mg

Tablets
Apothecon: *Sumycin*

250 mg
500 mg

Capsules
Lederle: *Achromycin V*

250 mg
500 mg

Capsules
Purepac

250 mg
250mg
500 mg

Capsules
Schein

250 mg

Capsules
Upjohn: *Panmycin*
—(continued)—

Tetracycline *(continued)*

250 mg
500 mg

Capsules
Warner Chilcott

Theophylline

300 mg

Tablets
Roberts: *Quibron-T Dividose*

300 mg

Tablets, Extended-release
Roberts: *Quibron-T/SR Dividose*

100 mg   **200 mg**   **300 mg**
†Also available: 450 mg

Tablets, Extended-release†
Key: *Theo-Dur*

50 mg   **75 mg**   **100 mg**

125 mg   **200 mg**   **300 mg**

Capsules, Extended-release
Rhône-Poulenc Rorer: *Slo-bid*

60 mg   **125 mg**   **250 mg**

Capsules, Extended-release
Rhône-Poulenc Rorer: *Slo-Phyllin*
—(continued)—

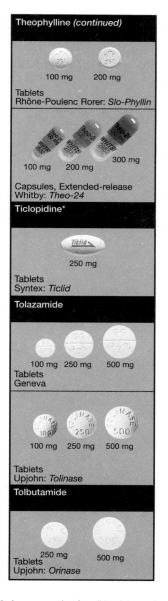

Theophylline *(continued)*

100 mg · 200 mg

Tablets
Rhône-Poulenc Rorer: *Slo-Phyllin*

100 mg · 200 mg · 300 mg

Capsules, Extended-release
Whitby: *Theo-24*

Ticlopidine*

250 mg

Tablets
Syntex: *Ticlid*

Tolazamide

100 mg · 250 mg · 500 mg

Tablets
Geneva

100 mg · 250 mg · 500 mg

Tablets
Upjohn: *Tolinase*

Tolbutamide

250 mg · 500 mg

Tablets
Upjohn: *Orinase*

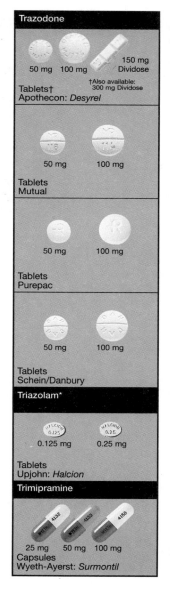

Trazodone

50 mg · 100 mg · 150 mg Dividose

†Also available:
300 mg Dividose

Tablets†
Apothecon: *Desyrel*

50 mg · 100 mg

Tablets
Mutual

50 mg · 100 mg

Tablets
Purepac

50 mg · 100 mg

Tablets
Schein/Danbury

Triazolam*

0.125 mg · 0.25 mg

Tablets
Upjohn: *Halcion*

Trimipramine

25 mg · 50 mg · 100 mg

Capsules
Wyeth-Ayerst: *Surmontil*

*Single source product for solid oral dosage forms in the U.S.

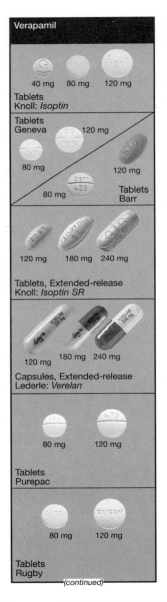

Verapamil

40 mg 80 mg 120 mg
Tablets
Knoll: *Isoptin*

Tablets
Geneva
80 mg 120 mg
80 mg 120 mg Tablets
Barr

120 mg 180 mg 240 mg

Tablets, Extended-release
Knoll: *Isoptin SR*

120 mg 180 mg 240 mg

Capsules, Extended-release
Lederle: *Verelan*

80 mg 120 mg

Tablets
Purepac

80 mg 120 mg

Tablets
Rugby

(continued)

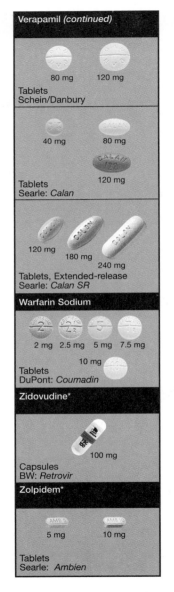

Verapamil *(continued)*

80 mg 120 mg
Tablets
Schein/Danbury

40 mg 80 mg

120 mg

Tablets
Searle: *Calan*

120 mg 180 mg 240 mg

Tablets, Extended-release
Searle: *Calan SR*

Warfarin Sodium

2 mg 2.5 mg 5 mg 7.5 mg

10 mg

Tablets
DuPont: *Coumadin*

Zidovudine*

100 mg

Capsules
BW: *Retrovir*

Zolpidem*

5 mg 10 mg

Tablets
Searle: *Ambien*

*Single source product for solid oral dosage forms in the U.S.

at evenly spaced times, day and night. For example, if you are to take 2 doses a day, the doses should be spaced about 12 hours apart. If this interferes with your sleep or other daily activities, or if you need help in planning the best times to take your medicine, check with your health care professional.

Dosing—The dose of fluoroquinolones will be different for different patients. *Follow your doctor's orders or the directions on the label.* The following information includes only the average doses of fluoroquinolones. Your dose may be different if you have kidney disease. *If your dose is different, do not change it* unless your doctor tells you to do so.

The number of tablets that you take depends on the strength of the medicine. Also, *the number of doses you take each day, the time allowed between doses, and the length of time you take the medicine depend on the medical problem for which you are using a fluoroquinolone.*

For ciprofloxacin
- For *oral* dosage form (tablets):

    —Adults: 250 to 750 milligrams (mg) every twelve hours for five to fourteen days, depending on the medical problem being treated.

    —Children up to 18 years of age: This medicine is not recommended in infants, children, or teenagers.

- For *injection* dosage form:

    —Adults: 200 to 400 mg every twelve hours.

    —Children up to 18 years of age: This medicine is not recommended in infants, children, or teenagers.

For enoxacin
- For *oral* dosage form (tablets):

    —Adults: 200 to 400 mg every twelve hours for seven to fourteen days, depending on the medical problem being treated. Gonorrhea is usually treated with a single, oral dose of 400 mg.

—Children up to 18 years of age: This medicine is not recommended in infants, children, or teenagers.

For lomefloxacin

- For *oral* dosage form (tablets):

—Adults: 400 mg once a day for ten to fourteen days, depending on the medical problem being treated.

—Children up to 18 years of age: This medicine is not recommended in infants, children, or teenagers.

For norfloxacin

- For *oral* dosage form (tablets):

—Adults: 400 mg every twelve hours for three to twenty-one days, depending on the medical problem being treated. Gonorrhea is usually treated with a single, oral dose of 800 mg.

—Children up to 18 years of age: This medicine is not recommended in infants, children, or teenagers.

For ofloxacin

- For *oral* dosage form (tablets):

—Adults: 200 to 400 mg every twelve hours for three to ten days, depending on the medical problem being treated. Gonorrhea is usually treated with a single, oral dose of 400 mg.

—Children up to 18 years of age: This medicine is not recommended in infants, children, or teenagers.

- For *injection* dosage form:

—Adults: 200 to 400 mg every twelve hours for three to ten days, depending on the medical problem being treated. Gonorrhea is usually treated with a single, oral dose of 400 mg.

—Children up to 18 years of age: This medicine is not recommended in infants, children, or teenagers.

Missed dose—If you miss a dose of this medicine, take it as soon as possible. This will help to keep a constant amount of medicine in the blood or urine. However, if it is almost time for your next dose, skip the missed dose and go back to your regular dosing schedule. Do not double doses.

Storage—To store this medicine:

- Keep out of the reach of children.
- Store away from heat and direct light.
- Do not store in the bathroom, near the kitchen sink, or in other damp places. Heat or moisture may cause the medicine to break down.
- Do not keep outdated medicine or medicine no longer needed. Be sure that any discarded medicine is out of the reach of children.

Precautions While Using This Medicine

If your symptoms do not improve within a few days, or if they become worse, check with your doctor.

If you are taking aluminum- or magnesium-containing antacids or sucralfate, do not take them at the same time that you take this medicine. It is best to take these medicines at least 2 hours before or 2 hours after taking norfloxacin or ofloxacin, at least 4 hours before or 2 hours after taking ciprofloxacin or lomefloxacin, and at least 8 hours before or 2 hours after taking enoxacin. These medicines may keep fluoroquinolones from working properly.

Some people who take fluoroquinolones may become more sensitive to sunlight than they are normally. Exposure to sunlight, even for brief periods of time, may cause severe sunburn; skin rash, redness, itching, or discoloration; or vision changes. When you begin taking this medicine:

- Stay out of direct sunlight, especially between the hours of 10:00 a.m. and 3:00 p.m., if possible.

- Wear protective clothing, including a hat and sunglasses.
- Apply a sun block product that has a skin protection factor (SPF) of at least 15. Some patients may require a product with a higher SPF number, especially if they have a fair complexion. If you have any questions about this, check with your health care professional.
- Do not use a sunlamp or tanning bed or booth.

If you have a severe reaction from the sun, check with your doctor.

Fluoroquinolones may also cause some people to become dizzy, lightheaded, drowsy, or less alert than they are normally. *Make sure you know how you react to this medicine before you drive, use machines, or do anything else that could be dangerous if you are dizzy or are not alert.* If these reactions are especially bothersome, check with your doctor.

Side Effects of This Medicine

Along with its needed effects, a medicine may cause some unwanted effects. Although not all of these side effects may occur, if they do occur they may need medical attention.

Check with your doctor immediately if any of the following side effects occur:

> *Rare*
>> Agitation; confusion; fever; hallucinations (seeing, hearing, or feeling things that are not there); pain at site of injection; peeling of the skin; shakiness or tremors; shortness of breath; skin rash, itching, or redness; swelling of face or neck

Other side effects may occur that usually do not need medical attention. These side effects may go away during

treatment as your body adjusts to the medicine. However, check with your doctor if any of the following side effects continue or are bothersome:

More common

Abdominal or stomach pain or discomfort; diarrhea; dizziness; drowsiness; headache; lightheadedness; nausea or vomiting; nervousness; trouble in sleeping

Less frequent or rare

Increased sensitivity of skin to sunlight

Other side effects not listed above may also occur in some patients. If you notice any other effects, check with your doctor.

FLUOXETINE   Systemic

A commonly used brand name in the U.S. and Canada is Prozac.

Description

Fluoxetine (floo-OX-uh-teen) is used to treat mental depression. It is also used to treat obsessive-compulsive disorder.

This medicine is available only with your doctor's prescription, in the following dosage form:

Oral

- Capsules (U.S. and Canada)
- Oral Solution (U.S. and Canada)

Before Using This Medicine

There have been recent suggestions that the use of fluoxetine may be related to increased thoughts about suicide in a very small number of patients. More study is needed to determine if the medicine caused this effect. Be sure you discuss this, and any possible precautions you should take, with your doctor before taking fluoxetine.

In deciding to use a medicine, the risks of taking the medicine must be weighed against the good it will do. This is a decision you and your doctor will make. For fluoxetine, the following should be considered:

Allergies—Tell your doctor if you have ever had any unusual or allergic reaction to fluoxetine. Also tell your health care professional if you are allergic to any other substances, such as foods, preservatives, or dyes.

Pregnancy—Studies have not been done in pregnant women. However, fluoxetine has not been shown to cause birth defects or other problems in animal studies.

Breast-feeding—Fluoxetine passes into breast milk and may cause unwanted effects, such as vomiting, watery stools, crying, and sleep problems in nursing babies. It may be necessary for you to take another medicine or to stop breast-feeding during treatment. Be sure you have discussed the risks and benefits of the medicine with your doctor.

Children—Studies on this medicine have been done only in adult patients, and there is no specific information comparing use of fluoxetine in children with use in other age groups.

Older adults—Many medicines have not been tested in older people. Therefore, it may not be known whether they work exactly the same way they do in younger adults or if they cause different side effects or problems in older people. In studies done to date that included elderly people, fluoxetine did not cause different side effects or problems in older people than it did in younger adults.

Other medicines—Although certain medicines should not be used together at all, in other cases two different medi-

cines may be used together even if an interaction might occur. In these cases, your doctor may want to change the dose, or other precautions may be necessary. When you are taking fluoxetine, it is especially important that your health care professional know if you are taking any of the following:

- Anticoagulants (blood thinners) or
- Digitalis glycosides (heart medicine)—Higher or lower blood levels of these medicines or fluoxetine may occur; your doctor may need to change the dose of either medicine
- Central nervous system (CNS) depressants (medicines that cause drowsiness)—The CNS depressant effects may be increased
- Monoamine oxidase (MAO) inhibitors (furazolidone [e.g., Furoxone], isocarboxazid [e.g., Marplan], pargyline [e.g., Eutonyl], phenelzine [e.g., Nardil], procarbazine [e.g., Matulane], tranylcypromine [e.g., Parnate])—Taking fluoxetine while you are taking or within 2 weeks of taking MAO inhibitors may cause confusion, agitation, restlessness, stomach or intestinal symptoms, sudden high body temperature, extremely high blood pressure, and severe convulsions; at least 14 days should be allowed between stopping treatment with an MAO inhibitor and starting treatment with fluoxetine; if you have been taking fluoxetine, at least 5 weeks should be allowed before starting treatment with an MAO inhibitor
- Phenytoin—Taking this medicine with fluoxetine may result in higher blood levels of phenytoin, which increases the chance of serious side effects.
- Tryptophan—Taking this medicine with fluoxetine may result in increased agitation or restlessness, and stomach or intestinal problems

Other medical problems—The presence of other medical problems may affect the use of fluoxetine. Make sure you tell your doctor if you have any other medical problems, especially:

- Diabetes—The amount of insulin or oral antidiabetic medicine that you need to take may change

- Kidney disease or
- Liver disease—Higher blood levels of fluoxetine may occur, increasing the chance of side effects
- Seizure disorders (history of)—The risk of seizures may be increased

---

Proper Use of This Medicine

Take this medicine only as directed by your doctor, to benefit your condition as much as possible. Do not take more of it, do not take it more often, and do not take it for a longer time than your doctor ordered.

If this medicine upsets your stomach, it may be taken with food.

Sometimes fluoxetine must be taken for up to 4 weeks or longer before you begin to feel better. Your doctor should check your progress at regular visits during this time.

Dosing—The dose of fluoxetine will be different for different patients. *Follow your doctor's orders or the directions on the label.* The following information includes only the average doses of fluoxetine. *If your dose is different, do not change it* unless your doctor tells you to do so:

The number of capsules or teaspoonfuls of solution that you take depends on the strength of the medicine. Also, *the number of doses you take each day, the time allowed between doses, and the length of time you take the medicine depend on the medical problem for which you are taking fluoxetine.*

- For *oral* dosage forms (capsules or solution):
    - —For depression or obsessive-compulsive disorder:
        - Adults—At first, usually 20 milligrams (mg) a day, taken as a single dose in the morning.
        - Children—Use and dose must be determined by your doctor.

Missed dose—If you miss a dose of this medicine, it is not necessary to make up the missed dose. Skip the missed dose and continue with your next scheduled dose. Do not double doses.

Storage—To store this medicine:

- Keep out of the reach of children.
- Store away from heat and direct light.
- Do not store in the bathroom, near the kitchen sink, or in other damp places. Heat or moisture may cause the medicine to break down.
- Do not keep outdated medicine or medicine no longer needed. Be sure that any discarded medicine is out of the reach of children.

Precautions While Using This Medicine

It is important that your doctor check your progress at regular visits, to allow dosage adjustments and help reduce any side effects.

This medicine will add to the effects of alcohol and other CNS depressants (medicines that slow down the nervous system, possibly causing drowsiness). Some examples of CNS depressants are antihistamines or medicine for hay fever, other allergies, or colds; sedatives, tranquilizers, or sleeping medicine; prescription pain medicine or narcotics; barbiturates; medicine for seizures; muscle relaxants; or anesthetics, including some dental anesthetics. *Check with your doctor before taking any of the above while you are using this medicine.*

If you develop a skin rash or hives, stop taking fluoxetine and check with your doctor as soon as possible.

For diabetic patients:

- This medicine may affect blood sugar levels. If you notice a change in the results of your blood or urine sugar tests or if you have any questions, check with your doctor.

This medicine may cause some people to become drowsy. *Make sure you know how you react to fluoxetine before you drive, use machines, or do anything else that could be dangerous if you are not alert.*

Dizziness, lightheadedness, or fainting may occur, especially when you get up from a lying or sitting position. Getting up slowly may help. If this problem continues or gets worse, check with your doctor.

This medicine may cause dryness of the mouth. For temporary relief, use sugarless gum or candy, melt bits of ice in your mouth, or use a saliva substitute. However, if your mouth continues to feel dry for more than 2 weeks, check with your medical doctor or dentist. Continuing dryness of the mouth may increase the chance of dental disease, including tooth decay, gum disease, and fungus infections.

Side Effects of This Medicine

Along with its needed effects, a medicine may cause some unwanted effects. Although not all of these side effects may occur, if they do occur they may need medical attention.

Check with your doctor as soon as possible if any of the following side effects occur:

Less common

Chills or fever; joint or muscle pain; skin rash, hives, or itching; trouble in breathing

Rare

Convulsions (seizures); signs of hypoglycemia (low blood sugar), including anxiety or nervousness, chills, cold sweats, confusion, cool, pale skin, difficulty in concentration, drowsiness, excessive hunger, fast heartbeat, headache, shakiness or unsteady walk, or unusual tiredness or weakness; skin rash or hives that may occur with burning or tingling in fingers, hands, or arms, chills or fever, joint or muscle pain, swelling of feet or lower legs, swollen glands, or trouble in breathing

Symptoms of overdose

Agitation and restlessness; convulsions (seizures); nausea and vomiting (severe); unusual excitement

Other side effects may occur that usually do not need medical attention. These side effects may go away during treatment as your body adjusts to the medicine. However, check with your doctor if any of the following side effects continue or are bothersome:

More common

Anxiety and nervousness; diarrhea; drowsiness; headache; increased sweating; nausea; trouble in sleeping

Less common

Abnormal dreams; change in taste; changes in vision; chest pain; constipation; cough; decreased appetite or weight loss; decreased sexual drive or ability; decrease in concentration; dizziness or lightheadedness; dryness of mouth; fast or irregular heartbeat; feeling of warmth or heat; flushing or redness of skin, especially on face and neck; frequent urination; increased appetite; menstrual pain; stomach cramps, gas, or pain; stuffy nose; tiredness or weakness; tremor; vomiting

Other side effects not listed above may also occur in some patients. If you notice any other effects, check with your doctor.

GABAPENTIN Systemic

A commonly used brand name in the U.S. and Canada is Neurontin. Another commonly used name is GBP.

Description

Gabapentin (GA-ba-pen-tin) is used to help control some types of seizures in the treatment of epilepsy. This medicine cannot cure epilepsy and will only work to control seizures for as long as you continue to take it.

Gabapentin is available only with your doctor's prescription, in the following dosage form:

Oral
- Capsules (U.S. and Canada)

Before Using This Medicine

In deciding to use a medicine, the risks of taking the medicine must be weighed against the good it will do. This is a decision you and your doctor will make. For gabapentin, the following should be considered:

Allergies—Tell your doctor if you have ever had any unusual or allergic reaction to gabapentin. Also tell your health care professional if you are allergic to any other substances, such as foods, preservatives, or dyes.

Pregnancy—Gabapentin has not been studied in pregnant women. However, studies in pregnant animals have shown that gabapentin may cause bone or kidney problems in offspring when given to the mother in doses as large as the largest human dose. Before taking this medicine, make sure your doctor knows if you are pregnant or if you may become pregnant.

Breast-feeding—It is not known whether gabapentin passes into breast milk. Although most medicines pass into breast milk in small amounts, many of them may be used safely while breast-feeding. Mothers who are taking this medicine and who wish to breast-feed should discuss this with their doctor.

Children—This medicine has not been studied in children younger than 12 years of age, and there is no specific information comparing use of gabapentin in children with use in other age groups.

Teenagers—This medicine has been tested in a small number of patients 12 to 18 years of age. In effective doses, gabapentin has not been shown to cause different side effects or problems than it does in adults.

Older adults—Gabapentin is removed from the body more slowly in elderly people than in younger people. Higher blood levels may occur, which may increase the chance of unwanted effects. Your doctor may give you a different gabapentin dose than a younger person would receive.

Other medicines—Although certain medicines should not be used together at all, in other cases two different medicines may be used together even if an interaction might occur. In these cases, your doctor may want to change the dose, or other precautions may be necessary. When you are taking gabapentin, it is especially important that your health care professional know if you are taking any of the following:

- Antacids (e.g., Maalox)—Lower blood levels of gabapentin may occur, so gabapentin may not work properly; gabapentin should be taken at least 2 hours after any antacid is taken.

Other medical problems—The presence of other medical problems may affect the use of gabapentin. Make sure you tell your doctor if you have any other medical problems, especially:

- Kidney disease—Higher blood levels of gabapentin may occur, which may increase the chance of unwanted effects; your doctor may need to change your dose

Proper Use of This Medicine

Take this medicine only as directed by your doctor, to help your condition as much as possible. Do not take more or less of it, and do not take it more or less often than your doctor ordered.

Gabapentin may be taken with or without food or on a full or empty stomach. However, if your doctor tells you to take the medicine a certain way, take it exactly as directed.

When taking gabapentin 3 times a day, do not allow more than 12 hours to pass between any 2 doses.

If you have trouble swallowing capsules, you may open the gabapentin capsule and mix the medicine with applesauce or juice. Mix only one dose at a time just before taking it. *Do not mix any doses to save for later,* because the medicine may change over time and may not work properly.

Dosing—The dose of gabapentin will be different for different patients. *Follow your doctor's orders or the directions on the label.* The following information includes only the average doses of gabapentin. *If your dose is different, do not change it* unless your doctor tells you to do so.

The number of capsules that you take depends on the strength of the medicine.

- For *oral* dosage form (capsules):
  —For epilepsy:
    - Adults and teenagers 12 years of age and older—300 milligrams (mg) at bedtime the first day, a total of 600 mg divided into two smaller doses the second day, then a total of 900 mg divided into three smaller doses each day. Your doctor may increase the dose gradually if needed. However, the dose is usually not more than 3600 mg a day.
    - Children up to 12 years of age—Use and dose must be determined by the doctor.

Missed dose—If you miss a dose of this medicine, take it as soon as possible. However, if it is less than 2 hours until your next dose, take the missed dose right away, and take the next dose 1 to 2 hours later. Then go back to your regular dosing schedule. Do not double doses.

Storage—To store this medicine:

- Keep out of the reach of children.
- Store away from heat and direct light.
- Do not store in the bathroom, near the kitchen sink, or in other damp places. Heat or moisture may cause the medicine to break down.
- Do not keep outdated medicine or medicine no longer needed. Be sure that any discarded medicine is out of the reach of children.

Precautions While Using This Medicine

It is important that your doctor check your progress at regular visits, especially for the first few months you take gabapentin. This is necessary to allow dose adjustments and to reduce any unwanted effects.

This medicine will add to the effects of alcohol and other CNS depressants (medicines that slow down the nervous system, possibly causing drowsiness). Some examples of CNS depressants are antihistamines or medicine for hay fever, other allergies, or colds; sedatives, tranquilizers, or sleeping medicine; prescription pain medicine or narcotics; barbiturates; other medicines for seizures; muscle relaxants; or anesthetics, including some dental anesthetics. *Check with your medical doctor or dentist before taking any of the above while you are taking gabapentin.*

Gabapentin may cause blurred vision, double vision, clumsiness, unsteadiness, dizziness, drowsiness, or trouble in thinking. *Make sure you know how you react to this medicine before you drive, use machines, or do anything else that could be dangerous if you are not alert, well-coordi-*

nated, or able to think or see well. If these reactions are especially bothersome, check with your doctor.

Before you have any medical tests, tell the doctor in charge that you are taking gabapentin. The results of dipstick tests for protein in the urine may be affected by this medicine.

Do not stop taking gabapentin without first checking with your doctor. Stopping the medicine suddenly may cause your seizures to return or to occur more often. Your doctor may want you to gradually reduce the amount you are taking before stopping completely.

Side Effects of This Medicine

Along with its needed effects, a medicine may cause some unwanted effects. Although not all of these side effects may occur, if they do occur they may need medical attention.

Check with your doctor as soon as possible if any of the following side effects occur:

More common

Clumsiness or unsteadiness; continuous, uncontrolled back and forth and/or rolling eye movements

Less common

Depression, irritability, or other mood or mental changes; loss of memory

Rare

Fever or chills, cough or hoarseness, lower back or side pain, painful or difficult urination

Symptoms of overdose

Double vision; severe diarrhea; severe dizziness; severe drowsiness; severe slurred speech; sluggishness

Other side effects may occur that usually do not need medical attention. These side effects may go away during

treatment as your body adjusts to the medicine. However, check with your doctor if any of the following side effects continue or are bothersome:

More common

Blurred or double vision; dizziness; drowsiness; muscle ache or pain; swelling of hands, feet, or lower legs; trembling or shaking; unusual tiredness or weakness

Less common

Diarrhea; dryness of mouth or throat; frequent urination; headache; indigestion; low blood pressure; nausea; noise in ears; runny nose; slurred speech; trouble in thinking; trouble in sleeping; vomiting; weakness or loss of strength; weight gain

Other side effects not listed above may also occur in some patients. If you notice any other effects, check with your doctor.

GRANISETRON Systemic†

A commonly used brand name in the U.S. is Kytril.

---

†Not commercially available in Canada.

Description

Granisetron (gra-NI-se-tron) is used to prevent the nausea and vomiting that may occur after treatment with anticancer medicines.

Granisetron is to be given only by or under the immediate supervision of your doctor. It is available in the following dosage form:

Parenteral

• Injection (U.S.)

Before Receiving This Medicine

In deciding to use a medicine, the risks of taking the medicine must be weighed against the good it will do. This is a decision you and your doctor will make. For granisetron, the following should be considered:

Allergies—Tell your doctor if you have ever had any unusual or allergic reaction to granisetron or ondansetron. Also tell your health care professional if you are allergic to any other substances, such as foods, preservatives, or dyes.

Pregnancy—Granisetron has not been studied in pregnant women. However, granisetron has not been shown to cause birth defects or other problems in animal studies.

Breast-feeding—It is not known whether granisetron passes into breast milk. Although most medicines pass into breast milk in small amounts, many of them may be used safely while breast-feeding. Mothers who are taking this medicine and who wish to breast-feed should discuss this with their doctor.

Children—This medicine has been tested in children 2 years of age and older and, in effective doses, has not been shown to cause different side effects or problems than it does in adults.

Older adults—This medicine has been tested in a limited number of patients 65 years of age or older and has not been shown to cause different side effects or problems in older people than it does in younger adults.

Other medicines—Although certain medicines should not be used together at all, in other cases two different medicines may be used together even if an interaction might occur. In these cases, your doctor may want to change the dose, or other precautions may be necessary. Tell your health care professional if you are taking any other prescription or nonprescription (over-the-counter [OTC]) medicine.

Other medical problems—The presence of other medical problems may affect the use of granisetron. Make sure you tell your doctor if you have any other medical problems.

Proper Use of This Medicine

Dosing—The dose of granisetron will be different for different patients. The following information includes only the average doses of granisetron.

- For *injection* dosage form:

  —For prevention of nausea and vomiting caused by anticancer medicine:

  - Adults and children 2 years of age or older—Dose is based on body weight and must be determined by your doctor. It is usually 10 micrograms (mcg) per kilogram (kg) (4.5 mcg per pound) of body weight. It is injected into a vein over a period of five minutes, beginning within thirty minutes before the anticancer medicine is given.
  - Children up to 2 years of age—Dose must be determined by your doctor.

Precautions While Receiving This Medicine

Check with your doctor if your nausea and vomiting does not stop within 10 minutes after receiving granisetron.

Side Effects of This Medicine

Along with its needed effects, a medicine may cause some unwanted effects. Although not all of these side effects

may occur, if they do occur they usually do not need medical attention. These side effects may go away during treatment as your body adjusts to the medicine. However, check with your doctor if any of the following side effects continue or are bothersome:

More common
    Headache

Less common or rare
    Constipation; diarrhea; drowsiness; unusual tiredness or
    weakness

Additional Information

Once a medicine has been approved for marketing for a certain use, experience may show that it is also useful for other medical problems. Although this use is not included in product labeling, granisetron is used in certain patients to prevent the nausea and vomiting that may occur after cancer radiation treatment in patients undergoing bone marrow transplantation.

Other than the above information, there is no additional information relating to proper use, precautions, or side effects for this use.

GUANETHIDINE   Systemic

Some commonly used brand names are:

In the U.S.—
    Ismelin
    Generic name product may also be available.

In Canada—
    Apo-Guanethidine
    Ismelin

Description

Guanethidine (gwahn-ETH-i-deen) belongs to the general class of medicines called antihypertensives. It is used to treat high blood pressure (hypertension).

High blood pressure adds to the work load of the heart and arteries. If it continues for a long time, the heart and arteries may not function properly. This can damage the blood vessels of the brain, heart, and kidneys, resulting in a stroke, heart failure, or kidney failure. High blood pressure may also increase the risk of heart attacks. These problems may be less likely to occur if blood pressure is controlled.

Guanethidine works by controlling nerve impulses along certain nerve pathways. As a result, it relaxes the blood vessels so that blood passes through them more easily. This helps to lower blood pressure.

Guanethidine is available only with your doctor's prescription, in the following dosage form:

Oral
- Tablets (U.S. and Canada)

Before Using This Medicine

In deciding to use a medicine, the risks of taking the medicine must be weighed against the good it will do. This is a decision you and your doctor will make. For guanethidine, the following should be considered:

Allergies—Tell your doctor if you have ever had any unusual or allergic reaction to guanethidine. Also tell your health care professional if you are allergic to any other substance, such as foods, preservatives, or dyes.

Pregnancy—Studies on effects in pregnancy have not been done in either humans or animals.

Breast-feeding—Small amounts of guanethidine pass into breast milk. However, this medicine has not been reported to cause problems in nursing babies.

Children—Although there is no specific information comparing use of guanethidine in children with use in other age groups, this medicine is not expected to cause different side effects or problems in children than it does in adults.

Older adults—Many medicines have not been studied specifically in older people. Therefore, it may not be known whether they work exactly the same way they do in younger adults. Although there is no specific information comparing use of guanethidine in the elderly with use in other age groups, dizziness, lightheadedness, or fainting may be more likely to occur in the elderly, who are more sensitive to the effects of guanethidine.

Other medicines—Although certain medicines should not be used together at all, in other cases two different medicines may be used together even if an interaction might occur. In these cases, your doctor may want to change the dose, or other precautions may be necessary. When you are taking guanethidine, it is especially important that your health care professional knows if you are taking any of the following:

- Antidiabetics, oral (diabetes medicine you take by mouth)—Effects may be increased by guanethidine

- Loxapine (e.g., Loxitane) or

- Thioxanthenes (chlorprothixene [e.g., Taractan], thiothixene [e.g., Navane]) or

- Tricyclic antidepressants (amitriptyline [e.g., Elavil], amoxapine [e.g., Asendin], clomipramine [e.g., Anafranil], desipramine [e.g., Pertofrane], doxepin [e.g., Sinequan], imipramine [e.g., Tofranil], nortriptyline [e.g., Aventyl], protriptyline [e.g., Vivactil], trimipramine [e.g., Surmontil]) or

- Trimeprazine (e.g., Temaril)—May decrease the effects of guanethidine on blood pressure

- Minoxidil (e.g., Loniten)—Effects on blood pressure may be greatly increased
- Monoamine oxidase (MAO) inhibitors (furazolidone [e.g., Furoxone], isocarboxazid [e.g., Marplan], phenelzine [e.g., Nardil], procarbazine [e.g., Matulane], selegiline [e.g., Eldepryl], tranylcypromine [e.g., Parnate])—Taking guanethidine while you are taking or within 2 weeks of taking MAO inhibitors may cause a severe increase in blood pressure

Other medical problems—The presence of other medical problems may affect the use of guanethidine. Make sure you tell your doctor if you have any other medical problems, especially:

- Asthma (history of) or
- Diarrhea or
- Pheochromocytoma or
- Stomach ulcer (history of)—May be worsened by guanethidine
- Diabetes mellitus (sugar diabetes)—Effects of medicine used to treat this may be increased by guanethidine
- Fever—Effects of guanethidine may be increased
- Heart or blood vessel disease or
- Heart attack or stroke (recent)—Lowering blood pressure may make problems resulting from these conditions worse
- Kidney disease—May be worsened. Also, effects of guanethidine may be increased because of slower removal of this medicine from the body
- Liver disease—Effects of guanethidine may be increased because of slower removal from the body

---

Proper Use of This Medicine

In addition to the use of the medicine your doctor has prescribed, treatment for your high blood pressure may include weight control and care in the types of foods you eat, especially foods high in sodium. Your doctor will tell you which of these are most important for you. You should check with your doctor before changing your diet.

Many patients who have high blood pressure will not notice any signs of the problem. In fact, many may feel normal. It is very important that you *take your medicine exactly as directed* and that you keep your appointments with your doctor even if you feel well.

Remember that guanethidine will not cure your high blood pressure but it does help control it. Therefore, you must continue to take it as directed if you expect to lower your blood pressure and keep it down. *You may have to take high blood pressure medicine for the rest of your life.* If high blood pressure is not treated, it can cause serious problems such as heart failure, blood vessel disease, stroke, or kidney disease.

To help you remember to take your medicine, try to get into the habit of taking it at the same time each day.

Dosing—The dose of guanethidine will be different for different patients. *Follow your doctor's orders or the directions on the label.* The following information includes only the average doses of guanethidine. *If your dose is different, do not change it* unless your doctor tells you to do so.

The number of tablets that you take depends on the strength of the medicine.

- For *oral* dosage form (tablets):

    —For high blood pressure:

    - Adults—At first, 10 or 12.5 milligrams (mg) once a day. Then, your doctor may increase your dose to 25 to 50 mg once a day.

    - Children—The dose is based on body weight. The usual dose is 200 micrograms (mcg) per kilogram (kg) (90.9 mcg per pound) of body weight a day. Then, your doctor may increase your dose as needed.

Missed dose—If you miss a dose of guanethidine, take it as soon as possible. However, if it is almost time for your next dose, skip the missed dose and go back to your regular dosing schedule. Do not double doses.

Storage—To store this medicine:

- Keep out of the reach of children.
- Store away from heat and direct light.
- Do not store in the bathroom, near the kitchen sink, or in other damp places. Heat or moisture may cause the medicine to break down.
- Do not keep outdated medicine or medicine no longer needed. Be sure that any discarded medicine is out of the reach of children.

Precautions While Using This Medicine

It is important that your doctor check your progress at regular visits to make sure that this medicine is working properly.

Dizziness, lightheadedness, or fainting may occur, especially when you get up from a lying or sitting position. This is more likely to occur in the morning. *Getting up slowly may help.* When you get up from lying down, sit on the edge of the bed with your feet dangling for 1 or 2 minutes. Then stand up slowly. If the problem continues or gets worse, check with your doctor.

The dizziness, lightheadedness, or fainting is also more likely to occur if you drink alcohol, stand for long periods of time, exercise, or if the weather is hot. *While you are taking this medicine, be careful in the amount of alcohol you drink. Also, use extra care during exercise or hot weather or if you must stand for long periods of time.*

Do not take other medicines unless they have been discussed with your doctor. This especially includes over-the-counter (nonprescription) medicines for appetite control, asthma, colds, cough, hay fever, or sinus problems, since they may tend to increase your blood pressure.

Before having any kind of surgery (including dental surgery) or emergency treatment, tell the medical doctor or dentist in charge that you are taking this medicine.

Tell your doctor if you get a fever since that may change the amount of medicine you have to take.

Side Effects of This Medicine

Along with its needed effects, a medicine may cause some unwanted effects. Although not all of these side effects may occur, if they do occur they may need medical attention.

Check with your doctor as soon as possible if any of the following side effects occur:

More common

Swelling of feet or lower legs

Less common or rare

Chest pain; shortness of breath

Other side effects may occur that usually do not need medical attention. These side effects may go away during treatment as your body adjusts to the medicine. However, check with your doctor if any of the following side effects continue or are bothersome:

More common

Diarrhea or increase in bowel movements; dizziness, lightheadedness, or fainting, especially when getting up from a lying or sitting position; sexual problems in males; slow heartbeat; stuffy nose; unusual tiredness or weakness

Less common or rare

> Blurred vision; drooping eyelids; dryness of mouth; head-
> ache; loss of hair on scalp; muscle pain or tremors;
> nausea or vomiting; nighttime urination; skin rash

Other side effects not listed above may also occur in some
patients. If you notice any other effects, check with your
doctor.

HALOPERIDOL   Systemic

Some commonly used brand names are:

In the U.S.—
Haldol
Haldol Decanoate

Generic name product may also be available.

In Canada—

Apo-Haloperidol	Novo-Peridol
Haldol	Peridol
Haldol LA	PMS Haloperidol

Generic name product may also be available.

Description

Haloperidol (ha-loe-PER-i-dole) is used to treat nervous,
mental, and emotional conditions. It is also used to control
the symptoms of Tourette's disorder. Haloperidol may also
be used for other conditions as determined by your doctor.

Haloperidol is available only with your doctor's prescription, in the following dosage forms:

Oral

- Solution (U.S. and Canada)
- Tablets (U.S. and Canada)

Parenteral

- Injection (U.S. and Canada)

Before Using This Medicine

In deciding to use a medicine, the risks of taking the medicine must be weighed against the good it will do. This is a decision you and your doctor will make. For haloperidol, the following should be considered:

Allergies—Tell your doctor if you have ever had any unusual or allergic reaction to haloperidol. Also tell your health care professional if you are allergic to any other substances, such as foods, preservatives, or dyes.

Pregnancy—Haloperidol has not been studied in pregnant women. However, studies in animals given 2 to 20 times the usual maximum human dose of haloperidol have shown reduced fertility, delayed delivery, cleft palate, and an increase in the number of stillbirths and newborn deaths.

Breast-feeding—Haloperidol passes into breast milk. Animal studies have shown that haloperidol in breast milk causes drowsiness and unusual muscle movements in the nursing offspring. Breast-feeding is not recommended during treatment with haloperidol.

Children—Side effects, especially muscle spasms of the neck and back, twisting movements of the body, trembling of fingers and hands, and inability to move the eyes are more likely to occur in children, who usually are more sensitive than adults to the effects of haloperidol.

Older adults—Constipation, dizziness or fainting, drowsiness, dryness of mouth, trembling of the hands and fingers, and symptoms of tardive dyskinesia (such as rapid, worm-like movements of the tongue or any other uncontrolled movements of the mouth, tongue, or jaw, and/or arms and legs) are especially likely to occur in elderly patients, who are usually more sensitive than younger adults to the effects of haloperidol.

Other medicines—Although certain medicines should not be used together at all, in other cases 2 different medicines may be used together even if an interaction might occur. In these cases, your doctor may want to change the dose, or other precautions may be necessary. When you are taking haloperidol, it is especially important that your health care professional know if you are taking any of the following:

- Amoxapine (e.g., Asendin) or
- Metoclopramide (e.g., Reglan) or
- Metyrosine (e.g., Demser) or
- Other antipsychotics (medicine for mental illness) or
- Pemoline (e.g., Cylert) or
- Pimozide (e.g., Orap) or_
- Promethazine (e.g., Phenergan) or
- Rauwolfia alkaloids (alseroxylon [e.g., Rauwiloid], deserpidine [e.g., Harmonyl], rauwolfia serpentina [e.g., Raudixin], reserpine [e.g., Serpasil]) or
- Trimeprazine (e.g., Temaril)—Taking these medicines with haloperidol may increase the frequency and severity of certain side effects
- Central nervous system (CNS) depressants (medicine that causes drowsiness) or
- Tricyclic antidepressants (medicine for depression)—Taking these medicines with haloperidol may result in increased CNS and other depressant effects, and in an increased chance of low blood pressure (hypotension)
- Epinephrine (e.g., Adrenalin)—Severe low blood pressure or irregular heartbeat may occur
- Levodopa (e.g., Dopar, Larodopa)—Haloperidol may interfere with the effects of this medicine
- Lithium (e.g., Eskalith, Lithane)—Although lithium and haloperidol are sometimes used together, their use must be closely monitored by your doctor, who may change the amount of medicine you need to take

Other medical problems—The presence of other medical problems may affect the use of haloperidol. Make sure you tell your doctor if you have any other medical problems, especially:

- Alcohol abuse—The risk of heat stroke may be increased
- Difficult urination or
- Glaucoma or
- Heart or blood vessel disease or
- Lung disease or
- Parkinson's disease—Haloperidol may make the condition worse
- Epilepsy—The risk of seizures may be increased
- Kidney disease or
- Liver disease—Higher blood levels of haloperidol may occur, increasing the chance of side effects
- Overactive thyroid—Serious unwanted effects may occur

Proper Use of This Medicine

If this medicine upsets your stomach, it may be taken with food or milk to lessen stomach irritation.

For patients taking the *liquid form of this medicine*:

- This medicine is to be taken by mouth even if it comes in a dropper bottle. Each dose is to be measured with the specially marked dropper provided with your prescription. Do not use other droppers since they may not deliver the correct amount of medicine.
- This medicine is best taken alone. However, if necessary, it may be mixed with water. If this is done, the mixture should be taken immediately after mixing. Haloperidol should not be taken in tea or coffee, since they cause the medicine to separate out of solution.

Take this medicine only as directed by your doctor. Do not take more of it, do not take it more often, and do not take it for a longer time than your doctor ordered. This is particularly important for children or elderly patients, since they may react very strongly to this medicine.

Continue taking this medicine for the full time of treatment. *Sometimes haloperidol must be taken for several days to several weeks before its full effect is reached.*

Dosing—The dose of haloperidol will be different for different patients. *Follow your doctor's orders or the directions on the label.* The following information includes only the average doses of haloperidol. *If your dose is different, do not change it* unless your doctor tells you to do so.

The number of tablets or teaspoonfuls of solution that you take or injections that you receive depends on the strength of the medicine. Also, *the number of doses you take each day, the time allowed between doses, and the length of time you take the medicine depend on the medical problem for which you are using haloperidol.*

- For *oral* dosage forms (solution and tablets):

—Adults and adolescents: To start, 500 micrograms to 5 milligrams two or three times a day. Your doctor may increase your dose if needed. However, the dose is usually not more than 100 milligrams a day.

—Children 3 to 12 years of age or weighing 15 to 40 kilograms (33 to 88 pounds): Dose is based on body weight. The usual dose is 25 to 150 micrograms per kilogram (11 to 68 micrograms per pound) a day, taken in smaller doses two or three times a day.

—Children up to 3 years of age: Dose must be determined by the doctor.

—Older adults: To start, 500 micrograms to 2 milligrams two or three times a day. The doctor may increase your dose if needed.

- For *short-acting injection* dosage form:

—Adults and adolescents: To start, 2 to 5 milligrams, usually injected into a muscle. The dose may be repeated every one to eight hours, depending on your condition.

—Children: Dose must be determined by the doctor.

- For *long-acting or depot injection* dosage form:

  —Adults and adolescents: To start, the dose is usually 10 to 15 times the daily oral dose you were taking, injected into a muscle once a month. The doctor may adjust how much of this medicine you need and how often you will need it, depending on your condition.

  —Children: Dose must be determined by the doctor.

Missed dose—If you miss a dose of this medicine, take it as soon as possible. Then take any remaining doses for that day at regularly spaced intervals. Do not double doses.

Storage—To store this medicine:

- Keep out of the reach of children.
- Store away from heat and direct light.
- Do not store the tablet form of this medicine in the bathroom, near the kitchen sink, or in other damp places. Heat or moisture may cause the medicine to break down.
- Keep the liquid form of this medicine from freezing.
- Do not keep outdated medicine or medicine no longer needed. Be sure that any discarded medicine is out of the reach of children.

Precautions While Using This Medicine

Your doctor should check your progress at regular visits, especially during the first few months of treatment with this medicine. The amount of haloperidol you take may be changed often to meet the needs of your condition. This also helps prevent side effects.

Do not stop taking this medicine without first checking with your doctor. Your doctor may want you to reduce gradually the amount you are taking before stopping completely. This will allow your body time to adjust and help avoid a worsening of your medical condition.

This medicine will add to the effects of alcohol and other CNS depressants (medicines that slow down the nervous system, possibly causing drowsiness). Some examples of CNS depressants are antihistamines or medicine for hay fever, other allergies, or colds; sedatives, tranquilizers, or sleeping medicine; prescription pain medicine or narcotics; barbiturates; medicine for seizures; muscle relaxants; or anesthetics, including some dental anesthetics. *Check with your doctor before taking any of the above while you are taking this medicine.*

This medicine may cause some people to become dizzy, drowsy, or less alert than they are normally, especially as the amount of medicine is increased. Even if you take haloperidol at bedtime, you may feel drowsy or less alert on arising. *Make sure you know how you react to this medicine before you drive, use machines, or do anything else that could be dangerous if you are dizzy or are not alert.*

Although not a problem for many patients, dizziness, light-headedness, or fainting may occur, especially when you get up from a lying or sitting position. Getting up slowly may help. However, if the problem continues or gets worse, check with your doctor.

This medicine will often make you sweat less, causing your body temperature to increase. *Use extra care not to become overheated during exercise or hot weather while you are taking this medicine, since overheating may result in heat stroke.* Also, hot baths or saunas may make you feel dizzy or faint while you are taking this medicine.

Before using any prescription or over-the-counter (OTC) medicine for colds or allergies, check with your doctor. These medicines may increase the chance of heat stroke or other unwanted effects, such as dizziness, dry mouth, blurred vision, and constipation, while you are taking haloperidol.

Before having any kind of surgery, dental treatment, or emergency treatment, tell the medical doctor or dentist in charge that you are using this medicine. Taking haloperidol together with medicines that are used during surgery or dental or emergency treatments may increase the CNS depressant effects.

Haloperidol may cause your skin to be more sensitive to sunlight than it is normally. Exposure to sunlight, even for brief periods of time, may cause a skin rash, itching, redness or other discoloration of the skin, or a severe sunburn. When you begin taking this medicine:

- Stay out of direct sunlight, especially between the hours of 10:00 a.m. and 3:00 p.m., if possible.
- Wear protective clothing, including a hat. Also, wear sunglasses.
- Apply a sun block product that has a skin protection factor (SPF) of at least 15. Some patients may require a product with a higher SPF number, especially if they have a fair complexion. If you have any questions about this, check with your health care professional.
- Apply a sun block lipstick that has an SPF of at least 15 to protect your lips.
- Do not use a sunlamp or tanning bed or booth.

If you have a severe reaction from the sun, check with your doctor.

Haloperidol may cause dryness of the mouth. For temporary relief, use sugarless candy or gum, melt bits of ice in your mouth, or use a saliva substitute. However, if your mouth continues to feel dry for more than 2 weeks, check with your medical doctor or dentist. Continuing dryness of the mouth may increase the chance of dental disease, including tooth decay, gum disease, and fungus infections.

If you are *receiving this medicine by injection:*

- The effects of the long-acting injection form of this

medicine may last for up to 6 weeks. *The precautions and side effects information for this medicine applies during this time.*

Side Effects of This Medicine

Along with its needed effects, haloperidol can sometimes cause serious side effects. Tardive dyskinesia (a movement disorder) may occur and may not go away after you stop using the medicine. Signs of tardive dyskinesia include fine, worm-like movements of the tongue, or other uncontrolled movements of the mouth, tongue, cheeks, jaw, or arms and legs. Other serious but rare side effects may also occur. These include severe muscle stiffness, fever, unusual tiredness or weakness, fast heartbeat, difficult breathing, increased sweating, loss of bladder control, and seizures (neuroleptic malignant syndrome). *You and your doctor should discuss the good this medicine will do as well as the risks of taking it.*

Stop taking haloperidol and get emergency help immediately if any of the following side effects occur:

Rare

Convulsions (seizures); difficult or fast breathing; fast heartbeat or irregular pulse; fever (high); high or low blood pressure; increased sweating; loss of bladder control; muscle stiffness (severe); unusually pale skin; unusual tiredness or weakness

Check with your doctor as soon as possible if any of the following side effects occur:

More common

Difficulty in speaking or swallowing; inability to move eyes; loss of balance control; mask-like face; muscle spasms, especially of the neck and back; restlessness or need to keep moving (severe); shuffling walk; stiffness of arms and legs; trembling and shaking of fingers

and hands; twisting movements of body; weakness of
arms and legs

Less common

Decreased thirst; difficulty in urination; dizziness, lightheadedness, or fainting; hallucinations (seeing or hearing things that are not there); lip smacking or
puckering; puffing of cheeks; rapid or worm-like movements of tongue; skin rash; uncontrolled chewing
movements; uncontrolled movements of arms and legs

Rare

Confusion; hot, dry skin, or lack of sweating; increased
blinking or spasms of eyelid; muscle weakness; sore
throat and fever; uncontrolled twisting movements of
neck, trunk, arms, or legs; unusual bleeding or bruising;
unusual facial expressions or body positions; yellow
eyes or skin

Symptoms of overdose

Difficulty in breathing (severe); dizziness (severe); drowsiness (severe); muscle trembling, jerking, stiffness, or
uncontrolled movements (severe); unusual tiredness or
weakness (severe)

Other side effects may occur that usually do not need
medical attention. These side effects may go away during
treatment as your body adjusts to the medicine. However,
check with your doctor if any of the following side effects
continue or are bothersome:

More common

Blurred vision; changes in menstrual period; constipation;
dryness of mouth; swelling or pain in breasts (in females); unusual secretion of milk; weight gain

Less common

Decreased sexual ability; drowsiness; increased sensitivity
of skin to sun (skin rash, itching, redness or other discoloration of skin, or severe sunburn); nausea or
vomiting

Some side effects, such as trembling of fingers and hands,
or uncontrolled movements of the mouth, tongue, and jaw,

may occur after you have stopped taking this medicine. If you notice any of these effects, check with your doctor as soon as possible.

Other side effects not listed above may also occur in some patients. If you notice any other effects, check with your doctor.

Additional Information

Once a medicine has been approved for marketing for a certain use, experience may show that it is also useful for other medical problems. Although these uses are not included in product labeling, haloperidol is used in certain patients with the following medical conditions:

- Huntington's chorea (an hereditary movement disorder)
- Infantile autism
- Nausea and vomiting caused by cancer chemotherapy

Other than the above information, there is no additional information relating to proper use, precautions, or side effects for these uses.

HEADACHE MEDICINES, ERGOT DERIVATIVE–CONTAINING   Systemic

Some commonly used brand names are:

In the U.S.—

Cafergot[3]	Ergomar[2]
Cafertine[3]	Ergostat[2]
Cafetrate[3]	Gotamine[3]
D.H.E. 45[1]	Migergot[5]
Ercaf[3]	Wigraine[3]
Ergo-Caff[3]	

In Canada—

Cafergot[3]	Dihydroergotamine-Sandoz[1]
Cafergot-PB[5]	Ergodryl[8]

In Canada (cont'd)—

Ergomar[2]

Gravergol[7]

Gynergen[2]

Medihaler Ergotamine[2]

Megral[6]

Wigraine[4]

Note: For quick reference, the following ergot derivative–containing headache medicines are numbered to match the corresponding brand names.

This information applies to the following medicines:

1. Dihydroergotamine (dye-hye-droe-er-GOT-a-meen)
2. Ergotamine (er-GOT-a-meen)
3. Ergotamine and Caffeine (kaf-EEN)‡
4. Ergotamine, Caffeine, and Belladonna Alkaloids (bell-a-DON-a AL-ka-loids)*
5. Ergotamine, Caffeine, Belladonna Alkaloids, and Pentobarbital (pen-toe-BAR-bi-tal)*
6. Ergotamine, Caffeine, and Cyclizine (SYE-kli-zeen)*
7. Ergotamine, Caffeine, and Dimenhydrinate (dye-men-HYE-dri-nate)*
8. Ergotamine, Caffeine, and Diphenhydramine (dye-fen-HYE-dra-mine)*

---

*Not commercially available in the U.S.

‡Generic name product may also be available in the U.S.

Description

Dihydroergotamine and ergotamine belong to the group of medicines known as ergot alkaloids. They are used to treat severe, throbbing headaches, such as migraine and cluster headaches. Dihydroergotamine and ergotamine are not ordinary pain relievers. They will not relieve any kind of pain other than throbbing headaches. Because these medicines can cause serious side effects, they are usually used for patients whose headaches are not relieved by acetaminophen, aspirin, or other pain relievers.

Dihydroergotamine and ergotamine may cause blood vessels in the body to constrict (become narrower). This effect can lead to serious side effects that are caused by a decrease in the flow of blood (blood circulation) to many parts of the body.

The caffeine present in many ergotamine-containing combinations helps ergotamine work better and faster by causing more of it to be quickly absorbed into the body. The belladonna alkaloids, cyclizine, dimenhydrinate, and diphenhydramine in some combinations help to relieve nausea and vomiting, which often occur together with the headaches. Cyclizine, dimenhydinate, diphenhydramine, and pentobarbital also help the patient relax and even sleep. This also helps relieve headaches.

Dihydroergotamine is also used for other conditions, as determined by your doctor.

These medicines are available only with your doctor's prescription, in the following dosage forms:

Oral

Ergotamine
  * Inhalation aerosol (Canada)
  * Sublingual tablets (U.S. and Canada)
  * Tablets (Canada)
Ergotamine and Caffeine
  * Tablets (U.S. and Canada)
Ergotamine, Caffeine, and Belladonna Alkaloids
  * Tablets (Canada)
Ergotamine, Caffeine, Belladonna Alkaloids, and Pentobarbital
  * Tablets (Canada)
Ergotamine, Caffeine, and Cyclizine
  * Tablets (Canada)
Ergotamine, Caffeine, and Dimenhydrinate
  * Capsules (Canada)
Ergotamine, Caffeine, and Diphenhydramine
  * Capsules (Canada)

Parenteral

Dihydroergotamine
  * Injection (U.S. and Canada)

Rectal

Ergotamine and Caffeine
  * Suppositories (U.S. and Canada)
Ergotamine, Caffeine, and Belladonna Alkaloids
  * Suppositories (Canada)

Ergotamine, Caffeine, Belladonna Alkaloids, and Pentobarbital
  • Suppositories (Canada)

Before Using This Medicine

In deciding to use a medicine, the risks of taking the medicine must be weighed against the good it will do. This is a decision you and your doctor will make. For these headache medicines, the following should be considered:

Allergies—Tell your doctor if you have ever had any unusual or allergic reaction to atropine, belladonna, pentobarbital or other barbiturates, caffeine, cyclizine, dimenhydrinate, diphenhydramine, or an ergot medicine. Also tell your health care professional if you are allergic to any other substances, such as foods, preservatives, or dyes.

Pregnancy—Use of dihydroergotamine or ergotamine by pregnant women may cause serious harm, including death of the fetus and miscarriage. Therefore, *these medicines should not be used during pregnancy.*

Breast-feeding—
  • *For dihydroergotamine and ergotamine:* These medicines pass into the breast milk and may cause unwanted effects, such as vomiting, diarrhea, weak pulse, changes in blood pressure, or convulsions (seizures) in nursing babies. Large amounts of these medicines may also decrease the flow of breast milk.
  • *For caffeine:* Caffeine passes into the breast milk. Large amounts of it may cause the baby to appear jittery or to have trouble in sleeping.
  • *For belladonna alkaloids, cyclizine, dimenhydrinate, and diphenhydramine:* These medicines have drying effects. Therefore, it is possible that they may reduce the amount of breast milk in some people. Dimenhy-

drinate passes into the breast milk. Cyclizine may also pass into the breast milk.

- *For pentobarbital:* Pentobarbital passes into the breast milk. Large amounts of it may cause unwanted effects such as drowsiness in nursing babies.

Be sure that you discuss these possible problems with your doctor before taking any of these medicines.

Children—

- *For dihydroergotamine and ergotamine:* These medicines are used to relieve severe, throbbing headaches in children 6 years of age or older. They have not been shown to cause different side effects or problems in children than they do in adults. However, these medicines can cause serious side effects in any patient. Therefore, it is especially important that you discuss with the child's doctor the good that this medicine may do as well as the risks of using it.

- *For belladonna alkaloids:* Young children, especially children with spastic paralysis or brain damage, may be especially sensitive to the effects of belladonna alkaloids. This may increase the chance of side effects during treatment.

- *For cyclizine, dimenhydrinate, diphenhydramine, and pentobarbital:* Although these medicines often cause drowsiness, some children become excited after taking them.

Older adults—

- *For dihydroergotamine and ergotamine:* The chance of serious side effects caused by decreases in blood flow is increased in elderly people receiving these medicines.

- *For belladonna alkaloids, cyclizine, dimenhydrinate, diphenhydramine, and pentobarbital:* Elderly people are more sensitive than younger adults to the effects of these medicines. This may increase the chance of side effects such as excitement, depression, dizziness, drowsiness, and confusion.

Other medicines—Although certain medicines should not be used together at all, in other cases two different medicines may be used together even if an interaction might occur. In these cases, your doctor may want to change the dose, or other precautions may be necessary. Many medicines can add to or decrease the effects of the belladonna alkaloids, caffeine, cyclizine, dimenhydrinate, diphenhydramine, or pentobarbital present in some of these headache medicines. Therefore, you should tell your health care professional if you are taking *any* other prescription or nonprescription (over-the-counter [OTC]) medicine. This is especially important if any medicine you take causes excitement, trouble in sleeping, dryness of the mouth, dizziness, or drowsiness.

When you are taking dihydroergotamine or ergotamine, it is especially important that your health care professional know if you are taking any of the following:

- Cocaine or
- Epinephrine by injection [e.g., Epi-Pen] or
- Other ergot medicines (ergoloid mesylates [e.g., Hydergine], ergonovine [e.g., Ergotrate], methylergonovine [e.g., Methergine], methysergide [e.g., Sansert])—The chance of serious side effects caused by dihydroergotamine or ergotamine may be increased

Other medical problems—The presence of other medical problems may affect the use of these headache medicines. Make sure you tell your doctor if you have any other medical problems, especially:

- Agoraphobia (fear of open or public places) or
- Panic attacks or
- Stomach ulcer or
- Trouble in sleeping (insomnia)—Caffeine can make your condition worse
- Diarrhea—Rectal dosage forms (suppositories) will not be effective if you have diarrhea

- Difficult urination or
- Enlarged prostate or
- Glaucoma (not well controlled) or
- Heart or blood vessel disease or
- High blood pressure (not well controlled) or
- Infection or
- Intestinal blockage or other intestinal problems or
- Itching (severe) or
- Kidney disease or
- Liver disease or
- Mental depression or
- Overactive thyroid or
- Urinary tract blockage—The chance of side effects may be increased

Also, tell your doctor if you need, or if you have recently had, an angioplasty (a procedure done to improve the flow of blood in a blocked blood vessel) or surgery on a blood vessel. The chance of serious side effects caused by dihydroergotamine or ergotamine may be increased.

Proper Use of This Medicine

Use this medicine only as directed by your doctor. Do not use more of it, and do not use it more often, than directed. If the amount you are to use does not relieve your headache, check with your doctor. Taking too much dihydroergotamine or ergotamine, or taking it too often, may cause serious effects, especially in elderly patients. Also, if a headache medicine (especially ergotamine) is used too often for migraines, it may lose its effectiveness or even cause a type of physical dependence. If this occurs, your headaches may actually get worse.

This medicine works best if you:

- *Use it at the first sign of headache or migraine attack. If you get warning signals of a coming migraine, take it before the headache actually starts.*

- *Lie down in a quiet, dark room until you are feeling better.*

Your doctor may direct you to take another medicine to help prevent headaches. *It is important that you follow your doctor's directions, even if your headaches continue to occur.* Headache-preventing medicines may take several weeks to start working. Even after they do start working, your headaches may not go away completely. However, your headaches should occur less often, and they should be less severe and easier to relieve. This can reduce the amount of dihydroergotamine, ergotamine, or pain relievers that you need. If you do not notice any improvement after several weeks of headache-preventing treatment, check with your doctor.

For patients using *dihydroergotamine:*

- Dihydroergotamine is given only by injection. Your health care professional will teach you how to inject yourself with the medicine. Be sure to follow the directions carefully. Check with your health care professional if you have any problems using the medicine.

For patients using *ergotamine inhalation* [e.g., Medihaler Ergotamine]:

- This medicine comes with patient directions. Read them carefully before using the medicine, and check with your health care professional if you have any questions.
- To use the inhaler—Remove the cap, then shake the container well. After breathing out, place the mouthpiece of the inhaler in your mouth. Aim it at the back of the throat. Breathe in; at the same time, press the vial down into the adapter. After inhaling the medicine, hold your breath as long as you can.

For patients using the *sublingual (under-the-tongue) tablets of ergotamine:*

- To use—Place the tablet under your tongue and let it remain there until it disappears. The sublingual tablet should not be chewed or swallowed, because it works faster when it is absorbed into the body through the lining of the mouth. Do not eat, drink, or smoke while the tablet is under your tongue.

For patients using *rectal suppository forms of a headache medicine:*

- If the suppository is too soft to use, chill it in the refrigerator for 30 minutes or run cold water over it before removing the foil wrapper.
- If you have been directed to use part of a suppository, you should divide the suppository into pieces that all contain the same amount of medicine. To do this, use a sharp knife and carefully cut the suppository lengthwise (from top to bottom) into pieces that are the same size. The suppository will be easier to cut if it has been kept in the refrigerator.
- To insert the suppository—First remove the foil wrapper and moisten the suppository with cold water. Lie down on your side and use your finger to push the suppository well up into the rectum.

Dosing—The dose of these headache medicines will be different for different patients. *Follow your doctor's orders or the directions on the label.* The following information includes only the average doses of these medicines. *If your dose is different, do not change it* unless your doctor tells you to do so.

For dihydroergotamine

- Adults: For relieving a migraine or cluster headache—1 mg. If your headache is not better, and no side effects are occurring, a second 1-mg dose may be used at least one hour later.
- Children 6 years of age and older: For relieving a migraine headache—It is not likely that a child will

be receiving dihydrogergotamine at home. If a child needs the medicine, the dose will have to be determined by the doctor.

For ergotamine

- Some headache medicines contain only ergotamine. Some of them contain other medicines along with the ergotamine. The number of tablets, capsules, or suppositories that you need for each dose depends on the amount of ergotamine in them. The size of each dose, and the number of doses that you take, also depend on the reason you are taking the medicine and on how you react to the medicine.

- For *oral* (capsule or tablet) and *sublingual* (under-the-tongue tablet) dosage forms:

  —Adults:

  • For relieving a migraine or cluster headache— 1 or 2 mg of ergotamine. If your headache is not better, and no side effects are occurring, a second dose and even a third dose may be taken; however, the doses should be taken at least 30 minutes apart. People who usually need more than one dose of the medicine, and who do not get side effects from it, may be able to take a larger first dose of not more than 3 mg of ergotamine. This may provide better relief of the headache with only one dose. *The medicine should not be taken more often than 2 times a week, at least five days apart.*

  • For preventing cluster headaches—The dose of ergotamine, and the number of doses you need every day, will depend on how many headaches you usually get each day. For some people, 1 or 2 mg of ergotamine once a day may be enough. Other people may need to take 1 or 2 mg of ergotamine 2 or 3 times a day.

  • For all uses—*Do not take more than 6 mg of ergotamine a day in the form of capsules or tablets.*

—Children 6 years of age and older: For relieving migraine headaches—1 mg of ergotamine. If the headache is not better, and no side effects are occurring, a second dose and even a third dose may be taken; however, the doses should be taken at least 30 minutes apart. *Children should not take more than 3 mg of ergotamine a day in the form of capsules or tablets. Also, this medicine should not be taken more often than 2 times a week, at least five days apart.*

• For *rectal suppository* dosage forms:

—Adults: For relieving migraine or cluster headaches—Usually 1 mg of ergotamine, but the dose may range from half of this amount to up to 2 mg. If your headache is not better, and no side effects are occurring, a second dose and even a third dose may be used; however, the doses should be taken at least 30 minutes apart. People who usually need more than one dose of the medicine, and who do not get side effects from it, may be able to use a larger first dose of not more than 3 mg. This may provide better relief of the headache with only one dose. *Adults should not use more than 4 mg of ergotamine a day in suppository form. Also, this medicine should not be used more often than 2 times a week, at least five days apart.*

—Children 6 years of age and older: For relieving migraine headaches—One-half or 1 mg of ergotamine. *Children should not receive more than 1 mg a day of ergotamine in suppository form. Also, this medicine should not be used more often than 2 times a week, at least five days apart.*

• For the *oral inhalation* dosage form:

—Adults: For relieving a migraine or cluster headache—1 spray (1 inhalation). Another inhalation may be used at least 5 minutes later, if needed. Up to a total of 6 inhalations a day may be used, at least 5 minutes apart. *This medicine should not be used more often than 2 times a week, at least five days apart.*

—Children: To be determined by the doctor.

Storage—To store this medicine:

- Keep out of the reach of children since overdose is especially dangerous in children.

- Store away from heat and direct light.

- Do not store in the bathroom, near the kitchen sink, or in other damp places. Heat or moisture may cause the medicine to break down.

- Suppositories should be stored in a cool place, but not allowed to freeze. Some manufacturers recommend keeping them in a refrigerator; others do not. Follow the directions on the package. However, cutting the suppository into smaller pieces, if you need to do so, will be easier if the suppository is kept in the refrigerator.

- Do not puncture, break, or burn the ergotamine inhalation aerosol container, even after it is empty.

- Do not keep outdated medicine or medicine no longer needed. Be sure that any discarded medicine is out of the reach of children.

Precautions While Using This Medicine

Check with your doctor:

- If your migraine headaches are worse than they were before you started using this medicine, or your headache medicine stops working as well as it did when you first started using it. This may mean that you are in danger of becoming dependent on the headache medicine. *Do not try to get better relief by increasing the dose.*

- If your migraine headaches are occurring more often than they did before you started using this medicine. This is especially important if a new headache occurs within 1 day after you took your last dose of headache medicine, or if you are having headaches every day. This may mean that you are dependent on the headache medicine. *Continuing to take this medicine will cause even more headaches later on.* Your doctor can give you advice on how to relieve the headaches.

Drinking alcoholic beverages can make headaches worse or cause new headaches to occur. People who suffer from severe headaches should probably avoid alcoholic beverages, especially during a headache.

Smoking may increase some of the harmful effects of dihydroergotamine or ergotamine. It is best to avoid smoking for several hours after taking these medicines.

Dihydroergotamine and ergotamine may make you more sensitive to cold temperatures, especially if you have blood circulation problems. They tend to decrease blood flow in the skin, fingers, and toes. Dress warmly during cold weather and be careful during prolonged exposure to cold temperatures. This is especially important for older patients, who are more likely than younger adults to already have problems with their circulation.

If you have a serious infection or illness of any kind, check with your doctor before using this medicine, since you may be more sensitive to its effects.

For patients using *ergotamine inhalation* [e.g., Medihaler Ergotamine]:

- Cough, hoarseness, or throat irritation may occur. Gargling and rinsing your mouth after each dose may help prevent the hoarseness and irritation. However, check with your doctor if these or any other side effects continue or are bothersome.

For patients taking one of the combination medicines that contains *caffeine:*

- Caffeine may interfere with the results of a test that uses dipyridamole (e.g., Persantine) to help find out how well your blood is flowing through certain blood vessels. You should not have any caffeine for at least 12 hours before the test.

- Caffeine may also interfere with some other laboratory tests. Before having any other laboratory tests, tell the person in charge if you have taken a medicine that contains caffeine.

For patients taking one of the combination medicines that contains *belladonna alkaloids, cyclizine, dimenhydrinate, diphenhydramine, or pentobarbital:*

- These medicines may cause some people to have blurred vision or to become drowsy, dizzy, lightheaded, or less alert than they are normally. These effects may be especially severe if you also take CNS depressants (medicines that slow down the nervous system, possibly causing drowsiness) together with one of these combination medicines. Some examples of CNS depressants are antihistamines or medicine for hay fever, other allergies, or colds; sedatives, tranquilizers, or sleeping medicine; prescription pain medicine or narcotics; barbiturates; medicine for seizures; muscle relaxants; and antiemetics (medicines that prevent or relieve nausea or vomiting). If you are not able to lie down for a while, *make sure you know how you react to this medicine or combination of medicines before you drive, use machines, or do anything else that could be dangerous if you are dizzy or are not alert and able to see well.*

- Belladonna alkaloids, cyclizine, dimenhydrinate, and diphenhydramine may cause dryness of the mouth, nose, and throat. For temporary relief of mouth dryness, use sugarless candy or gum, melt bits of ice in your mouth, or use a saliva substitute.

- Belladonna alkaloids may interfere with certain laboratory tests that check the amount of acid in your stomach. They should not be taken for 24 hours before the test.

- Cyclizine, dimenhydrinate, and diphenhydramine may interfere with skin tests that show whether you are allergic to certain substances. They should not be taken for 3 days before the test.

Side Effects of This Medicine

Along with its needed effects, a medicine may cause some unwanted effects. Although not all of these side effects may occur, if they do occur they may need medical attention.

Check with your doctor immediately if the following side effects occur, because they may mean that you are developing a problem with blood circulation:

Less common or rare

Anxiety or confusion (severe); change in vision; chest pain; increase in blood pressure; pain in arms, legs, or lower back, especially if pain occurs in your calves or heels while you are walking; pale, bluish-colored, or cold hands or feet (not caused by cold temperatures and occurring together with other side effects listed in this section); red or violet-colored blisters on the skin of the hands or feet

Also check with your doctor immediately if any of the following side effects occur, because they may mean that you have taken an overdose of the medicine:

Less common or rare

Convulsions (seizures); diarrhea, nausea, vomiting, or stomach pain or bloating (severe) occurring together with other signs of overdose or of problems with blood circulation; dizziness, drowsiness, or weakness (severe), occurring together with other signs of overdose or of problems with blood circulation; fast or slow heartbeat; diarrhea; headaches more often and/or more severe than before; problems with moving bowels, occurring together with pain or discomfort in the rectum (with rectal suppositories only); shortness of breath; unusual excitement

The following side effects may go away after a little while. *Do not take any more medicine while they are present.* If any of them occur together with other signs of problems with blood circulation, *check with your doctor right away.* Even if any of the following side effects occur without other signs of problems with blood circulation, *check with your doctor if any of them continue for more than one hour:*

More common

Itching of skin; coldness, numbness, or tingling in fingers, toes, or face; weakness in legs

Also, check with your doctor as soon as possible if you notice any of the following side effects:

More common

Swelling of face, fingers, feet, or lower legs

Other side effects may occur that usually do not need medical attention. These side effects may go away after a little while. However, check with your doctor if any of the following side effects continue or are bothersome:

More common

Diarrhea, nausea, or vomiting (occurring without other signs of overdose or problems with blood circulation); dizziness or drowsiness (occurring without other signs of overdose or problems with blood circulation, especially with combinations containing cyclizine, dimenhydrinate, diphenhydramine, or pentobarbital); nervousness or restlessness; dryness of mouth (especially with combi-

      nations containing belladonna alkaloids, cyclizine, di-
      menhydrinate, or diphenhydramine)

After you stop taking this medicine, your body may need
time to adjust. The length of time this takes depends on
the amount of medicine you were taking and how long
you took it. During this time check with your doctor if
your headaches begin again or worsen.

Other side effects not listed above may also occur in some
patients. If you notice any other effects, check with your
doctor.

Additional Information

Once a medicine has been approved for marketing for a
certain use, experience may show that it is also useful for
other medical problems. Although this use is not specifically included in product labeling, dihydroergotamine is
sometimes used together with another medicine (heparin)
to help prevent blood clots that may occur after certain
kinds of surgery. It is also used to prevent or treat low
blood pressure in some patients.

For patients receiving this medicine for *preventing blood
clots:*

- You may need to receive this medicine two or three
  times a day for several days in a row. This may
  increase the chance of problems caused by decreased
  blood flow. Your health care professional will be following your progress, to make sure that this medicine
  is not causing problems with blood circulation.

For patients using this medicine to *prevent or treat low
blood pressure:*

- Take this medicine every day as directed by your
  doctor.
- The dose of dihydroergotamine will depend on
  whether the medicine is going to be injected under

the skin or into a muscle, and, sometimes, on the weight of the patient. For these reasons, the dose will have to be determined by your doctor.

- Your doctor will need to check your progress at regular visits, to make sure that the medicine is working properly without causing side effects.

- This medicine is less likely to cause problems with blood circulation in patients with low blood pressure than it is in patients with normal or high blood pressure.

- In patients being treated for low blood pressure, an increase in blood pressure is the wanted effect, not a side effect that may need medical attention.

Other than the above information, there is no additional information relating to proper use, precautions, or side effects for these uses.

HISTAMINE H$_2$-RECEPTOR ANTAGONISTS   Systemic

Some commonly used brand names are:

In the U.S.—

Axid[3]   Tagamet[1]
Pepcid[2]   Zantac[4]
Pepcid I.V.[2]

In Canada—

Apo-Cimetidine[1]   Pepcid I.V.[2]
Apo-Ranitidine[4]   Peptol[1]
Axid[3]   Tagamet[1]
Novocimetine[1]   Zantac[4]
Pepcid[2]   Zantac-C[4]

Note: For quick reference, the following histamine H$_2$-receptor antagonists are numbered to match the corresponding brand names.

This information applies to the following medicines:

1. Cimetidine (sye-MET-i-deen)§
2. Famotidine (fa-MOE-ti-deen)

3. Nizatidine (ni-ZA-ti-deen)
4. Ranitidine (ra-NIT-ti-deen)

§Generic name product may also be available in Canada.

Description

Histamine H₂-receptor antagonists, also known as H₂-blockers, are used to treat duodenal ulcers and prevent their return. They are also used to treat gastric ulcers and in some conditions, such as Zollinger-Ellison disease, in which the stomach produces too much acid. H₂-blockers may also be used for other conditions as determined by your doctor.

H₂-blockers work by decreasing the amount of acid produced by the stomach.

They are available only with your doctor's prescription, in the following dosage forms:

Oral

Cimetidine
- Oral solution (U.S. and Canada)
- Tablets (U.S. and Canada)

Famotidine
- Oral suspension (U.S.)
- Tablets (U.S. and Canada)

Nizatidine
- Capsules (U.S. and Canada)

Ranitidine
- Capsules (U.S. and Canada)
- Syrup (U.S. and Canada)
- Tablets (U.S. and Canada)

Parenteral

Cimetidine
- Injection (U.S. and Canada)

Famotidine
- Injection (U.S. and Canada)

Ranitidine
- Injection (U.S. and Canada)

Before Using This Medicine

In deciding to use a medicine, the risks of taking the medicine must be weighed against the good it will do. This is a decision you and your doctor will make. For H_2-blockers, the following should be considered:

Allergies—Tell your doctor if you have ever had any unusual or allergic reaction to cimetidine, famotidine, nizatidine, or ranitidine.

Pregnancy—H_2-blockers have not been studied in pregnant women. In animal studies, famotidine and ranitidine have not been shown to cause birth defects or other problems. However, one study in rats suggested that cimetidine may affect male sexual development. More studies are needed to confirm this. Also, studies in rabbits with very high doses have shown that nizatidine causes miscarriages and low birth weights. Make sure your doctor knows if you are pregnant or if you may become pregnant before taking H_2-blockers.

Breast-feeding—Cimetidine, famotidine, nizatidine, and ranitidine pass into the breast milk and may cause unwanted effects, such as decreased amount of stomach acid and increased excitement, in the nursing baby. It may be necessary for you to take another medicine or to stop breast-feeding during treatment. Be sure you have discussed the risks and benefits of the medicine with your doctor.

Children—This medicine has been tested in children and, in effective doses, has not been shown to cause different side effects or problems than it does in adults when used for short periods of time.

Older adults—Confusion and dizziness may be especially likely to occur in elderly patients, who are usually more sensitive than younger adults to the effects of H_2-blockers.

Other medicines—Although certain medicines should not be used together at all, in other cases two different medicines may be used together even if an interaction might occur. In these cases, your doctor may want to change the dose, or other precautions may be necessary. When you are taking or receiving H₂-blockers it is especially important that your health care professional know if you are taking any of the following:

- Aminophylline (e.g., Somophyllin) or
- Anticoagulants (blood thinners) or
- Caffeine (e.g., NoDoz) or
- Metoprolol (e.g., Lopressor) or
- Oxtriphylline (e.g., Choledyl) or
- Phenytoin (e.g., Dilantin) or
- Propranolol (e.g., Inderal) or
- Theophylline (e.g., Somophyllin-T) or
- Tricyclic antidepressants (amitriptyline [e.g., Elavil], amoxapine [e.g., Asendin], clomipramine [e.g., Anafranil], desipramine [e.g., Pertofrane], doxepin [e.g., Sinequan], imipramine [e.g., Tofranil], nortriptyline [e.g., Aventyl], protriptyline [e.g., Vivactil], trimipramine [e.g., Surmontil])— Use of these medicines with cimetidine has been shown to increase the effects of cimetidine. This is less of a problem with ranitidine and has not been reported for famotidine or nizatidine. However, all of the H₂-blockers are similar, so drug interactions may occur with any of them
- Ketoconazole—H₂-blockers may decrease the effects of ketoconazole; H₂-blockers should be taken at least 2 hours after ketoconazole

Other medical problems—The presence of other medical problems may affect the use of H₂-blockers. Make sure you tell your doctor if you have any other medical problems, especially:

- Kidney disease or
- Liver disease—The H₂-blocker may build up in the bloodstream, which may increase the risk of side effects

---

Proper Use of This Medicine

For patients taking:

- One dose a day—Take it at bedtime, unless otherwise directed.

- Two doses a day—Take one in the morning and one at bedtime.
- Several doses a day—Take them with meals and at bedtime for best results.

It may take several days before this medicine begins to relieve stomach pain. To help relieve this pain, antacids may be taken with the H$_2$-blocker, unless your doctor has told you not to use them. However, you should wait one-half to one hour between taking the antacid and the H$_2$-blocker.

Take this medicine for the full time of treatment, even if you begin to feel better. Also, it is important that you keep your appointments with your doctor for check-ups so that your doctor will be better able to tell you when to stop taking this medicine.

Dosing—The dose of histamine H$_2$-receptor antagonists (also called H$_2$-blockers) will be different for different patients. *Follow your doctor's orders or the directions on the label.* The following information includes only the average doses of these medicines. *If your dose is different, do not change it unless your doctor tells you to do so.*

The number of capsules or tablets or teaspoonfuls of solution, suspension, or syrup that you take depends on the strength of the medicine. Also, the number of doses you take each day, the time allowed between doses, and the length of time you take the medicine depend on the medical problem for which you are taking the H$_2$-receptor antagonist.

For cimetidine

- For *oral* dosage forms (solution and tablets):

  —To treat duodenal or gastric ulcers:

  - Older adults, adults, and teenagers—300 milligrams (mg) four times a day, with meals and at bedtime. Some people may take 400 or 600 mg

two times a day, on waking up and at bedtime. Others may take 800 mg at bedtime.
• Children—20 to 40 mg per kilogram (kg) (9.1 to 18.2 mg per pound) of body weight a day, divided into four doses, taken with meals and at bedtime.

—To prevent duodenal ulcers:

• Older adults, adults, and teenagers—300 mg two times a day, on waking up and at bedtime. Instead some people may take 400 mg at bedtime.
• Children—Dose must be determined by your doctor.

—To treat conditions in which the stomach produces too much acid:

• Adults—300 mg four times a day, with meals and at bedtime. Your doctor may change the dose if needed.
• Children—Dose must be determined by your doctor.

—To treat gastroesophageal reflux disease:

• Adults—800 to 1600 mg a day, divided into smaller doses. Treatment usually lasts for 12 weeks.
• Children—Dose must be determined by your doctor.

• For *injectable* dosage form:

—To treat duodenal ulcers, gastric ulcers or conditions in which the stomach produces too much acid:

• Older adults, adults, and teenagers—300 mg injected into muscle, every six to eight hours. Or, 300 mg injected slowly into a vein every six to eight hours. Instead, 900 mg may be injected slowly into a vein around the clock at the rate of 37.5 mg per hour. Some people may need 150 mg at first, before beginning the around-the-clock treatment.

• Children—5 to 10 mg per kg (2.3 to 4.5 mg per pound) of body weight injected into a vein or muscle, every six to eight hours. Or, 5 to 10 mg per kg (2.3 to 4.6 mg per pound) of body weight injected slowly into a vein every six to eight hours.

—To prevent stress-related bleeding:

• Older adults, adults, and teenagers—50 mg per hour injected slowly around the clock for up to 7 days.

• Children—Dose must be determined by your doctor.

For famotidine

• For *oral* dosage forms (solution and tablets):

—To treat duodenal ulcers:

Older adults, adults, and teenagers—40 milligrams (mg) once a day at bedtime. Some people may take 20 mg two times a day.

• Children—Dose must be determined by your doctor.

—To prevent duodenal ulcers:

• Older adults, adults, and teenagers—20 mg once a day at bedtime.

• Children—Dose must be determined by your doctor.

—To treat gastric ulcers:

• Older adults, adults, and teenagers—40 mg once a day at bedtime.

• Children—Dose must be determined by your doctor.

—To treat conditions in which the stomach produces too much acid:

• Older adults, adults, and children—20 mg every six hours. Your doctor may change the dose if needed.

• Children—Dose must be determined by your doctor.

—To treat gastroesophageal reflux disease:

• Older adults, adults, and teenagers—20 mg two times a day, usually for up to 6 weeks.

• Children weighing more than 10 kg (4.5 pounds): 1 to 2 mg per kilogram (kg) (0.5 to 0.9 mg per pound) of body weight a day divided into two doses.

• Children weighing less than 10 kg (4.5 pounds): 1 to 2 mg per kg (0.5 to 0.9 mg per pound) of body weight a day, divided into three doses.

• For *injectable* dosage form:

—To treat duodenal ulcers, gastric ulcers, or conditions in which the stomach produces too much acid:

• Older adults, adults, and teenagers—20 mg injected into a vein, every twelve hours. Or, 20 mg injected slowly into a vein every twelve hours.

• Children—Dose must be determined by your doctor.

For nizatidine

• For *oral* dosage form (capsules):

—To treat duodenal or gastric ulcers:

• Older adults, adults, and teenagers—300 milligrams (mg) once a day at bedtime. Some people may take 150 mg two times a day.

• Children—Dose must be determined by your doctor.

—To prevent duodenal ulcers:

• Adults and teenagers—150 mg once a day at bedtime.

• Children—Dose must be determined by your doctor.

—To treat gastroesophageal reflux disease:

• Adults and teenagers—150 mg two times a day.

• Children—Dose must be determined by your doctor.

For ranitidine

- For *oral* dosage form (capsules, syrup, or tablets):

    —To treat duodenal ulcers:

    - Older adults, adults, teenagers—150 milligrams (mg) two times a day. Some people may take 300 mg once a day at bedtime.
    - Children—2 to 4 mg per kilogram (kg) (1 to 2 mg per pound) of body weight two times a day. However, your dose will not be more than 300 mg a day.

    —To prevent duodenal ulcers:

    - Older adults, adults, teenagers—150 mg at bedtime.
    - Children—Dose must be detemined by your doctor.

    —To treat gastric ulcers:

    - Older adults, adults, teenagers—150 mg two times a day.
    - Children—2 to 4 mg per kg (1 to 2 mg per pound) of body weight two times a day. However, your dose will not be more than 300 mg a day.

    —To treat some conditions in which the stomach produces too much acid:

    - Older adults, adults, teenagers—150 mg two times a day. Your doctor may change the dose if needed.
    - Children—Dose must be determined by your doctor.

    —To treat gastroesophageal reflux disease:

    - Older adults, adults, and teenagers—150 mg two times a day. Your dose may be increased if needed.
    - Children—2 to 8 mg per kg (1 to 3.6 mg per pound) of body weight a day, three times a day. However, most children will usually take not more than 300 mg a day.

- For *injectable* dosage form:
  - —To treat duodenal ulcers, gastric ulcers, or conditions in which the stomach produces too much acid:
    - Older adults, adults, and teenagers—50 mg injected into a muscle every six to eight hours. Or, 50 mg injected slowly into a vein every six to eight hours. Instead, you may receive 6.25 mg per hour injected slowly around the clock. However, most people will usually not need more than 400 mg a day.
  - —To treat duodenal or gastric ulcers:
    - Children—2 to 4 mg per kg (1 to 2 mg per pound) of body weight a day, injected slowly into a vein.

Missed dose—If you miss a dose of this medicine, take it as soon as possible. However, if it is almost time for your next dose, skip the missed dose and go back to your regular dosing schedule. Do not double doses.

Storage—To store this medicine:
- Keep out of the reach of children.
- Store away from heat and direct light.
- Do not store the tablet form of this medicine in the bathroom, near the kitchen sink, or in other damp places. Heat or moisture may cause the medicine to break down.
- Keep the liquid form of this medicine from freezing.
- Do not keep outdated medicine or medicine no longer needed. Be sure that any discarded medicine is out of the reach of children.

Precautions While Using This Medicine

Some tests may be affected by this medicine. Tell the doctor in charge that you are taking this medicine before:

- You have any skin tests for allergies.
- You have any tests to determine how much acid your stomach produces.

Remember that certain medicines, such as aspirin, and certain foods and drinks (e.g., citrus products, carbonated drinks, etc.) irritate the stomach and may make your problem worse.

Cigarette smoking tends to decrease the effect of H$_2$-blockers by increasing the amount of acid produced by the stomach. This is more likely to affect the stomach's nighttime production of acid. While taking H$_2$-blockers, stop smoking completely, or at least do not smoke after taking the last dose of the day.

Drinking alcoholic beverages while taking an H$_2$-receptor antagonist has been reported to increase the blood levels of alcohol. You should consult your health care professional for guidance.

Check with your doctor if your ulcer pain continues or gets worse.

Side Effects of This Medicine

Along with its needed effects, a medicine may cause some unwanted effects. Although not all of these side effects may occur, if they do occur they may need medical attention.

Check with your doctor as soon as possible if any of the following side effects occur:

Rare

> Burning, itching, redness, skin rash; confusion; fast, pounding, or irregular heartbeat; fever; slow heartbeat; sore throat and fever; swelling; tightness in chest; unusual bleeding or bruising; unusual tiredness or weakness

Other side effects may occur that usually do not need medical attention. These side effects may go away during treatment as your body adjusts to the medicine. However, check with your doctor if any of the following side effects continue or are bothersome:

Less common or rare

Blurred vision; constipation; decreased sexual ability (especially in patients with Zollinger-Ellison disease who have received high doses of cimetidine for at least 1 year); decrease in sexual desire; diarrhea; dizziness; drowsiness; dryness of mouth or skin; headache; increased sweating; joint or muscle pain; loss of appetite; loss of hair (temporary); nausea or vomiting; ringing or buzzing in ears; skin rash; swelling of breasts or breast soreness in females and males

Not all of the side effects listed above have been reported for each of these medicines, but they have been reported for at least one of them. All of the H$_2$-blockers are similar, so any of the above side effects may occur with any of these medicines.

Other side effects not listed above may also occur in some patients. If you notice any other effects, check with your doctor.

Additional Information

Once a medicine has been approved for marketing for a certain use, experience may show that it is also useful for other medical problems. Although these uses are not included in product labeling, H$_2$-blockers are used in certain patients with the following medical conditions:

- Damage to the stomach and/or intestines due to stress or trauma
- Hives
- Pancreatic problems

- Stomach or intestinal ulcers (sores) resulting from damage caused by medication used to treat rheumatoid arthritis

Other than the above information, there is no additional information relating to proper use, precautions, or side effects for these uses.

HMG-CoA REDUCTASE INHIBITORS   Systemic

Some commonly used brand names are:

In the U.S.—

Lescol[1]   Pravachol[3]

Mevacor[2]   Zocor[4]

In Canada—

Mevacor[2]   Zocor[4]

Pravachol[3]

Other commonly used names are:

Epistatin[4]   Mevinolin[2]

Eptastatin[3]   Synvinolin[4]

Note: For quick reference, the following HMG-CoA reductase inhibitors are numbered to match the corresponding brand names.

This information applies to the following medicines:

1. Fluvastatin (FLOO-va-sta-tin)†
2. Lovastatin (LOE-va-sta-tin)
3. Pravastatin (PRA-va-stat-in)
4. Simvastatin (SIM-va-stat-in)

---

†Not commercially available in Canada.

Description

Fluvastatin, lovastatin, pravastatin, and simvastatin are used to lower levels of cholesterol and other fats in the blood. This may help prevent medical problems caused by cholesterol clogging the blood vessels.

These medicines belong to the group of medicines called 3-hydroxy-3-methylglutaryl coenzyme A (HMG-CoA) reductase inhibitors. They work by blocking an enzyme that is needed by the body to make cholesterol. Thus, less cholesterol is made.

HMG-CoA reductase inhibitors are available only with your doctor's prescription, in the following dosage forms:

Oral

Fluvastatin
- Capsules (U.S.)

Lovastatin
- Tablets (U.S. and Canada)

Pravastatin
- Tablets (U.S. and Canada)

Simvastatin
- Tablets (U.S and Canada)

Before Using This Medicine

In deciding to use a medicine, the risks of taking the medicine must be weighed against the good it will do. This is a decision you and your doctor will make. For HMG-CoA reductase inhibitors, the following should be considered:

Allergies—Tell your doctor if you have ever had any unusual or allergic reaction to HMG-CoA reductase inhibitors. Also tell your health care professional if you are allergic to any other substances, such as foods, preservatives, or dyes.

Diet—Before prescribing medicines to lower your cholesterol, your doctor will probably try to control your condition by prescribing a personal diet for you. Such a diet will be lower in total fat, particularly saturated fat, and dietary cholesterol. Many people are able to control their condition by carefully following their doctor's orders for proper diet and exercise. *Medicine is prescribed only when* *additional help is needed* and is effective only when a schedule of diet and exercise is properly followed.

Also, this medicine is less effective if you are greatly overweight. It may be very important for you to go on a reducing diet. However, check with your doctor before going on any diet.

Pregnancy—HMG-CoA reductase inhibitors should not be used during pregnancy or by women who plan to become pregnant in the near future. These medicines block formation of cholesterol, which is necessary for the fetus to develop properly. HMG-CoA reductase inhibitors may cause birth defects or other problems in the baby if taken during pregnancy. An effective form of birth control should be used during treatment with these medicines. *Check with your doctor immediately if you think you have become pregnant while taking this medicine.* Be sure you have discussed this with your doctor.

Breast-feeding—These medicines are not recommended for use during breast-feeding because they may cause unwanted effects in nursing babies.

Children—Studies on this medicine have been done only in adult patients, and there is no specific information comparing use of HMG-CoA reductase inhibitors in children with use in other age groups. However, lovastatin and simvastatin have been used in a limited number of children under 18 years of age. Early information seems to show that these medicines may be effective in children, but their long-term safety has not been studied.

Older adults—This medicine has been tested in a limited number of patients 65 years of age or older and has not been shown to cause different side effects or problems in older people than it does in younger adults.

Other medicines—Although certain medicines should not be used together at all, in other cases two different medicines may be used together even if an interaction might

occur. In these cases, your doctor may want to change the dose, or other precautions may be necessary. When you are taking HMG-CoA reductase inhibitors, it is especially important that your health care professional know if you are taking any of the following:

- Cyclosporine (e.g., Sandimmune) or
- Gemfibrozil (e.g., Lopid) or
- Niacin—Use of these medicines with an HMG-CoA reductase inhibitor may increase the risk of developing muscle problems and kidney failure

Other medical problems—The presence of other medical problems may affect the use of HMG-CoA reductase inhibitors. Make sure you tell your doctor if you have any other medical problems, especially:

- Alcohol abuse (or history of) or
- Liver disease—Use of this medicine may make liver problems worse
- Convulsions (seizures), not well-controlled, or
- Organ transplant with therapy to prevent transplant rejection or
- If you have recently had major surgery—Patients with these conditions may be at risk of developing problems that may lead to kidney failure

---

Proper Use of This Medicine

Use this medicine only as directed by your doctor. Do not use more or less of it, and do not use it more often or for a longer time than your doctor ordered.

Remember that this medicine will not cure your condition but it does help control it. Therefore, you must continue to take it as directed if you expect to keep your cholesterol levels down.

Follow carefully the special diet your doctor gave you. This is the most important part of controlling your condition, and is necessary if the medicine is to work properly.

For patients taking *lovastatin:*
- This medicine works better when it is taken with food. If you are taking this medicine once a day, take it with the evening meal. If you are taking more than one dose a day, take each dose with a meal or snack.

Dosing—The dose of these medicines will be different for different patients. *Follow your doctor's orders or the directions on the label.* The following information includes only the average doses of these medicines. *If your dose is different, do not change it* unless your doctor tells you to do so.

The number of capsules or tablets that you take depends on the strength of the medicine.

For fluvastatin
- For *oral* dosage form (capsules):
  —For high cholesterol:
    - Adults—20 to 40 milligrams (mg) once a day in the evening.
    - Children—Use and dose must be determined by your doctor.

For lovastatin
- For *oral* dosage form (tablets):
  —For high cholesterol:
    - Adults—20 to 80 milligrams (mg) a day taken as a single dose or divided into smaller doses. Take with meals.
    - Children—Use and dose must be determined by your doctor.

For pravastatin
- For *oral* dosage form (tablets):
  —For high cholesterol:
    - Adults—10 to 40 mg once a day at bedtime.
    - Children—Use and dose must be determined by your doctor.

For simvastatin
- For *oral* dosage form (tablets):
  - —For high cholesterol:
    - Adults—5 to 40 mg once a day in the evening.
    - Children—Use and dose must be determined by your doctor.

Missed dose—If you miss a dose of this medicine, take it as soon as possible. However, if it is almost time for your next dose, skip the missed dose and go back to your regular dosing schedule. Do not double doses.

Storage—To store this medicine:
- Keep out of the reach of children.
- Store away from heat and direct light.
- Do not store in the bathroom, near the kitchen sink, or in other damp places. Heat or moisture may cause the medicine to break down.
- Keep the medicine from freezing. Do not refrigerate.
- Do not keep outdated medicine or medicine no longer needed. Be sure that any discarded medicine is out of the reach of children.

Precautions While Using This Medicine

It is very important that your doctor check your progress at regular visits. This will allow your doctor to see if the medicine is working properly to lower your cholesterol levels and that it does not cause unwanted effects.

Check with your doctor immediately if you think that you may be pregnant. HMG-CoA reductase inhibitors may cause birth defects or other problems in the baby if taken during pregnancy.

Do not stop taking this medicine without first checking with your doctor. When you stop taking this medicine, your blood cholesterol levels may increase again. Your doctor may want you to follow a special diet to help prevent this from happening.

Before having any kind of surgery (including dental surgery) or emergency treatment, tell the medical doctor or dentist in charge that you are taking this medicine.

Side Effects of This Medicine

Along with its needed effects, a medicine may cause some unwanted effects. Although not all of these side effects may occur, if they do occur they may need medical attention.

Check with your doctor as soon as possible if any of the following side effects occur:

> *Less common or rare*
>> Fever; muscle aches or cramps; severe stomach pain; unusual tiredness or weakness

Other side effects may occur that usually do not need medical attention. These side effects may go away during treatment as your body adjusts to the medicine. However, check with your doctor if any of the following side effects continue or are bothersome:

> *More common*
>> Constipation; diarrhea; dizziness; gas; headache; heartburn; nausea; skin rash; stomach pain
>
> *Rare*
>> Decreased sexual ability; trouble in sleeping

Other side effects not listed above may also occur in some patients. If you notice any other effects, check with your doctor.

HYDRALAZINE Systemic

Some commonly used brand names are:

In the U.S.—
Apresoline
Generic name product may also be available.

In Canada—
Apresoline
Novo-Hylazin

Description

Hydralazine (hye-DRAL-a-zeen) belongs to the general class of medicines called antihypertensives. It is used to treat high blood pressure (hypertension).

High blood pressure adds to the work load of the heart and arteries. If it continues for a long time, the heart and arteries may not function properly. This can damage the blood vessels of the brain, heart, and kidneys, resulting in a stroke, heart failure, or kidney failure. High blood pressure may also increase the risk of heart attacks. These problems may be less likely to occur if blood pressure is controlled.

Hydralazine works by relaxing blood vessels and increasing the supply of blood and oxygen to the heart while reducing its work load.

Hydralazine may also be used for other conditions as determined by your doctor.

Hydralazine is available only with your doctor's prescription, in the following dosage forms:

Oral
• Tablets (U.S. and Canada)

Parenteral
• Injection (U.S. and Canada)

Before Using This Medicine

In deciding to use a medicine, the risks of taking the medicine must be weighed against the good it will do. This is a decision you and your doctor will make. For hydralazine, the following should be considered:

Allergies—Tell your doctor if you have ever had any unusual or allergic reaction to hydralazine. Also tell your health care professional if you are allergic to any other substance, such as foods, preservatives, or dyes.

Pregnancy—Hydralazine has not been studied in pregnant women. However, blood problems have been reported in infants of mothers who took hydralazine during pregnancy. In addition, studies in mice have shown that hydralazine causes birth defects (cleft palate, defects in head and face bones). These birth defects may also occur in rabbits, but do not occur in rats. Before taking this medicine, make sure your doctor knows if you are pregnant or if you may become pregnant.

Breast-feeding—It is not known whether hydralazine passes into breast milk.

Children—Although there is no specific information comparing use of hydralazine in children with use in other age groups, this medicine is not expected to cause different side effects or problems in children than it does in adults.

Older adults—Many medicines have not been studied specifically in older people. Therefore, it may not be known whether they work exactly the same way they do in younger adults. Although there is no specific information comparing use of hydralazine in the elderly with use in other age groups, this medicine is not expected to cause different side effects or problems in older people than it does in younger adults. However, dizziness or lightheadedness may be more likely to occur in the elderly, who are more sensitive to the effects of hydralazine.

Other medicines—Although certain medicines should not be used together at all, in other cases two different medicines may be used together even if an interaction might occur. In these cases, your doctor may want to change the dose, or other precautions may be necessary. When you are taking hydralazine, it is especially important that your health care professional know if you are taking the following:

- Diazoxide (e.g., Proglycem)—Effect on blood pressure may be increased

Other medical problems—The presence of other medical problems may affect the use of hydralazine. Make sure you tell your doctor if you have any other medical problems, especially:

- Heart or blood vessel disease or
- Stroke—Lowering blood pressure may make problems resulting from these conditions worse
- Kidney disease—Effects may be increased because of slower removal of hydralazine from the body

---

Proper Use of This Medicine

For patients taking this medicine *for high blood pressure:*

- In addition to the use of the medicine your doctor has prescribed, treatment for your high blood pressure may include weight control and care in the types of foods you eat, especially foods high in sodium. Your doctor will tell you which of these are most important for you. You should check with your doctor before changing your diet.

- Many patients who have high blood pressure will not notice any signs of the problem. In fact, many may feel normal. It is very important that you *take your medicine exactly as directed* and that you keep your appointments with your doctor even if you feel well.

- Remember that hydralazine will not cure your high blood pressure, but it does help control it. Therefore, you must continue to take it as directed if you expect to lower your blood pressure and keep it down. *You may have to take high blood pressure medicine for the rest of your life.* If high blood pressure is not treated, it can cause serious problems such as heart failure, blood vessel disease, stroke, or kidney disease.

To help you remember to take your medicine, try to get into the habit of taking it at the same time each day.

Dosing—The dose of hydralazine will be different for different patients. *Follow your doctor's orders or the directions on the label.* The following information includes only the average doses of hydralazine. *If your dose is different, do not change it* unless your doctor tells you to do so.

The number of tablets that you take depends on the strength of the medicine.

* For *oral* dosage form (tablets):
    —For high blood pressure:
      * Adults—10 to 50 milligrams (mg) four times a day.
      * Children—Dose is based on body weight or size. The usual dose is 0.75 to 7.5 mg per kilogram (kg) (0.34 to 3.4 mg per pound) of body weight a day. This is divided into two to four doses.
* For *injection* dosage form:
    —For high blood pressure:
      * Adults—10 to 40 mg injected into a muscle or a vein. Your doctor may repeat the dose as needed.
      * Children—Dose is based on body weight or size. The usual dose is 1.7 to 3.5 mg per kg (0.77 to 1.6 mg per pound) of body weight a day. This is divided into four to six doses and injected into a muscle or a vein.

Missed dose—If you miss a dose of this medicine, take it as soon as possible. However, if it is almost time for your next dose, skip the missed dose and go back to your regular dosing schedule. Do not double doses.

Storage—To store this medicine:
- Keep out of the reach of children.
- Store away from heat and direct light.
- Do not store in the bathroom, near the kitchen sink, or in other damp places. Heat or moisture may cause the medicine to break down.
- Do not keep outdated medicine or medicine no longer needed. Be sure that any discarded medicine is out of the reach of children.

Precautions While Using This Medicine

It is important that your doctor check your progress at regular visits to make sure that this medicine is working properly.

For patients taking this medicine *for high blood pressure:*

- *Do not take other medicines unless they have been discussed with your doctor.* This especially includes over-the-counter (nonprescription) medicines for appetite control, asthma, colds, cough, hay fever, or sinus, since they may tend to increase your blood pressure.

Hydralazine may cause some people to have headaches or to feel dizzy. *Make sure you know how you react to this medicine before you drive, use machines, or do anything else that could be dangerous if you are dizzy or are not alert.*

Side Effects of This Medicine

Along with its needed effects, a medicine may cause some unwanted effects. Although not all of these side effects may occur, if they do occur they may need medical attention.

In general, side effects with hydralazine are rare at lower doses. However, check with your doctor as soon as possible if any of the following occur:

Less common

> Blisters on skin; chest pain; general feeling of discomfort or illness or weakness; joint pain; numbness, tingling, pain, or weakness in hands or feet; skin rash or itching; sore throat and fever; swelling of feet or lower legs; swelling of the lymph glands

Other side effects may occur that usually do not need medical attention. These side effects may go away during treatment as your body adjusts to the medicine. However, check with your doctor if any of the following side effects continue or are bothersome:

More common

> Diarrhea; fast or irregular heartbeat; headache; loss of appetite; nausea or vomiting; pounding heartbeat

Less common

> Constipation; dizziness or lightheadedness; redness or flushing of face; shortness of breath; stuffy nose; watering or irritated eyes

Other side effects not listed above may also occur in some patients. If you notice any other effects, check with your doctor.

Additional Information

Once a medicine has been approved for marketing for a certain use, experience may show that it is also useful for other medical problems. Although this use is not specifically included in product labeling, hydralazine is used in certain patients with the following medical condition:

• Congestive heart failure

Other than the above information, there is no additional information relating to proper use, precautions, or side effects for this use.

INSULIN Systemic

Some commonly used brand names are:

In the U.S.—

Humulin 50/50[7]

Humulin 70/30[7]

Humulin L[9]

Humulin N[5]

Humulin R[2]

Humulin U Ultralente[11]

Lente Iletin I[8]

Lente Iletin II[8]

Lente Insulin[8]

Lente L[8]

Novolin 70/30[7]

Novolin L[9]

Novolin N[5]

Novolin R[2]

NPH Iletin I[4]

NPH Iletin II[4]

NPH Insulin[4]

NPH-N[4]

Regular (Concentrated)

Iletin II, U-500[1]

Regular Iletin I[1]

Regular Iletin II[1]

Regular Insulin[1]

Ultralente U[10]

Velosulin Human[2]

In Canada—

Humulin 10/90[7]

Humulin 20/80[7]

Humulin 30/70[7]

Humulin 40/60[7]

Humulin 50/50[7]

Humulin-L[9]

Humulin-N[5]

Humulin-R[2]

Humulin-U[11]

Insulin-Toronto[1]

Lente Iletin[8]

Lente Iletin II[8]

Lente Insulin[8]

Novolin ge 10/90[7]

Novolin ge 20/80[7]

Novolin ge 30/70[7]

Novolin ge 40/60[7]

Novolin ge 50/50[7]

Novolin ge Lente[9]

Novolin ge NPH[5]

Novolin ge Toronto[2]

Novolin ge Ultralente[11]

NPH Iletin[4]

NPH Iletin II[4]

NPH Insulin[4]

Regular Iletin[1]

Regular Iletin II[1]

Semilente Insulin[12]

Ultralente Insulin[10]

Velosulin Human[2]

Other commonly used names are:

lente insulin[8]

NPH insulin[4]

PZI insulin[13]

regular insulin[1]

semilente insulin[12]

ultralente insulin[10]

Note: For quick reference, the following insulins are numbered to match the corresponding brand names.

This information applies to the following medicines:

1. Insulin (IN-su-lin)
2. Insulin Human

 3. Buffered Insulin Human*†
 4. Isophane (EYE-so-fayn) Insulin
 5. Isophane Insulin, Human
 6. Isophane Insulin and Insulin*†
 7. Isophane Insulin, Human and Insulin Human
 8. Insulin Zinc
 9. Insulin Zinc, Human
10. Extended Insulin Zinc
11. Extended Insulin Zinc, Human
12. Prompt Insulin Zinc*
13. Protamine Zinc Insulin*†

---

*Not commercially available in the U.S.
†Not commercially available in Canada.

Description

Insulin (IN-su-lin) is a hormone that helps the body turn the food we eat into energy. This occurs whether we make our own insulin in the pancreas gland or take it by injection.

Diabetes mellitus (sugar diabetes) is a condition where the body does not make enough insulin to meet its needs or does not properly use the insulin it makes.

Insulin can be obtained from beef or pork pancreas glands or from new processes that produce human insulin. All types of insulin must be injected because, if taken by mouth, insulin is destroyed by chemical reactions in the stomach.

One or more injections of insulin a day may be needed to control your diabetes. Insulin is usually injected before meals or at bedtime. Your doctor will discuss the number of injections you will need, the kind of insulin to use, the correct dose, and the right time to take it.

A prescription is not necessary to purchase most insulin. However, your doctor must first determine your insulin needs and provide you with special instructions for control of your diabetes. Insulin is available in the following dosage forms:

Parenteral

Insulin
- Injection (U.S. and Canada)

Insulin Human
- Injection (U.S. and Canada)

Buffered Insulin Human
- Injection

Isophane Insulin
- Injection (U.S. and Canada)

Isophane Insulin and Insulin
- Injection

Isophane Insulin, Human
- Injection (U.S. and Canada)

Isophane Insulin, Human, and Insulin Human
- Injection (U.S. and Canada)

Insulin Zinc
- Injection (U.S. and Canada)

Insulin Zinc, Human
- Injection (U.S. and Canada)

Extended Insulin Zinc
- Injection (U.S. and Canada)

Extended Insulin Zinc, Human
- Injection (U.S. and Canada)

Prompt Insulin Zinc
- Injection (Canada)

Protamine Zinc Insulin
- Injection

Before Using This Medicine

In deciding to use a medicine, the risks of taking the medicine must be weighed against the good it will do. This is a decision you and your doctor will make. For insulin, the following should be considered:

Allergies—Tell your doctor if you have ever had any unusual or allergic reaction to insulin. Also tell your health care professional if you are allergic to any other substances, such as foods, preservatives, or dyes.

Diet—If you have insulin-dependent diabetes (type I), your doctor will prescribe both insulin and a personalized meal plan for you. Such a diet is low in fat and simple sugars such as table sugar, and sweet foods and beverages. This meal plan is also high in complex carbohydrates (starchy foods) such as cereals, grains, bread, pasta or noodles, starchy vegetables, and dried beans, peas, or lentils. The daily number of calories in this meal plan should be adjusted by your doctor or a registered dietitian to help you reach and maintain a healthy body weight. In addition, meals and snacks are arranged to meet the energy needs of your body at different times of the day. *It is very important that you carefully follow your meal plan.*

Pregnancy—Your requirements for insulin change during pregnancy. Because it is especially important for the health of both you and the baby that your blood sugar be closely controlled, be sure to tell your doctor if you suspect you are pregnant or if you are planning to become pregnant.

Breast-feeding—Insulin does not pass into breast milk and will not affect the nursing infant.

Other medicines—Although certain medicines should not be used together at all, in other cases two different medicines may be used together even if an interaction might occur. In these cases, your doctor may want to change the dose, or other precautions may be necessary. When using insulin, it is especially important that your health care professional know if you are taking any of the following:

- Beta-blockers—Beta-blockers may increase the risk of developing either high or low blood sugar levels. Also, they can mask symptoms of low blood sugar (such as rapid pulse). Because of this, a person with diabetes might not recognize low blood sugar and might not take immediate steps to treat it. Beta-blockers can also cause a low blood sugar level to last longer than it would have normally

Corticosteroids (e.g., prednisone or other cortisone-like medicines)—Your dose of either medicine may need to be adjusted because the corticosteroids may interfere with
insulin and thus increase your blood sugar

Other medical problems—The presence of other medical
problems may affect the dose of insulin you need. Be
sure to tell your doctor if you have any other medical
problems, especially:

- Infections or
- Kidney disease or
- Liver disease or
- Thyroid disease—These conditions may change your daily
  insulin dose

Proper Use of This Medicine

Make sure you have the type and strength of insulin that
your doctor ordered for you. You may find that keeping
an insulin label with you is helpful when buying insulin
supplies. The concentration (strength) of insulin is measured by units, and is sometimes expressed in terms such
as U-100 insulin.

Insulin doses are measured and given with specially
marked insulin syringes. These syringes come in 3 sizes:
30 units, 50 units, and 100 units. Your insulin syringe will
allow you to measure the units of insulin that have been
prescribed for you, and allow you to easily read the measuring scale.

There are several important steps that will help you suc-
cessfully prepare your insulin injection. To draw the insulin up into the syringe correctly, you need to follow
these steps:

- Wash your hands.
- If your insulin is the intermediate- or long-acting kind
  (cloudy), be sure that it is completely mixed. Mix the

insulin by slowly rolling the bottle between your hands or gently tipping the bottle over a few times.

- Never shake the bottle vigorously (hard).
- Do not use the insulin if it looks lumpy or grainy, seems unusually thick, sticks to the bottle, or seems to be even a little discolored. Do not use the insulin if it contains crystals or if the bottle looks frosted. Regular insulin (short-acting) should be used only if it is clear and colorless.
- Remove the colored protective cap on the bottle. Do *not* remove the rubber stopper.
- Wipe the top of the bottle with an alcohol swab.
- Remove the needle cover of the insulin syringe.
- Draw air into the syringe by pulling back on the plunger. The amount of air should be equal to your insulin dose.
- Gently push the needle through the top of the rubber stopper.
- Push plunger in all the way, to inject air into the bottle.
- Turn the bottle with syringe upside down in one hand. Be sure the tip of the needle is covered by the insulin. With your other hand, draw the plunger back slowly to draw the correct dose of insulin into the syringe.
- Check the insulin in the syringe for air bubbles. To remove air bubbles, push the insulin slowly back into the bottle and draw up your dose again.
- Check your dose again.
- Remove the needle from the bottle and re-cover the needle.

If you are mixing more than 1 type of insulin in the same syringe, you also need to know about the following:

- When mixing regular insulin with another type of insulin, *always* draw the regular insulin into the syringe first. When mixing 2 types of insulins other than regular insulin, it does not matter in what order you draw them.

- After you decide on a certain order for drawing up your insulin, you should use the same order each time.

- Some mixtures of insulins have to be injected immediately. Others may be stable for longer periods of time, which means that you can wait before you inject the mixture. Check with your health care professional to find out which type you have.

- If your mixture is stable and you mixed it ahead of time, gently turn the filled syringe back and forth to remix the insulins before you inject them. Do not shake the syringe.

After you have your syringe prepared, you are ready to inject the insulin into your body. To do this:

- Clean the site where the injection is to be made with an alcohol swab, and let the area dry.

- Inject the insulin into fatty tissue. Injection sites include your thighs, abdomen (stomach area), upper arms, or buttocks. Generally, insulin is absorbed into the bloodstream most evenly from the abdomen. If you are either thin or greatly overweight, you may be given special instructions for giving yourself insulin injections.

- Pinch up a large area of skin and hold it firmly. With your other hand, hold the syringe like a pencil. Push the needle straight into the pinched-up skin at a 90-degree angle. Be sure the needle is all the way in. Drawing back on the syringe each time to check for blood (also called routine aspiration) is not necessary.

- Push the plunger all the way down, using less than 5 seconds to inject the dose. Hold an alcohol swab near the needle and pull the needle straight out of the skin.

- Press the swab against the injection site for several seconds. Do not rub.

For patients using *disposable syringes:*

- Manufacturers of disposable syringes recommend that they be used only once, because the sterility of a reused syringe cannot be guaranteed. However, some patients prefer to reuse a syringe until its needle becomes dull. Most insulins have chemicals added that keep them from growing the bacteria that are usually found on the skin. Because of this, some patients may decide to reuse a disposable syringe. However, the syringe should be thrown away when the needle becomes dull, has been bent, or has come into contact with any surface other than the cleaned and swabbed area of skin. Also, if you plan to reuse a syringe, the needle must be recapped after each use. Check with your health care professional to find out the best way to reuse syringes.
- Laws in some states require that used insulin syringes and needles be destroyed. Be careful when you recap, bend, or break a needle, because these actions increase the chances of a needle-stick injury. It is best to put used syringes and needles in a disposable container that is puncture-resistant or to use a needle-clipping device. The chances of a syringe being reused by someone else is lower if the plunger is taken out of the barrel and broken in half when you dispose of a syringe.

For patients using *a glass syringe and metal needle:*

- This type of syringe and needle may be used repeatedly if it is sterilized each time. You should get an instruction sheet that tells you how to do this. If you need more information on this, ask your health care professional.

For patients using *an insulin-infusion pump:*

- Regular insulin is the only insulin product that should be used with insulin infusion pumps.

- Do not use the insulin injection if it looks lumpy, cloudy, unusually thick, or even slightly discolored, or if it contains crystals. Use the insulin only if it is clear and colorless.

- Do not mix the buffered regular insulin injection with any other insulin. If you do, crystals may form that will block the pump catheter. Also, the potency of the insulin may change.

- It is important to follow the pump manufacturer's directions on how to load the syringe and/or pump reservoir. Your correct insulin dose may not be given if loading is not done correctly.

- Check the infusion tubing and infusion-site dressing often for improper insulin infusion, as your health care professional recommends.

Dosing—The dose of these medicines will be different for different patients. *Follow your doctor's orders or the directions on the label.* The following information applies to the average doses of these medicines. *If your dose is different, do not change it* unless your doctor tells you to do so.

The number of injections that you receive depends on the strength or type of the medicine. Also, *the number of doses you receive each day, the time allowed between doses, and the length of time you receive the medicine depend on the amount of sugar in your blood or urine.*

For regular insulin (R)—crystalline zinc, human buffered, and human regular insulins

- For *injection* dosage form:

  —For treating sugar diabetes (diabetes mellitus):

   • Adults and teenagers—The dose is based on your blood sugar and must be determined by your doctor. The medicine is injected under the skin fifteen or thirty minutes before meals up to four times a day.

• Children—Dose is based on your blood sugar and body size, and must be determined by your doctor.

—For treating uncontrolled diabetes (diabetic ketoacidosis):

• Adults—The dose is based on your blood sugar and body weight, and must be determined by your doctor. The usual dose is 0.1 USP Units per kilogram (kg) (0.05 USP Units per pound) of body weight injected slowly into a vein each hour.

• Children—The dose is based on your blood sugar and body size, and must be determined by your doctor.

For isophane insulin (NPH)—isophane and human isophane insulins

• For *injection* dosage form:

—For treating sugar diabetes (diabetes mellitus):

• Adults and teenagers—The dose is based on your blood sugar and must be determined by your doctor. The medicine is injected under the skin thirty to sixty minutes before breakfast. You may need a dose before another meal or at bedtime.

• Children—Dose is based on your blood sugar and body size, and must be determined by your doctor.

For isophane insulin/insulin (NPH/R)—human isophane/regular insulin

• For *injection* dosage form:

—For treating sugar diabetes (diabetes mellitus):

• Adults and teenagers—The dose is based on your blood sugar and must be determined by your doctor. The medicine is injected under the skin fifteen to thirty minutes before breakfast.

• Children—Dose is based on your blood sugar and body size, and must be determined by your doctor.

For insulin zinc (L)—lente and human lente insulins
- For *injection* dosage form:
  - —For treating sugar diabetes (diabetes mellitus):
    - Adults and teenagers—The dose is based on your blood sugar and must be determined by your doctor. The medicine is injected under the skin thirty to sixty minutes before breakfast. You may need a dose before another meal or at bedtime.
    - Children—Dose is based on your blood sugar and body size, and must be determined by your doctor.

For insulin zinc extended (U)—ultralente and human ultralente insulins
- For *injection* dosage form:
  - —For treating sugar diabetes (diabetes mellitus):
    - Adults and teenagers—The dose is based on your blood sugar and must be determined by your doctor. The medicine is injected under the skin thirty to sixty minutes before breakfast.
    - Children—Dose is based on your blood sugar and body size, and must be determined by your doctor.

For prompt insulin zinc (S)—semilente and human semilente insulins
- For *injection* dosage form:
  - —For treating sugar diabetes (diabetes mellitus):
    - Adults and teenagers—The dose is based on your blood sugar and must be determined by your doctor. The medicine is injected under the skin thirty to sixty minutes before breakfast. You may need a dose thirty minutes before another meal or at bedtime.
    - Children—Dose is based on your blood sugar and body size, and must be determined by your doctor.

For protamine zinc insulin (PZI)—protamine zinc insulin
- For *injection* dosage form:
  —For treating sugar diabetes (diabetes mellitus):
  - Adults and teenagers—The dose is based on your blood sugar and must be determined by your doctor. The medicine is injected under the skin thirty to sixty minutes before breakfast.
  - Children—Dose is based on your blood sugar and body size, and must be determined by your doctor.

Storage—Storage and expiration date:
- When buying insulin, always check the package expiration date to make sure the insulin will be used before it expires.
- This expiration date applies *only* when the insulin has been stored in the refrigerator. Expiration is much shorter if the insulin is left unrefrigerated. Do not use insulin after the expiration date stated on the label even if the bottle has never been opened. Check with your pharmacist about a possible exchange of bottles.
- An unopened bottle of insulin should be refrigerated until needed. It should never be frozen. Remove the insulin from the refrigerator and allow it to reach room temperature before injecting.
- An insulin bottle in use may be kept at room temperature for up to 1 month. Insulin that has been kept at room temperature for longer than a month should be thrown away.
- Do not expose insulin to extremely hot temperatures or to sunlight. Do not leave insulin in the hot summer sun or in a hot closed car. Extreme heat will cause insulin to become less effective much more quickly.

Precautions While Using This Medicine

It is very important that your doctor check your progress at regular visits, especially during the first few weeks of insulin treatment.

It is very important to follow carefully any instructions from your health care team about:

- Alcohol—Drinking alcohol may cause severe low blood sugar. Discuss this with your health care team.

- Tobacco—If you have been smoking for a long time and suddenly stop, your dosage of insulin may need to be reduced. If you decide to quit, tell your doctor first.

- Meal plan—To be successful in your treatment, you must closely follow the diet your doctor or dietitian prescribed for you. Do not miss or delay your meals.

- Exercise—Ask your doctor what kind of exercise to do, the best time to do it, and how much you should do daily.

- Blood tests—This is the best way to tell whether your diabetes is being controlled properly. Blood sugar testing is a useful guide to help you and your health care team adjust your insulin dose, meal plan, and exercise schedule.

- Urine ketone tests—You will also be asked at certain times to test for acetone, which is an acid that may be released from your bloodstream into your urine when your blood glucose is too high.

- Injection sites—If you carefully select and rotate the sites where you give your insulin injections, you may be able to prevent skin problems. Also, the insulin may be better absorbed into the bloodstream.

- Other medicines—Do not take other medicines unless they have been discussed with your doctor. This especially includes nonprescription medicines such as aspirin, and those for appetite control, asthma, colds, cough, hay fever, or sinus problems.

Insulin can cause low blood sugar (also called insulin reaction or hypoglycemia). Symptoms of low blood sugar are:

Anxious feeling
Cold sweats
Confusion

Cool pale skin
Difficulty in concentration
Drowsiness
Excessive hunger
Headache
Nausea
Nervousness
Rapid pulse
Shakiness
Unusual tiredness or weakness
Vision changes

- Different people may feel different symptoms of low blood sugar (hypoglycemia). It is important that you learn the symptoms of low blood sugar that you usually have so that you can treat it quickly.

- The symptoms of hypoglycemia (low blood sugar) may develop quickly and may result from:

  —delaying or missing a scheduled meal or snack.

  —exercising more than usual.

  —drinking a significant amount of alcohol.

  —taking certain medicines.

  —using too much insulin.

  —sickness (especially with vomiting or diarrhea).

- Eating some form of quick-acting sugar when symptoms of hypoglycemia first appear will usually prevent them from getting worse. Good sources of sugar include:

  Glucose tablets or gel that you can buy
  A restaurant sugar packet
  Fruit juice (4 to 6 ounces or one-half cup)
  Corn syrup (1 tablespoon)
  Honey (1 tablespoon)
  Regular (non-diet) soft drinks (4 to 6 ounces or one-half cup)
  Sugar cubes (6 one-half-inch sized) or table sugar (dissolved in water)

- Do not use chocolate because its fat slows down the sugar entering into the bloodstream.

- If a snack is not scheduled for an hour or more you should also eat some crackers and cheese, or half a sandwich, or ice cream, or a peanut butter cookie, or drink an 8 ounce glass of milk.

- Symptoms of low blood sugar must be treated before they lead to unconsciousness (passing out). Glucagon is also used in emergency situations such as unconsciousness. Have a glucagon kit available, along with a syringe and needle, and know how to prepare and use it. Members of your household should know how and when to use it, also. Check the expiration date of the glucagon and remind yourself when to buy a new kit. If your kit has expired, ask your pharmacist to exchange it for a new one.

Hyperglycemia (high blood sugar) is another problem related to uncontrolled diabetes. If you have any symptoms of high blood sugar, you need to contact your health care team right away. If it is not treated, severe hyperglycemia can lead to ketoacidosis (diabetic coma) and death. The symptoms of hyperglycemia appear more slowly than those of low blood sugar and usually include:

Increased urination
Unusual thirst
Dry mouth
Drowsiness
Flushed, dry skin
Fruit-like breath odor
Loss of appetite
Stomach ache, nausea, or vomiting
Tiredness
Troubled breathing (rapid and deep)
Increased blood sugar level

- Symptoms of ketoacidosis (diabetic coma) that need immediate hospitalization include:

  Flushed, dry skin
  Fruit-like breath odor
  Stomach ache, nausea, or vomiting
  Troubled breathing (rapid and deep)

- Hyperglycemia (high blood sugar) symptoms may occur if you:

  —have a fever, diarrhea, or infection.

  —do not take enough insulin.

  —skip a dose of insulin.

  —do not exercise as much as usual.

  —overeat or do not follow your meal plan.

- Your doctor may recommend changes in your insulin dose or meal plan to avoid hyperglycemia. Symptoms of high blood sugar must be corrected before they progress to more serious conditions. Check with your doctor often to make sure you are controlling your blood sugar.

In case of emergency—There may be a time when you need emergency help for a problem caused by your diabetes. You need to be prepared for these emergencies. It is a good idea to:

- Wear a medical identification (I.D.) bracelet or neck chain at all times. Also, carry an I.D. card in your wallet or purse that says that you have diabetes and lists all of your medicines. •

- Keep an extra supply of insulin and syringes with needles on hand.

- Have a glucagon kit and a syringe and needle available and know how to prepare and use it if severe hypoglycemia (low blood sugar) occurs.

- Keep some kind of quick-acting sugar handy to treat hypoglycemia (low blood sugar) symptoms.

In case of illness:

- When you become ill with a cold, fever, or the flu, you need to take your usual insulin dose, even if you feel too sick to eat. This is especially true if you have nausea, vomiting, or diarrhea. Infection usually increases your need for insulin. Call your doctor for specific instructions.

- Continue taking your insulin and try to stay on your regular meal plan. However, if you have trouble eating solid food, drink fruit juices, non-diet soft drinks, or clear soups, or eat small amounts of bland foods. A dietitian or your doctor can give you a list of foods and the amounts to use for sick days.

- Test your blood sugar level at least every 4 hours while you are awake and check your urine for acetone. If acetone is present, call your doctor at once. If you have severe or prolonged vomiting, check with your doctor. Even when you start feeling better, let your doctor know how you are doing.

Travel—If you take a few special precautions when you travel, you are less likely to have problems related to your diabetes during trips away from home. It is a good idea to:

- Carry a recent prescription from your doctor for your diabetes medicine and also for the type of syringe and needles you use.

- Do not make major changes in your meal plan or medicine schedule without advice from your health care team.

- Carry your diabetic supplies on your person or in a purse or briefcase to reduce the possibility of loss.

- Carry snack foods with you in case of delays between meals.

- Make allowances for changing time zones and keep your meal times as close to usual as possible.

- In hot climates, use an insulated container for your insulin.

- When traveling to foreign countries, it is advisable to pack enough diabetic supplies to last until you return home and to have extra or reserve supplies kept separate from your main supplies.

- Carry a letter from your doctor with all the details of your diabetes and medicines you need, including your need for syringes.
- When carrying a large quantity of diabetic supplies, divide them throughout your hand-carried luggage to avoid problems if something is lost, and to avoid possible freezing in airplane storage areas.

IPRATROPIUM   Inhalation

A commonly used brand name in the U.S. and Canada is Atrovent.

Description

Ipratropium is a bronchodilator (medicine that opens up narrowed breathing passages). It is taken by inhalation to help control the symptoms of lung diseases, such as bronchial asthma, chronic bronchitis, and emphysema. When ipratropium is used regularly every day, it may be used alone or with other bronchodilators to help decrease coughing, wheezing, shortness of breath, and troubled breathing by increasing the flow of air into the lungs.

When ipratropium inhalation is used to treat acute attacks of asthma, it is used only in a nebulizer and must be used in combination with other bronchodilators.

Ipratropium is available only with your doctor's prescription, in the following dosage forms:

Inhalation
- Inhalation aerosol (U.S. and Canada)
- Inhalation solution (U.S. and Canada)

Before Using This Medicine

In deciding to use a medicine, the risks of using the medicine must be weighed against the good it will do. This is

a decision you and your doctor will make. For ipratropium, the following should be considered:

Allergies—Tell your doctor if you have ever had any unusual or allergic reaction to ipratropium, atropine, belladonna, hyoscyamine, or scopolamine, or to other inhalation aerosol medicines.

Pregnancy—Ipratropium has not been studied in pregnant women. However, it has not been shown to cause birth defects or other problems in animal studies.

Breast-feeding—It is not known whether ipratropium passes into the breast milk. Although most medicines pass into breast milk in small amounts, many of them may be used safely while breast-feeding. Mothers who are using this medicine and who wish to breast-feed should discuss this with their doctor.

Children—Although there is no specific information comparing the use of ipratropium in children up to 5 years of age with other age groups, this medicine is not expected to cause different side effects or problems in children than it does in adults.

Older adults—Ipratropium inhalation has been tested in a small number of patients 65 years of age or older. This medicine is not expected to cause different side effects or problems in older people than it does in younger adults.

Other medicines—Although certain medicines should not be used together at all, in other cases two different medicines may be used together even if an interaction might occur. In these cases, your doctor may want to change the dose, or other precautions may be necessary. When you are taking ipratropium, it is especially important that your health care professional know if you are taking any other prescription or nonprescription (over-the-counter [OTC]) medicine.

Other medical problems—The presence of other medical problems may affect the use of ipratropium. Make sure you tell your doctor if you have any other medical problem, especially:

- Difficult urination—Ipratropium may make the condition worse
- Glaucoma—Ipratropium may make the condition worse if it gets into the eyes

---

Proper Use of This Medicine

Ipratropium is used to help control the symptoms of lung diseases, such as chronic bronchitis, emphysema, and asthma. However, for treatment of bronchospasm or asthma attacks that have already started, ipratropium inhalation solution is used only in a nebulizer and in combination with other bronchodilators.

It is very important that you use ipratropium only as directed. Do not use more of it and do not use it more often than your doctor ordered. To do so may increase the chance of side effects.

Keep the spray or solution away from the eyes because this medicine may cause irritation or blurred vision. Closing your eyes while you are inhaling ipratropium may help keep the medicine out of your eyes. Rinsing your eyes with cool water may help if any medicine does get into your eyes.

Ipratropium usually comes with patient directions. Read them carefully before using this medicine.

For patients using *ipratropium inhalation aerosol:*

- If you do not understand the directions or you are not sure how to use the inhaler, ask your health care professional to show you how to use it. Also, ask your health care professional to check regularly how you use the inhaler to make sure you are using it properly.
- When you use the inhaler for the first time, or if you

have not used it for a while, the inhaler may not
deliver the right amount of medicine with the first
puff. Therefore, before using the inhaler, test it to
make sure it works properly.

- *To test the inhaler:*

  —Insert the metal canister firmly into the clean
  mouthpiece according to the manufacturer's instructions. Check to make sure it is placed properly into
  the mouthpiece.

  —Take the cover off the mouthpiece and shake the
  inhaler three or four times.

  —Hold the inhaler well away from you against a
  light background and press the top of the canister,
  spraying the medicine into the air. If you see a fine
  mist, you will know the inhaler is working properly
  to provide the right amount of medicine when you
  use it. If you do not see a fine mist, try a second
  time.

- *To use the inhaler:*

  —Using your thumb and one or two fingers, hold
  the inhaler upright, with the mouthpiece end down
  and pointing toward you.

  —Take the cover off the mouthpiece. Check the
  mouthpiece for any foreign object. Then, gently
  shake the inhaler and canister three or four times.

  —Hold the mouthpiece away from your mouth and
  breathe out slowly and completely.

  —Use the inhalation method recommended by
  your doctor.

    - Open-mouth method—Place the mouthpiece
      about 1 or 2 inches (2 fingerwidths) in front of
      your widely opened mouth. Make sure the in-
      haler is aimed into your mouth so the spray
      does not hit the roof of your mouth or your
      tongue.

    - Closed-mouth method—Place the mouthpiece

in your mouth between your teeth and over your tongue with your lips closed tightly around it. Make sure your tongue or teeth are not blocking the opening.

—Tilt your head back a little. Start to breathe in slowly and deeply through your mouth and, at the same time, press the top of the canister once to get one puff of medicine. Continue to breathe in slowly until you have taken a full breath. Try to inhale for 3 to 4 seconds. It is important to press down on the top of the canister and breathe in at the same time so the medicine is pulled into your lungs. This step may be difficult at first. If you are using the closed-mouth method and you see a fine mist coming from your mouth or nose, the inhaler is not being used correctly.

—After inhaling the spray into your lungs, hold your breath as long as you can up to 10 seconds. This gives the medicine time to settle into your airways and lungs.

—Take the mouthpiece away from your mouth and breathe out slowly.

—If your doctor has told you to inhale more than one puff of medicine at each dose, gently shake the inhaler again, and take the second puff following exactly the same steps you used for the first puff.

—When you are finished, wipe off the mouthpiece and replace the cover to keep the mouthpiece clean and free of foreign objects.

• Your doctor may want you to use a spacer device with the inhaler. A spacer makes the inhaler easier to use. With a spacer, more of the medicine is able to reach your lungs and less of it stays in the mouth and throat.

  —*To use a spacer device with the inhaler:*

  • Attach the spacer to the inhaler according to

the manufacturer's directions. There are different types of spacers available, but the method of breathing remains the same with most spacers.

• Gently shake the inhaler and spacer three or four times.

• Hold the mouthpiece of the spacer away from your mouth and breathe out slowly to the end of a normal breath.

• Place the mouthpiece into your mouth between your teeth and over your tongue with your lips closed around it.

• Press down on the canister top once to release one puff of medicine into the spacer. Within one or two seconds, start to breathe in slowly and deeply through your mouth for 5 to 10 seconds. Count the seconds while inhaling. Do not breathe in through your nose.

• Then hold your breath as long as you can up to 10 seconds.

• Breathe out slowly. Do not remove the mouthpiece from your mouth. Breathe in and out slowly three or four times to be sure the spacer device is emptied.

• If your doctor has told you to take more than one puff of medicine at each dose, gently shake the inhaler and spacer again and take the second puff, following exactly the same steps you used for the first puff.

• When you are finished, remove the spacer device from the inhaler and replace the cover of the mouthpiece.

• Clean the inhaler, mouthpiece, and spacer at least twice a week to prevent build-up of medicine and blockage of the mouthpiece.

—*To clean the inhaler:*

• Remove the metal canister from the inhaler and set aside.

• Wash the mouthpiece and cover, the plastic case, and the spacer with soap and hot water. Rinse well with warm, running water.

• Shake off the excess water and let the inhaler parts air dry completely before replacing the metal canister and cover.

• The metal canister stem may get dirty or blocked. While the canister is out of the mouthpiece, check the two small holes in the stem of the canister.

• If the holes seem blocked, rinse them with clear, lukewarm water.

• Let the canister dry completely before you put it back into the dry mouthpiece.

• Replace the cover to keep the mouthpiece clean.

• *To check how full the canister is:*

—Place only the canister in a container of water.

—If the canister floats at the top of the water, it is empty and needs replacing. If it sinks to the bottom of the water, it is full. When the canister stands upright in the water, it is about one-half full.

—Take the canister out of the water and let it dry completely before putting it back into the dry mouthpiece.

For patients using *ipratropium inhalation solution:*

• Use this medicine only in a power-operated nebulizer with an adequate flow rate and equipped with a face mask or mouthpiece. Your doctor will tell you which nebulizer to use. Make sure you understand exactly how to use it. If you have any questions about this, check with your doctor.

• *To prepare the medicine for use in the nebulizer:*

—*If you are using the single-dose vial of ipratropium:*

- Break away one vial by pulling it firmly from the strip.

- Twist off the top to open the vial. Use the contents of the vial as soon as possible after opening it.

- Squeeze the contents of the vial into the cup of the nebulizer. If your doctor has told you to use less than a full vial of solution, use a syringe to withdraw the correct amount of solution from the vial and add it to the nebulizer cup. Be sure to throw away the syringe after one use.

—*If you are using the multiple-dose bottle of ipratropium:*

- Use a syringe to withdraw the correct amount of solution from the bottle and add it to the nebulizer cup. Do not use the same syringe more than once.

- If you have been told to dilute the ipratropium inhalation solution in the nebulizer cup with the sodium chloride solution provided, use a new syringe to add the sodium chloride solution to the cup as directed by your health care professional.

- If your doctor told you to use another inhalation solution with the ipratropium inhalation solution, add that solution also to the nebulizer cup.

- *To use the nebulizer:*

  —Gently shake the nebulizer cup to mix the solutions well.

  —Connect the nebulizer tube to the air or oxygen pump and begin the treatment. Adjust the mask, if you are using one, to prevent mist from getting into your eyes.

  —Use the method of breathing your doctor told you

to use to take the treatment. One way is to breathe slowly and deeply through the mask or mouthpiece. Another way is to breathe in and out normally with the mouthpiece in your mouth, taking a deep breath every one or two minutes. Continue to breathe in the medicine as instructed until no more mist is formed in the nebulizer cup or until you hear a sputtering (spitting or popping) sound.

—When you have finished, replace the caps on the solutions. Store the bottles of solution in the refrigerator until the next treatment.

—Clean the nebulizer according to the manufacturer's directions.

For patients using *ipratropium* regularly (for example, every day):

 • *In order for ipratropium to work properly, it must be inhaled every day in regularly spaced doses as ordered by your doctor.*

Dosing—The dose of ipratropium will be different for different patients. *Follow your doctor's orders or the directions on the label.* The following information includes only the average doses of ipratropium. *If your dose is different, do not change it* unless your doctor tells you to do so.

 • For symptoms of lung diseases, such as bronchial asthma, chronic bronchitis, or emphysema:

   —For *inhalation aerosol* dosage form:

     • Adults and children 12 years of age and older—18 to 40 micrograms (mcg) (1 or 2 puffs) three or four times a day, at regularly spaced times.

     • Children up to 12 years of age—Use and dose must be determined by your doctor.

   —For *inhalation solution* dosage form:

     • Adults and children 12 years of age and older—250 to 500 mcg mixed, if necessary, with the sodium chloride solution provided with this medicine, to make 3 to 5 milliliters (mL) of solution. This mixture is used in a nebulizer three or four times a day, every six to eight hours.

• Children 5 to 12 years of age—125 to 250 mcg mixed, if necessary, with the sodium chloride solution provided with this medicine, to make 3 to 5 milliliters (mL) of solution. This mixture is used in a nebulizer three or four times a day, every four to six hours as needed.

• Children up to 5 years of age—Use and dose must be determined by your doctor.

Missed dose—If you use ipratropium inhalation regularly and you miss a dose of this medicine, use it as soon as possible. Then use any remaining doses for that day at regularly spaced times.

Storage—To store this medicine:

• Keep out of the reach of children.
• Store away from heat.
• Store the solution form of this medicine away from direct light. Store the aerosol form of this medicine away from direct sunlight.
• Keep the medicine from freezing.
• Store any opened bottles of the solution form of this medicine in the refrigerator.
• Do not puncture, break, or burn the aerosol container, even if it is empty.
• Do not keep outdated medicine or medicine no longer needed. Be sure that any discarded medicine is out of the reach of children.

Precautions While Using This Medicine

Check with your doctor at once if your symptoms do not improve within 30 minutes after using a dose of this medicine or if your condition gets worse.

For patients using *ipratropium inhalation solution:*

*   *If you are also using cromolyn inhalation solution, do not mix that solution with the ipratropium inhalation solution from the 20-mL multiple-dose vial for use in a nebulizer.* To do so will cause the solution to become cloudy and prevent the cromolyn from working properly. However, if your condition requires you to use cromolyn inhalation solution with ipratropium inhalation solution, it may be mixed with ipratropium inhalation solution from the 2-mL single-dose vial.

Ipratropium may cause dryness of the mouth or throat. For temporary relief of mouth dryness, use sugarless candy or gum, melt bits of ice in your mouth, or use a saliva substitute. However, if your mouth continues to feel dry for more than 2 weeks, check with your medical doctor or dentist. Continuing dryness of the mouth may increase the chance of dental disease, including tooth decay, gum disease, and fungus infections.

Side Effects of This Medicine

Along with its needed effects, a medicine may cause some unwanted effects. Although not all of these side effects may occur, if they do occur they may require medical attention.

Check with your doctor as soon as possible if any of the following side effects occur:

Less common

Increased wheezing, tightness in chest, or difficulty in breathing

Rare

Difficulty in swallowing; severe eye pain; skin rash or hives; swelling of tongue or lips; ulcers or sores in mouth and on lips

Other side effects may occur that usually do not need medical attention. These side effects may go away during

treatment as your body adjusts to the medicine. However, check with your doctor if any of the following side effects continue or are bothersome:

More common

Cough or dryness of mouth or throat; headache or dizziness; nervousness; stomach upset or nausea

Less common or rare

Blurred vision or other changes in vision; constipation (continuing); difficult urination; metallic or unpleasant taste; pounding heartbeat; stuffy nose; trembling; trouble in sleeping; unusual tiredness or weakness

Other side effects not listed above may also occur in some patients. If you notice any other effects, check with your doctor.

KETOROLAC Systemic

Some commonly used brand names are:

In the U.S.—
Toradol*IM*   Toradol*ORAL*

In Canada—
Toradol   Toradol*IM*

Description

Ketorolac (kee-TOE-role-ak) is used to relieve pain. It belongs to the group of medicines called anti-inflammatory analgesics. Ketorolac is not a narcotic and is not habit-forming. It will not cause physical or mental dependence, as narcotics can. However, ketorolac is sometimes used together with a narcotic to provide better pain relief than either medicine used alone.

Ketorolac is available only with your doctor's prescription, in the following dosage forms:

Oral
- Tablets (U.S. and Canada)

Parenteral
- Injection (U.S. and Canada)

Before Using This Medicine

In deciding to use a medicine, the risks of taking the medicine must be weighed against the good it will do. This is a decision you and your doctor will make. For ketorolac, the following should be considered:

Allergies—Tell your doctor if you have ever had any unusual or allergic reaction to ketorolac or to any of the following medicines:

Aspirin or other salicylates
Diclofenac (e.g., Voltaren)
Diflunisal (e.g., Dolobid)
Etodolac (e.g., Lodine)
Fenoprofen (e.g., Nalfon)
Floctafenine (e.g., Idarac)
Flurbiprofen, oral (e.g., Ansaid)
Ibuprofen (e.g., Motrin)
Indomethacin (e.g., Indocin)
Ketoprofen (e.g., Orudis)
Meclofenamate (e.g., Meclomen)
Mefenamic acid (e.g., Ponstel)
Nabumetone (e.g., Relafen)
Naproxen (e.g., Naprosyn)
Oxaprozin (e.g., Daypro)
Oxyphenbutazone (e.g., Tandearil)
Phenylbutazone (e.g., Butazolidin)
Piroxicam (e.g., Feldene)
Sulindac (e.g., Clinoril)
Suprofen (e.g., Suprol)
Tenoxicam (e.g., Mobiflex)
Tiaprofenic acid (e.g., Surgam)
Tolmetin (e.g., Tolectin)
Zomepirac (e.g., Zomax)

Also tell your health care professional if you are allergic to any other substances, such as foods, preservatives, or dyes.

Pregnancy—Studies on birth defects with ketorolac have not been done in pregnant women. However, it crosses the placenta. There is a chance that regular use of ketorolac during the last few months of pregnancy may cause unwanted effects on the heart or blood flow of the fetus or newborn baby. Ketorolac has not been shown to cause birth defects in animal studies. However, animal studies have shown that, if taken late in pregnancy, ketorolac may increase the length of pregnancy, prolong labor, or cause other problems during delivery.

Breast-feeding—Small amounts of ketorolac pass into the breast milk. Mothers who are taking this medicine and who wish to breast-feed should discuss this with their doctor.

Children—Studies on this medicine have been done only in adult patients, and there is no specific information comparing use of ketorolac in children with use in other age groups.

Older adults—Stomach or intestinal problems, swelling of the face, feet, or lower legs, or sudden decrease in the amount of urine, may be especially likely to occur in elderly patients, who are usually more sensitive than younger adults to the effects of anti-inflammatory analgesics such as ketorolac. Also, elderly people are more likely than younger adults to get very sick if the medicine causes stomach problems. Studies in older adults have shown that ketorolac stays in the body longer than it does in younger people. Your doctor will consider this when deciding on how much ketorolac should be given for each dose and how often it should be given.

Other medicines—Although certain medicines should not be used together at all, in other cases two different medicines may be used together even if an interaction might

occur. In these cases, your doctor may want to change the dose, or other precautions may be necessary. When you are using ketorolac, it is especially important that your health care professional know if you are taking any of the following:

- Anticoagulants (blood thinners) or
- Cefamandole (e.g., Mandol) or
- Cefoperazone (e.g., Cefobid) or
- Cefotetan (e.g., Cefotan) or
- Heparin or
- Moxalactam (e.g., Moxam) or
- Plicamycin (e.g., Mithracin) or
- Valproic acid (e.g., Depakene)—Use of any of these medicines together with ketorolac may increase the chance of bleeding
- Aspirin or other salicylates or
- Other medicine for inflammation or pain, except narcotics— The chance of serious side effects may be increased
- Lithium (e.g., Lithane) or
- Methotrexate (e.g., Mexate)—Higher blood levels of lithium or methotrexate and an increased chance of side effects may occur
- Probenecid (e.g., Benemid)—Higher blood levels of ketorolac and an increased chance of side effects may occur

Other medical problems—The presence of other medical problems may affect the use of ketorolac. Make sure you tell your doctor if you smoke tobacco or if you have any other medical problems, especially:

- Alcohol abuse or
- Diabetes mellitus (sugar diabetes) or
- Edema (swelling of face, fingers, feet or lower legs caused by too much fluid in the body) or
- Kidney disease or
- Liver disease (severe) or
- Systemic lupus erythematosus (SLE)—The chance of serious side effects may be increased
- Asthma or
- Colitis, stomach ulcer, or other stomach problems or
- Heart disease or

- High blood pressure—Ketorolac may make your condition worse
- Hemophilia or other bleeding problems—Ketorolac may increase the chance of serious bleeding

---

Proper Use of This Medicine

For patients taking *ketorolac tablets:*

- To lessen stomach upset, ketorolac tablets should be taken with food (a meal or a snack) or with an antacid. However, your doctor may want you to take the first few doses 30 minutes before meals or 2 hours after meals. This helps the medicine work a little faster when you first begin to take it.
- Take this medicine with a full glass of water. Also, do not lie down for about 15 to 30 minutes after taking it. This helps to prevent irritation that may lead to trouble in swallowing.

For patients using *ketorolac injection*:

- Medicines given by injection are sometimes used at home. If you will be using ketorolac at home, your health care professional will teach you how the injections are to be given. You will also have a chance to practice giving injections. *Be certain that you understand exactly how the medicine is to be injected.*

For safe and effective use of this medicine, do not use more of it, do not use it more often, and do not use it for a longer time than ordered by your doctor. Using too much of this medicine increases the chance of unwanted effects, especially in elderly patients.

Dosing—The dose of ketorolac will be different for different patients. *Follow your doctor's orders or the directions on the label.* The following information includes only the average doses of ketorolac. *If your dose is different, do not change it* unless your doctor tells you to do so.

- For *oral* dosage form (tablets):
  —For pain:
  - Adults—One 10-milligram (mg) tablet four times a day, four to six hours apart. Your doctor may want you to take two tablets for the first dose only. This helps the medicine start working a little faster.
  - Children—Use and dose must be determined by your doctor.
- For *injection* dosage form:
  —For pain:
  - Adults—15 or 30 mg four times a day, at least 4 to 6 hours apart. This amount of medicine may be contained in 1 mL or in one-half (0.5) mL of the injection, depending on the strength. Sometimes, larger amounts are used for the first dose only. This helps the medicine start working a little faster.
  - Children—Use and dose must be determined by your doctor.

Missed dose—If you have been directed to use this medicine according to a regular schedule, and you miss a dose, use it as soon as possible. However, if it is almost time for your next dose, skip the missed dose and go back to your regular dosing schedule. Do not double doses.

Storage—To store this medicine:

- Keep out of the reach of children.
- Store away from heat and direct light.
- Do not store ketorolac tablets in the bathroom, near the kitchen sink, or in other damp places. Heat or moisture may cause the medicine to break down.
- Keep the injection form of ketorolac from freezing. Do not store it in the refrigerator.
- Do not keep outdated medicine or medicine no longer

needed. Be sure that any discarded medicine is out of the reach of children.

Precautions While Using This Medicine

Taking certain other medicines together with ketorolac may increase the chance of unwanted effects. The risk will depend on how much of each medicine you take every day, and on how long you take the medicines together. Therefore, do not take acetaminophen (e.g., Tylenol) or aspirin or other salicylates together with ketorolac for more than a few days, unless otherwise directed by your medical doctor or dentist. Also, *do not take any of the following medicines together with ketorolac, unless your medical doctor or dentist has directed you to do so and is following your progress*:

Diclofenac (e.g., Voltaren)
Diflunisal (e.g., Dolobid)
Etodolac (e.g., Lodine)
Fenoprofen (e.g., Nalfon)
Floctafenine (e.g., Idarac)
Flurbiprofen, oral (e.g., Ansaid)
Ibuprofen (e.g., Motrin)
Indomethacin (e.g., Indocin)
Ketoprofen (e.g., Orudis)
Meclofenamate (e.g., Meclomen)
Mefenamic acid (e.g., Ponstel)
Nabumetone (e.g., Relafen)
Naproxen (e.g., Naprosyn)
Oxaprozin (e.g., Daypro)
Phenylbutazone (e.g., Butazolidin)
Piroxicam (e.g., Feldene)
Sulindac (e.g., Clinoril)
Tenoxicam (e.g., Mobiflex)
Tiaprofenic acid (e.g., Surgam)
Tolmetin (e.g., Tolectin)

Ketorolac may cause some people to become dizzy or drowsy. If either of these side effects occurs, *do not drive,*

*use machines, or do anything else that could be dangerous
if you are not alert.*

Side Effects of This Medicine

Along with its needed effects, a medicine may cause some
unwanted effects. Although not all of these side effects
may occur, if they do occur they may need medical
attention.

*Stop using this medicine and check with your doctor imme-
diately if any of the following side effects occur:*

Rare

Bleeding or crusting sores on lips; blue lips and fingernails; chest pain; convulsions; fainting; shortness of
breath, fast, irregular, noisy or troubled breathing, tightness in chest, and/or wheezing; vomiting of blood or
material that looks like coffee grounds

Also, check with your doctor as soon as possible if any
of the following side effects occur:

Less common

Swelling of face, fingers, lower legs, ankles, and/or feet;
weight gain (unusual)

Rare

Abdominal or stomach pain, cramping, or burning (severe); bleeding from rectum or bloody or black, tarry
stools; bloody or cloudy urine; bruising (not at place
of injection) or small red spots on skin; burning, red,
tender, thick, scaly, or peeling skin; decrease in amount
of urine (sudden); fever with or without chills or sore
throat; hallucinations (seeing, hearing, or feeling things
that are not there); hives or itching of skin; increased
blood pressure; increased sweating; muscle cramps or
pain; nausea, heartburn, and/or indigestion (severe and
continuing); nosebleeds; pain in lower back and/or side;
puffiness or swelling of the eyelids or around the eyes;
skin rash; sores, ulcers, or white spots on lips or in

mouth; swollen and/or painful glands; swollen tongue; thirst (continuing); unusual tiredness or weakness

Other side effects may occur that usually do not need medical attention. These side effects may go away during treatment as your body adjusts to the medicine. However, check with your doctor if any of the following side effects continue or are bothersome:

More common

Abdominal or stomach pain (mild or moderate); bruising at place of injection; drowsiness; indigestion; nausea

Less common or rare

Bloating or gas; burning or pain at place of injection; constipation; diarrhea; dizziness; feeling of fullness in abdominal or stomach area; headache; increased sweating; vomiting

Other side effects not listed above may also occur in some patients. If you notice any other effects, check with your doctor.

LEVODOPA   Systemic

Some commonly used brand names are:

In the U.S.—

Dopar[2]

Larodopa[2]

Sinemet[1]

Sinemet CR[1]

In Canada—

Larodopa[2]

Sinemet[1]

Sinemet CR[1]

Note: For quick reference, the following levodopa are numbered to match the corresponding brand names.

This information applies to the following medicines:

1. Carbidopa and Levodopa (KAR-bi-doe-pa and LEE-voe-doe-pa)
2. Levodopa

Description

Levodopa is used alone or in combination with carbidopa to treat Parkinson's disease, sometimes referred to as shaking palsy or paralysis agitans. Some patients require the combination of medicine, while others benefit from levodopa alone. By improving muscle control, this medicine allows more normal movements of the body.

Levodopa alone or in combination is available only with your doctor's prescription. It is available in the following dosage forms:

Oral

Carbidopa and Levodopa
- Tablets (U.S. and Canada)
- Extended-release tablets (U.S. and Canada)

Levodopa
- Capsules (U.S.)
- Tablets (U.S. and Canada)

Before Using This Medicine

In deciding to use a medicine, the risks of taking the medicine must be weighed against the good it will do. This is a decision you and your doctor will make. For levodopa and for carbidopa and levodopa combination, the following should be considered:

Allergies—Tell your doctor if you have ever had any unusual or allergic reaction to levodopa alone or in combination with carbidopa. Also tell your health care professional if you are allergic to any other substances, such as foods, preservatives, or dyes.

Diet—Since protein may interfere with the body's response to levodopa, high protein diets should be avoided. Intake of normal amounts of protein should be spaced equally throughout the day.

For patients taking levodopa by itself:
- Pyridoxine (vitamin B_6) has been found to reduce the effects of levodopa when levodopa is taken by itself. This does not happen with the combination of carbi-

dopa and levodopa. *If you are taking levodopa by itself, do not take vitamin products containing vitamin B_6 during treatment, unless prescribed by your doctor.*

- Large amounts of pyridoxine are also contained in some foods such as avocado, bacon, beans, beef liver, dry skim milk, oatmeal, peas, pork, sweet potato, tuna, and certain health foods. Check with your doctor about how much of these foods you may have in your diet while you are taking levodopa. Also, ask your health care professional for help when selecting vitamin products.

Pregnancy—Studies have not been done in pregnant women. However, studies in animals have shown that levodopa affects the baby's growth both before and after birth if given during pregnancy in doses many times the human dose. Also, studies in rabbits have shown that levodopa, alone or in combination with carbidopa, causes birth defects.

Breast-feeding—Levodopa and carbidopa pass into the breast milk and may cause unwanted side effects in the nursing baby. Also, levodopa may reduce the flow of breast milk.

Children—Studies on this medicine have been done only in adult patients, and there is no specific information comparing use of levodopa or carbidopa in children with use in other age groups.

Older adults—Elderly people are especially sensitive to the effects of levodopa. This may increase the chance of side effects during treatment.

Other medicines—Although certain medicines should not be used together at all, in other cases two different medicines may be used together even if an interaction might occur. In these cases, your doctor may want to change the dose, or other precautions may be necessary. When you are taking levodopa or carbidopa and levodopa combination, it is especially important that your health care professional know if you are taking any of the following:

- Cocaine—Cocaine use by individuals taking levodopa, alone or in combination with carbidopa, may cause an irregular heartbeat

- Ethotoin (e.g., Peganone) or

- Haloperidol (e.g., Haldol) or

- Mephenytoin (e.g., Mesantoin) or

- Phenothiazines (acetophenazine [e.g., Tindal], chlorpromazine [e.g., Thorazine], fluphenazine [e.g., Prolixin], mesoridazine [e.g., Serentil], perphenazine [e.g., Trilafon], prochlorperazine [e.g., Compazine], promazine [e.g., Sparine], promethazine [e.g., Phenergan], thioridazine [e.g., Mellaril], trifluoperazine [e.g., Stelazine], triflupromazine [e.g., Vesprin], trimeprazine [e.g., Temaril]) or

- Phenytoin (e.g., Dilantin)—Taking these medicines with levodopa may lessen the effects of levodopa

- Monoamine oxidase (MAO) inhibitors (furazolidone [e.g., Furoxone], isocarboxazid [e.g., Marplan], phenelzine [e.g., Nardil], procarbazine [e.g., Matulane], tranylcypromine [e.g., Parnate])—Taking levodopa while you are taking or within 2 weeks of taking monoamine oxidase (MAO) inhibitors may cause sudden extremely high blood pressure; at least 14 days should be allowed between stopping treatment with one medicine and starting treatment with the other medicine

- Pyridoxine (vitamin B$_6$, e.g., Hexa-Betalin), present in some foods and vitamin formulas (for levodopa used alone)— Pyridoxine reverses the effects of levodopa

- Selegiline—Dosage of levodopa or carbidopa and levodopa combination may need to be decreased

Other medical problems—The presence of other medical problems may affect the use of levodopa. Make sure you tell your doctor if you have any other medical problems, especially:

- Diabetes mellitus (sugar diabetes)—The amount of insulin or antidiabetic medicine that you need to take may change

- Emphysema, asthma, bronchitis, or other chronic lung disease or

- Glaucoma or
- Heart or blood vessel disease or
- Hormone problems or
- Melanoma (a type of skin cancer) (or history of) or
- Mental illness—Levodopa may make the condition worse
- Kidney disease or
- Liver disease—Higher blood levels of levodopa may occur, increasing the chance of side effects
- Seizure disorders, such as epilepsy (history of)—The risk of seizures may be increased
- Stomach ulcer (history of)—The ulcer may occur again

Proper Use of This Medicine

It is best not to take this medicine with or after food, especially high-protein food, since food may decrease levodopa's effect. However, *to lessen possible stomach upset, your doctor may want you to take food shortly after taking this medicine (about 15 minutes after)*. If stomach upset is severe or continues, check with your doctor.

Take this medicine only as directed. Do not take more or less of it, and do not take it more often than your doctor ordered.

For patients taking *carbidopa and levodopa extended-release tablets*:

- Swallow the tablet whole without crushing or chewing, unless your doctor tells you not to. If your doctor tells you to, you may break the tablet in half.

Some people must take this medicine for several weeks or months before full benefit is received. *Do not stop taking it even if you do not think it is working*. Instead, check with your doctor.

Dosing—The dose of levodopa or carbidopa and levodopa combination will be different for different patients. *Follow your doctor's orders or the directions on the label.* The

following information includes only the average doses of
levodopa or carbidopa and levodopa combination. *If your
dose is different, do not change it* unless your doctor tells
you to do so.

The number of capsules or tablets that you take depends
on the strength of the medicine. Also, *the number of doses
you take each day, the time allowed between doses, and
the length of time you take the medicine depend on your
special needs*.

For levodopa

• For Parkinson's disease:

—For *oral* dosage form (capsules and tablets):

• Adults and teenagers—At first, 250 milligrams
(mg) two to four times a day. Your doctor may
increase your dose if needed. However, the dose
is usually not more than 8000 mg a day.

• Children up to 12 years of age—Use and dose
must be determined by your doctor.

For levodopa and carbidopa combination

• For Parkinson's disease:

—For *oral tablet* dosage form:

• Adults—At first, 1 tablet three or four times a
day. Your doctor may need to change your dose,
depending on how you respond to this combination medicine.

• Children and teenagers—Use and dose must be
determined by your doctor.

—For *oral extended-release tablet* dosage form:

• Adults—At first, 1 tablet two times a day. However, you may need to take more than this. Your
doctor will decide the right dose for you, depending on your condition and the other medicines you may be taking for Parkinson's disease.

• Children and teenagers—Use and dose must be
determined by your doctor.

Missed dose—If you miss a dose of this medicine, take it as soon as possible. However, if your next scheduled dose is within 2 hours, skip the missed dose and go back to your regular dosing schedule. Do not double doses.

Storage—To store this medicine:

- Keep out of the reach of children.
- Store away from heat and direct light.
- Do not store in the bathroom, near the kitchen sink, or in other damp places. Heat or moisture may cause the medicine to break down.
- Do not keep outdated medicine or medicine no longer needed. Be sure that any discarded medicine is out of the reach of children.

Precautions While Using This Medicine

Before having any kind of surgery (including dental surgery) or emergency treatment, tell the medical doctor or dentist in charge that you are taking this medicine.

For *diabetic patients*:

- This medicine may cause test results for urine sugar or ketones to be wrong. Check with your doctor before depending on home tests using the paper-strip or tablet method.

This medicine may cause some people to become drowsy or less alert than they are normally. *Make sure you know how you react to this medicine before you drive, use machines, or do anything else that could be dangerous if you are not alert.*

Dizziness, lightheadedness, or fainting may occur, especially when you get up from a lying or sitting position. Getting up slowly may help. If the problem continues or gets worse, check with your doctor.

For patients taking levodopa by itself:

- Pyridoxine (vitamin B$_6$) has been found to reduce the effects of levodopa when levodopa is taken by itself. This does not happen with the combination of carbidopa and levodopa. *If you are taking levodopa by itself, do not take vitamin products containing vitamin B$_6$ during* treatment, unless prescribed by your doctor.

- Large amounts of pyridoxine are also contained in some foods such as avocado, bacon, beans, beef liver, dry skim milk, oatmeal, peas, pork, sweet potato, tuna, and certain health foods. Check with your doctor about how much of these foods you may have in your diet while you are taking levodopa. Also, ask your health care professional for help when selecting vitamin products.

As your condition improves and your body movements become easier, *be careful not to overdo physical activities. Injuries resulting from falls may occur.* Physical activities must be increased gradually to allow your body to adjust to changing balance, circulation, and coordination. *This is especially important in the elderly.*

After taking this medicine for long periods of time, such as a year or more, some patients suddenly lose the ability to move. Their muscles do not seem to work. This loss of movement may last from a few minutes to several hours. The patient then is able to move as before. This condition may unexpectedly occur again and again. If you should have this problem, sometimes called the ''on-off'' effect, check with your doctor.

Side Effects of This Medicine

Along with its needed effects, a medicine may cause some unwanted effects. Although not all of these side effects

may occur, if they do occur they may need medical attention.

Check with your doctor as soon as possible if any of the following side effects occur:

More common

Mental depression; mood or mental changes (such as aggressive behavior); unusual and uncontrolled movements of the body

Less common—more common when levodopa is used alone

Difficult urination; dizziness or lightheadedness when getting up from a lying or sitting position; irregular heartbeat; nausea or vomiting (severe or continuing); spasm or closing of eyelids (not more common when levodopa is used alone)

Rare

High blood pressure; stomach pain; unusual tiredness or weakness

Other side effects may occur that usually do not need medical attention. These side effects may go away during treatment as your body adjusts to the medicine. However, check with your doctor if any of the following side effects continue or are bothersome:

More common

Anxiety, confusion, or nervousness (especially in elderly patients receiving other medicine for Parkinson's disease)

Less common

Constipation (more common when levodopa is used alone); diarrhea; dryness of mouth; flushing of skin; headache; loss of appetite; muscle twitching; nightmares (more common when levodopa is used alone); trouble in sleeping

This medicine may sometimes cause the urine and sweat to be darker in color than usual. The urine may at first be reddish, then turn to nearly black after being exposed to air. Some bathroom cleaning products will produce a similar effect when in contact with urine containing this medicine. This is to be expected during treatment with this medicine.

Other side effects not listed above may also occur in some patients. If you notice any other effects, check with your doctor.

LITHIUM   Systemic

Some commonly used brand names are:

In the U.S.—

Cibalith-S	Lithobid
Eskalith	Lithonate
Eskalith CR	Lithotabs
Lithane	

Generic name product may also be available.

In Canada—

Carbolith	Lithane
Duralith	Lithizine

Description

Lithium (LITH-ee-um) is used to treat the manic stage of bipolar disorder (manic-depressive illness). Manic-depressive patients experience severe mood changes, ranging from an excited or manic state (for example, unusual anger or irritability or a false sense of well-being) to depression or sadness. Lithium is used to reduce the frequency and severity of manic states. Lithium may also reduce the frequency and severity of depression in bipolar disorder.

It is not known how lithium works to stabilize a person's mood. However, it does act on the central nervous system. It helps you to have more control over your emotions and helps you cope better with the problems of living.

It is important that you and your family understand all the effects of lithium. These effects depend on your individual condition and response and the amount of lithium you use. You also must know when to contact your doctor if there are problems with the medicine's use. Lithium may also be used for other conditions as determined by your doctor.

This medicine is available only with your doctor's prescription, in the following dosage forms:

Oral
- Capsules (U.S. and Canada)
- Slow-release capsules (Canada)
- Syrup (U.S.)
- Tablets (U.S. and Canada)
- Extended-release tablets (U.S. and Canada)

Before Using This Medicine

In deciding to use a medicine, the risks of taking the medicine must be weighed against the good it will do. This is a decision you and your doctor will make. For lithium, the following should be considered:

Allergies—Tell your doctor if you have ever had any unusual or allergic reaction to lithium. Also tell your health care professional if you are allergic to any other substances, such as foods, preservatives, or dyes.

Diet—Make certain your health care professional knows if you are on a low-sodium or low-salt diet. Too little salt in your diet could lead to serious side effects.

Pregnancy—Lithium is not recommended for use during pregnancy, especially during the first 3 months. Studies have shown that lithium may rarely cause thyroid problems and heart or blood vessel defects in the baby. It has also been shown to cause muscle weakness and severe drowsiness in newborn babies of mothers taking lithium near time of delivery.

Breast-feeding—Lithium passes into the breast milk. It has been reported to cause unwanted effects such as muscle weakness, lowered body temperature, and heart problems in nursing babies. Before taking this medicine, be sure you have discussed with your doctor the risks and benefits of breast-feeding.

Children—Lithium may cause weakened bones in children during treatment.

Older adults—Unusual thirst, an increase in amount of urine, diarrhea, drowsiness, loss of appetite, muscle weakness, trembling, slurred speech, nausea or vomiting, goiter, or symptoms of underactive thyroid are especially likely to occur in elderly patients, who are often more sensitive than younger adults to the effects of lithium.

Other medicines—Although certain medicines should not be used together at all, in other cases two different medicines may be used together even if an interaction might occur. In these cases, your doctor may want to change the dose, or other precautions may be necessary. When you are taking lithium, it is especially important that your health care professional know if you are taking any of the following:

- Antipsychotics (medicine for mental illness)—Blood levels of both medicines may change, increasing the chance of serious side effects
- Diuretics (water pills) or
- Inflammation or pain medicine, except narcotics—Higher blood levels of lithium may occur, increasing the chance of serious side effects
- Medicine for asthma, bronchitis, emphysema, sinusitis, or cystic fibrosis that contains the following:
  Calcium iodide or
  Iodinated glycerol or
  Potassium iodide—Unwanted effects on the thyroid gland may occur

Other medical problems—The presence of other medical problems may affect the use of lithium. Make sure you tell your doctor if you have any other medical problems, especially:

- Brain disease or
- Schizophrenia—You may be especially sensitive to lithium, and mental effects (such as increased confusion) may occur
- Diabetes mellitus (sugar diabetes)—Lithium may increase the blood levels of insulin; the dose of insulin you need to take may change
- Difficult urination or
- Infection (severe, occurring with fever, prolonged sweating, diarrhea, or vomiting) or
- Kidney disease—Higher blood levels of lithium may occur, increasing the chance of serious side effects
- Epilepsy or
- Goiter or other thyroid disease, or
- Heart disease or
- Parkinson's disease or
- Psoriasis—Lithium may make the condition worse
- Leukemia (history of)—Lithium may cause the leukemia to occur again

Proper Use of This Medicine

Take this medicine after a meal or snack. Doing so will reduce stomach upset, tremors, or weakness and may also prevent a laxative effect.

For patients taking the *long-acting or slow-release form* of lithium:

- Swallow the tablet or capsule whole.
- Do not break, crush, or chew before swallowing.

For patients taking the *syrup form* of lithium:

- Dilute the syrup in fruit juice or another flavored beverage before taking.

During treatment with lithium, drink 2 or 3 quarts of water or other fluids each day, and use a normal amount of salt in your food, unless otherwise directed by your doctor.

Take this medicine exactly as directed. Do not take more or less of it, do not take it more or less often, and do not take it for a longer time than your doctor ordered. To do so may increase the chance of unwanted effects.

Sometimes lithium must be taken for 1 to several weeks before you begin to feel better.

In order for lithium to work properly, it must be taken every day in regularly spaced doses as ordered by your doctor. This is necessary to keep a constant amount of lithium in your blood. To help keep the amount constant, do not miss any doses and *do not stop taking the medicine even if you feel better.*

Dosing—The dose of lithium will be different for different patients. *Follow your doctor's orders or the directions on the label.* The following information includes only the average doses of lithium. *If your dose is different, do not change it* unless your doctor tells you to do so.

The number of capsules or tablets or teaspoonfuls of syrup that you take depends on the strength of the medicine. Also, *the number of doses you take each day, the time allowed between doses, and the length of time you take the medicine depend on the medical problem for which you are using lithium.*

- For *short-acting oral* dosage forms (capsules, tablets, syrup):

  —Adults and adolescents: To start, 300 to 600 milligrams three times a day.

  —Children up to 12 years of age: The dose is based on body weight. To start, the usual dose is 15 to 20 milligrams per kilogram of body weight (6.8 to 9 milligrams per pound) a day, given in smaller doses two or three times during the day.

- For *long-acting oral* dosage forms (slow-release capsules, extended-release tablets):

—Adults and adolescents: 300 to 600 milligrams three times a day, or 450 to 900 milligrams two times a day.

—Children up to 12 years of age: Dose must be determined by the doctor.

Missed dose—If you miss a dose of this medicine, take it as soon as possible. However, if it is within 4 hours (about 6 hours for extended-release tablets or slow-release capsules) of your next dose, skip the missed dose and go back to your regular dosing schedule. Do not double doses.

Storage—To store this medicine:

- Keep out of the reach of children.
- Store away from heat and direct light.
- Do not store in the bathroom, near the kitchen sink, or in other damp places. Heat or moisture may cause the medicine to break down.
- Keep the syrup form of this medicine from freezing.
- Do not keep outdated medicine or medicine no longer needed. Be sure that any discarded medicine is out of the reach of children.

Precautions While Using This Medicine

Your doctor should check your progress at regular visits to make sure that the medicine is working properly and that possible side effects are avoided. Laboratory tests may be necessary.

Lithium may not work properly if you drink large amounts of caffeine-containing coffee, tea, or colas.

This medicine may cause some people to become dizzy, drowsy, or less alert than they are normally. *Make sure you know how you react to this medicine before you drive, use machines, or do anything else that could be dangerous if you are dizzy or are not alert.*

Use extra care in hot weather and during activities that cause you to sweat heavily, such as hot baths, saunas, or exercising. The loss of too much water and salt from your body could lead to serious side effects from this medicine.

If you have an infection or illness that causes heavy sweating, vomiting, or diarrhea, check with your doctor. The loss of too much water and salt from your body could lead to serious side effects from lithium.

Do not go on a diet to lose weight and do not make a major change in your diet without first checking with your doctor. Improper dieting could cause the loss of too much water and salt from your body and could lead to serious side effects from this medicine.

For patients taking the *slow-release capsules or the extended-release tablets:*

- Do not use this medicine interchangeably with other lithium products.

It is important that you and your family know the early symptoms of lithium overdose or toxicity and when to call the doctor.

Side Effects of This Medicine

Along with its needed effects, a medicine may cause some unwanted effects. Although not all of these side effects may occur, if they do occur they may need medical attention.

Check with your doctor immediately if any of the following side effects occur:

   Early symptoms of overdose or toxicity

> Diarrhea; drowsiness; loss of appetite; muscle weakness; nausea or vomiting; slurred speech; trembling

Late symptoms of overdose or toxicity

> Blurred vision; clumsiness or unsteadiness; confusion; convulsions (seizures); dizziness; increase in amount of urine; trembling (severe)

Check with your doctor as soon as possible if any of the following side effects occur:

Less common

> Fainting; fast or slow heartbeat; irregular pulse; troubled breathing (especially during hard work or exercise); unusual tiredness or weakness; weight gain

Rare

> Blue color and pain in fingers and toes; coldness of arms and legs; dizziness; eye pain; headache; noises in the ears; vision problems

Signs of low thyroid function

> Dry, rough skin; hair loss; hoarseness; mental depression; sensitivity to cold; swelling of feet or lower legs; swelling of neck; unusual excitement

Other side effects may occur that usually do not need medical attention. These side effects may go away during treatment as your body adjusts to the medicine. However, check with your doctor if any of the following side effects continue or are bothersome:

More common

> Increased frequency of urination or loss of bladder control—more common in women than in men, usually beginning 2 to 7 years after start of treatment; increased thirst; nausea (mild); trembling of hands (slight)

Less common

> Acne or skin rash; bloated feeling or pressure in the stomach; muscle twitching (slight)

Other side effects not listed above may also occur in some patients. If you notice any other effects, check with your doctor.

Additional Information

Once a medicine has been approved for marketing for a certain use, experience may show that it is also useful for other medical problems. Although these uses are not included in product labeling, lithium is used in certain patients with the following medical conditions:

- Cluster headaches
- Mental depression
- Neutropenia (a blood condition in which there is a decreased number of a certain type of white blood cells)

Other than the above information, there is no additional information relating to proper use, precautions, or side effects for these uses.

LOXAPINE   Systemic

Some commonly used brand names are:

In the U.S.—

Loxitane   Loxitane IM

Loxitane C

Generic name product may also be available.

In Canada—

Loxapac

Description

Loxapine (LOX-a-peen) is used to treat nervous, mental, and emotional conditions.

Loxapine is available only with your doctor's prescription, in the following dosage forms:

Oral

- Solution (U.S. and Canada)
- Capsules (U.S.)
- Tablets (Canada)

Parenteral
- Injection (U.S. and Canada)

Before Using This Medicine

In deciding to use a medicine, the risks of taking the medicine must be weighed against the good it will do. This is a decision you and your doctor will make. For loxapine, the following should be considered:

Allergies—Tell your doctor if you have ever had any unusual or allergic reaction to loxapine or amoxapine. Also tell your health care professional if you are allergic to any other substances, such as foods, preservatives, or dyes.

Pregnancy—Loxapine has not been shown to cause birth defects or other problems in humans. However, animal studies have shown unwanted effects in the fetus.

Breast-feeding—It is not known if loxapine passes into breast milk.

Children—Studies on this medicine have been done only in adult patients, and there is no specific information comparing use of loxapine in children with use in other age groups.

Older adults—Elderly patients are usually more sensitive than younger adults to the effects of loxapine. Constipation, dizziness or fainting, drowsiness, dry mouth, trembling of the hands and fingers, and symptoms of tardive dyskinesia (such as rapid, worm-like movements of the tongue or any other uncontrolled movements of the mouth, tongue, or jaw, and/or arms and legs) are especially likely to occur in elderly patients.

Other medicines—Although certain medicines should not be used together at all, in other cases two different medicines may be used together even if an interaction might

occur. In these cases, your doctor may want to change the dose, or other precautions may be necessary. When you are taking loxapine, it is especially important that your health care professional know if you are taking any of the following:

- Amoxapine (e.g., Asendin) or
- Methyldopa (e.g., Aldomet) or
- Metoclopramide (e.g., Reglan) or
- Metyrosine (e.g., Demser) or
- Other antipsychotics (medicine for mental illness) or
- Pemoline (e.g., Cylert) or
- Pimozide (e.g., Orap) or
- Promethazine (e.g., Phenergan) or
- Rauwolfia alkaloids (alseroxylon [e.g., Rauwiloid], deserpidine [e.g., Harmonyl], rauwolfia serpentina [e.g., Raudixin], reserpine [e.g., Serpasil]) or
- Trimeprazine (e.g., Temaril)—Taking these medicines with loxapine may increase the chance and seriousness of some side effects
- Central nervous system (CNS) depressants (medicine that causes drowsiness) or
- Tricyclic antidepressants (medicine for depression)—Taking these medicines with loxapine may increase the CNS depressant effects
- Guanadrel (e.g., Hylorel) or
- Guanethidine (e.g., Ismelin)—Loxapine may decrease the effects of these medicines

Other medical problems—The presence of other medical problems may affect the use of loxapine. Make sure you tell your doctor if you have any other medical problems, especially:

- Alcohol abuse—CNS depressant effects may be increased
- Difficult urination or
- Enlarged prostate or
- Glaucoma (or predisposition to) or
- Parkinson's disease—Loxapine may make the condition worse
- Heart or blood vessel disease—An increased risk of low blood pressure (hypotension) or changes in the rhythm of your heart may occur

- Liver disease—Higher blood levels of loxapine may occur, increasing the chance of side effects
- Seizure disorders—Loxapine may increase the risk of seizures

---

Proper Use of This Medicine

This medicine may be taken with food or a full glass (8 ounces) of water or milk to reduce stomach irritation.

For patients taking the *oral solution*:

- Measure the solution only with the dropper provided by the manufacturer. This will give a more accurate dose.

The liquid medicine must be mixed with orange juice or grapefruit juice just before you take it to make it easier to take.

Do not take more of this medicine, do not take it more often, and do not take it for a longer time than your doctor ordered. To do so may increase the chance of unwanted effects.

Dosing—The dose of loxapine will be different for different patients. *Follow your doctor's orders or the directions on the label.* The following information includes only the average doses of loxapine. *If your dose is different, do not change it* unless your doctor tells you to do so.

The number of capsules or tablets or amount of solution that you take depends on the strength of the medicine. Also, *the number of doses you take each day, the time allowed between doses, and the length of time you take the medicine depend on the medical problem for which you are taking loxapine.*

- For *oral* dosage forms (capsules, oral solution, or tablets):

—Adults: To start, 10 milligrams taken two times a day. Your doctor may increase your dose if needed.

—Children up to 16 years of age: The dose must be determined by the doctor.

• For *injection* dosage form:

—Adults: 12.5 to 50 milligrams every four to six hours, injected into a muscle.

—Children up to 16 years of age: The dose must be determined by the doctor.

Missed dose—If you miss a dose of this medicine, take it as soon as possible. However, if it is within one hour of your next dose, skip the missed dose and go back to your regular dosing schedule. Do not double doses.

Storage—To store this medicine:

• Keep out of the reach of children.

• Store away from heat and direct light.

• Do not store the capsule or tablet form of this medicine in the bathroom, near the kitchen sink, or in other damp places. Heat or moisture may cause the medicine to break down.

• Keep the liquid form of this medicine from freezing.

• Do not keep outdated medicine or medicine no longer needed. Be sure that any discarded medicine is out of the reach of children.

Precautions While Using This Medicine

Your doctor should check your progress at regular visits, especially during the first few months of treatment with this medicine. The amount of loxapine you take may be changed often to meet the needs of your condition and to help avoid side effects.

Do not stop taking this medicine without first checking with your doctor. Your doctor may want you to reduce gradually the amount you are taking before stopping completely. This will allow your body time to adjust and to keep your condition from becoming worse.

This medicine will add to the effects of alcohol and other CNS depressants (medicines that slow down the nervous system, possibly causing drowsiness). Some examples of CNS depressants are antihistamines or medicine for hay fever, other allergies, or colds; sedatives, tranquilizers, or sleeping medicine; prescription pain medicine or narcotics; barbiturates; medicine for seizures; or anesthetics, including some dental anesthetics. *Check with your doctor before taking any of the above while you are taking this medicine.*

Do not take this medicine within two hours of taking antacids or medicine for diarrhea. Taking loxapine and antacids or medicine for diarrhea too close together may make this medicine less effective.

This medicine may cause some people to become drowsy or less alert than they are normally, especially as the amount of medicine is increased. Even if you take this medicine at bedtime, you may feel drowsy or less alert on arising. *Make sure you know how you react to this medicine before you drive, use machines, or do anything else that could be dangerous if you are not alert.*

Although it is not a problem for most patients, dizziness, lightheadedness, or fainting may occur, especially when you get up from a lying or sitting position. Getting up slowly may help. However, if the problem continues or gets worse, check with your doctor.

Loxapine may cause your skin to be more sensitive to sunlight than it is normally. Exposure to sunlight, even for brief periods of time, may cause a skin rash, itching, redness or other discoloration of the skin, or a severe sunburn. When you begin taking this medicine:

- Stay out of direct sunlight, especially between the hours of 10:00 a.m. and 3:00 p.m., if possible.
- Wear protective clothing, including a hat. Also, wear sunglasses.
- Apply a sun block product that has a skin protection factor (SPF) of at least 15. Some patients may require a product with a higher SPF number, especially if they have a fair complexion. If you have any questions about this, check with your health care professional.
- Apply a sun block lipstick that has an SPF of at least 15 to protect your lips.
- Do not use a sunlamp or tanning bed or booth.

If you have a severe reaction from the sun, check with your doctor.

Loxapine may cause dryness of the mouth. For temporary relief, use sugarless candy or gum, melt bits of ice in your mouth, or use a saliva substitute. However, if your mouth continues to feel dry for more than 2 weeks, check with your medical doctor or dentist. Continuing dryness of the mouth may increase the chance of dental disease, including tooth decay, gum disease, and fungus infections.

Before having any kind of surgery, dental treatment, or emergency treatment, tell the medical doctor or dentist in charge that you are taking this medicine. Taking loxapine together with medicines that are used during surgery or dental or emergency treatments may increase the CNS depressant effects.

Side Effects of This Medicine

Along with its needed effects, loxapine can sometimes cause serious side effects. Tardive dyskinesia (a movement disorder) may occur and may not go away after you stop using the medicine. Signs of tardive dyskinesia include fine, worm-like movements of the tongue, or other uncontrolled movements of the mouth, tongue, cheeks, jaw, or arms and legs. Other serious but rare side effects may also occur. These include severe muscle stiffness, fever, unusual tiredness or weakness, fast heartbeat, difficult breathing, increased sweating, loss of bladder control, and seizures (neuroleptic malignant syndrome). *You and your doctor should discuss the good this medicine will do as well as the risks of taking it.*

Stop taking loxapine and get emergency help immediately if any of the following side effects occur:

> *Rare*
>> Convulsions (seizures); difficult or fast breathing; fast heartbeat or irregular pulse; fever (high); high or low blood pressure; increased sweating; loss of bladder control; muscle stiffness (severe); unusually pale skin; unusual tiredness or weakness

Check with your doctor immediately if any of the following side effects occur:

> *More common*
>> Lip smacking or puckering; puffing of cheeks; rapid or fine, worm-like movements of tongue; uncontrolled chewing movements; uncontrolled movements of arms or legs

Also, check with your doctor as soon as possible if any of the following side effects occur:

> *More common (occurring with increase of dosage)*
>> Difficulty in speaking or swallowing; loss of balance control; mask-like face; restlessness or desire to keep moving; shuffling walk; slowed movements; stiffness of arms and legs; trembling and shaking of fingers and hands

> *Less common*
>> Constipation (severe); difficult urination; inability to move eyes; muscle spasms, especially of the neck and back; skin rash; twisting movements of the body

Rare

   Sore throat and fever; increased blinking or spasms of
   eyelid; uncontrolled twisting movements of neck, trunk,
   arms, or legs; unusual bleeding or bruising; unusual
   facial expressions or body positions; yellow eyes or
   skin

Symptoms of overdose

   Dizziness (severe); drowsiness (severe); muscle trembling,
   jerking, stiffness, or uncontrolled movements (severe);
   troubled breathing (severe); unusual tiredness or weakness (severe)

Other side effects may occur that usually do not need
medical attention. These side effects may go away during
treatment as your body adjusts to the medicine. However,
check with your doctor if any of the following side effects
continue or are bothersome:

More common

   Blurred vision; confusion; dizziness, lightheadedness, or
   fainting; drowsiness; dryness of mouth

Less common

   Constipation (mild); decreased sexual ability; enlargement
   of breasts (males and females); headache; increased
   sensitivity of skin to sun; missing menstrual periods;
   nausea or vomiting; trouble in sleeping; unusual secretion of milk; weight gain

Certain side effects of this medicine may occur after you
have stopped taking it. Check with your doctor as soon as
possible if you notice any of the following effects after
you have stopped taking loxapine:

   Dizziness; nausea and vomiting; rapid or worm-like movements of the tongue; stomach upset or pain; trembling of
   fingers and hands; uncontrolled chewing movements

Other side effects not listed above may also occur in some
patients. If you notice any other effects, check with your
doctor.

Additional Information

Once a medicine has been approved for marketing for a certain use, experience may show that it is also useful for other medical problems. Although this use is not included in product labeling, loxapine is used in certain patients with the following medical condition:

- Anxiety associated with mental depression

Other than the above information, there is no additional information relating to proper use, precautions, or side effects for this use.

MAPROTILINE Systemic

A commonly used brand name in the U.S. and Canada is Ludiomil.
Generic name product may also be available in the U.S.

Description

Maprotiline (ma-PROE-ti-leen) is used to relieve mental depression, including anxiety that sometimes occurs with depression.

Maprotiline is available only with your doctor's prescription, in the following dosage form:

Oral
- Tablets (U.S. and Canada)

Before Using This Medicine

In deciding to use a medicine, the risks of taking the medicine must be weighed against the good it will do. This is a decision you and your doctor will make. For maprotiline, the following should be considered:

Allergies—Tell your doctor if you have ever had any unusual or allergic reaction to maprotiline or tricyclic antidepressants. Also tell your health care professional if you are allergic to any other substances, such as foods, preservatives, or dyes.

Pregnancy—Maprotiline has not been studied in pregnant women. However, this medicine has not been shown to cause birth defects or other problems in animal studies.

Breast-feeding—Maprotiline passes into the breast milk. However, this medicine has not been reported to cause problems in nursing babies.

Children—Studies on this medicine have been done only in adult patients, and there is no specific information comparing use of maprotiline in children with use in other age groups.

Older adults—Drowsiness, dizziness or lightheadedness; confusion; vision problems; dryness of mouth; constipation; and difficulty in urinating may be especially likely to occur in elderly patients, who are usually more sensitive than younger adults to the effects of maprotiline.

Other medicines—Although certain medicines should not be used together at all, in other cases two different medicines may be used together even if an interaction might occur. In these cases, your doctor may want to change the dose, or other precautions may be necessary. When you are taking maprotiline, it is especially important that your health care professional know if you are taking any of the following:

- Amphetamines or
- Appetite suppressants (diet pills) or
- Medicine for asthma or other breathing problems or
- Medicine for colds, sinus problems, or hay fever or other allergies (including nose drops or sprays)—Using these medicines with maprotiline may cause serious unwanted effects on your heart and blood pressure

- Central nervous system (CNS) depressants (medicines that cause drowsiness)—Taking these medicines with maprotiline may increase the CNS depressant effects
- Monoamine oxidase (MAO) inhibitors (furazolidone [e.g., Furoxone], isocarboxazid [e.g., Marplan], phenelzine [e.g., Nardil], procarbazine [e.g., Matulane], selegiline [e.g., Eldepryl], tranylcypromine [e.g., Parnate])—Taking maprotiline while you are taking or within 2 weeks of taking monoamine oxidase (MAO) inhibitors may cause very serious side effects, such as sudden high body temperature, extremely high blood pressure, and severe convulsions; at least 14 days should be allowed between stopping treatment with one medicine and starting treatment with the other

Other medical problems—The presence of other medical problems may affect the use of maprotiline. Make sure you tell your doctor if you have any other medical problems, especially:

- Alcohol abuse or
- Seizure disorders (including epilepsy)—The risk of seizures may be increased
- Asthma or
- Difficult urination or
- Enlarged prostate or
- Glaucoma or
- Mental illness (severe) or
- Stomach or intestinal problems—Maprotiline may make the condition worse
- Heart or blood vessel disease or
- Overactive thyroid—Serious effects on your heart may occur
- Liver disease—Higher blood levels of maprotiline may occur, increasing the chance of side effects

---

Proper Use of This Medicine

Take this medicine only as directed by your doctor to benefit your condition as much as possible. Do not take more of it, do not take it more often, and do not take it for a longer time than your doctor ordered.

Sometimes this medicine must be taken for up to two or three weeks before you begin to feel better. Your doctor should check your progress at regular visits.

Dosing—The dose of maprotiline will be different for different patients. *Follow your doctor's orders or the directions on the label.* The following information includes only the average doses of maprotiline. *If your dose is different, do not change it* unless your doctor tells you to do so.

The number of tablets that you take depends on the strength of the medicine. Also, *the number of doses you take each day, the time allowed between doses, and the length of time you take the medicine depend on the medical problem for which you are taking maprotiline.*

- For *oral* dosage form (tablets):
  - —For depression:
    - Adults—At first, 25 milligrams (mg) taken one to three times a day. Your doctor may increase your dose as needed. However, the dose is usually not more than 150 mg a day, unless you are in the hospital. Some hospitalized patients may need higher doses.
    - Children—Use and dose must be determined by your doctor.

Missed dose—If you miss a dose of this medicine and your dosing schedule is:

- One dose a day at bedtime—Do not take the missed dose in the morning since it may cause disturbing side effects during waking hours. Instead, check with your doctor.
- More than one dose a day—Take the missed dose as soon as possible. Then go back to your regular dosing schedule. However, if it is almost time for your next

dose, skip the missed dose and go back to your regular dosing schedule. Do not double doses. If you have any questions about this, check with your doctor.

Storage—To store this medicine:

- Keep out of the reach of children.
- Store away from heat and direct light.
- Do not store in the bathroom, near the kitchen sink, or in other damp places. Heat or moisture may cause the medicine to break down.
- Do not keep outdated medicine or medicine no longer needed. Be sure that any discarded medicine is out of the reach of children.

Precautions While Using This Medicine

It is very important that your doctor check your progress at regular visits. This will allow your dosage to be changed if necessary and will help to reduce side effects.

This medicine will add to the effects of alcohol and other CNS depressants (medicines that slow down the nervous system, possibly causing drowsiness). Some examples of CNS depressants are antihistamines or medicine for hay fever, other allergies, or colds; sedatives, tranquilizers, or sleeping medicine; prescription pain medicine or narcotics; barbiturates; medicine for seizures; or anesthetics, including some dental anesthetics. *Check with your doctor before taking any of the above while you are using this medicine.*

This medicine may cause blurred vision, especially during the first few weeks of treatment. It may also cause some people to become drowsy or less alert than they are normally. *If these effects occur, do not drive, use machines, or do anything else that could be dangerous if you are not alert or able to see well.*

Dizziness, lightheadedness, or fainting may occur, especially when you get up from a lying or sitting position. Getting up slowly may help. If this problem continues or gets worse, check with your doctor.

Maprotiline may cause dryness of the mouth. For temporary relief, use sugarless gum or candy, melt bits of ice in your mouth, or use a saliva substitute. However, if your mouth continues to feel dry for more than 2 weeks, check with your medical doctor or dentist. Continuing dryness of the mouth may increase the chance of dental disease, including tooth decay, gum disease, and fungus infections.

Before having any kind of surgery, dental treatment, or emergency treatment, tell the medical doctor or dentist in charge that you are using this medicine. Taking maprotiline together with medicines that are used during surgery or dental or emergency treatments may increase the CNS depressant effects.

Do not stop taking this medicine without first checking with your doctor. Your doctor may want you to reduce gradually the amount you are taking before stopping completely. This will allow your body to adjust properly and will reduce the possibility of unwanted effects.

Side Effects of This Medicine

Along with its needed effects, a medicine may cause some unwanted effects. Although not all of these side effects may occur, if they do occur, they may need medical attention.

Check with your doctor as soon as possible if any of the following side effects occur:

> *More common*
> > Skin rash, redness, swelling, or itching

> *Less common*
> > Constipation (severe); nausea or vomiting; shakiness or trembling; seizures (convulsions); unusual excitement; weight loss

Rare

> Breast enlargement—in males and females; confusion (especially in the elderly); difficulty in urinating; fainting; hallucinations (seeing, hearing, or feeling things that are not there); inappropriate secretion of milk—in females; irregular heartbeat (pounding, racing, skipping); sore throat and fever; swelling of testicles; yellow eyes or skin

Symptoms of overdose

> Convulsions (seizures); dizziness (severe); drowsiness (severe); fast or irregular heartbeat; fever; muscle stiffness or weakness (severe); restlessness or agitation; trouble in breathing; vomiting

Other side effects may occur that usually do not need medical attention. These side effects may go away during treatment as your body adjusts to the medicine. However, check with your doctor if any of the following side effects continue or are bothersome:

More common

> Blurred vision; decreased sexual ability; dizziness or lightheadedness (especially in the elderly); drowsiness; dryness of mouth; headache; increased or decreased sexual drive; tiredness or weakness

Less common

> Constipation (mild); diarrhea; heartburn; increased appetite and weight gain; increased sensitivity of skin to sunlight; increased sweating; trouble in sleeping; weight loss

After you stop taking this medicine, your body will need time to adjust. This usually takes about 3 to 10 days. Continue to follow the precautions listed above during this period of time.

Other side effects not listed above may also occur in some patients. If you notice any other effects, check with your doctor.

Additional Information

Once a medicine has been approved for marketing for a certain use, experience may show that it is also useful for other medical problems. Although this use in not included in product labeling, maprotiline is used in certain patients with the following medical condition:

- Chronic neurogenic pain (a certain type of pain that is continuing)

Other than the above information, there is no additional information relating to proper use, precautions, or side effects for these uses.

MESALAMINE   Oral

Some commonly used brand names are:

In the U.S.—
Asacol   Pentasa

In Canada—
Asacol   Pentasa
Mesasal   Salofalk

Other commonly used names are: 5-aminosalicylic acid, 5-ASA, and mesalazine.

Description

Mesalamine (me-SAL-a-meen) is used to treat inflammatory bowel disease, such as ulcerative colitis. It works inside the bowel by helping to reduce the inflammation and other symptoms of the disease.

Mesalamine is available only with your doctor's prescription. It is available in the following dosage forms:

Oral
- Extended-release capsules (U.S. and Canada)
- Delayed-release tablets (U.S. and Canada)
- Extended-release tablets (Canada)

Before Using This Medicine

In deciding to use a medicine, the risks of taking the medicine must be weighed against the good it will do. This is a decision you and your doctor will make. For mesalamine, the following should be considered:

Allergies—Tell your doctor if you have ever had any unusual or allergic reaction to mesalamine, olsalazine, sulfasalazine, or any salicylates (for example, aspirin). Also tell your health care professional if you are allergic to any other substances, such as foods, preservatives, or dyes.

Pregnancy—Mesalamine has not been studied in pregnant women. However, mesalamine has not been shown to cause birth defects or other problems in animal studies.

Breast-feeding—Mesalamine may pass into the breast milk. However, this medicine has not been reported to cause problems in nursing babies.

Children—Studies on this medicine have been done only in adult patients, and there is no specific information comparing use of mesalamine in children with use in other age groups.

Older adults—Many medicines have not been studied specifically in older people. Therefore, it may not be known whether they work exactly the same way they do in younger adults or if they cause different side effects or problems in older people. There is no information comparing use of mesalamine in the elderly with use in other age groups.

Other medicines—Although certain medicines should not be used together at all, in other cases two different medicines may be used together even if an interaction might occur. In these cases, your doctor may want to change the dose, or other precautions may be necessary. Tell your health care professional if you are using any other prescription or nonprescription (over-the-counter [OTC]) medicine.

Other medical problems—The presence of other medical problems may affect the use of mesalamine. Make sure you tell your doctor if you have any other medical problems, especially:

- Kidney disease—The use of mesalamine may cause further damage to the kidneys
- Narrowing of the tube where food passes out of the stomach—May delay release of mesalamine into the body

---

Proper Use of This Medicine

Swallow the capsule or tablet whole. Do not break, crush, or chew it before swallowing.

Take this medicine before meals and at bedtime with a full glass (8 ounces) of water, unless otherwise directed by your doctor.

Keep taking this medicine for the full time of treatment, even if you begin to feel better after a few days. *Do not miss any doses.*

Do not change to another brand without checking with your doctor. The doses are different for different brands. If you refill your medicine and it looks different, check with your pharmacist.

Dosing—The dose of mesalamine will be different for different patients. *Follow your doctor's orders or the directions on the label.* The following information includes only the average doses of mesalamine. *If your dose is different, do not change it* unless your doctor tells you to do so.

The number of capsules or tablets that you take depends on the brand and strength of the medicine.

- For inflammatory bowel disease:

  —For *long-acting oral* dosage form (extended-release capsules or tablets):

  - Adults—1 gram four times a day for up to eight weeks.

  - Children—Use and dose must be determined by your doctor.

  —For *long-acting oral* dosage form (delayed-release tablets):

  - Adults—

    —For *Asacol:* 800 milligrams (mg) three times a day for six weeks.

    —For *Mesasal:* A total of 1.5 to 3 grams a day, divided into smaller doses that are taken at separate times.

    —For *Salofalk:* 1 gram three or four times a day.

  - Children—Use and dose must be determined by your doctor.

Missed dose—If you miss a dose of this medicine, take it as soon as possible. However, if it is almost time for your next dose, skip the missed dose and go back to your regular dosing schedule. Do not double doses.

Storage—To store this medicine:

- Keep out of the reach of children.

- Store away from heat and direct light.

- Do not store in the bathroom, near the kitchen sink, or in other damp places. Heat or moisture may cause the medicine to break down.

- Keep the medicine from freezing. Do not refrigerate.

- Do not keep outdated medicine or medicine no longer needed. Be sure that any discarded medicine is out of the reach of children.

Precautions While Using This Medicine

It is important that your doctor check your progress at regular visits.

For patients taking the capsule form of this medicine:

- You may sometimes notice what looks like small beads in your stool. These are just the empty shells that are left after the medicine has been absorbed into your body.

For patients taking the tablet form of this medicine:

- You may sometimes notice what looks like a tablet in your stool. This is just the empty shell that is left after the medicine has been absorbed into your body.

Side Effects of This Medicine

Along with its needed effects, a medicine may cause some unwanted effects. Although not all of these side effects may occur, if they do occur they may need medical attention.

Stop taking this medicine and check with your doctor immediately if any of the following side effects occur:

Less common

Abdominal or stomach cramps or pain (severe); bloody diarrhea; fever; headache (severe); skin rash and itching

Rare

Anxiety; back or stomach pain (severe); blue or pale skin; chest pain, possibly moving to the left arm, neck, or shoulder; chills; fast heartbeat; nausea or vomiting; shortness of breath; swelling of the stomach; unusual tiredness or weakness; yellow eyes or skin

Symptoms of overdose

Confusion; diarrhea (severe or continuing); dizziness or lightheadedness; drowsiness (severe); fast or deep

> breathing; headache (severe or continuing); hearing loss
> or ringing or buzzing in ears (continuing); nausea or
> vomiting (continuing)

Other side effects may occur that usually do not need
medical attention. These side effects may go away during
treatment as your body adjusts to the medicine. However,
check with your doctor if any of the following side effects
continue or are bothersome:

More common

> Abdominal or stomach cramps or pain (mild); diarrhea
> (mild); dizziness; headache (mild); runny or stuffy nose
> or sneezing

Less common

> Acne; back or joint pain; gas or flatulence; indigestion;
> loss of appetite; loss of hair

Other side effects not listed above may also occur in some
patients. If you notice any other effects, check with your
doctor.

Additional Information

Once a medicine has been approved for marketing for a
certain use, experience may show that it is also useful for
other medical problems. Although this use is not included
in product labeling, mesalamine may be used to treat mild
or moderate Crohn's disease and help prevent it from occurring again.

Other than the above information, there is no additional
information relating to proper use, precautions, or side effects for this use.

METHYLDOPA   Systemic

Some commonly used brand names are:

In the U.S.—
  Aldomet
  Generic name product may also be available.

In Canada—
  Aldomet   Dopamet
  Apo-Methyldopa   Novomedopa
  Generic name product may also be available.

Description

Methyldopa (meth-ill-DOE-pa) belongs to the general class of medicines called antihypertensives. It is used to treat high blood pressure (hypertension).

High blood pressure adds to the work load of the heart and arteries. If it continues for a long time, the heart and arteries may not function properly. This can damage the blood vessels of the brain, heart, and kidneys, resulting in a stroke, heart failure, or kidney failure. High blood pressure may also increase the risk of heart attacks. These problems may be less likely to occur if blood pressure is controlled.

Methyldopa works by controlling impulses along certain nerve pathways. As a result, it relaxes blood vessels so that blood passes through them more easily. This helps to lower blood pressure.

Methyldopa is available only with your doctor's prescription, in the following dosage forms:

Oral
  • Oral suspension (U.S.)
  • Tablets (U.S. and Canada)

Parenteral
  • Injection (U.S. and Canada)

Before Using This Medicine

In deciding to use a medicine, the risks of taking the medicine must be weighed against the good it will do. This is a decision you and your doctor will make. For methyldopa, the following should be considered:

Allergies—Tell your doctor if you have ever had any unusual or allergic reaction to methyldopa. Also tell your health care professional if you are allergic to any other substances, such as foods, sulfites or other preservatives, or dyes. Some methyldopa products may contain sulfites. Your health care professional can help you avoid products that may cause a problem.

Pregnancy—Methyldopa has not been studied in pregnant women in the first and second trimesters (the first 6 months of pregnancy). However, studies in pregnant women during the third trimester (the last 3 months of pregnancy) have not shown that methyldopa causes birth defects or other problems.

Breast-feeding—Although methyldopa passes into breast milk, it has not been reported to cause problems in nursing babies.

Children—Although there is no specific information comparing use of methyldopa in children with use in other age groups, this medicine is not expected to cause different side effects or problems in children than it does in adults.

Older adults—Dizziness or lightheadedness and drowsiness may be more likely to occur in the elderly, who are more sensitive to the effects of methyldopa.

Other medicines—Although certain medicines should not be used together at all, in other cases two different medicines may be used together even if an interaction might occur. In these cases, your doctor may want to change the dose, or other precautions may be necessary. When you

are taking methyldopa, it is especially important that your health care professional know if you are taking any of the following:

- Monoamine oxidase (MAO) inhibitors (furazolidone [e.g., Furoxone], isocarboxazid [e.g., Marplan], phenelzine [e.g., Nardil], procarbazine [e.g., Matulane], selegiline [e.g., Eldepryl], tranylcypromine [e.g., Parnate])—Taking methyldopa while you are taking or within 2 weeks of taking MAO inhibitors may cause nervousness in patients receiving MAO inhibitors; headache, severe high blood pressure, and hallucinations have been reported

Other medical problems—The presence of other medical problems may affect the use of methyldopa. Make sure you tell your doctor if you have any other medical problems, especially:

- Angina (chest pain)—Methyldopa may worsen the condition
- Kidney disease or
- Liver disease—Effects of methyldopa may be increased because of slower removal from the body
- Mental depression (history of)—Methyldopa can cause mental depression
- Parkinson's disease—Methyldopa may worsen condition
- Pheochromocytoma—Methyldopa may interfere with tests for the condition; in addition, there have been reports of increased blood pressure
- If you have taken methyldopa in the past and developed liver problems

---

Proper Use of This Medicine

In addition to the use of the medicine your doctor has prescribed, treatment for your high blood pressure may include weight control and care in the types of foods you eat, especially foods high in sodium. Your doctor will tell you which of these are most important for you. You should check with your doctor before changing your diet.

Many patients who have high blood pressure will not notice any signs of the problem. In fact, many may feel normal. It is very important that you *take your medicine exactly as directed* and that you keep your appointments with your doctor even if you feel well.

Remember that methyldopa will not cure your high blood pressure, but it does help control it. Therefore, you must continue to take it as directed if you expect to lower your blood pressure and keep it down. *You may have to take high blood pressure medicine for the rest of your life.* If high blood pressure is not treated, it can cause serious problems such as heart failure, blood vessel disease, stroke, or kidney disease.

To help you remember to take your medicine, try to get into the habit of taking it at the same time each day.

Dosing—The dose of methyldopa will be different for different patients. *Follow your doctor's orders or the directions on the label.* The following information includes only the average doses of methyldopa. *If your dose is different, do not change it* unless your doctor tells you to do so.

The number of tablets or teaspoonfuls of suspension that you take depends on the strength of the medicine.

- For *oral* dosage form (suspension or tablets):
  - —For high blood pressure:
    - Adults—250 milligrams (mg) to 2 grams a day. This is divided into two to four doses.
    - Children—Dose is based on body weight or size and must be determined by your doctor. The usual dose is 10 mg per kilogram (kg) (4.5 mg per pound) of body weight a day. This is divided into two to four doses. Your doctor may increase the dose as needed.
- For *injection* dosage form:
  - —For high blood pressure:
    - Adults—250 to 500 mg mixed in 100 milliliters (mL) of solution (5% dextrose) and slowly injected into a vein every six hours as needed.

• Children—Dose is based on body weight and must be determined by your doctor. The usual dose is 5 to 10 mg per kg (2.3 to 4.5 mg per pound) of body weight. This is mixed in a solution (5% dextrose) and slowly injected into a vein every six hours as needed.

Missed dose—If you miss a dose of this medicine, take it as soon as possible. However, if it is almost time for your next dose, skip the missed dose and go back to your regular dosing schedule. Do not double doses.

Storage—To store this medicine:
• Keep out of the reach of children.
• Store away from heat and direct light.
• Do not store in the bathroom, near the kitchen sink, or in other damp places. Heat or moisture may cause the medicine to break down.
• Keep the oral liquid form of this medicine from freezing.
• Do not keep outdated medicine or medicine no longer needed. Be sure that any discarded medicine is out of the reach of children.

Precautions While Using This Medicine

It is important that your doctor check your progress at regular visits to make sure that this medicine is working properly.

Do not take other medicines unless they have been discussed with your doctor. This especially includes over-the-counter (nonprescription) medicines for appetite control, asthma, colds, cough, hay fever, or sinus problems, since they may tend to increase your blood pressure.

If you have a fever and there seems to be no reason for it, check with your doctor. This is especially important during the first few weeks you take methyldopa, since fever may be a sign of a serious reaction to this medicine.

Before having any kind of surgery (including dental surgery) or emergency treatment, make sure the medical doctor or dentist in charge knows that you are taking this medicine.

Methyldopa may cause some people to become drowsy or less alert than they are normally. This is more likely to happen when you begin to take it or when you increase the amount of medicine you are taking. *Make sure you know how you react to this medicine before you drive, use machines, or do anything else that could be dangerous if you are not alert.*

Dizziness, lightheadedness, or fainting may occur, especially when you get up from a lying or sitting position. Getting up slowly may help, but if the problem continues or gets worse, check with your doctor.

Methyldopa may cause dryness of the mouth. For temporary relief, use sugarless candy or gum, melt bits of ice in your mouth, or use a saliva substitute. However, if your mouth continues to feel dry for more than 2 weeks, check with your medical doctor or dentist. Continuing dryness of the mouth may increase the chance of dental disease, including tooth decay, gum disease, and fungus infections.

Tell the doctor in charge that you are taking this medicine before you have any medical tests. The results of some tests may be affected by this medicine.

Side Effects of This Medicine

Along with its needed effects, a medicine may cause some unwanted effects. Although not all of these side effects may occur, if they do occur, they may need medical attention.

Check with your doctor immediately if the following side effect occurs:

Less common

Fever, shortly after starting to take this medicine

Check with your doctor as soon as possible if any of the following side effects occur:

More common

Swelling of feet or lower legs

Less common

Mental depression or anxiety; nightmares or unusually vivid dreams

Rare

Dark or amber urine; diarrhea or stomach cramps (severe or continuing); fever, chills, trouble breathing, and fast heartbeat; general feeling of discomfort or illness or weakness; joint pain; pale stools; skin rash or itching; stomach pain (severe) with nausea and vomiting; tiredness or weakness after having taken this medicine for several weeks (continuing); yellow eyes or skin

Other side effects may occur that usually do not need medical attention. These side effects may go away during treatment as your body adjusts to the medicine. However, check with your doctor if any of the following side effects continue or are bothersome:

More common

Drowsiness; dryness of mouth; headache

Less common

Decreased sexual ability or interest in sex; diarrhea; dizziness or lightheadedness when getting up from a lying or sitting position; nausea or vomiting; numbness, tingling, pain, or weakness in hands or feet; slow heartbeat; stuffy nose; swelling of breasts or unusual milk production

Other side effects not listed above may also occur in some patients. If you notice any other effects, check with your doctor.

METOCLOPRAMIDE   Systemic

Some commonly used brand names are:

In the U.S.—

Clopra   Reclomide
Octamide   Reglan
Octamide PFS

Generic name product may also be available.

In Canada—

Apo-Metoclop   Maxeran
Emex   Reglan

Description

Metoclopramide (met-oh-KLOE-pra-mide) is a medicine that increases the movements or contractions of the stomach and intestines. When given by injection it is used to help diagnose certain problems of the stomach and/or intestines. It is also used by injection to prevent the nausea and vomiting that may occur after treatment with anticancer medicines. Another medicine may be used with metoclopramide to prevent side effects that may occur when metoclopramide is used with anticancer medicines.

When taken by mouth, metoclopramide is used to treat the symptoms of a certain type of stomach problem called diabetic gastroparesis. It relieves symptoms such as nausea, vomiting, continued feeling of fullness after meals, and loss of appetite. Metoclopramide is also used, for a short time, to treat symptoms such as heartburn in patients who suffer esophageal injury from a backward flow of gastric acid into the esophagus.

Metoclopramide may also be used for other conditions as determined by your doctor.

Metoclopramide is available only with your doctor's prescription. It is available in the following dosage forms:

Oral
- Tablets (U.S. and Canada)
- Syrup (U.S. and Canada)

Parenteral
- Injection (U.S. and Canada)

Before Using This Medicine

In deciding to use a medicine, the risks of taking the medicine must be weighed against the good it will do. This is a decision you and your doctor will make. For metoclopramide, the following should be considered:

Allergies—Tell your doctor if you have ever had any unusual or allergic reaction to metoclopramide, procaine, or procainamide. Also tell your health care professional if you are allergic to any other substances, such as foods, preservatives, or dyes.

Pregnancy—Not enough studies have been done in humans to determine metoclopramide's safety during pregnancy. However, metoclopramide has not been shown to cause birth defects or other problems in animal studies.

Breast-feeding—Although metoclopramide passes into the breast milk, it has not been shown to cause problems in nursing babies.

Children—Muscle spasms, especially of jaw, neck, and back, and tic-like (jerky) movements of head and face may be especially likely to occur in children, who are usually more sensitive than adults to the effects of metoclopramide. Premature and full-term infants may develop blood problems if given high doses of metoclopramide.

Older adults—Shuffling walk and trembling and shaking of hands may be especially likely to occur in elderly patients after they have taken metoclopramide over a long time.

Other medicines—Although certain medicines should not be used together at all, in other cases two different medicines may be used together even if an interaction might occur. In these cases, your doctor may want to change the dose, or other precautions may be necessary. When you are taking metoclopramide, it is especially important that your health care professional know if you are taking the following:

- Central nervous system (CNS) depressants (medicine that causes drowsiness)—Use with metoclopramide may cause severe drowsiness

Other medical problems—The presence of other medical problems may affect the use of metoclopramide. Make sure you tell your doctor if you have any other medical problems, especially:

- Abdominal or stomach bleeding or
- Asthma or
- High blood pressure or
- Intestinal blockage or
- Parkinson's disease—Metoclopramide may make these conditions worse
- Epilepsy—Metoclopramide may increase the risk of having a seizure
- Kidney disease (severe) or
- Liver disease (severe)—Higher blood levels of metoclopramide may result, possibly increasing the chance of side effects

---

Proper Use of This Medicine

Take this medicine 30 minutes before meals and at bedtime, unless otherwise directed by your doctor.

Take metoclopramide only as directed. Do not take more of it, do not take it more often, and do not take it for a longer time than your doctor ordered. To do so may increase the chance of side effects.

Dosing—The dose of metoclopramide will be different for different patients. *Follow your doctor's orders or the directions on the label.* The following information includes only the average doses of metoclopramide. *If your dose is different, do not change it* unless your doctor tells you to do so.

The number of tablets or teaspoonfuls of syrup that you take depends on the strength of the medicine. Also, *the number of doses you take each day, the time allowed between doses, and the length of time you take the medicine depend on the medical problem for which you are taking metoclopramide.*

- For *oral* dosage forms (syrup or tablets):

  —To treat the symptoms of a stomach problem called diabetic gastroparesis:

  - Adults and teenagers—10 milligrams (mg) thirty minutes before symptoms are likely to begin or before each meal and at bedtime. The dose may be taken up to four times a day. However, most people usually will not take more than 500 micrograms (mcg) per kilogram (kg) (227 mcg per pound) of body weight a day.

  - Children—Dose must be determined by your doctor.

  —For heartburn:

  - Adults and teenagers—10 to 15 mg thirty minutes before symptoms are likely to begin or before each meal and at bedtime. The dose may be taken up to four times a day. However, most people usually will not take more than 500 mcg per kg (227 mcg per pound) of body weight a day.

  - Children—Dose must be determined by your doctor.

  —To increase movements or contractions of the stomach and intestines:

  - Children 5 to 14 years of age—2.5 to 5 mg three times a day, thirty minutes before meals.

> Some children may receive 100 to 200 mcg per kg (45.5 to 90.9 mcg per pound) of body weight, thirty minutes before meals and at bedtime.

- For *injection* dosage form:

—To increase movements or contractions of the stomach and intestine:

- Adults and teenagers—10 mg injected into a vein.

- Children—Dose is based on body weight and must be determined by your doctor. The usual dose is 1 mg per kilogram (kg) (0.45 mg per pound) of body weight injected into a vein. Your doctor may repeat this dose after sixty minutes if needed.

—To prevent nausea and vomiting caused by anticancer medicines:

- Adults and teenagers—Dose is based on body weight and must be determined by your doctor. The usual dose is 1 to 2 mg per kg (0.45 to 0.9 mg per pound) of body weight, injected slowly into a vein, thirty minutes before you take your anticancer medicine. Your doctor may repeat this dose every two or three hours if needed. Some people may need a larger dose to start.

- Children—1 mg per kg (0.45 mg per pound) of body weight injected into a vein. Your doctor may repeat this dose after sixty minutes if needed.

—To prevent vomiting after surgery:

- Adults and teenagers—10 to 20 mg injected into a muscle near the end of surgery.

- Children—Dose must be determined by your doctor.

Missed dose—If you miss a dose of this medicine, take it as soon as possible. However, if it is almost time for your next dose, skip the missed dose and go back to your regular dosing schedule. Do not double doses.

Storage—To store this medicine:

- Keep out of the reach of children.
- Store away from heat and direct light.
- Do not store the tablet form of this medicine in the bathroom, near the kitchen sink, or in other damp places. Heat or moisture may cause the medicine to break down.
- Keep the syrup form of this medicine from freezing.
- Do not keep outdated medicine or medicine no longer needed. Be sure that any discarded medicine is out of the reach of children.

Precautions While Using This Medicine

This medicine will add to the effects of alcohol and other CNS depressants (medicines that slow down the nervous system, possibly causing drowsiness). Some examples of CNS depressants are antihistamines or medicine for hay fever, other allergies, or colds; sedatives, tranquilizers, or sleeping medicine; prescription pain medicine or narcotics; barbiturates; medicine for seizures; muscle relaxants; or anesthetics, including some dental anesthetics. *Check with your doctor before taking any of the above while you are using this medicine.*

This medicine may cause some people to become dizzy, lightheaded, drowsy, or less alert than they are normally. *Make sure you know how you react to this medicine before you drive, use machines, or do anything else that could be dangerous if you are dizzy or are not alert.*

Side Effects of This Medicine

Along with its needed effects, a medicine may cause some unwanted effects. Although not all of these side effects

may occur, if they do occur they may need medical attention.

Check with your doctor as soon as possible if any of the following side effects occur:

Rare

Chills; difficulty in speaking or swallowing; dizziness or fainting; fast or irregular heartbeat; fever; general feeling of tiredness or weakness; headache (severe or continuing); increase in blood pressure; lip smacking or puckering; loss of balance control; mask-like face; rapid or worm-like movements of tongue; shuffling walk; sore throat; stiffness of arms or legs; trembling and shaking of hands and fingers; uncontrolled chewing movements; uncontrolled movements of arms and legs

With high doses—may occur within minutes of receiving a dose of metoclopramide and last for 2 to 24 hours

Aching or discomfort in lower legs; panic-like sensation; sensation of crawling in legs; unusual nervousness, restlessness, or irritability

Symptoms of overdose—may also occur rarely with usual doses, especially in children and young adults, and with high doses used to treat the nausea and vomiting caused by anticancer medicines

Confusion; drowsiness (severe)

Other side effects may occur that usually do not need medical attention. These side effects may go away during treatment as your body adjusts to the medicine. However, check with your doctor if any of the following side effects continue or are bothersome:

More common

Diarrhea—with high doses; drowsiness; restlessness

Less common or rare

Breast tenderness and swelling; changes in menstruation; constipation; depression; increased flow of breast milk; nausea; skin rash; trouble in sleeping; unusual dryness of mouth; unusual irritability

Other side effects not listed above may also occur in some patients. If you notice any other effects, check with your doctor.

Additional Information

Once a medicine has been approved for marketing for a certain use, experience may show that it is also useful for other medical problems. Although these uses are not included in product labeling, metoclopramide is used in certain patients with the following medical conditions:

- Failure of the stomach to empty its contents
- Nausea and vomiting caused by other medicines
- Persistent hiccups
- Prevention of aspirating fluid into the lungs during surgery
- Vascular headaches

Other than the above information, there is no additional information relating to proper use, precautions, or side effects for these uses.

METRONIDAZOLE   Systemic

Some commonly used brand names are:

In the U.S.—

Flagyl	Metric 21
Flagyl I.V.	Metro I.V.
Flagyl I.V. RTU	Protostat

Generic name product may also be available.

In Canada—

Apo-Metronidazole	Novonidazol
Flagyl	Trikacide

Generic name product may also be available.

Description

Metronidazole (me-troe-NI-da-zole) is used to treat infections. It may also be used for other problems as determined by your doctor. It will not work for colds, flu, or other virus infections.

Metronidazole is available only with your doctor's prescription, in the following dosage forms:

Oral
- Capsules (Canada)
- Tablets (U.S. and Canada)

Parenteral
- Injection (U.S. and Canada)

Before Using This Medicine

In deciding to use a medicine, the risks of taking the medicine must be weighed against the good it will do. This is a decision you and your doctor will make. For metronidazole, the following should be considered:

Allergies—Tell your doctor if you have ever had any unusual or allergic reaction to metronidazole. Also tell your health care professional if you are allergic to any other substances, such as foods, preservatives, or dyes.

Pregnancy—Studies have not been done in humans. Metronidazole has not been shown to cause birth defects in animal studies; however, use is not recommended during the first trimester of pregnancy.

Breast-feeding—Use is not recommended in nursing mothers since metronidazole passes into the breast milk and may cause unwanted effects in the baby. However, in some infections your doctor may want you to stop breast-feeding and take this medicine for a short time. During this time the breast milk should be squeezed out or sucked out with a breast pump and thrown away. One or two days after you finish taking this medicine, you may go back to breast-feeding.

Children—Metronidazole has been used in children and, in effective doses, has not been shown to cause different side effects or problems in children than it does in adults.

Older adults—Many medicines have not been studied specifically in older people. Therefore, it may not be known whether they work exactly the same way they do in younger adults or if they cause different side effects or problems in older people. There is no specific information comparing use of metronidazole in the elderly with use in other age groups.

Other medicines—Although certain medicines should not be used together at all, in other cases two different medicines may be used together even if an interaction might occur. In these cases, your doctor may want to change the dose, or other precautions may be necessary. When you are taking metronidazole, it is especially important that your health care professional knows if you are taking any of the following:

- Anticoagulants (blood thinners)—Patients taking anticoagulants with metronidazole may have an increased chance of bleeding
- Disulfiram (e.g., Antabuse)—Patients taking disulfiram with metronidazole may have an increase in side effects affecting the central nervous system

Other medical problems—The presence of other medical problems may affect the use of metronidazole. Make sure you tell your doctor if you have any other medical problems, especially:

- Blood disease or a history of blood disease—Metronidazole may make the condition worse
- Central nervous system (CNS) disease, including epilepsy—Metronidazole may increase the chance of seizures (convulsions) or other CNS side effects
- Heart disease—Metronidazole by injection may make heart disease worse

• Liver disease, severe—Patients with severe liver disease may have an increase in side effects

---

Proper Use of This Medicine

If this medicine upsets your stomach, it may be taken with meals or a snack. If stomach upset (nausea, vomiting, stomach pain, or diarrhea) continues, check with your doctor.

To help clear up your infection completely, *keep taking this medicine for the full time of treatment,* even if you begin to feel better after a few days. If you stop taking this medicine too soon, your symptoms may return.

In some kinds of infections, this medicine works best when there is a constant amount in the blood. *To help keep the amount constant, do not miss any doses. Also, it is best to take the doses at evenly spaced times, day and night.* For example, if you are to take 4 doses a day, the doses should be spaced about 6 hours apart. If this interferes with your sleep or other daily activities, or if you need help in planning the best times to take your medicine, check with your health care professional.

Dosing—The dose of metronidazole will be different for different patients. *Follow your doctor's orders or the directions on the label.* The following information includes only the average doses of metronidazole. *If your dose is different, do not change it* unless your doctor tells you to do so.

The number of capsules or tablets that you take depends on the strength of the medicine. Also, *the number of doses you take each day, the time allowed between doses, and the length of time you take the medicine depend on the medical problem for which you are taking metronidazole.*

- *For oral* dosage forms (capsules, tablets):
    —For bacterial infections:
    - Adults and teenagers—Dose is based on body weight. The usual dose is 7.5 milligrams (mg) per kilogram (kg) (3.4 mg per pound) of body weight, up to a maximum dose of 1 gram, every six hours for at least seven days.
    - Children—Dose is based on body weight. The usual dose is 7.5 mg per kg (3.4 mg per pound) of body weight every six hours; or 10 mg per kg (4.5 mg per pound) every eight hours.
    —For amebiasis infections:
    - Adults and teenagers—500 to 750 mg three times a day for five to ten days.
    - Children—Dose is based on body weight. The usual dose is 11.6 to 16.7 mg per kg (5.3 to 7.6 mg per pound) of body weight three times a day for ten days.
    —For trichomoniasis infections:
    - Adults and teenagers—A single dose of 2 grams; or 1 gram two times a day for one day; or 250 mg three times a day for seven days.
    - Children—Dose is based on body weight. The usual dose is 5 mg per kg (2.3 mg per pound) of body weight three times a day for seven days.
- For *injection* dosage form:
    —For bacterial infections:
    - Adults and children over 1 week of age—Dose is based on body weight. The usual dose is 15 mg per kg (6.8 mg per pound) of body weight one time to start, then 7.5 mg per kg (3.4 mg per pound) of body weight injected into a vein every six hours for at least seven days.
    - Preterm infants—Dose is based on body weight. The usual dose is 15 mg per kg (6.8 mg per

pound) of body weight one time to start, then 7.5 mg per kg (3.4 mg per pound) of body weight, injected into a vein, every twelve hours starting forty-eight hours after the first dose.

• Full-term infants—Dose is based on body weight. The usual dose is 15 mg per kg (6.8 mg per pound) of body weight one time to start, then 7.5 mg per kg (3.4 mg per pound) of body weight, injected into a vein, every twelve hours starting twenty-four hours after the first dose.

—For treatment before and during bowel surgery:

• Adults and teenagers—Dose is based on body weight. The usual dose is 15 mg per kg (6.8 mg per pound), injected into a vein, one hour before surgery, then 7.5 mg per kg (3.4 mg per pound) of body weight, injected into a vein, six hours and twelve hours after the first dose.

• Children—Use and dose must be determined by your doctor.

Missed dose—If you miss a dose of this medicine, take it as soon as possible. This will help to keep a constant amount of medicine in the blood. However, if it is almost time for your next dose, skip the missed dose and go back to your regular dosing schedule. Do not double doses.

Storage—To store this medicine:

• Keep out of the reach of children.

• Store away from heat and direct light.

• Do not store the capsule or tablet form of this medicine in the bathroom, near the kitchen sink, or in other damp places. Heat or moisture may cause the medicine to break down.

• Do not keep outdated medicine or medicine no longer needed. Be sure that any discarded medicine is out of the reach of children.

Precautions While Using This Medicine

If your symptoms do not improve within a few days, or if they become worse, check with your doctor.

Drinking alcoholic beverages while taking this medicine may cause stomach pain, nausea, vomiting, headache, or flushing or redness of the face. Other alcohol-containing preparations (for example, elixirs, cough syrups, tonics) may also cause problems. These problems may last for at least a day after you stop taking metronidazole. Also, this medicine may cause alcoholic beverages to taste different. Therefore, *you should not drink alcoholic beverages or take other alcohol-containing preparations while you are taking this medicine and for at least a day after stopping it.*

Metronidazole may cause dryness of the mouth, an unpleasant or sharp metallic taste, and a change in taste sensation. For temporary relief of dry mouth, use sugarless candy or gum, melt bits of ice in your mouth, or use a saliva substitute. However, if your mouth continues to feel dry for more than 2 weeks, check with your medical doctor or dentist. Continuing dryness of the mouth may increase the chance of dental disease, including tooth decay, gum disease, and fungus infections.

This medicine may also cause some people to become dizzy or lightheaded. *Make sure you know how you react to this medicine before you drive, use machines, or do anything else that could be dangerous if you are dizzy or are not alert.* If these reactions are especially bothersome, check with your doctor.

If you are taking this medicine for trichomoniasis (an infection of the sex organs in males and females), your doctor may want to treat your sexual partner at the same time you are being treated, even if he or she has no symptoms. Also, it may be desirable to use a condom (prophylactic) during intercourse. These measures will help keep you from getting the infection back again from your partner. If you have any questions about this, check with your doctor.

Side Effects of This Medicine

Along with its needed effects, a medicine may cause some unwanted effects. Although not all of these side effects may occur, if they do occur they may need medical attention.

Check with your doctor immediately if any of the following side effects occur:

> *Less common*
> Numbness, tingling, pain, or weakness in hands or feet
> *Rare*
> Convulsions (seizures)

Also, check with your doctor as soon as possible if any of the following side effects occur:

> *Less common*
> Any vaginal irritation, discharge, or dryness not present before use of this medicine; clumsiness or unsteadiness; mood or other mental changes; skin rash, hives, redness, or itching; sore throat and fever; stomach and back pain (severe)
>
> *For injection form*
> Pain, tenderness, redness, or swelling over vein in which the medicine is given

Other side effects may occur that usually do not need medical attention. These side effects may go away during treatment as your body adjusts to the medicine. However, check with your doctor if any of the following side effects continue or are bothersome:

> *More common*
> Diarrhea; dizziness or lightheadedness; headache; loss of appetite; nausea or vomiting; stomach pain or cramps

Less common or rare
> Change in taste sensation; dryness of mouth; unpleasant or sharp metallic taste

In some patients metronidazole may cause dark urine. This is only temporary and will go away when you stop taking this medicine.

Other side effects not listed above may also occur in some patients. If you notice any other effects, check with your doctor.

Additional Information

Once a medicine has been approved for marketing for a certain use, experience may show that it is also useful for other medical problems. Although these uses are not included in product labeling, metronidazole is used in certain patients with the following medical conditions:

- Antibiotic-associated colitis
- Bacterial vaginosis
- Balantidiasis
- Dental infections
- Gastritis or ulcer due to *Helicobacter pylori*
- Giardiasis
- Inflammatory bowel disease

For patients taking this medicine for *giardiasis*:

- After treatment, it is important that your doctor check whether or not the infection in your intestinal tract has been cleared up completely.

Other than the above information, there is no additional information relating to proper use, precautions, or side effects for this use.

MISOPROSTOL Systemic

A commonly used brand name in the U.S. and Canada is Cytotec.

Description

Misoprostol (mye-soe-PROST-ole) is taken to prevent stomach ulcers in patients taking anti-inflammatory drugs, including aspirin. Misoprostol may also be used for other conditions as determined by your doctor.

Misoprostol helps the stomach protect itself against acid damage. It also decreases the amount of acid produced by the stomach.

This medicine is available only with your doctor's prescription, in the following dosage form:

Oral
- Tablets (U.S. and Canada)

Before Using This Medicine

In deciding to use a medicine, the risks of taking the medicine must be weighed against the good it will do. This is a decision you and your doctor will make. For misoprostol, the following should be considered:

Allergies—Tell your doctor if you have ever had any unusual or allergic reaction to misoprostol. Also tell your health care professional if you are allergic to any other substances, such as foods, preservatives, or dyes.

Pregnancy—*Misoprostol must not be used during pregnancy*. It has been shown to cause contractions and bleeding of the uterus. Misoprostol may also cause miscarriage.

Before starting to take this medicine you must have had a negative pregnancy test within the previous 2 weeks.

Also, you must start taking misoprostol only on the second or third day of your next normal menstrual period. In addition, it will be necessary that you use an effective form of birth control while taking this medicine. Be sure that you have discussed this with your doctor before taking this medicine.

Breast-feeding—It is not known whether misoprostol passes into breast milk. However, misoprostol is not recommended for use during breast-feeding because it may cause diarrhea in nursing babies.

Children—Studies on this medicine have been done only in adult patients, and there is no specific information comparing use of misoprostol in children with use in other age groups.

Older adults—This medicine has been tested and has not been shown to cause different side effects or problems in older people than it does in younger adults.

Other medicines—Although certain medicines should not be used together at all, in other cases two different medicines may be used together even if an interaction might occur. In these cases, your doctor may want to change the dose, or other precautions may be necessary. Tell your health care professional if you are taking any other prescription or nonprescription (over-the-counter [OTC]) medicine.

Other medical problems—The presence of other medical problems may affect the use of misoprostol. Make sure you tell your doctor if you have any other medical problems, especially:

- Blood vessel disease—Medicines similar to misoprostol have been shown to make this condition worse
- Epilepsy (uncontrolled)—Medicines similar to misoprostol have been shown to cause convulsions (seizures)

Proper Use of This Medicine

Misoprostol is best taken with or after meals and at bedtime, unless otherwise directed by your doctor.

Dosing—The dose of misoprostol will be different for different patients. *Follow your doctor's orders or the directions on the label.* The following information includes only the average doses of misoprostol. *If your dose is different, do not change it* unless your doctor tells you to do so.

- To prevent stomach ulcers in patients taking anti-inflammatory medicines including aspirin:

  —For *oral* dosage form (tablets):

  - Adults—200 micrograms (mcg) four times a day, with or after meals and at bedtime. Or, your dose may be 400 mcg two times day with the last dose taken at bedtime. Your doctor may reduce the dose to 100 mcg if you are sensitive to high doses.

  - Children and teenagers—Dose must be determined by your doctor.

Missed dose—If you miss a dose of this medicine, take it as soon as possible. However, if it is almost time for your next dose, skip the missed dose and go back to your regular dosing schedule. Do not double doses.

Storage—To store this medicine:

- Keep out of the reach of children.
- Store away from heat and direct light.
- Do not store in the bathroom, near the kitchen sink, or in other damp places. Heat or moisture may cause the medicine to break down.
- Do not keep outdated medicine or medicine no longer needed. Be sure that any discarded medicine is out of the reach of children.

Precautions While Using This Medicine

Misoprostol may cause miscarriage if taken during pregnancy. Therefore, if you suspect that you may have become pregnant, stop taking this medicine immediately and check with your doctor.

This medicine may cause diarrhea in some people. The diarrhea will usually disappear within a few days as your body adjusts to the medicine. However, check with your doctor if the diarrhea is severe and/or does not stop after a week. Your doctor may have to lower the dose of misoprostol you are taking.

Side Effects of This Medicine

Along with its needed effects, a medicine may cause some unwanted effects. Some side effects may occur that usually do not need medical attention. These side effects may go away during treatment as your body adjusts to the medicine. However, check with your doctor if any of the following side effects continue or are bothersome:

More common
    Abdominal or stomach pain (mild); diarrhea

Less common or rare
    Bleeding from vagina; constipation; cramps in lower abdomen or stomach area; gas; headache; nausea and/or vomiting

Other side effects not listed above may also occur in some patients. If you notice any other effects, check with your doctor.

Additional Information

Once a medicine has been approved for marketing for a certain use, experience may show that it is also useful for

other medical problems. Although this use is not included in product labeling, misoprostol is used in certain patients with the following medical condition:

- Duodenal ulcers

For patients taking this medicine for *duodenal ulcers*:

- Antacids may be taken with misoprostol, if needed, to help relieve stomach pain, unless you are otherwise directed by your doctor. However, do not take magnesium-containing antacids, since they may cause diarrhea or worsen the diarrhea that is sometimes caused by misoprostol.

- Take this medicine for the full time of treatment, even if you begin to feel better. Also, it is important that you keep your appointments with your doctor so that your doctor will be better able to tell you when to stop taking this medicine.

- *Misoprostol is not normally taken for more than 4 weeks when used to treat duodenal ulcers.* However, your doctor may order treatment for a second 4-week period if needed.

Other than the above information, there is no additional information relating to proper use, precautions, or side effects for these uses.

NARCOTIC ANALGESICS—For Pain Relief   Systemic

Some commonly used brand names are:

In the U.S.—

Astramorph[9]	Dilaudid[5]
Astramorph PF[9]	Dilaudid-HP[5]
Buprenex[1]	Dolene[15]
Darvon[15]	Dolophine[8]
Darvon-N[15]	Doraphen[15]
Demerol[7]	Doxaphene[15]

In the U.S. (cont'd)—

Duramorph[9]
Levo-Dromoran[6]
Methadose[8]
M S Contin[9]
MSIR[9]
Nubain[10]
Numorphan[13]
Pantopon[11]
Profene[15]
Pro Pox[15]

Propoxycon[15]
RMS Uniserts[9]
Roxanol[9]
Roxanol 100[9]
Roxanol SR[9]
Stadol[2]
Roxicodone[12]
Talwin[14]
Talwin-Nx[14]

In Canada—

Darvon-N[15]
Demerol[7]
Dilaudid[5]
Dilaudid-HP[5]
Epimorph[9]
Hycodan[4]#
Levo-Dromoran[6]
Morphine H.P.[9]
Morphitec[9]
M.O.S.[9]
M.O.S.-S.R.[9]
M S Contin[9]

Novopropoxyn[15]
Nubain[10]
Numorphan[13]
Pantopon[11]
Paveral[3]
Robidone[4]
Roxanol[9]
642[15]
Stadol[2]
Statex[9]
Supeudol[12]
Talwin[14]

Other commonly used names are:

dextropropoxyphene[15]
dihydromorphinone[5]
levorphan[6]

papaveretum[11]
pethidine[7]

Note: For quick reference, the following narcotic analgesics are numbered to match the corresponding brand names.

This information applies to the following medicines:

1. Buprenorphine (byoo-pre-NOR-feen)
2. Butorphanol (byoo-TOR-fa-nole)
3. Codeine (KOE-deen)‡§
4. Hydrocodone (hye-droe-KOE-done)*
5. Hydromorphone (hye-droe-MOR-fone)‡
6. Levorphanol (lee-VOR-fa-nole)‡
7. Meperidine (me-PER-i-deen)‡§
8. Methadone (METH-a-done)‡**
9. Morphine (MOR-feen)‡§
10. Nalbuphine (NAL-byoo-feen)‡
11. Opium Injection (OH-pee-um)
12. Oxycodone (ox-i-KOE-done)
13. Oxymorphone (ox-i-MOR-fone)

14. Pentazocine (pen-TAZ-oh-seen)
15. Propoxyphene (proe-POX-i-feen)‡

This information does *not* apply to Opium Tincture or Paregoric.

---

  *Not commercially available in the U.S.

  ‡Generic name product may also be available in the U.S.

  §Generic name product may also be available in Canada.

  #For Canadian product only. In the U.S., *Hycodan* also contains homatropine; in Canada, *Hycodan* contains only hydrocodone.

  **In Canada, methadone is available only through doctors who have received special approval to prescribe it.

Description

Narcotic (nar-KOT-ik) analgesics (an-al-JEE-zicks) are used to relieve pain. Some of these medicines are also used just before or during an operation to help the anesthetic work better. Codeine and hydrocodone are also used to relieve coughing. Methadone is also used to help some people control their dependence on heroin or other narcotics. Narcotic analgesics may also be used for other conditions as determined by your doctor.

Narcotic analgesics act in the central nervous system (CNS) to relieve pain. Some of their side effects are also caused by actions in the CNS.

If a narcotic is used for a long time, it may become habit-forming (causing mental or physical dependence). Physical dependence may lead to withdrawal side effects when you stop taking the medicine.

These medicines are available only with your medical doctor's or dentist's prescription. For some of them, prescriptions cannot be refilled and you must obtain a new prescription from your medical doctor or dentist each time you need the medicine. In addition, other rules and regulations may apply when methadone is used to treat narcotic dependence.

These medicines are available in the following dosage forms:

Oral
  Codeine
  - Oral solution (U.S. and Canada)
  - Tablets (U.S. and Canada)

  Hydrocodone
  - Syrup (Canada)
  - Tablets (Canada)

  Hydromorphone
  - Tablets (U.S. and Canada)

  Levorphanol
  - Tablets (U.S. and Canada)

  Meperidine
  - Syrup (U.S.)
  - Tablets (U.S. and Canada)

  Methadone
  - Oral concentrate (U.S.)
  - Oral solution (U.S.)
  - Tablets (U.S.)
  - Dispersible tablets (U.S.)

  Morphine
  - Oral solution (U.S. and Canada)
  - Syrup (Canada)
  - Tablets (U.S. and Canada)
  - Extended-release tablets (U.S. and Canada)

  Oxycodone
  - Oral solution (U.S.)
  - Tablets (U.S. and Canada)

  Pentazocine
  - Tablets (Canada)

  Pentazocine and Naloxone
  - Tablets (U.S.)

  Propoxyphene
  - Capsules (U.S. and Canada)
  - Oral suspension (U.S.)
  - Tablets (U.S. and Canada)

Parenteral
  Buprenorphine
  - Injection (U.S.)

  Butorphanol
  - Injection (U.S. and Canada)

  Codeine
  - Injection (U.S. and Canada)

Hydromorphone
  • Injection (U.S. and Canada)
Levorphanol
  • Injection (U.S. and Canada)
Meperidine
  • Injection (U.S. and Canada)
Methadone
  • Injection (U.S.)
Morphine
  • Injection (U.S. and Canada)
Nalbuphine
  • Injection (U.S. and Canada)
Opium
  • Injection (U.S. and Canada)
Oxymorphone
  • Injection (U.S. and Canada)
Pentazocine
  • Injection (U.S. and Canada)

Rectal

Hydromorphone
  • Suppositories (U.S. and Canada)
Morphine
  • Suppositories (U.S. and Canada)
Oxycodone
  • Suppositories (Canada)
Oxymorphone
  • Suppositories (U.S. and Canada)

Before Using This Medicine

In deciding to use a medicine, the risks of taking the medicine must be weighed against the good it will do. This is a decision you and your doctor will make. For narcotic analgesics, the following should be considered:

Allergies—Tell your doctor if you have ever had any unusual or allergic reaction to any of the narcotic analgesics. Also tell your health care professional if you are allergic to any other substances, such as foods, preservatives, or dyes.

Pregnancy—Although studies on birth defects with narcotic analgesics have not been done in pregnant women, these medicines have not been reported to cause birth defects. However, hydrocodone, hydromorphone, and morphine caused birth defects in animals when given in very large doses. Buprenorphine and codeine did not cause birth defects in animal studies, but they caused other unwanted effects. Butorphanol, nalbuphine, pentazocine, and propoxyphene did not cause birth defects in animals. There is no information about whether other narcotic analgesics cause birth defects in animals.

Too much use of a narcotic during pregnancy may cause the baby to become dependent on the medicine. This may lead to withdrawal side effects after birth. Also, some of these medicines may cause breathing problems in the newborn infant if taken just before delivery.

Breast-feeding—Most narcotic analgesics have not been reported to cause problems in nursing babies. However, when the mother is taking large amounts of methadone (in a methadone maintenance program), the nursing baby may become dependent on the medicine. Also, butorphanol, codeine, meperidine, morphine, opium, and propoxyphene pass into the breast milk.

Children—Breathing problems may be especially likely to occur in children younger than 2 years of age. These children are usually more sensitive than adults to the effects of narcotic analgesics. Also, unusual excitement or restlessness may be more likely to occur in children receiving these medicines.

Older adults—Elderly people are especially sensitive to the effects of narcotic analgesics. This may increase the chance of side effects, especially breathing problems, during treatment.

Other medicines—Although certain medicines should not be used together at all, in other cases two different medi-

cines may be used together even if an interaction might occur. In these cases, your doctor may want to change the dose, or other precautions may be necessary. When you are taking a narcotic analgesic, it is especially important that your health care professional know if you are taking any of the following:

- Carbamazepine (e.g., Tegretol)—Propoxyphene may increase the blood levels of carbamazepine, which increases the chance of serious side effects
- Central nervous system (CNS) depressants or
- Monoamine oxidase (MAO) inhibitors (furazolidone [e.g., Furoxone], isocarboxazid [e.g., Marplan], pargyline [e.g., Eutonyl], phenelzine [e.g., Nardil], procarbazine [e.g., Matulane], tranylcypromine [e.g., Parnate] (taken currently or within the past 2 weeks) or
- Tricyclic antidepressants (amitriptyline [e.g., Elavil], amoxapine [e.g., Asendin], clomipramine [e.g., Anafranil], desipramine [e.g., Pertofrane], doxepin [e.g., Sinequan], imipramine [e.g., Tofranil], nortriptyline [e.g., Aventyl], protriptyline [e.g., Vivactil], trimipramine [e.g., Surmontil])—The chance of side effects may be increased; the combination of meperidine (e.g., Demerol) and MAO inhibitors is especially dangerous
- Naltrexone (e.g., Trexan)—Narcotics will not be effective in people taking naltrexone
- Rifampin (e.g., Rifadin)—Rifampin decreases the effects of methadone and may cause withdrawal symptoms in people who are dependent on methadone
- Zidovudine (e.g., AZT, Retrovir)—Morphine may increase the blood levels of zidovudine and increase the chance of serious side effects

Other medical problems—The presence of other medical problems may affect the use of narcotic analgesics. Make sure you tell your doctor if you have any other medical problems, especially:

- Alcohol abuse, or history of, or
- Drug dependence, especially narcotic abuse, or history of, or
- Emotional problems—The chance of side effects may be increased; also, withdrawal symptoms may occur if a nar-

cotic you are dependent on is replaced by buprenorphine, butorphanol, nalbuphine, or pentazocine
- Brain disease or head injury or
- Emphysema, asthma, or other chronic lung disease or
- Enlarged prostate or problems with urination or
- Gallbladder disease or gallstones—Some of the side effects of narcotic analgesics can be dangerous if these conditions are present
- Colitis or
- Heart disease or
- Kidney disease or
- Liver disease or
- Underactive thyroid—The chance of side effects may be increased
- Convulsions (seizures), history of—Some of the narcotic analgesics can cause convulsions

---

Proper Use of This Medicine

Some narcotic analgesics given by injection may be given at home to patients who do not need to be in the hospital. If you are using an injection form of this medicine at home, *make sure you clearly understand and carefully follow your doctor's instructions.*

To take the *syrup form of meperidine:*
- Unless otherwise directed by your medical doctor or dentist, *take this medicine mixed with a half glass (4 ounces) of water* to lessen the numbing effect of the medicine on your mouth and throat.

To take the *oral liquid forms of methadone:*
- *This medicine may have to be mixed with water or another liquid before you take it.* Read the label carefully for directions. If you have any questions about this, check with your health care professional.

To take the *dispersible tablet form of methadone:*
- *These tablets must be stirred into water or fruit juice just before each dose is taken. Read the label care-*

fully for directions. If you have any questions about this, check with your health care professional.

To take *oral liquid forms of morphine:*

• This medicine may be mixed with a glass of fruit juice just before you take it, if desired, to improve the taste.

To take *long-acting morphine tablets:*

• *These tablets must be swallowed whole.* Do not break, crush, or chew them before swallowing.

To use *suppositories:*

• If the suppository is too soft to insert, chill it in the refrigerator for 30 minutes or run cold water over it before removing the foil wrapper.

• To insert the suppository: First remove the foil wrapper and moisten the suppository with cold water. Lie down on your side and use your finger to push the suppository well up into the rectum.

Take this medicine only as directed by your medical doctor or dentist. Do not take more of it, do not take it more often, and do not take it for a longer time than your medical doctor or dentist ordered. This is especially important for young children and elderly patients, who are especially sensitive to the effects of narcotic analgesics. If too much is taken, the medicine may become habit-forming (causing mental or physical dependence) or lead to medical problems because of an overdose.

If you think this medicine is not working properly after you have been taking it for a few weeks, *do not increase the dose.* Instead, check with your doctor.

Missed dose—If your medical doctor or dentist has ordered you to take this medicine according to a regular schedule and you miss a dose, take it as soon as you remember. However, if it is almost time for your next dose, skip the missed dose and go back to your regular dosing schedule. *Do not double doses.*

Storage—To store this medicine:

- Keep out of the reach of children. Overdose is very dangerous in young children.

- Store away from heat and direct light.

- Do not store tablets or capsules in the bathroom, near the kitchen sink, or in other damp places. Heat or moisture may cause the medicine to break down.

- Store hydromorphone, oxycodone, or oxymorphone suppositories in the refrigerator.

- Keep liquid (including injections) and suppository forms of the medicine from freezing.

- Do not keep outdated medicine or medicine no longer needed. Be sure that any discarded medicine is out of the reach of children.

Precautions While Using This Medicine

If you will be taking this medicine for a long time (for example, for several months at a time), your doctor should check your progress at regular visits.

Narcotic analgesics will add to the effects of alcohol and other CNS depressants (medicines that slow down the nervous system, possibly causing drowsiness). Some examples of CNS depressants are antihistamines or medicine for hay fever, other allergies, or colds; sedatives, tranquilizers, or sleeping medicine; other prescription pain medicines including other narcotics; barbiturates; medicine for seizures; muscle relaxants; or anesthetics, including some dental anesthetics. *Do not drink alcoholic beverages, and check with your medical doctor or dentist before taking any of the medicines listed above, while you are using this medicine.*

This medicine may cause some people to become drowsy, dizzy, or lightheaded, or to feel a false sense of well-being. *Make sure you know how you react to this medicine before you drive, use machines, or do anything else that could be dangerous if you are dizzy or are not alert and clearheaded.*

Dizziness, lightheadedness, or fainting may occur, especially when you get up suddenly from a lying or sitting position. Getting up slowly may help lessen this problem.

Nausea or vomiting may occur, especially after the first couple of doses. This effect may go away if you lie down for a while. However, if nausea or vomiting continues, check with your medical doctor or dentist. Lying down for a while may also help relieve some other side effects, such as dizziness or lightheadedness, that may occur.

Before having any kind of surgery (including dental surgery) or emergency treatment, tell the medical doctor or dentist in charge that you are taking this medicine.

Narcotic analgesics may cause dryness of the mouth. For temporary relief, use sugarless candy or gum, melt bits of ice in your mouth, or use a saliva substitute. However, if dry mouth continues for more than 2 weeks, check with your dentist. Continuing dryness of the mouth may increase the chance of dental disease, including tooth decay, gum disease, and fungus infections.

If you have been taking this medicine regularly for several weeks or more, *do not suddenly stop using it without first checking with your doctor.* Your doctor may want you to reduce gradually the amount you are taking before stopping completely, in order to lessen the chance of withdrawal side effects.

If you think you or someone else may have taken an overdose, get emergency help at once. Taking an overdose of this medicine or taking alcohol or CNS depressants with this medicine may lead to unconsciousness or death. Signs of overdose include convulsions (seizures), confusion, severe nervousness or restlessness, severe dizziness, severe drowsiness, slow or troubled breathing, and severe weakness.

Side Effects of This Medicine

Along with its needed effects, a medicine may cause some unwanted effects. Although not all of these side effects may occur, if they do occur they may need medical attention.

Get emergency help immediately if any of the following symptoms of overdose occur:

> Cold, clammy skin; confusion; convulsions (seizures); dizziness (severe); drowsiness (severe); low blood pressure; nervousness or restlessness (severe); pinpoint pupils of eyes; slow heartbeat; slow or troubled breathing; weakness (severe)

Also, check with your doctor as soon as possible if any of the following side effects occur:

Less common or rare

> Dark urine (for propoxyphene only); fast, slow, or pounding heartbeat; feelings of unreality; hallucinations (seeing, hearing, or feeling things that are not there); hives, itching, or skin rash; increased sweating (more common with hydrocodone, meperidine, and methadone); irregular breathing; mental depression or other mood or mental changes; pale stools (for propoxyphene only); redness or flushing of face (more common with hydrocodone, meperidine, and methadone); ringing or buzzing in the ears; shortness of breath, wheezing, or troubled breathing; swelling of face; trembling or uncontrolled muscle movements; unusual excitement or restlessness (especially in children); yellow eyes or skin (for propoxyphene only)

Other side effects may occur that usually do not need medical attention. These side effects may go away during treatment as your body adjusts to the medicine. However, check with your doctor if any of the following side effects continue or are bothersome:

More common

Dizziness, lightheadedness, or feeling faint; drowsiness; nausea or vomiting

Less common or rare

Blurred or double vision or other changes in vision; constipation (more common with long-term use and with codeine); decrease in amount of urine; difficult or painful urination; dry mouth; false sense of well-being; frequent urge to urinate; general feeling of discomfort or illness; headache; loss of appetite; nervousness or restlessness; nightmares or unusual dreams; redness, swelling, pain, or burning at place of injection; stomach cramps or pain; trouble in sleeping; unusual tiredness or weakness

After you stop using this medicine, your body may need time to adjust. The length of time this takes depends on the amount of medicine you were using and how long you used it. During this period of time check with your doctor if you notice any of the following side effects:

Body aches; diarrhea; fast heartbeat; fever, runny nose, or sneezing; gooseflesh; increased sweating; increased yawning; loss of appetite; nausea or vomiting; nervousness, restlessness, or irritability; shivering or trembling; stomach cramps; trouble in sleeping; unusually large pupils of eyes; weakness

Other side effects not listed above may also occur in some patients. If you notice any other effects, check with your doctor.

NARCOTIC ANALGESICS AND ACETAMINOPHEN   Systemic

Some commonly used brand names are:

In the U.S.—

Acetaco[1]	Myapap with Codeine[1]
Aceta with Codeine[1]	Norcet[4]
Allay[4]	Norcet 7.5[4]
Amacodone[4]	Percocet[6]
Anexsia[4]	Phenaphen with Codeine
Anexsia 7.5[4]	No.2[1]#
Anodynos DHC[4]	Phenaphen with Codeine
Anolor DH 5[4]	No.3[1]#
Bancap-HC[4]	Phenaphen with Codeine
Capital with Codeine[1]	No.4[1]#
Codalan No.1[2]	Phenaphen-650 with Codeine[1]
Codalan No.2[2]	Polygesic[4]
Codalan No.3[2]	Propacet 100[8]
Co-Gesic[4]	Propain-HC[4]
Compal[3]	Pro Pox with APAP[8]
Darvocet-N 50[8]	Proval[1]
Darvocet-N 100[8]	Pyregesic-C[1]
Demerol-APAP[5]	Rogesic No.3[4]
Dolacet[4]	Roxicet[6]
Dolene-AP-65[8]	Roxicet 5/500[6]
Doxapap-N[8]	Senefen III[4]
D-Rex 65[8]	Talacen[7]
Duocet[4]	Tylaprin with Codeine[1]
Duradyne DHC[4]	Tylenol with Codeine[1]
E-Lor[8]	Tylenol with Codeine No.1[1]
Genagesic[8]	Tylenol with Codeine No.2[1]
HY-5[4]	Tylenol with Codeine No.3[1]
Hycomed[4]	Tylenol with Codeine No.4[1]
Hycopap[4]	Tylox[6]
Hyco-Pap[4]	Ty-Pap with Codeine[1]
Hydrocet[4]	Ty-Tab with Codeine No.2[1]
Hydrogesic[4]	Ty-Tab with Codeine No.3[1]
HY-PHEN[4]	Ty-Tab with Codeine No.4[1]
Lorcet-HD[4]	Ultragesic[4]
Lorcet Plus[4]	Vapocet[4]
Lortab[4]	Vicodin[4]
Lortab 5[4]	Vicodin ES[4]
Lortab 7[4]	Wygesic[8]
Megagesic[4]	Zydone[4]
M-Gesic[1]	

In Canada—

Atasol-8[2]

Atasol-15[2]

Atasol-30[2]

Codamin #2[2]

Codamin #3[2]

Codaminophen[2]

Empracet-30[1]

Empracet-60[1]

Emtec-30[1]

Endocet[6]

Exdol-8[2]

Exdol-15[2]

Exdol-30[2]

Lenoltec with Codeine No.1[2]

Lenoltec with Codeine No.2[2]

Lenoltec with Codeine No.3[2]

Lenoltec with Codeine No.4[1]

Novogesic C8[2]

Novogesic C15[2]

Novogesic C30[2]

Oxycocet[6]

Percocet[6]

Percocet-Demi[6]

Rounox and Codeine 15[1]

Rounox and Codeine 30[1]

Rounox and Codeine 60[1]

Tylenol No.1[2]

Tylenol No.1 Forte[2]

Tylenol with Codeine[2]

Tylenol with Codeine No.2[2]

Tylenol with Codeine No.3[2]

Tylenol with Codeine No.4[1]

Veganin[2]

Other commonly used names are:

APAP with codeine[1]

drocode, acetaminophen, and
caffeine[3]

hydrocodone with APAP[4]

oxycodone with APAP[6]

propoxyphene with APAP[8]

Note: For quick reference, the following narcotic analgesics and acetaminophen
      combinations are numbered to match the corresponding brand names.

This information applies to the following medicines:

1. Acetaminophen (a-seat-a-MIN-oh-fen) and Codeine (KOE-deen)‡
2. Acetaminophen, Codeine, and Caffeine (kaf-EEN)§
3. Dihydrocodeine (dye-hye-droe-KOE-deen), Acetaminophen, and Caffeine†
4. Hydrocodone (hye-droe-KOE-done) and Acetaminophen†‡
5. Meperidine (me-PER-i-deen) and Acetaminophen†
6. Oxycodone (ox-i-KOE-done) and Acetaminophen‡
7. Pentazocine (pen-TAZ-oh-seen) and Acetaminophen†
8. Propoxyphene (proe-POX-i-feen) and Acetaminophen†‡

---

†Not commercially available in Canada.

‡Generic name product may also be available in the U.S.

§Generic name product may also be available in Canada.

#In Canada, *Phenaphen with Codeine* is different from the product
with that name in the U.S. The Canadian product contains phenobarbital,
ASA, and codeine.

Description

Combination medicines containing narcotic (nar-KOT-ik)
analgesics (an-al-JEE-zicks) and acetaminophen are used

to relieve pain. A narcotic analgesic and acetaminophen used together may provide better pain relief than either medicine used alone. In some cases, relief of pain may come at lower doses of each medicine.

Narcotic analgesics act in the central nervous system (CNS) to relieve pain. Many of their side effects are also caused by actions in the CNS. When narcotics are used for a long time, your body may get used to them so that larger amounts are needed to relieve pain. This is called tolerance to the medicine. Also, when narcotics are used for a long time or in large doses, they may become habit-forming (causing mental or physical dependence). Physical dependence may lead to withdrawal symptoms when you stop taking the medicine.

Acetaminophen does not become habit-forming when taken for a long time or in large doses, but it may cause other unwanted effects, including liver damage, if too much is taken.

In the U.S., these medicines are available only with your medical doctor's or dentist's prescription. In Canada, some acetaminophen, codeine, and caffeine combinations are available without a prescription.

These medicines are available in the following dosage forms:

Oral

Acetaminophen and Codeine
- Capsules (U.S.)
- Elixir (U.S. and Canada)
- Oral suspension (U.S.)
- Tablets (U.S. and Canada)

Acetaminophen, Codeine, and Caffeine
- Capsules (Canada)
- Tablets (U.S. and Canada)

Dihydrocodeine, Acetaminophen, and Caffeine
- Capsules (U.S.)

Hydrocodone and Acetaminophen
- Capsules (U.S.)

- Oral solution (U.S.)
- Tablets (U.S.)

Meperidine and Acetaminophen
- Tablets (U.S.)

Oxycodone and Acetaminophen
- Capsules (U.S.)
- Oral solution (U.S.)
- Tablets (U.S. and Canada)

Pentazocine and Acetaminophen
- Tablets (U.S.)

Propoxyphene and Acetaminophen
- Capsules (U.S.)
- Tablets (U.S.)

Before Using This Medicine

In deciding to use a medicine, the risks of taking the medicine must be weighed against the good it will do. This is a decision you and your doctor will make. For narcotic analgesic and acetaminophen combinations, the following should be considered:

Allergies—Tell your doctor if you have ever had any unusual or allergic reaction to acetaminophen or to a narcotic analgesic. Also tell your health care professional if you are allergic to any other substances, such as foods, preservatives, or dyes.

Pregnancy—

- *For acetaminophen:* Although studies on birth defects with acetaminophen have not been done in pregnant women, it has not been reported to cause birth defects or other problems.

- *For narcotic analgesics:* Although studies on birth defects with narcotic analgesics have not been done in pregnant women, they have not been reported to cause birth defects. However, hydrocodone caused birth defects in animal studies when very large doses were used. Codeine did not cause birth defects in animals, but it caused slower development of bones and other toxic or harmful effects in the fetus. Pentazocine and propoxyphene did not cause birth defects in animals. There is no information about whether dihydrocodeine, meperidine, or oxycodone cause birth defects in animals.

Too much use of a narcotic during pregnancy may cause the fetus to become dependent on the medicine. This may lead to withdrawal side effects in the newborn baby. Also, some of these medicines may cause breathing problems in the newborn baby if taken just before or during delivery.

• *For caffeine:* Studies in humans have not shown that caffeine (contained in some of these combination medicines) causes birth defects. However, studies in animals have shown that caffeine causes birth defects when given in very large doses (amounts equal to those present in 12 to 24 cups of coffee a day).

Breast-feeding—Acetaminophen, codeine, meperidine, and propoxyphene pass into the breast milk. It is not known whether other narcotic analgesics pass into the breast milk. However, these medicines have not been reported to cause problems in nursing babies.

Children—Breathing problems may be especially likely to occur when narcotic analgesics are given to children younger than 2 years of age. These children are usually more sensitive than adults to the effects of narcotic analgesics. Also, unusual excitement or restlessness may be more likely to occur in children receiving these medicines.

Acetaminophen has been tested in children and has not been shown to cause different side effects or problems in children than it does in adults.

Older adults—Elderly people are especially sensitive to the effects of narcotic analgesics. This may increase the chance of side effects, especially breathing problems, during treatment.

Acetaminophen has been tested and has not been shown to cause different side effects or problems in older people than it does in younger adults.

Other medicines—Although certain medicines should not be used together at all, in other cases two different medicines may be used together even if an interaction might occur. In these cases, your doctor may want to change the dose, or other precautions may be necessary. When you are taking a narcotic analgesic and acetaminophen combination, it is especially important that your health care professional know if you are taking any of the following:

- Carbamazepine (e.g., Tegretol)—Propoxyphene may increase the blood levels of carbamazepine, which increases the chance of serious side effects
- Central nervous system (CNS) depressants or
- Monoamine oxidase (MAO) inhibitors (furazolidone [e.g., Furoxone], isocarboxazid [e.g., Marplan], pargyline [e.g., Eutonyl], phenelzine [e.g., Nardil], procarbazine [e.g., Matulane], tranylcypromine [e.g., Parnate]) (taken currently or within the past 2 weeks) or
- Tricyclic antidepressants (amitriptyline [e.g., Elavil], amoxapine [e.g., Asendin], clomipramine [e.g., Anafranil], desipramine [e.g., Pertofrane], doxepin [e.g., Sinequan], imipramine [e.g., Tofranil], nortriptyline [e.g., Aventyl], protriptyline [e.g., Vivactil], trimipramine [e.g., Surmontil])—Taking these medicines together with a narcotic analgesic may increase the chance of serious side effects
- Naltrexone (e.g., Trexan)—Naltrexone keeps narcotic analgesics from working to relieve pain; people taking naltrexone should take pain relievers that do not contain a narcotic
- Zidovudine (e.g., AZT, Retrovir)—Acetaminophen may increase the blood levels of zidovudine, which increases the chance of serious side effects

Other medical problems—The presence of other medical problems may affect the use of narcotic analgesic and acetaminophen combinations. Make sure you tell your doctor if you have any other medical problems, especially:

- Alcohol and/or other drug abuse, or history of, or
- Brain disease or head injury or
- Colitis or
- Convulsions (seizures), history of, or
- Emotional problems or mental illness or
- Emphysema, asthma, or other chronic lung disease or
- Hepatitis or other liver disease or
- Kidney disease or
- Underactive thyroid—The chance of serious side effects may be increased

- Enlarged prostate or problems with urination or
- Gallbladder disease or gallstones—Some of the effects of narcotic analgesics may be especially serious in people with these medical problems

- Heart disease—Caffeine (present in some of these combination medicines) can make some kinds of heart disease worse

Proper Use of This Medicine

Take this medicine only as directed by your medical doctor or dentist. Do not take more of it, do not take it more often, and do not take it for a longer time than your medical doctor or dentist ordered. This is especially important for young children and elderly patients, who may be more sensitive than other people to the effects of narcotic analgesics. If too much of a narcotic analgesic is taken, it may become habit-forming (causing mental or physical dependence) or lead to medical problems because of an overdose. Taking too much acetaminophen may cause liver damage.

If you think that this medicine is not working properly after you have been taking it for a few weeks, *do not increase the dose*. Instead, check with your medical doctor or dentist.

Missed dose—If your medical doctor or dentist has ordered you to take this medicine according to a regular schedule and you miss a dose, take it as soon as you remember. However, if it is almost time for your next dose, skip the missed dose and go back to your regular dosing schedule. *Do not double doses.*

Storage—To store this medicine:

- Keep out of the reach of children. Overdose is very dangerous in young children.
- Store away from heat and direct light.
- Do not store tablets or capsules in the bathroom, near the kitchen sink, or in other damp places. Heat or moisture may cause the medicine to break down.
- Keep the liquid forms of this medicine from freezing.
- Do not keep outdated medicine or medicine no longer needed. Be sure that any discarded medicine is out of the reach of children.

Precautions While Using This Medicine

If you will be taking this medicine for a long time (for example, for several months at a time), or in high doses, your doctor should check your progress at regular visits.

Check the labels of all nonprescription (over-the-counter [OTC]) and prescription medicines you now take. If any contain acetaminophen or a narcotic be especially careful, since taking them while taking this medicine may lead to overdose. If you have any questions about this, check with your medical doctor, dentist, or pharmacist.

The narcotic analgesic in this medicine will add to the effects of alcohol and other CNS depressants (medicines that slow down the nervous system, possibly causing drowsiness). Some examples of CNS depressants are antihistamines or medicine for hay fever, other allergies, or colds; sedatives, tranquilizers, or sleeping medicine; other prescription pain medicine or narcotics; barbiturates; medicine for seizures; muscle relaxants; or anesthetics, including some dental anesthetics. Also, there may be a greater risk of liver damage if large amounts of alcoholic beverages are used while you are taking acetaminophen. *Do not drink alcoholic beverages, and check with your medical doctor or dentist before taking any of the medicines listed above, while you are using this medicine.*

Too much use of the acetaminophen in this combination medicine together with certain other medicines may increase the chance of unwanted effects. The risk will depend on how much of each medicine you take every day, and on how long you take the medicines together. If your doctor directs you to take these medicines together on a regular basis, follow his or her directions carefully. However, do not take this medicine together with any of the following medicines for more than a few days, unless your doctor has directed you to do so and is following your progress:

Aspirin or other salicylates
Diclofenac (e.g., Voltaren)
Diflunisal (e.g., Dolobid)
Fenoprofen (e.g., Nalfon)
Floctafenine (e.g., Idarac)
Flurbiprofen, oral (e.g., Ansaid)
Ibuprofen (e.g., Motrin)
Indomethacin (e.g., Indocin)
Ketoprofen (e.g., Orudis)
Ketorolac (e.g., Toradol)
Meclofenamate (e.g., Meclomen)
Mefenamic acid (e.g., Ponstel)
Naproxen (e.g., Naprosyn)
Phenylbutazone (e.g., Butazolidin)
Piroxicam (e.g., Feldene)
Sulindac (e.g., Clinoril)
Tiaprofenic acid (e.g., Surgam)
Tolmetin (e.g., Tolectin)

This medicine may cause some people to become drowsy, dizzy, or lightheaded, or to feel a false sense of well-being. *Make sure you know how you react to this medicine before you drive, use machines, or do anything else that could be dangerous if you are dizzy or are not alert and clearheaded.*

Dizziness, lightheadedness, or fainting may occur, especially when you get up suddenly from a lying or sitting position. Getting up slowly may help lessen this problem.

Nausea or vomiting may occur, especially after the first couple of doses. This effect may go away if you lie down for a while. However, if nausea or vomiting continues, check with your medical doctor or dentist. Lying down for a while may also help relieve some other side effects, such as dizziness or lightheadedness, that may occur.

Before having any kind of surgery (including dental surgery) or emergency treatment, tell the medical doctor or dentist in charge that you are taking this medicine.

Narcotic analgesics may cause dryness of the mouth. For temporary relief, use sugarless candy or gum, melt bits of ice in your mouth, or use a saliva substitute. However, if dry mouth continues for more than 2 weeks, check with your dentist. Continuing dryness of the mouth may increase the chance of dental disease, including tooth decay, gum disease, and fungus infections.

If you have been taking this medicine regularly for several weeks or more, *do not suddenly stop taking it without first checking with your doctor.* Your doctor may want you to reduce gradually the amount you are taking before stopping completely, to lessen the chance of withdrawal side effects. This will depend on which of these medicines you have been taking, and the amount you have been taking every day.

If you think you or someone else may have taken an overdose of this medicine, get emergency help at once. Taking an overdose of this medicine or taking alcohol or CNS depressants with this medicine may lead to unconsciousness or death. Signs of overdose of narcotics include convulsions (seizures), confusion, severe nervousness or restlessness, severe dizziness, severe drowsiness, shortness of breath or troubled breathing, and severe weakness. Signs of severe acetaminophen overdose may not occur until several days after the overdose is taken.

Side Effects of This Medicine

Along with its needed effects, a medicine may cause some unwanted effects. Although not all of these side effects may occur, if they do occur they may need medical attention.

Get emergency help immediately if any of the following symptoms of overdose occur:

>Cold, clammy skin; confusion (severe); convulsions (seizures); diarrhea; dizziness (severe); drowsiness (severe); increased sweating; low blood pressure; nausea or vomiting (continuing); nervousness or restlessness (severe); pinpoint pupils of eyes; shortness of breath or unusually slow or troubled breathing; slow heartbeat; stomach cramps or pain; weakness (severe)

Also, check with your doctor as soon as possible if any of the following side effects occur:

Less common or rare

>Black, tarry stools; bloody or cloudy urine; confusion; dark urine; difficult or painful urination; fast, slow, or pounding heartbeat; frequent urge to urinate; hallucinations (seeing, hearing, or feeling things that are not there); increased sweating; irregular breathing or wheezing; mental depression; pain in lower back and/ or side (severe and/or sharp); pale stools; pinpoint red spots on skin; redness or flushing of face; ringing or buzzing in ears; skin rash, hives, or itching; sore throat and fever; sudden decrease in amount of urine; swelling of face; trembling or uncontrolled muscle movements;

unusual bleeding or bruising; unusual excitement (especially in children); yellow eyes or skin

Other side effects may occur that usually do not need medical attention. These side effects may go away during treatment as your body adjusts to the medicine. However, check with your medical doctor or dentist if any of the following side effects continue or are bothersome:

More common

Dizziness, lightheadedness, or feeling faint; drowsiness; nausea or vomiting; unusual tiredness or weakness

Less common or rare

Blurred or double vision or other changes in vision; constipation (more common with long-term use and with codeine or meperidine); dry mouth; false sense of well-being; general feeling of discomfort or illness; headache; loss of appetite; nervousness or restlessness; nightmares or unusual dreams; trouble in sleeping

Although not all of the side effects listed above have been reported for all of these combination medicines, they have been reported for at least one of them. However, since all of the narcotic analgesics are very similar, any of the above side effects may occur with any of these medicines.

After you stop using this medicine, your body may need time to adjust. The length of time this takes depends on which of these medicines you were taking, the amount of medicine you were using, and how long you used it. During this time check with your doctor if you notice any of the following side effects:

Body aches; diarrhea; fast heartbeat; fever, runny nose, or sneezing; gooseflesh; increased sweating; increased yawning; loss of appetite; nausea or vomiting; nervousness, restlessness, or irritability; shivering or trembling; stomach cramps; trouble in sleeping; weakness

Other side effects not listed above may also occur in some patients. If you notice any other effects, check with your doctor.

NARCOTIC ANALGESICS AND ASPIRIN Systemic

Some commonly used brand names are:

In the U.S.—

Azdone[5]	Emcodeine No.4[2]
Bexophene[10]	Empirin with Codeine No.2[2]
Cotanal-65[10]	Empirin with Codeine No.3[2]
Damason-P[6]	Empirin with Codeine No.4[2]
Darvon Compound[10]	Lortab ASA[5]
Darvon Compound-65[10]	Margesic A-C[10]
Darvon with A.S.A.[9]	Percodan[7]
Darvon-N with A.S.A.[9]	Percodan-Demi[7]
Doraphen Compound-65[10]	Pro Pox Plus[10]
Doxaphene Compound[10]	Roxiprin[7]
Emcodeine No.2[2]	Synalgos-DC[1]
Emcodeine No.3[2]	Talwin Compound[8]

In Canada—

A.C.&C[3]	Novopropoxyn Compound[10]
Anacin with Codeine[3]	Oxycodan[7]
Ancasal 8[3]	Percodan[7]
Ancasal 15[3]	Percodan-Demi[7]
Ancasal 30[3]	692[10]
C2 Buffered with Codeine[4]	222 Forte[3]
C2 with Codeine[3]	222[3]
Coryphen with Codeine[2]	282[3]
Darvon-N Compound[10]	292[3]
Darvon-N with A.S.A.[9]	293[3]
Endodan[7]	

Other commonly used names are:

dihydrocodeine compound[1]	propoxyphene hydrochloride
drocode and aspirin[1]	compound[10]

Note: For quick reference, the following narcotic analgesics and aspirin combinations are numbered to match the corresponding brand names.

This information applies to the following medicines:

1. Aspirin, Caffeine, and Dihydrocodeine (dye-hye-droe-KOE-deen)†‡
2. Aspirin (AS-pir-in) and Codeine (KOE-deen)‡#
3. Aspirin, Codeine, and Caffeine (kaf-EEN)*#
4. Aspirin, Codeine, and Caffeine, Buffered*#
5. Hydrocodone (hye-droe-KOE-done) and Aspirin†
6. Hydrocodone, Aspirin, and Caffeine†

7. Oxycodone (ox-i-KOE-done) and Aspirin‡#
8. Pentazocine (pen-TAZ-oh-seen) and Aspirin†
9. Propoxyphene (proe-POX-i-feen) and Aspirin#
10. Propoxyphene, Aspirin, and Caffeine‡#

---

*Not commercially available in the U.S.
†Not commercially available in Canada.
‡Generic name product may also be available in the U.S.
§Generic name product may also be available in Canada.
#In Canada, *Aspirin* is a brand name. Acetylsalicylic acid is the generic name in Canada. ASA, a synonym for acetylsalicylic acid, is the term that commonly appears on Canadian product labels.

Description

Combination medicines containing narcotic (nar-KOT-ik) analgesics (an-al-JEE-zicks) and aspirin are used to relieve pain. A narcotic analgesic and aspirin used together may provide better pain relief than either medicine used alone. In some cases, relief of pain may come at lower doses of each medicine.

Narcotic analgesics act in the central nervous system (CNS) to relieve pain. Many of their side effects are also caused by actions in the CNS. When narcotics are used for a long time, your body may get used to them so that larger amounts are needed to relieve pain. This is called tolerance to the medicine. Also, when narcotics are used for a long time or in large doses, they may become habit-forming (causing mental or physical dependence). Physical dependence may lead to withdrawal symptoms when you stop taking the medicine.

Aspirin does not become habit-forming when taken for a long time or in large doses, but it may cause other unwanted effects if too much is taken.

In the U.S., these medicines are available only with your medical doctor's or dentist's prescription. In Canada, some strengths of aspirin, codeine, and caffeine combination are available without a prescription.

These medicines are available in the following dosage forms:

Oral

Aspirin, Caffeine, and Dihydrocodeine
- Capsules (U.S.)

Aspirin and Codeine
- Tablets (U.S. and Canada)

Aspirin, Codeine, and Caffeine
- Tablets (Canada)

Aspirin, Codeine, and Caffeine, Buffered
- Tablets (Canada)

Hydrocodone and Aspirin
- Tablets (U.S.)

Hydrocodone, Aspirin, and Caffeine
- Tablets (U.S.)

Oxycodone and Aspirin
- Tablets (U.S. and Canada)

Pentazocine and Aspirin
- Tablets (U.S.)

Propoxyphene and Aspirin
- Capsules (U.S. and Canada)
- Tablets (U.S.)

Propoxyphene, Aspirin, and Caffeine
- Capsules (U.S. and Canada)
- Tablets (Canada)

Before Using This Medicine

In deciding to use a medicine, the risks of taking the medicine must be weighed against the good it will do. This is a decision you and your doctor will make. For narcotic analgesic and aspirin combinations, the following should be considered:

Allergies—Tell your doctor if you have ever had any unusual or allergic reaction to a narcotic analgesic, aspirin or other salicylates, including methyl salicylate (oil of wintergreen), or any of the following medicines:

Diclofenac (e.g., Voltaren)

Diflunisal (e.g., Dolobid)
Fenoprofen (e.g., Nalfon)
Floctafenine (e.g., Idarac)
Flurbiprofen, oral (e.g., Ansaid)
Ibuprofen (e.g., Motrin)
Indomethacin (e.g., Indocin)
Ketoprofen (e.g., Orudis)
Ketorolac (e.g., Toradol)
Meclofenamate (e.g., Meclomen)
Mefenamic acid (e.g., Ponstel)
Naproxen (e.g., Naprosyn)
Oxyphenbutazone (e.g., Tandearil)
Phenylbutazone (e.g., Butazolidin)
Piroxicam (e.g., Feldene)
Sulindac (e.g., Clinoril)
Suprofen (e.g., Suprol)
Tiaprofenic acid (e.g., Surgam)
Tolmetin (e.g., Tolectin)
Zomepirac (e.g., Zomax)

Also tell your health care professional if you are allergic to any other substances, such as foods, preservatives, or dyes.

Pregnancy—

- *For aspirin:* Studies in humans have not shown that aspirin causes birth defects. However, studies in animals have shown that aspirin causes birth defects.

  Some reports have suggested that too much use of aspirin late in pregnancy may cause a decrease in the newborn's weight and possible death of the fetus or newborn baby. However, the mothers in these reports had been taking much larger amounts of aspirin than are usually recommended. Studies of mothers taking aspirin in the doses that are usually recommended did not show these effects. However, regular use of aspirin late in pregnancy may cause unwanted effects on the heart or blood flow in the fetus or in the newborn baby. Also, use of aspirin during the last 2 weeks of pregnancy may cause bleeding problems in the fetus before or during delivery or in the newborn baby.

Too much use of aspirin during the last 3 months of pregnancy may increase the length of pregnancy, prolong labor, cause other problems during delivery, or cause severe bleeding in the mother before, during, or after delivery. *Do not take aspirin during the last 3 months of pregnancy unless it has been ordered by your doctor.*

- *For narcotic analgesics:* Although studies on birth defects with narcotic analgesics have not been done in pregnant women, they have not been reported to cause birth defects. However, hydrocodone caused birth defects in animal studies when given in very large doses. Codeine did not cause birth defects in animals, but it caused slower development of bones and other toxic or harmful effects on the fetus. Pentazocine and propoxyphene did not cause birth defects in animals. There is no information about whether dihydrocodeine or oxycodone causes birth defects in animals.

Too much use of a narcotic during pregnancy may cause the fetus to become dependent on the medicine. This may lead to withdrawal side effects in the newborn baby. Also, some of these medicines may cause breathing problems in the newborn baby if taken just before or during delivery.

- *For caffeine:* Studies in humans have not shown that caffeine (contained in some of these combination medicines) causes birth defects. However, studies in animals have shown that caffeine causes birth defects when given in very large doses (amounts equal to those present in 12 to 24 cups of coffee a day).

Breast-feeding—These combination medicines have not been reported to cause problems in nursing babies. However, aspirin, caffeine, codeine, and propoxyphene pass into the breast milk. It is not known whether dihydrocodeine, hydrocodone, oxycodone, or pentazocine passes into the breast milk.

Children—*Do not give a medicine containing aspirin to a child or a teenager with a fever or other symptoms of a virus infection, especially flu or chickenpox, without first discussing its use with your child's doctor.* This is very important because aspirin may cause a serious illness called Reye's syndrome in children with fever caused by a virus infection, especially flu or chickenpox. Children who do not have a virus infection may also be more sensitive to the effects of aspirin, especially if they have a fever or have lost large amounts of body fluid because of vomiting, diarrhea, or sweating. This may increase the chance of side effects during treatment.

The narcotic analgesic in this combination medicine can cause breathing problems, especially in children younger than 2 years of age. These children are usually more sensitive than adults to the effects of narcotic analgesics. Also, unusual excitement or restlessness may be more likely to occur in children receiving these medicines.

Older adults—Elderly people are especially sensitive to the effects of aspirin and of narcotic analgesics. This may increase the chance of side effects, especially breathing problems caused by narcotic analgesics, during treatment.

Other medicines—Although certain medicines should not be used together at all, in other cases two different medicines may be used together even if an interaction might occur. In these cases, your doctor may want to change the dose, or other precautions may be necessary. When you are taking a narcotic analgesic and aspirin combination, it is especially important that your health care professional know if you are taking any of the following:

- Anticoagulants (blood thinners) or
- Carbenicillin by injection (e.g., Geopen) or
- Cefamandole (e.g., Mandol) or
- Cefoperazone (e.g., Cefobid) or
- Cefotetan (e.g., Cefotan) or
- Dipyridamole (e.g., Persantine) or

- Divalproex (e.g., Depakote) or
- Heparin or
- Medicine for inflammation or pain, except narcotics, or
- Moxalactam (e.g., Moxam) or
- Pentoxifylline (e.g., Trental) or
- Plicamycin (e.g., Mithracin) or
- Ticarcillin (e.g., Ticar) or
- Valproic acid (e.g., Depakene)—Taking these medicines together with aspirin may increase the chance of bleeding
- Antidiabetics, oral (diabetes medicine you take by mouth)—Aspirin may increase the effects of the antidiabetic medicine; a change in the dose of the antidiabetic medicine may be needed if aspirin is taken regularly
- Carbamazepine (e.g., Tegretol)—Propoxyphene can increase the blood levels of carbamazepine, which increases the chance of serious side effects
- Central nervous system (CNS) depressants or
- Diarrhea medicine or
- Methotrexate (e.g., Mexate) or
- Tricyclic antidepressants (amitriptyline [e.g., Elavil], amoxapine [e.g., Asendin], clomipramine [e.g., Anafranil], desipramine [e.g., Pertofrane], doxepin [e.g., Sinequan], imipramine [e.g., Tofranil], nortriptyline [e.g., Aventyl], protriptyline [e.g., Vivactil], trimipramine [e.g., Surmontil]) or
- Vancomycin (e.g., Vancocin)—The chance of side effects may be increased
- Naltrexone (e.g., Trexan)—Naltrexone keeps narcotic analgesics from working to relieve pain; people taking naltrexone should use pain relievers that do not contain a narcotic
- Probenecid (e.g., Benemid) or
- Sulfinpyrazone (e.g., Anturane)—Aspirin can keep these medicines from working as well for treating gout; also, use of sulfinpyrazone and aspirin together may increase the chance of bleeding
- Urinary alkalizers (medicine that makes the urine less acid, such as acetazolamide [e.g., Diamox], calcium- and/or magnesium-containing antacids, dichlorphenamide [e.g., Daranide], methazolamide [e.g., Neptazane], potassium or sodium citrate and/or citric acid, sodium bicarbonate [bak-

ing soda])—These medicines may make aspirin less effective by causing it to be removed from the body more quickly

- Zidovudine (e.g., AZT, Retrovir)—Higher blood levels of zidovudine and an increased chance of serious side effects may occur

Other medical problems—The presence of other medical problems may affect the use of narcotic analgesic and aspirin combinations. Make sure you tell your doctor if you have any other medical problems, especially:

- Alcohol and/or other drug abuse, or history of, or
- Asthma, allergies, and nasal polyps (history of) or
- Brain disease or head injury or
- Colitis or
- Convulsions (seizures), history of, or
- Emotional problems or mental illness or
- Emphysema or other chronic lung disease or
- Kidney disease or
- Liver disease or
- Underactive thyroid—The chance of serious side effects may be increased

- Anemia or
- Overactive thyroid or
- Stomach ulcer or other stomach problems—Aspirin may make these conditions worse

- Enlarged prostate or problems with urination or
- Gallbladder disease or gallstones—Narcotic analgesics have side effects that may be dangerous if these medical problems are present

- Gout—Aspirin can make this condition worse and can also lessen the effects of some medicines used to treat gout

- Heart disease—Large amounts of aspirin and caffeine (present in some of these combination medicines) can make some kinds of heart disease worse

- Hemophilia or other bleeding problems or
- Vitamin K deficiency—Aspirin increases the chance of serious bleeding

Proper Use of This Medicine

Take this medicine with food or a full glass (8 ounces) of water to lessen stomach irritation.

Do not take this medicine if it has a strong vinegar-like odor. This odor means the aspirin in it is breaking down. If you have any questions about this, check with your health care professional.

Take this medicine only as directed by your medical doctor or dentist. Do not take more of it, do not take it more often, and do not take it for a longer time than your medical doctor or dentist ordered. This is especially important for children and elderly patients, who are usually more sensitive to the effects of these medicines. If too much of a narcotic analgesic is taken, it may become habit-forming (causing mental or physical dependence) or lead to medical problems because of an overdose. Also, taking too much aspirin may cause stomach problems or lead to medical problems because of an overdose.

If you think that this medicine is not working as well after you have been taking it for a few weeks, *do not increase the dose.* Instead, check with your medical doctor or dentist.

Missed dose—If your medical doctor or dentist has ordered you to take this medicine according to a regular schedule and you miss a dose, take it as soon as you remember. However, if it is almost time for your next dose, skip the missed dose and go back to your regular dosing schedule. *Do not double doses.*

Storage—To store this medicine:

- Keep out of the reach of children. Overdose is very dangerous in young children.
- Store away from heat and direct light.
- Do not store this medicine in the bathroom, near the kitchen sink, or in other damp places. Heat or moisture may cause the medicine to break down.

- Do not keep outdated medicine or medicine no longer needed. Be sure that any discarded medicine is out of the reach of children.

Precautions While Using This Medicine

If you will be taking this medicine for a long time (for example, for several months at a time), your doctor should check your progress at regular visits.

Check the labels of all nonprescription (over-the-counter [OTC]) and prescription medicines you now take. If any contain a narcotic, aspirin, or other salicylates, be especially careful, since taking them while taking this medicine may lead to overdose. If you have any questions about this, check with your medical doctor, dentist, or pharmacist.

This medicine will add to the effects of alcohol and other CNS depressants (medicines that slow down the nervous system, possibly causing drowsiness). Some examples of CNS depressants are antihistamines or medicine for hay fever, other allergies, or colds; sedatives, tranquilizers, or sleeping medicine; other prescription pain medicine or narcotics; barbiturates; medicine for seizures; muscle relaxants; or anesthetics, including some dental anesthetics. Also, stomach problems may be more likely to occur if you drink alcoholic beverages while you are taking aspirin. *Do not drink alcoholic beverages, and check with your medical doctor or dentist before taking any of the medicines listed above, while you are using this medicine.*

Taking acetaminophen or certain other medicines together with the aspirin in this combination medicine may increase the chance of unwanted effects. The risk will depend on how much of each medicine you take every day, and on how long you take the medicines together. If your doctor directs you to take these medicines together on a regular basis, follow his or her directions carefully. However, do not take acetaminophen or any of the following medicines together with this combination medicine for more than a few days, unless your doctor has directed you to do so and is following your progress:

Diclofenac (e.g., Voltaren)
Diflunisal (e.g., Dolobid)
Fenoprofen (e.g., Nalfon)
Floctafenine (e.g., Idarac)
Flurbiprofen, oral (e.g., Ansaid)
Ibuprofen (e.g., Motrin)
Indomethacin (e.g., Indocin)
Ketoprofen (e.g., Orudis)
Ketorolac (e.g., Toradol)
Meclofenamate (e.g., Meclomen)
Mefenamic acid (e.g., Ponstel)
Naproxen (e.g., Naprosyn)
Phenylbutazone (e.g., Butazolidin)
Piroxicam (e.g., Feldene)
Sulindac (e.g., Clinoril)
Tiaprofenic acid (e.g., Surgam)
Tolmetin (e.g., Tolectin)

This medicine may cause some people to become drowsy, dizzy, or lightheaded, or to feel a false sense of well-being. *Make sure you know how you react to this medicine before you drive, use machines, or do anything else that could be dangerous if you are dizzy or are not alert and clearheaded.*

Dizziness, lightheadedness, or fainting may occur, especially when you get up suddenly from a lying or sitting position. Getting up slowly may help lessen this problem.

Nausea or vomiting may occur, especially after the first couple of doses. This effect may go away if you lie down for a while. However, if nausea or vomiting continues, check with your doctor. Lying down for a while may also help some other side effects, such as dizziness or lightheadedness.

Before having any kind of surgery (including dental surgery) or emergency treatment, tell the medical doctor or dentist in charge that you are taking this medicine.

Do not take this medicine for 5 days before any surgery, including dental surgery, unless otherwise directed by your medical doctor or dentist. Taking aspirin during this time may cause bleeding problems.

If you are taking one of the combination medicines containing buffered aspirin, and you are also taking a tetracycline antibiotic, do not take the two medicines within 3 to 4 hours of each other. Taking them too close together may prevent the tetracycline from being absorbed by your body. If you have any questions about this, check with your health care professional.

For *diabetic patients:*
* False urine sugar test results may occur if you are regularly taking 8 or more 325-mg (5-grain) or 5 or more 500-mg doses of aspirin a day. Smaller amounts or occasional use of aspirin usually will not affect urine sugar tests. If you have any questions about this, check with your health care professional, especially if your diabetes is not well controlled.

Narcotic analgesics may cause dryness of the mouth. For temporary relief, use sugarless candy or gum, melt bits of ice in your mouth, or use a saliva substitute. However, if dry mouth continues for more than 2 weeks, check with your dentist. Continuing dryness of the mouth may increase the chance of dental disease, including tooth decay, gum disease, and fungus infections.

If you have been taking this medicine regularly for several weeks or more, *do not suddenly stop using it without first checking with your doctor.* Depending on which of these medicines you have been taking, and the amount you have been taking every day, your doctor may want you to reduce gradually the amount you are taking before stopping completely, to lessen the chance of withdrawal side effects.

If you think you or someone else may have taken an overdose of this medicine, get emergency help at once. Taking an overdose of this medicine or taking alcohol or CNS depressants with this medicine may lead to unconsciousness or death. Signs of overdose of this medicine include convulsions (seizures); hearing loss; confusion; ringing or buzzing in the ears; severe excitement, nervousness, or restlessness; severe dizziness, severe drowsiness, shortness of breath or troubled breathing, and severe weakness.

Side Effects of This Medicine

Along with its needed effects, a medicine may cause some unwanted effects. Although not all of these side effects may occur, if they do occur they may need medical attention.

Get emergency help immediately if any of the following symptoms of overdose occur:

> Any loss of hearing; bloody urine; cold, clammy skin; confusion (severe); convulsions (seizures); diarrhea (severe or continuing); dizziness or lightheadedness (severe); drowsiness (severe); excitement, nervousness, or restlessness (severe); fever; hallucinations (seeing, hearing, or feeling things that are not there); headache (severe or continuing); increased sweating; increased thirst; low blood pressure; nausea or vomiting (severe or continuing); pinpoint pupils of eyes; ringing or buzzing in the ears; shortness of breath or unusually slow or troubled breathing; slow heartbeat; stomach pain (severe or continuing); uncontrollable flapping movements of the hands (especially in elderly patients); vision problems; weakness (severe)

Also, check with your doctor as soon as possible if any of the following side effects occur:

Less common or rare

Bloody or black, tarry stools; confusion; dark urine; fast, slow, or pounding heartbeat; increased sweating (more common with hydrocodone); irregular breathing; mental depression; pale stools; redness or flushing of face (more common with hydrocodone); skin rash, hives, or itching; stomach pain (severe); swelling of face; tightness in chest or wheezing; trembling or uncontrolled muscle movements; unusual excitement (especially in children); unusual tiredness or weakness; vomiting of blood or material that looks like coffee grounds; yellow eyes or skin

Other side effects may occur that usually do not need medical attention. These side effects may go away during treatment as your body adjusts to the medicine. However, check with your doctor if any of the following side effects continue or are bothersome:

More common

Dizziness, lightheadedness, or feeling faint; drowsiness; heartburn or indigestion; nausea or vomiting; stomach pain (mild)

Less common or rare

Blurred or double vision or other changes in vision; constipation (more common with long-term use and with codeine); difficult, painful, or decreased urination; dryness of mouth; false sense of well-being; frequent urge to urinate; general feeling of discomfort or illness; headache; loss of appetite; nervousness or restlessness; nightmares or unusual dreams; trouble in sleeping; unusual tiredness; unusual weakness

Although not all of the side effects listed above have been reported for all of these medicines, they have been reported for at least one of them. However, since all of the narcotic analgesics are very similar, any of the above side effects may occur with any of these medicines.

After you stop using this medicine, your body may need time to adjust. The length of time this takes depends on which of these medicines you were taking, the amount of medicine you were using, and how long you used it. During this period of time check with your doctor if you notice any of the following side effects:

> Body aches; diarrhea; fever, runny nose, or sneezing; goose-flesh; increased sweating; increased yawning; loss of appetite; nausea or vomiting; nervousness, restlessness, or irritability; shivering or trembling; stomach cramps; trouble in sleeping; weakness

Other side effects not listed above may also occur in some patients. If you notice any other effects, check with your medical doctor or dentist.

NEDOCROMIL   Inhalation

A commonly used brand name in the U.S. and Canada is Tilade.

Description

Nedocromil (ne-DOK-roe-mil) is used to prevent the symptoms of asthma. When it is used regularly, nedocromil lessens the number and severity of asthma attacks by reducing inflammation in the lungs. Nedocromil is also used just before exposure to conditions or substances (for example, allergens, chemicals, cold air, or air pollutants) that cause reactions, to prevent bronchospasm (wheezing or difficulty in breathing). In addition, nedocromil is used to prevent bronchospasm following exercise. This medicine will not help an asthma or bronchospasm attack that has already started.

Nedocromil may be used alone or with other asthma medicines, such as bronchodilators (medicines that open up narrowed breathing passages) and corticosteroids (cortisone-like medicines).

Nedocromil works by acting on certain inflammatory cells in the lungs to prevent them from releasing substances that cause asthma symptoms and/or bronchospasm.

This medicine is available only with your doctor's prescription, in the following dosage form:

Inhalation
- Inhalation aerosol (U.S. and Canada)

Before Using This Medicine

In deciding to use a medicine, the risks of using the medicine must be weighed against the good it will do. This is a decision you and your doctor will make. For nedocromil, the following should be considered:

Allergies—Tell your doctor if you have ever had any unusual or allergic reaction to nedocromil or to any other inhalation aerosol medicine.

Pregnancy—Nedocromil has not been studied in pregnant women. However, nedocromil has not been shown to cause birth defects or other problems in animal studies.

Breast-feeding—It is not known whether nedocromil passes into breast milk. Although most medicines pass into breast milk in small amounts, many of them may be used safely while breast-feeding. Mothers who are using this medicine and who wish to breast-feed should discuss this with their doctor.

Children—Nedocromil has been tested in a limited number of children 6 years of age and older. In effective doses, it is not expected to cause different side effects or problems in children than it does in adults.

Older adults—Many medicines have not been studied specifically in older people. Therefore, it may not be known whether they work the same way they do in younger adults. Although there is no specific information comparing use of nedocromil in the elderly with use in other age groups, it is not expected to cause different side effects or problems in older people than it does in younger adults.

Proper Use of This Medicine

Nedocromil is used to help prevent symptoms of asthma or bronchospasm (wheezing or difficulty in breathing). When this medicine is used regularly, it decreases the number and severity of asthma attacks. Nedocromil will not relieve an asthma or bronchospasm attack that has already started.

Nedocromil inhalation aerosol usually comes with patient directions. Read them carefully before using this medicine. If you do not understand the directions or if you are not sure how to use the inhaler, ask your health care professional to show you what to do. Also, ask your health care professional to check regularly how you use the inhaler to make sure you are using it properly.

The nedocromil aerosol canister provides about 56 or 112 inhalations, depending on the size of the canister your doctor ordered. You should keep a record of the number of inhalations you use so you will know when the canister is almost empty. This canister, unlike other aerosol canisters, cannot be floated in water to test its fullness.

When you use the inhaler for the first time, or if you have not used it for several days, the inhaler may not deliver the right amount of medicine with the first puff. Therefore, before using the inhaler, test it to make sure it works properly.

To test the inhaler:

- Insert the metal canister firmly into the clean mouthpiece according to the manufacturer's instructions. Check to make sure the canister is placed properly into the mouthpiece.

- Take the cover off the mouthpiece and shake the inhaler well.
- Hold the canister well away from you against a light background, and press the top of the canister, spraying the medicine one time into the air. If you see a fine mist, you will know the inhaler is working properly to provide the right amount of medicine when you use it. If you do not see a fine mist, try a second time.

To use the inhaler:

- Using your thumb and one or two fingers, hold the inhaler upright with the mouthpiece end down and pointing toward you.
- Take the cover off the mouthpiece. Check the mouthpiece for any foreign objects. Do not use the inhaler with any other mouthpieces.
- Gently shake the inhaler three or four times.
- Hold the mouthpiece away from your mouth and breathe out slowly and completely to the end of a normal breath.
- Use the inhalation method recommended by your doctor.

  —Open-mouth method: Place the mouthpiece about 1 to 2 inches (2 fingerwidths) in front of your widely opened mouth. Make sure the inhaler is aimed into your mouth so the spray does not hit the roof of your mouth or your tongue. Close your eyes just before spraying to keep the spray out of your eyes.

  —Closed-mouth method: Place the mouthpiece in your mouth between your teeth and over your tongue with your lips closed tightly around it. Make sure your tongue or teeth are not blocking the opening.

- Tilt your head back a little. Start to breathe in slowly and deeply through your mouth and, at the same time, press the top of the canister once to get one puff of medicine. Continue to breathe in slowly for 3 to 4 seconds until you have taken a full breath. It is important to press down on the canister and breathe in slowly at the same time so the medicine is pulled into your lungs. This step may be difficult at first. If you are using the closed-mouth method and you see a fine mist coming from your mouth or nose, the inhaler is not being used correctly.

- Hold your breath as long as you can for up to 10 seconds (count slowly to 10). This gives the medicine time to get into your airways and lungs.
- Take the mouthpiece away from your mouth and breathe out slowly.
- If your doctor has told you to inhale more than one puff of medicine at each dose, wait 1 minute between puffs. Then, gently shake the inhaler again, and take the second puff following exactly the same steps you used for the first puff. Breathe in only one puff at a time.
- If your doctor has told you to use an inhaled bronchodilator before using nedocromil, you should wait at least 2 minutes after using the bronchodilator before using nedocromil. This allows the nedocromil to get deeper into your lungs.
- When you are finished, wipe off the mouthpiece and replace the cover to keep the mouthpiece clean and free of foreign objects.

Your doctor may want you to use a spacer device with the inhaler. A spacer makes the inhaler easier to use. It allows more of the medicine to reach your lungs and helps make sure that less of it stays in your mouth and throat.

To use a spacer device with the inhaler:

- Attach the spacer to the inhaler according to the manufacturer's directions. There are different types of spacers available, but the method of breathing remains the same with most spacers.

- Gently shake the inhaler and spacer three or four times.

- Hold the mouthpiece of the spacer away from your mouth and breathe out slowly to the end of a normal breath.

- Place the mouthpiece into your mouth between your teeth and over your tongue with your lips closed around it.

- Press down on the canister top once to release one puff of medicine into the spacer. Then, within one or two seconds, begin to breathe in slowly and deeply through your mouth for 5 to 10 seconds. Count the seconds while inhaling. Do not breathe in through your nose.

- Hold your breath as long as you can for up to 10 seconds (count slowly to ten).

- Breathe out slowly. Do not remove the mouthpiece from your mouth. Breathe in and out slowly two or three times to make sure the spacer device is emptied.

- If your doctor has told you to take more than one puff of medicine at each dose, wait a minute between puffs. Then, gently shake the inhaler and spacer again and take the second puff, following exactly the same steps you used for the first puff.

- When you have finished, remove the spacer device from the inhaler and replace the cover of the mouthpiece.

To clean the inhaler:

- Clean the inhaler often to prevent build-up of medicine and blocking of the mouthpiece. The mouthpiece can be washed every day and should be washed at least twice a week.

- Remove the metal canister from the inhaler and set it aside. Do not get the canister wet.

- Wash the mouthpiece in hot water.

- Shake off the excess water and let the mouthpiece air dry completely before replacing the metal canister and cover.

For patients using nedocromil regularly (for example, every day):

- *In order for nedocromil to work properly, it must be inhaled every day in regularly spaced doses as ordered by your doctor.*
- Usually about 2 to 4 weeks may pass before you begin to feel the full effects of this medicine.

Missed dose—If you are using nedocromil regularly and you miss a dose of this medicine, take it as soon as possible. Then take any remaining doses for that day at regularly spaced times.

Dosing—The dose of nedocromil will be different for different patients. *Follow your doctor's orders or the directions on the label.* The following information includes only the average doses of nedocromil. *If your dose is different, do not change it* unless your doctor tells you to do so:

- For *inhalation* dosage form (inhalation aerosol):

  —For prevention of asthma symptoms:

  - Adults and children 12 years of age or older— 3.5 or 4 milligrams (mg) (2 puffs) two to four times a day at regularly spaced times.
  - Children up to 12 years of age—Use and dose must be determined by the doctor.

  —For prevention of bronchospasm caused by exercise or a substance:

  - Adults and children 12 years of age or older— 4 mg (2 puffs) as a single dose up to thirty minutes before exercise or exposure to any condition or substance that may cause an attack.
  - Children up to 12 years of age—Use and dose must be determined by the doctor.

Storage—To store this medicine:
- Keep out of the reach of children.
- Store away from heat and direct sunlight.
- Keep the medicine from freezing.
- Do not puncture, break, or burn the aerosol container, even if it is empty.
- Do not keep outdated medicine or medicine no longer needed. Be sure that any discarded medicine is out of the reach of children.
- Always keep the dust cover on the mouthpiece when the inhaler is not in use.

Precautions While Using This Medicine

If your symptoms do not improve within 2 to 4 weeks, check with your doctor. Also, check with your doctor if your condition becomes worse.

You may also be taking a corticosteroid or a bronchodilator for asthma along with this medicine. *Do not stop taking the corticosteroid or bronchodilator even if your asthma seems better, unless you are told to do so by your doctor.*

Throat irritation and/or an unpleasant taste may occur after you use this medicine. Gargling and rinsing the mouth after each dose may help prevent these effects.

Side Effects of This Medicine

Along with its needed effects, a medicine may cause some unwanted effects. Although not all of these side effects may occur, if they do occur they may need medical attention.

Check with your doctor as soon as possible if any of the following side effects occur:

Less common

   Increased wheezing, tightness in chest, or difficulty in
   breathing

Other side effects may occur that usually do not need
medical attention. These side effects may go away during
treatment as your body adjusts to the medicine. However,
check with your doctor if any of the following side effects
continue or are bothersome:

Less common

   Cough; headache; nausea; runny or stuffy nose; throat
   irritation

After you use nedocromil inhalation aerosol, you may notice an unpleasant taste. This may be expected and will
usually go away after a while.

Other side effects not listed above may also occur in some
patients. If you notice any other effects, check with your
doctor.

NICOTINE   Systemic

Some commonly used brand names are:

In the U.S.—

Habitrol	Nicorette DS
Nicoderm	Nicotrol
Nicorette	ProStep

In Canada—

Habitrol	Nicorette
Nicoderm	Nicotrol

Description

Nicotine (NIK-o-teen), in a flavored chewing gum or a
skin patch, is used to help you stop smoking. It is used
for up to 12 to 20 weeks as part of a supervised stop-
smoking program. These programs may include education,

counseling, and psychological support. Using nicotine replacement products without taking part in a supervised stop-smoking program has not been shown to be effective.

- As you chew nicotine gum, nicotine passes through the lining of your mouth and into your body.
- When you wear a nicotine patch, nicotine passes through your skin into your bloodstream.

This nicotine takes the place of nicotine that you would otherwise get from smoking. In this way, the withdrawal effects of not smoking are less severe. Then, as your body adjusts to not smoking, the use of the nicotine gum is decreased gradually, or the strength of the patches is decreased over a few weeks. Finally, use is stopped altogether.

Children, pregnant women, and nonsmokers should not use nicotine gum or patches because of unwanted effects.

Nicotine gum and patches are available only with your doctor's prescription, in the following dosage forms:

Oral
- Chewing gum tablets (U.S. and Canada)

Topical
- Transdermal (stick-on) skin patch (U.S. and Canada)

Before Using This Medicine

In deciding to use a medicine, the risks of taking the medicine must be weighed against the good it will do. This is a decision you and your doctor will make. For nicotine gum, the following should be considered:

Allergies—Tell your doctor if you have ever had any unusual or allergic reaction to nicotine. Also tell your health care professional if you are allergic to any other substances, such as foods, preservatives, or dyes. If you plan to use the nicotine patches, tell your doctor if you have ever had a rash or irritation from adhesive tape or bandages.

Pregnancy—Nicotine, whether from smoking or from the gum or patches, is not recommended during pregnancy. Studies in humans show that miscarriages have occurred in pregnant women using nicotine replacement products. In addition, studies in animals have shown that nicotine can cause harmful effects in the fetus.

Breast-feeding—Nicotine passes into breast milk and may cause unwanted effects in the baby. It may be necessary for you to stop breast-feeding during treatment.

Children—Small amounts of nicotine can cause serious harm in children. Even used nicotine patches contain enough nicotine to cause problems in children.

Older adults—Nicotine gum and patches have been used in a limited number of patients 60 years of age or older, and have not been shown to cause different side effects or problems in older people than in younger adults.

Other medicines—Although certain medicines should not be used together at all, in other cases two different medicines may be used together even if an interaction might occur. In these cases, your doctor may want to change the dose, or other precautions may be necessary. When you are using nicotine gum or patches, it is especially important that your health care professional know if you are taking any of the following:

- Aminophylline (e.g., Somophyllin) or
- Insulin or
- Oxtriphylline (e.g., Choledyl) or
- Propoxyphene (e.g., Darvon) or
- Propranolol (e.g., Inderal) or
- Theophylline (e.g., Somophyllin-T)—Stopping smoking may increase the effects of these medicines; the amount of medicine you need to take may change

Other medical problems—The presence of other medical problems may affect the use of nicotine gum or patches.

Make sure you tell your doctor if you have any other medical problems, especially:

- Dental problems (with gum only) or
- Diabetes mellitus (sugar diabetes) or
- Heart or blood vessel disease or
- High blood pressure or
- Inflammation of mouth or throat (with gum only) or
- Irritated skin (with patches only) or
- Overactive thyroid or
- Pheochromocytoma (PCC) or
- Stomach ulcer or
- Temporomandibular (jaw) joint disorder (TMJ) (with gum only)—Nicotine gum or patches may make the condition worse

---

Proper Use of This Medicine

For patients using the *chewing gum tablets:*

- Nicotine gum usually comes with patient directions. *Read the directions carefully before using this medicine.*
- *When you feel the urge to smoke, chew one piece of gum very slowly* until you taste it or feel a slight tingling in your mouth. Stop chewing, and place (''park'') the chewing gum tablet between your cheek and gum until the taste or tingling is almost gone. Then chew slowly until you taste it again. Continue chewing and stopping (''parking'') in this way for about 30 minutes in order to get the full dose of nicotine.
- *Do not chew too fast*, do not chew more than one piece at a time, and do not chew a piece of gum too soon after another. To do so may cause unwanted side effects or an overdose. Also, slower chewing will reduce the possibility of belching.
- *Use nicotine gum exactly as directed by your doctor.* Remember that it is also important to participate in

a stop-smoking program during treatment. This may make it easier for you to stop smoking.

- As your urge to smoke becomes less frequent, *gradually reduce the number of pieces of gum you chew each day* until you are chewing one or two pieces a day. This may be possible within 2 to 3 months.

- *Remember to carry nicotine gum with you at all times* in case you feel the sudden urge to smoke. One cigarette may be enough to start you on the smoking habit again.

- Using hard sugarless candy between doses of gum may help to relieve the discomfort in your mouth.

For patients using the *transdermal system (skin patch):*

- *Use this medicine exactly as directed by your doctor.* It will work only if applied correctly. *This medicine usually comes with patient instructions. Read them carefully before using this product.* Remember that it is also important to participate in a stop-smoking program during treatment. This may make it easier for you to stop smoking.

- Do not remove the patch from its sealed pouch until you are ready to put it on your skin. The patch may not work as well if it is unwrapped too soon.

- Do not try to trim or cut the adhesive patch to adjust the dosage. Check with your doctor if you think the medicine is not working as it should.

- Apply the patch to a clean, dry area of skin on your upper arm, chest, or back. Choose an area that is not very oily, has little or no hair, and is free of scars, cuts, burns, or any other skin irritations.

- Press the patch firmly in place with the palm of your hand for about 10 seconds. Make sure there is good contact with your skin, especially around the edges of the patch.

- The patch should stay in place even when you are showering, bathing, or swimming. Apply a new patch if one falls off.

- Rinse your hands with plain water after you have finished applying the patch to your skin. Nicotine on your hands could get into your eyes and nose and cause stinging, redness, or more serious problems. Using soap to wash your hands will increase the amount of nicotine that passes through your skin.

- After 16 or 24 hours, depending on which product you are using, remove the patch. Choose a different place on your skin to apply the next patch. Do not put a new patch in the same place for at least one week. Do not leave the patch on for more than 24 hours. It will not work as well after that time and it may irritate your skin.

- After removing a used patch, fold the patch in half with the sticky sides together. Place the folded, used patch in its protective pouch or in aluminum foil. Make sure to dispose of it out of the reach of children and pets.

- Try to change the patch at the same time each day. If you want to change the time when you put on your patch, just remove the patch you are wearing and put on a new patch. After that, apply a fresh patch at the new time each day.

Dosing—The dose of nicotine will be different for different patients. *Follow your doctor's orders or the directions on the label*. The following information includes only the average doses of nicotine. *If your dose is different, do not change it* unless your doctor tells you to do so.

- For the *oral* dosage form (chewing gum tablets):

  —To help you stop smoking:

  - Adults and older children—The usual dose is 20 to 24 milligrams (mg) a day. However, the number of pieces of nicotine gum you chew each day depends on how often you have the urge to smoke, how fast you chew, and the strength of the gum. You should not chew more than 30 pieces of 2-mg strength gum or more than 15 pieces of 4-mg strength gum (a total of 60 mg) a day.

- Children up to 12 years of age—Use and dose must be determined by your doctor.

- For the *transdermal* (stick-on) skin patch:

  —To help you stop smoking:

  - Adults—The dose you receive will be based on your body weight, how often you have the urge to smoke, and the strength of the patch you use. This dose will be determined by your doctor.

  - Children—Use and dose must be determined by your doctor.

Storage—To store this medicine:

- Keep out of the reach of children because even small doses of nicotine can cause serious harm in children.

- Store away from heat and direct light.

- Do not store in the bathroom, near the kitchen sink, or in other damp places. Heat or moisture may cause the medicine to break down.

- Do not keep outdated medicine or medicine no longer needed. Be sure that any discarded medicine is out of the reach of children and pets.

Precautions While Using This Medicine

Your doctor should check your progress at regular visits to make sure that the nicotine gum or patches are working properly and that possible side effects are avoided.

Do not smoke during treatment with nicotine gum or patches because of the risk of nicotine overdose.

Nicotine should not be used in pregnancy. If there is a possibility you might become pregnant, you may want to use some type of birth control. If you think you may have become pregnant, stop taking this medicine immediately and check with your doctor.

Nicotine products must be kept out of the reach of children and pets. Even used nicotine patches contain enough nicotine to cause problems in children. If a child chews or swallows one or more pieces of nicotine gum, contact your doctor or poison control center at once. If a child puts on a nicotine patch or plays with a patch that is out of the sealed pouch, take it away from the child and contact your doctor or poison control center at once.

For patients using the *chewing gum tablets:*

- *Do not chew more than 30 2-mg pieces, or 15 4-mg pieces of gum a day.* Chewing too many pieces may be harmful because of the risk of overdose.
- *Do not use nicotine gum for longer than 6 months.* To do so may result in physical dependence on the nicotine.
- *If the gum sticks to your dental work, stop using it and check with your medical doctor or dentist.* Dentures or other dental work may be damaged because nicotine gum is stickier and harder to chew than ordinary gum.

For patients using the *transdermal system (skin patch):*

- Mild itching, burning, or tingling may occur when the patch is first applied, and should go away within an hour. After a patch is removed, the skin underneath it may be somewhat red. It should not remain red for more than a day. *If you get a skin rash from the patch, or if the skin becomes swollen or very red, call your doctor.* Do not put on a new patch. If you become allergic to the nicotine in the patch, you could get sick from using cigarettes or other products that contain nicotine.
- *Do not use nicotine patches for longer than 12 to 20 weeks* (depending on the product) if you have

stopped smoking, because continuing use of nicotine in any form can be harmful and addictive.

Side Effects of This Medicine

Along with its needed effects, a medicine may cause some unwanted effects. Although not all of these side effects may occur, if they do occur they may need medical attention.

Check with your doctor as soon as possible if any of the following side effects occur:

More common

Injury to mouth, teeth, or dental work—with chewing gum only

Rare

Hives, itching, rash, redness, or swelling; irregular heartbeat

Symptoms of overdose (may occur in the following order)

Nausea and/or vomiting; increased watering of mouth (severe); abdominal or stomach pain (severe); diarrhea (severe); cold sweat; headache (severe); dizziness (severe); drooling; disturbed hearing and vision; confusion; weakness (severe); fainting; low blood pressure; difficulty in breathing (severe); fast, weak, or irregular heartbeat; convulsions (seizures)

Other side effects may occur that usually do not need medical attention. These side effects may go away during treatment as your body adjusts to the medicine. However, check with your doctor if any of the following side effects continue or are bothersome:

More common

Belching—with chewing gum only; fast heartbeat; headache (mild); increased appetite; increased watering of mouth (mild)—with chewing gum only; jaw muscle ache—with chewing gum only; redness, itching, and/or burning at site of application of patch—usually stops within an hour; sore mouth or throat—with chewing gum only

Less common or rare

Constipation; coughing (increased); diarrhea; dizziness or lightheadedness (mild); drowsiness; dryness of mouth; hiccups—with chewing gum only; hoarseness—with chewing gum only; irritability or nervousness; loss of appetite; menstrual pain; muscle or joint pain; stomach upset or indigestion (mild); sweating (increased); trouble in sleeping or unusual dreams

Other side effects not listed above may also occur in some patients. If you notice any other effects, check with your doctor.

NITRATES—Lingual Aerosol Systemic

This information applies to nitroglycerin oral spray.
A commonly used brand name in the U.S. and Canada is Nitrolingual.
Another commonly used name is glyceryl trinitrate.

Description

Nitrates (NYE-trates) are used to treat the symptoms of angina (chest pain). Depending on the type of dosage form and how it is taken, nitrates are used to treat angina in three ways:

- to relieve an attack that is occurring by using the medicine when the attack begins;

- to prevent attacks from occurring by using the medicine just before an attack is expected to occur; or

- to reduce the number of attacks that occur by using the medicine regularly on a long-term basis.

When used as a lingual (in the mouth) spray, nitroglycerin is used either to relieve the pain of angina attacks or to prevent an expected angina attack.

Nitroglycerin works by relaxing blood vessels and increasing the supply of blood and oxygen to the heart while reducing its work load.

Nitroglycerin as discussed here is available only with your doctor's prescription, in the following dosage form:

Oral
- Lingual aerosol (U.S. and Canada)

Before Using This Medicine

In deciding to use a medicine, the risks of taking the medicine must be weighed against the good it will do. This is a decision you and your doctor will make. For nitroglycerin lingual aerosol, the following should be considered:

Allergies—Tell your doctor if you have ever had any unusual or allergic reaction to nitrates or nitrites. Also tell your health care professional if you are allergic to any other substances, such as certain foods, preservatives, or dyes.

Pregnancy—Studies on effects in pregnancy have not been done in either humans or animals.

Breast-feeding—It is not known whether this medicine passes into breast milk. Although most medicines pass into breast milk in small amounts, many of them may be used safely while breast-feeding. Mothers who are taking this medicine and who wish to breast-feed should discuss this with their doctor.

Children—Studies on this medicine have been done only in adult patients, and there is no specific information comparing use of nitroglycerin in children with use in other age groups.

Older adults—Dizziness or lightheadedness may be more likely to occur in the elderly, who may be more sensitive to the effects of nitrates.

Other medicines—Although certain medicines should not be used together at all, in other cases two different medicines may be used together even if an interaction might occur. In these cases, your doctor may want to change the dose, or other precautions may be necessary. When you are taking nitroglycerin, it is especially important that your health care professional know if you are taking any of the following:

- Antihypertensives (high blood pressure medicine) or
- Other heart medicine—May increase the effects of nitroglycerin on blood pressure

Other medical problems—The presence of other medical problems may affect the use of nitroglycerin. Make sure you tell your doctor if you have any other medical problems, especially:

- Anemia (severe)
- Glaucoma—May be worsened by nitroglycerin
- Head injury (recent) or
- Stroke (recent)—Nitroglycerin may increase pressure in the brain, which can make problems worse
- Heart attack (recent)—Nitroglycerin may lower blood pressure, which can aggravate problems associated with heart attack
- Kidney disease or
- Liver disease—Effects may be increased because of slower removal of nitroglycerin from the body
- Overactive thyroid

Proper Use of This Medicine

Use nitroglycerin spray exactly as directed by your doctor. It will work only if used correctly.

This medicine usually comes with patient instructions. Read them carefully before you actually need to use it. Then, if you need the medicine quickly, you will know how to use it.

To use nitroglycerin lingual spray:

- Remove the plastic cover. *Do not shake the container.*
- Hold the container upright. With the container held close to your mouth, press the button to spray onto or under your tongue. *Do not inhale the spray.*
- Release the button and close your mouth. Avoid swallowing immediately after using the spray.

For patients using nitroglycerin oral spray *to relieve the pain of an angina attack*:

- *When you begin to feel an attack of angina starting (chest pains or a tightness or squeezing in the chest), sit down. Then use 1 or 2 sprays as directed by your doctor.* This medicine works best when you are standing or sitting. However, since you may become dizzy, lightheaded, or faint soon after using a spray, it is safer to sit rather than stand while the medicine is working. If you become dizzy or faint while sitting, take several deep breaths and bend forward with your head between your knees.
- Remain calm and you should feel better in a few minutes.
- *This medicine usually gives relief in less than 5 minutes.* However, if the pain is not relieved, use a second spray. If the pain continues for another 5 minutes, a third spray may be used. *If you still have the chest pains after a total of 3 sprays in a 15-minute period, contact your doctor or go to a hospital emergency room immediately.*

For patients using nitroglycerin oral spray *to prevent an expected angina attack*:

- You may prevent anginal chest pains for up to 1 hour by using a spray 5 to 10 minutes before expected emotional stress or physical exertion that in the past seemed to bring on an attack.

Dosing—The dose of nitroglycerin lingual spray will be different for different patients. *Follow your doctor's orders or the directions on the label.* The following information includes only the average doses of nitroglycerin lingual spray. *If your dose is different, do not change it* unless your doctor tells you to do so.

- For *oral* dosage form (lingual spray):
  —For chest pain:
    - Adults—One or two sprays on or under the tongue. The dose may be repeated every five minutes as needed. If the chest pain is not relieved after a total of three sprays in a fifteen-minute period, call your doctor or go to the emergency room right away.

Storage—To store this medicine:

- Keep out of the reach of children.
- Store away from heat and direct light.
- Keep the medicine from freezing.
- Do not puncture, break, or burn the aerosol container, even after it is empty.
- Do not keep outdated medicine or medicine no longer needed. Be sure that any discarded medicine is out of the reach of children.

Precautions While Using This Medicine

If you have been using this medicine regularly for several weeks, do not suddenly stop using it. Stopping suddenly may bring on attacks of angina. Check with your doctor for the best way to reduce gradually the amount you are using before stopping completely.

Dizziness, lightheadedness, or faintness may occur, especially when you get up quickly from a lying or sitting position. Getting up slowly may help. If you feel dizzy, sit or lie down.

The dizziness, lightheadedness, or fainting is also more likely to occur if you drink alcohol, stand for long periods of time, exercise, or if the weather is hot. *While you are taking this medicine, be careful to limit the amount of alcohol you drink. Also, use extra care during exercise or hot weather or if you must stand for long periods of time.*

After using a dose of this medicine you may get a headache that lasts for a short time. This is a common side effect, which should become less noticeable after you have used the medicine for a while. If this effect continues or if the headaches are severe, check with your doctor.

Side Effects of This Medicine

Along with its needed effects, a medicine may cause some unwanted effects. Although not all of these side effects may occur, if they do occur they may need medical attention.

Check with your doctor as soon as possible if any of the following side effects occur:

  Rare
     Blurred vision; dryness of mouth; headache (severe or prolonged); skin rash

  Signs and symptoms of overdose (in the order in which they may occur)
     Bluish-colored lips, fingernails, or palms of hands; dizziness (extreme) or fainting; feeling of extreme pressure in head; shortness of breath; unusual tiredness or weakness; weak and fast heartbeat; fever; convulsions (seizures)

Other side effects may occur that usually do not need medical attention. These side effects may go away during treatment as your body adjusts to the medicine. However, check with your doctor if any of the following side effects continue or are bothersome:

More common

Dizziness or lightheadedness, especially when getting up from a lying or sitting position; fast pulse; flushing of face and neck; headache; nausea or vomiting; restlessness

Other side effects not listed above may also occur in some patients. If you notice any other effects, check with your doctor.

NITRATES—Sublingual, Chewable, or Buccal Systemic

Some commonly used brand names are:

In the U.S.—

Cardilate[1]
Isonate[2]
Isorbid[2]
Isordil[2]

Nitrogard[3]
Nitrostat[3]
Sorbitrate[2]

In Canada—

Apo-ISDN[2]
Cardilate[1]
Coronex[2]

Isordil[2]
Nitrogard SR[3]
Nitrostat[3]

Other commonly used names are:

Eritrityl tetranitrate[1]
Erythritol tetranitrate[1]

Glyceryl trinitrate[3]

Note: For quick reference, the following nitrates are numbered to match the corresponding brand names.

This information applies to the following medicines:

1. Erythrityl Tetranitrate (e-RI-thri-till tet-ra-NYE-trate)
2. Isosorbide Dinitrate (eye-soe-SOR-bide dye-NYE-trate)‡
3. Nitroglycerin (nye-troe-GLI-ser-in)‡§

Note: This information does *not* apply to amyl nitrite or pentaerythritol
     tetranitrate.

---

‡Generic name product may also be available in the U.S.
§Generic name product may also be available in Canada.

Description

Nitrates (NYE-trates) are used to treat the symptoms of
angina (chest pain). Depending on the type of dosage form
and how it is taken, nitrates are used to treat angina in
three ways:

- to relieve an attack that is occurring by using the
  medicine when the attack begins;
- to prevent attacks from occurring by using the medicine just before an attack is expected to occur; or
- to reduce the number of attacks that occur by using
  the medicine regularly on a long-term basis.

Nitrates are available in different forms. Sublingual nitrates are generally placed under the tongue where they
dissolve and are absorbed through the lining of the mouth.
Some can also be used buccally, being placed under the
lip or in the cheek. The chewable dosage forms, after
being chewed and held in the mouth before swallowing,
are absorbed in the same way. *It is important to remember
that each dosage form is different and that the specific
directions for each type must be followed if the medicine
is to work properly.*

Nitrates that are used *to relieve the pain* of an angina
attack include:

- sublingual nitroglycerin;
- buccal nitroglycerin;
- sublingual isosorbide dinitrate; and
- chewable isosorbide dinitrate.

Those that can be used *to prevent expected attacks* of
angina include:

- sublingual nitroglycerin;
- buccal nitroglycerin;
- sublingual erythrityl tetranitrate;
- sublingual isosorbide dinitrate; and
- chewable isosorbide dinitrate.

Products that are used regularly on a long-term basis *to reduce the number of attacks* that occur include:

- buccal nitroglycerin;
- oral/sublingual erythrityl tetranitrate; and
- chewable isosorbide dinitrate; and
- sublingual isosorbide dinitrate.

Nitrates work by relaxing blood vessels and increasing the supply of blood and oxygen to the heart while reducing its work load.

Nitrates may also be used for other conditions as determined by your doctor.

The nitrates discussed here are available only with your doctor's prescription, in the following dosage forms:

Buccal

Nitroglycerin
- Extended-release tablets (U.S. and Canada)

Chewable

Isosorbide dinitrate
- Tablets (U.S.)

Sublingual

Erythrityl tetranitrate
- Tablets (U.S. and Canada)
Isosorbide dinitrate
- Tablets (U.S. and Canada)
Nitroglycerin
- Tablets (U.S. and Canada)

Before Using This Medicine

In deciding to use a medicine, the risks of taking the medicine must be weighed against the good it will do. This is a decision you and your doctor will make. For nitrates, the following should be considered:

Allergies—Tell your doctor if you have ever had any unusual or allergic reaction to nitrates or nitrites. Also tell your health care professional if you are allergic to any other substances, such as certain foods, preservatives, or dyes.

Pregnancy—Nitrates have not been studied in pregnant women. However, studies in rabbits given large doses of isosorbide dinitrate have shown adverse effects on the fetus. Before taking these medicines, make sure your doctor knows if you are pregnant or if you may become pregnant.

Breast-feeding—It is not known whether these medicines pass into breast milk. Although most medicines pass into breast milk in small amounts, many of them may be used safely while breast-feeding. Mothers who are taking these medicines and who wish to breast-feed should discuss this with their doctor.

Children—Studies on these medicines have been done only in adult patients, and there is no specific information comparing use of nitrates in children with use in other age groups.

Older adults—Dizziness or lightheadedness may be more likely to occur in the elderly, who may be more sensitive to the effects of nitrates.

Other medicines—Although certain medicines should not be used together at all, in other cases two different medicines may be used together even if an interaction might occur. In these cases, your doctor may want to change the dose, or other precautions may be necessary. When you are taking nitrates, it is especially important that your health care professional know if you are taking any of the following:

- Antihypertensives (high blood pressure medicine) or
- Other heart medicine—May increase the effects of nitrates on blood pressure

Other medical problems—The presence of other medical problems may affect the use of nitroglycerin. Make sure you tell your doctor if you have any other medical problems, especially:

- Anemia (severe)
- Glaucoma—May be worsened by nitrates
- Head injury (recent) or
- Stroke (recent)—Nitrates may increase pressure in the brain, which can make problems worse
- Heart attack (recent)—Nitrates may lower blood pressure, which can aggravate problems associated with heart attack
- Kidney disease or
- Liver disease—Effects may be increased because of slower removal of nitroglycerin from the body
- Overactive thyroid

Proper Use of This Medicine

Take this medicine exactly as directed by your doctor. It will work only if taken correctly.

Sublingual tablets should not be chewed, crushed, or swallowed. They work much faster when absorbed through the lining of the mouth. Place the tablet under the tongue, between the lip and gum, or between the cheek and gum and let it dissolve there. Do not eat, drink, smoke, or use chewing tobacco while a tablet is dissolving.

Buccal extended-release tablets should not be chewed, crushed, or swallowed. They are designed to release a dose of nitroglycerin over a period of hours, not all at once.

- Allow the tablet to dissolve slowly in place between the upper lip and gum (above the front teeth), or between the cheek and upper gum. If food or drink is to be taken during the 3 to 5 hours when the tablet is dissolving, place the tablet between the *upper* lip and gum, above the front teeth. If you have dentures, you may place the tablet anywhere between the cheek and gum.

- Touching the tablet with your tongue or drinking hot liquids may cause the tablet to dissolve faster.

- Do not go to sleep while a tablet is dissolving because it could slip down your throat and cause choking.

- If you accidentally swallow the tablet, replace it with another one.

- Do not use chewing tobacco while a tablet is in place.

Chewable tablets must be chewed well and held in the mouth for about 2 minutes before you swallow them. This will allow the medicine to be absorbed through the lining of the mouth.

For patients using *nitroglycerin or isosorbide dinitrate to relieve the pain of an angina attack*:

- *When you begin to feel an attack of angina starting (chest pains or a tightness or squeezing in the chest), sit down. Then place a tablet in your mouth, either sublingually or buccally, or chew a chewable tablet.* This medicine works best when you are standing or sitting. However, since you may become dizzy, lightheaded, or faint soon after using a tablet, it is safer to sit rather than stand while the medicine is working. If you become dizzy or faint while sitting, take several deep breaths and bend forward with your head between your knees.

- Remain calm and you should feel better in a few minutes.

- *This medicine usually gives relief in 1 to 5 minutes.* However, if the pain is not relieved, and you are using:

  —Sublingual tablets, either sublingually or buccally: Use a second tablet. If the pain continues for another 5 minutes, a third tablet may be used. *If you still have the chest pains after a total of 3 tablets in a 15-minute period, contact your doctor or go to a hospital emergency room immediately.*

  —Buccal extended-release tablets: *Use a sublingual (under the tongue) nitroglycerin tablet and check with your doctor.* Do not use another buccal tablet since the effects of a buccal tablet last for several hours.

For patients using *nitroglycerin, erythrityl tetranitrate, or isosorbide dinitrate to prevent an expected angina attack:*

- You may prevent anginal chest pains for up to 1 hour (6 hours for the extended-release nitroglycerin tablet) by using a buccal or sublingual tablet or chewing a chewable tablet 5 to 10 minutes before expected emotional stress or physical exertion that in the past seemed to bring on an attack.

For patients using *isosorbide dinitrate or extended-release buccal nitroglycerin regularly on a long-term basis to reduce the number of angina attacks that occur:*

- Chewable or sublingual isosorbide dinitrate and buccal extended-release nitroglycerin tablets can be used either to prevent angina attacks or to help relieve an attack that has already started.

Dosing—The dose of nitrates will be different for different patients. *Follow your doctor's orders or the directions on the label.* The following information includes only the average doses of nitrates. *If your dose is different, do not change it* unless your doctor tells you to do so.

For erythrityl tetranitrate

- For angina (chest pain):

  —For *buccal or sublingual* dosage form (tablets):

  - Adults—5 to 10 milligrams (mg) three or four times a day.
  - Children—Dose must be determined by your doctor.

For isosorbide dinitrate

- For angina (chest pain):

  —For *chewable* dosage form (tablets):

  - Adults—5 mg every two to three hours, chewed well and held in mouth for one or two minutes.
  - Children—Dose must be determined by your doctor.

  —For *buccal or sublingual* dosage form (tablets):

  - Adults—2.5 to 5 mg every two to three hours.
  - Children—Dose must be determined by your doctor.

For nitroglycerin

- For angina (chest pain):

  —For *buccal* dosage form (extended-release tablets):

  - Adults—1 mg every five hours while awake. Your doctor may increase your dose.
  - Children—Dose must be determined by your doctor.

  —For *sublingual* dosage form (tablets):

  - Adults—150 to 600 micrograms (mcg) (0.15 to 0.6 mg) every five minutes. If you still have chest pain after a total of three tablets in fifteen minutes, call your doctor or go to the emergency room right away.

- Children—Dose must be determined by your doctor.

Missed dose—For patients using isosorbide dinitrate or extended-release buccal nitroglycerin regularly on a long-term basis to reduce the number of angina attacks that occur:

- If you miss a dose of this medicine, use it as soon as possible. However, if the next scheduled dose is within 2 hours, skip the missed dose and go back to your regular dosing schedule. Do not double doses.

Stability and proper storage—

For sublingual nitroglycerin

- Sublingual nitroglycerin tablets may lose some of their strength if they are exposed to air, heat, or moisture for long periods of time. However, if you screw the cap on tightly after each use and you properly store the bottle, the tablets should retain their strength until the expiration date on the bottle.

- Some people think they should test the strength of their sublingual nitroglycerin tablets by looking for a tingling or burning sensation, a feeling of warmth or flushing, or a headache after a tablet has been dissolved under the tongue. This kind of testing is not completely reliable since some patients may be unable to detect these effects. In addition, newer, stabilized sublingual nitroglycerin tablets are less likely to produce these detectable effects.

- To help keep the nitroglycerin tablets at full strength:
    —keep the medicine in the original glass, screw-cap bottle. For patients who wish to carry a small number of tablets with them for emergency use, a specially designed container is available. However, only containers specifically labeled as suitable for use with nitroglycerin sublingual tablets should be used.
    —remove the cotton plug that comes in the bottle and *do not* put it back.

—*put the cap on the bottle quickly and tightly after each use.*

—to select a tablet for use, pour several into the bottle cap, take one, and pour the others back into the bottle. Try not to hold them in the palm of your hand because they may pick up moisture and crumble.

—do not keep other medicines in the same bottle with the nitroglycerin since they will weaken the nitroglycerin effect.

—keep the medicine handy at all times but try not to carry the bottle close to the body. Medicine may lose strength because of body warmth. Instead, carry the tightly closed bottle in your purse or the pocket of a jacket or other loose-fitting clothing whenever possible.

—store the bottle of nitroglycerin tablets in a cool, dry place. Storage at average room temperature away from direct heat or direct sunlight is best. Do not store in the refrigerator or in a bathroom medicine cabinet because the moisture usually present in these areas may cause the tablets to crumble if the container is not tightly closed. Do not keep the tablets in your automobile glove compartment.

- Keep out of the reach of children.
- Do not keep outdated medicine or medicine no longer needed. Be sure that any discarded medicine is out of the reach of children.

For erythrityl tetranitrate, isosorbide dinitrate, and buccal extended-release nitroglycerin

- These forms of nitrates are more stable than sublingual nitroglycerin.
- Keep out of the reach of children.
- Store away from heat and direct light.
- Do not store in the bathroom, near the kitchen sink, or in other damp places. Heat or moisture may cause the medicine to break down.

- Do not keep outdated medicine or medicine no longer needed. Be sure that any discarded medicine is out of the reach of children.

Precautions While Using This Medicine

If you have been taking this medicine regularly for several weeks, do not suddenly stop using it. Stopping suddenly may bring on attacks of angina. Check with your doctor for the best way to reduce gradually the amount you are taking before stopping completely.

Dizziness, lightheadedness, or faintness may occur, especially when you get up quickly from a lying or sitting position. Getting up slowly may help. If you feel dizzy, sit or lie down.

The dizziness, lightheadedness, or fainting is also more likely to occur if you drink alcohol, stand for long periods of time, exercise, or if the weather is hot. *While you are taking this medicine, be careful to limit the amount of alcohol you drink. Also, use extra care during exercise or hot weather or if you must stand for long periods of time.*

After taking a dose of this medicine you may get a headache that lasts for a short time. This is a common side effect, which should become less noticeable after you have taken the medicine for a while. If this effect continues or if the headaches are severe, check with your doctor.

Side Effects of This Medicine

Along with its needed effects, a medicine may cause some unwanted effects. Although not all of these side effects may occur, if they do occur they may need medical attention.

Check with your doctor as soon as possible if any of the following side effects occur:

Rare

Blurred vision; dryness of mouth; headache (severe or prolonged); skin rash

Signs and symptoms of overdose (in the order in which they may occur)

Bluish-colored lips, fingernails, or palms of hands; dizziness (extreme) or fainting; feeling of extreme pressure in head; shortness of breath; unusual tiredness or weakness; weak and fast heartbeat; fever; convulsions (seizures)

Other side effects may occur that usually do not need medical attention. These side effects may go away during treatment as your body adjusts to the medicine. However, check with your doctor if any of the following side effects continue or are bothersome:

More common

Dizziness or lightheadedness, especially when getting up from a lying or sitting position; fast pulse; flushing of face and neck; headache; nausea or vomiting; restlessness

Other side effects not listed above may also occur in some patients. If you notice any other effects, check with your doctor.

NITRATES—Topical   Systemic

Some commonly used brand names are:

In the U.S.—

Deponit[2]	Nitrol[1]
Nitro-Bid[1]	Nitrong[1]
Nitrodisc[2]	Nitrostat[1]
Nitro-Dur[2]	NTS[2]
Nitro-Dur II[2]	Transderm-Nitro[2]

In Canada—

Nitro-Bid[1]

Nitrol[1]

Nitrong[1]

Transderm-Nitro[2]

Another commonly used name for nitroglycerin is glyceryl trinitrate.

Note: For quick reference, the following nitrates are numbered to match the corresponding brand names.

This information applies to the following medicines:

1. Nitroglycerin Ointment‡
2. Nitroglycerin Transdermal Patches‡

‡Generic name product may also be available in the U.S.

Description

Nitrates (NYE-trates) are used to treat the symptoms of angina (chest pain). Depending on the type of dosage form and how it is taken, nitrates are used to treat angina in three ways:

- to relieve an attack that is occurring by using the medicine when the attack begins;
- to prevent attacks from occurring by using the medicine just before an attack is expected to occur; or
- to reduce the number of attacks that occur by using the medicine regularly on a long-term basis.

When applied to the skin, nitrates are used to reduce the number of angina attacks that occur. The only nitrate available for this purpose is topical nitroglycerin (nye-troe-GLI-ser-in).

Topical nitroglycerin is absorbed through the skin. It works by relaxing blood vessels and increasing the supply of blood and oxygen to the heart while reducing its work load. This helps prevent future angina attacks from occurring.

Topical nitroglycerin may also be used for other conditions as determined by your doctor.

Nitroglycerin as discussed here is available only with your doctor's prescription, in the following dosage forms:

Topical
- Ointment (U.S. and Canada)
- Transdermal (stick-on) patch (U.S. and Canada)

Before Using This Medicine

In deciding to use a medicine, the risks of taking the medicine must be weighed against the good it will do. This is a decision you and your doctor will make. For nitroglycerin applied to the skin, the following should be considered:

Allergies—Tell your doctor if you have ever had any unusual or allergic reaction to nitrates or nitrites. Also tell your health care professional if you are allergic to any other substances, such as certain foods, preservatives, or dyes.

Pregnancy—Nitrates have not been studied in pregnant women. Before taking these medicines, make sure your doctor knows if you are pregnant or if you may become pregnant.

Breast-feeding—It is not known whether this medicine passes into breast milk. Although most medicines pass into breast milk in small amounts, many of them may be used safely while breast-feeding. Mothers who are taking these medicines and who wish to breast-feed should discuss this with their doctor.

Children—Studies on these medicines have been done only in adult patients, and there is no specific information comparing use of nitrates in children with use in other age groups.

Older adults—Dizziness or lightheadedness may be more likely to occur in the elderly, who may be more sensitive to the effects of nitrates.

Other medicines—Although certain medicines should not be used together at all, in other cases two different medicines may be used together even if an interaction might occur. In these cases, your doctor may want to change the dose, or other precautions may be necessary. When you are using nitroglycerin, it is especially important that your health care professional know if you are taking any of the following:

- Antihypertensives (high blood pressure medicine) or
- Other heart medicine—May increase the effects of nitroglycerin on blood pressure

Other medical problems—The presence of other medical problems may affect the use of nitroglycerin. Make sure you tell your doctor if you have any other medical problems, especially:

- Anemia (severe)
- Glaucoma—May be worsened by nitroglycerin
- Head injury (recent) or
- Stroke (recent)—Nitroglycerin may increase pressure in the brain, which can make problems worse
- Heart attack (recent)—Nitroglycerin may lower blood pressure, which can aggravate problems associated with heart attack
- Kidney disease or
- Liver disease—Effects may be increased because of slower removal of nitroglycerin from the body
- Overactive thyroid

Proper Use of This Medicine

Use nitroglycerin exactly as directed by your doctor. It will work only if applied correctly.

The ointment and transdermal forms of nitroglycerin are used to reduce the number of angina attacks. They will not relieve an attack that has already started because they work too slowly. Check with your doctor if you need a fast-acting medicine to relieve the pain of an angina attack.

This medicine usually comes with patient instructions. Read them carefully before using.

For patients using the *ointment* form of this medicine:

- Before applying a new dose of ointment, remove any ointment remaining on the skin from a previous dose. This will allow the fresh ointment to release the nitroglycerin properly.

- This medicine comes with dose-measuring papers. Use them to measure the length of ointment squeezed from the tube and to apply the ointment to the skin. *Do not rub or massage the ointment into the skin; just spread in a thin, even layer, covering an area of the same size each time it is applied.*

- Apply the ointment to skin that has little or no hair.

- Apply each dose of ointment to a different area of skin to prevent irritation or other skin problems.

- If your doctor has ordered an occlusive dressing (airtight covering, such as kitchen plastic wrap) to be applied over this medicine, make sure you know how to apply it. Since occlusive dressings increase the amount of medicine absorbed through the skin and the possibility of side effects, use them only as directed. If you have any questions about this, check with your health care professional.

For patients using the *transdermal (stick-on patch) system:*

- Do not try to trim or cut the adhesive patch to adjust the dosage. Check with your doctor if you think the medicine is not working as it should.

- Apply the patch to a clean, dry skin area with little or no hair and free of scars, cuts, or irritation. Remove the previous patch before applying a new one.

- Apply a new patch if the first one becomes loose or falls off.

- Apply each dose to a different area of skin to prevent skin irritation or other problems.

Dosing—The dose of nitroglycerin will be different for different patients. *Follow your doctor's orders or the directions on the label.* The following information includes only the average doses of nitrates. *If your dose is different, do not change it* unless your doctor tells you to do so.

For nitroglycerin

- For angina (chest pain):

—For *ointment* dosage form:

- Adults—15 to 30 milligrams (mg) (about one to two inches of ointment squeezed from tube) every six to eight hours.
- Children—Use and dose must be determined by your doctor.

—For *transdermal system (skin patch)* dosage form:

- Adults—Apply one transdermal dosage system (skin patch) to intact skin once a day. The patch is usually left on for 12 to 14 hours a day and then taken off. Follow your doctor's instructions for when to put on and take off the skin patch.
- Children—Use and dose must be determined by your doctor.

Missed dose—

- For patients using the *ointment* form of this medicine: If you miss a dose of this medicine, apply it as soon as possible unless the next scheduled dose is within 2 hours. Then go back to your regular dosing schedule. Do not increase the amount used.
- For patients using the *transdermal (stick-on patch) system*: If you miss a dose of this medicine, apply it as soon as possible. Then go back to your regular dosing schedule.

Storage—

- To store the *ointment* form of this medicine:
  —Keep out of the reach of children.

—Store the tube of nitroglycerin ointment in a cool place and keep it tightly closed.

—Do not keep outdated medicine or medicine no longer needed. Be sure that any discarded medicine is out of the reach of children.

• To store the *transdermal (stick-on patch) system*:

—Keep out of the reach of children.

—Store away from heat and direct light.

—Do not store in the bathroom, near the kitchen sink, or in other damp places. Heat or moisture may cause the medicine to break down.

—Do not keep outdated medicine or medicine no longer needed. Be sure that any discarded medicine is out of the reach of children.

Precautions While Using This Medicine

If you have been using nitroglycerin regularly for several weeks or more, do not suddenly stop using it. Stopping suddenly may bring on attacks of angina. Check with your doctor for the best way to reduce gradually the amount you are using before stopping completely.

Dizziness, lightheadedness, or faintness may occur, especially when you get up quickly from a lying or sitting position. Getting up slowly may help. If you feel dizzy, sit or lie down.

The dizziness, lightheadedness, or fainting is also more likely to occur if you drink alcohol, stand for long periods of time, exercise, or if the weather is hot. *While you are taking this medicine, be careful to limit the amount of alcohol you drink. Also, use extra care during exercise or hot weather or if you must stand for long periods of time.*

After using a dose of this medicine you may get a head-ache that lasts for a short time. This is a common side effect, which should become less noticeable after you have used the medicine for a while. If this effect continues, or if the headaches are severe, check with your doctor.

Side Effects of This Medicine

Along with its needed effects, a medicine may cause some unwanted effects. Although not all of these side effects may occur, if they do occur they may need medical attention.

Check with your doctor as soon as possible if any of the following side effects occur:

Rare

> Blurred vision; dryness of mouth; headache (severe or prolonged)

Signs and symptoms of overdose (in the order in which they may occur)

> Bluish-colored lips, fingernails, or palms of hands; dizziness (extreme) or fainting; feeling of extreme pressure in head; shortness of breath; unusual tiredness or weakness; weak and fast heartbeat; fever; convulsions (seizures)

Other side effects may occur that usually do not need medical attention. These side effects may go away during treatment as your body adjusts to the medicine. However, check with your doctor if any of the following side effects continue or are bothersome:

More common

> Dizziness or lightheadedness, especially when getting up from a lying or sitting position; fast pulse; flushing of face and neck; headache; nausea or vomiting; restlessness

Less common

> Sore, reddened skin

Other side effects not listed above may also occur in some patients. If you notice any other effects, check with your doctor.

NITROFURANTOIN   Systemic

Some commonly used brand names are:

In the U.S.—

Furadantin	Macrobid
Furalan	Macrodantin
Furatoin	Nitrofuracot

Generic name product may also be available.

In Canada—

Apo-Nitrofurantoin	Macrodantin

Description

Nitrofurantoin (nye-troe-fyoor-AN-toyn) belongs to the family of medicines called anti-infectives. It is used to treat infections of the urinary tract. It may also be used for other conditions as determined by your doctor.

Nitrofurantoin is available only with your doctor's prescription, in the following dosage forms:

Oral

- Capsules (U.S. and Canada)
- Extended-release Capsules (U.S.)
- Oral Suspension (U.S.)
- Tablets (U.S. and Canada)

Before Using This Medicine

In deciding to use a medicine, the risks of taking the medicine must be weighed against the good it will do. This is a decision you and your doctor will make. For nitrofurantoin, the following should be considered:

Allergies—Tell your doctor if you have ever had any unusual or allergic reaction to nitrofurantoin or to any related medicines such as furazolidone (e.g., Furoxone) or nitrofurazone (e.g., Furacin). Also tell your health care professional if you are allergic to any other substances, such as foods, preservatives, or dyes.

Pregnancy—Nitrofurantoin should not be used if you are within a week or two of your delivery date or during labor and delivery. It may cause problems in the infant.

Breast-feeding—Nitrofurantoin passes into the breast milk in small amounts and may cause problems in nursing babies, especially those with glucose-6-phosphate dehydrogenase (G6PD) deficiency.

Children—Infants up to 1 month of age should not be given this medicine because they are especially sensitive to the effects of nitrofurantoin.

Older adults—Elderly people may be more sensitive to the effects of nitrofurantoin. This may increase the chance of side effects during treatment.

Other medicines—Although certain medicines should not be used together at all, in other cases two different medicines may be used together even if an interaction might occur. In these cases, your doctor may want to change the dose, or other precautions may be necessary. When you are taking nitrofurantoin, it is especially important that your health care professional know if you are taking any of the following:

- Acetohydroxamic acid (e.g., Lithostat) or
- Antidiabetics, oral (diabetes medicine you take by mouth) or
- Dapsone or
- Furazolidone (e.g., Furoxone) or
- Methyldopa (e.g., Aldomet) or
- Primaquine or
- Procainamide (e.g., Pronestyl) or
- Quinidine (e.g., Quinidex) or
- Sulfonamides (sulfa medicine) or
- Sulfoxone (e.g., Diasone) or
- Vitamin K (e.g., AquaMEPHYTON, Synkayvite)—Patients

who take nitrofurantoin with any of these medicines may
have an increase in side effects affecting the blood

- Carbamazepine (e.g., Tegretol) or
- Chloroquine (e.g., Aralen) or
- Cisplatin (e.g., Platinol) or
- Cytarabine (e.g., Cytosar-U) or
- Diphtheria, tetanus, and pertussis (DTP) vaccine or
- Disulfiram (e.g., Antabuse) or
- Ethotoin (e.g., Peganone) or
- Hydroxychloroquine (e.g., Plaquenil) or
- Lindane, topical (e.g., Kwell) or
- Lithium (e.g., Lithane) or
- Mephenytoin (e.g., Mesantoin) or
- Mexiletine (e.g., Mexitil) or
- Other anti-infectives by mouth or by injection (medicine
  for infection) or
- Pemoline (e.g., Cylert) or
- Phenytoin (e.g., Dilantin) or
- Pyridoxine (e.g., Hexa-Betalin) (with long-term, high-dose
  use) or
- Vincristine (e.g., Oncovin)—Patients who take nitrofuran-
  toin with any of these medicines, or who have received a
  DTP vaccine within the last 30 days or are going to receive
  a DTP may have an increase in side effects affecting the
  nervous system
- Probenecid (e.g., Benemid) or
- Sulfinpyrazone (e.g., Anturane)—Patients who take nitrofurantoin with any of these medicines may have an increase
  in side effects
- Quinine (e.g., Quinamm)—Patients who take nitrofurantoin
  with quinine may have an increase in side effects affecting
  the blood and the nervous system

Other medical problems—The presence of other medical
problems may affect the use of nitrofurantoin. Make sure
you tell your doctor if you have any other medical problems, especially:

- Glucose-6-phosphate dehydrogenase (G6PD) deficiency—
  Nitrofurantoin may cause anemia in patients with G6PD
  deficiency

- Kidney disease (other than infection)—The chance of side effects of this medicine may be increased and the medicine may be less effective in patients with kidney disease
- Lung disease or
- Nerve damage—Patients with lung disease or nerve damage may have an increase in side effects when they take nitrofurantoin

---

Proper Use of This Medicine

Do not give this medicine to infants up to 1 month of age.

Nitrofurantoin is best taken with food or milk. This may lessen stomach upset and help your body absorb the medicine better.

For patients taking the *oral liquid form of this medicine:*

- Shake the oral liquid forcefully before each dose to help make it pour more smoothly and to be sure the medicine is evenly mixed.
- Use a specially marked measuring spoon or other device to measure each dose accurately. The average household teaspoon may not hold the right amount of liquid.
- Nitrofurantoin may be mixed with water, milk, fruit juices, or infants' formulas. If it is mixed with other liquids, take the medicine immediately after mixing. Be sure to drink all the liquid in order to get the full dose of medicine.

For patients taking the *extended-release capsule* form of this medicine:

- Swallow the capsules whole.
- Do not open, crush, or chew the capsules before swallowing them.

To help clear up your infection completely, *keep taking this medicine for the full time of treatment,* even if you begin to feel better after a few days. *Do not miss any doses.*

Dosing—The dose of nitrofurantoin will be different for different patients. *Follow your doctor's orders or the directions on the label.* The following information includes only the average doses of nitrofurantoin. *If your dose is different, do not change it* unless your doctor tells you to do so.

- For the *capsule, oral suspension, and tablet* dosage forms:

    —Adults and adolescents: 50 to 100 mg every six hours.

    —Children 1 month of age and older: Dose is based on body weight and will be determined by your doctor.

    —Children up to 1 month of age: Use is not recommended.

- For the *extended-release capsule* dosage form:

    —Adults and children 12 years of age and older: 100 mg every twelve hours for seven days.

    —Children up to 12 years of age: Dose must be determined by the doctor.

Missed dose—If you do miss a dose of this medicine, take it as soon as possible. However, if it is almost time for your next dose, skip the next dose and go back to your regular dosing schedule. Do not double doses.

Storage—To store this medicine:

- Keep out of the reach of children.
- Store away from heat and direct light.
- Do not store the capsule or tablet form of this medicine in the bathroom, near the kitchen sink, or in other damp places. Heat or moisture may cause the medicine to break down.

- Keep the oral liquid form of this medicine from freezing.
- Do not keep outdated medicine or medicine no longer needed. Be sure that any discarded medicine is out of the reach of children.

Precautions While Using This Medicine

It is important that your doctor check your progress at regular visits if you will be taking this medicine for a long time.

If your symptoms do not improve within a few days, or if they become worse, check with your doctor.

For *diabetic patients:*

- *This medicine may cause false test results with some urine sugar tests.* Check with your doctor before changing your diet or the dosage of your diabetes medicine.

Side Effects of This Medicine

Along with its needed effects, a medicine may cause some unwanted effects. Although not all of these side effects may occur, if they do occur they may need medical attention.

Check with your doctor immediately if any of the following side effects occur:

More common

Chest pain; chills; cough; fever; troubled breathing

Less common

Dizziness; drowsiness; headache; numbness, tingling, or burning of face or mouth; sore throat and fever; unusual muscle weakness; unusual tiredness or weakness

Rare

Itching; joint pain; pale skin; skin rash; yellow eyes or skin

Other side effects may occur that usually do not need medical attention. These side effects may go away during treatment as your body adjusts to the medicine. However, check with your doctor if any of the following side effects continue or are bothersome:

More common

Abdominal or stomach pain or upset; diarrhea; loss of appetite; nausea or vomiting

This medicine may cause the urine to become rust-yellow to brown. This side effect does not require medical attention.

Other side effects not listed above may also occur in some patients. If you notice any other effects, check with your doctor.

NONSTEROIDAL ANTI-INFLAMMATORY DRUGS   Systemic

Some commonly used brand names are:

In the U.S.—

Advil[7]	Daypro[14]
Advil Caplets[7]	Dolgesic[7]
Advil, Children's[7]	Dolobid[2]
Aleve[13]	Excedrin IB[7]
Anaprox[13]	Excedrin IB Caplets[7]
Anaprox DS[13]	Feldene[16]
Ansaid[6]	Genpril[7]
Bayer Select Ibuprofen Caplets[7]	Genpril Caplets[7]
	Haltran[7]
Cataflam[1]	Ibifon 600 Caplets[7]
Clinoril[17]	Ibren[7]
Cotylbutazone[15]	Ibu[7]
Cramp End[7]	Ibu-200[7]

In the U.S. (cont'd)—

Ibu-4[7]
Ibu-6[7]
Ibu-8[7]
Ibuprin[7]
Ibuprohm[7]
Ibuprohm Caplets[7]
Ibu-Tab[7]
Indocin[8]
Indocin SR[8]
Lodine[3]
Meclomen[10]
Medipren[7]
Medipren Caplets[7]
Midol IB[7]
Motrin[7]
Motrin, Children's[7]
Motrin-IB[7]

Motrin-IB Caplets[7]
Nalfon[4]
Nalfon 200[4]
Naprosyn[13]
Nuprin[7]
Nuprin Caplets[7]
Orudis[9]
Oruvail[9]
Pamprin-IB[7]
Ponstel[11]
Relafen[12]
Rufen[7]
Tolectin 200[20]
Tolectin 400[20]
Tolectin 600[20]
Trendar[7]
Voltaren[1]

In Canada—

Actiprofen Caplets[7]
Advil[7]
Advil Caplets[7]
Albert Tiafen[19]
Alka Butazolidin[15]
Anaprox[13]
Anaprox DS[13]
Ansaid[6]
Apo-Diclo[1]
Apo-Diflunisal[2]
Apo-Flurbiprofen[6]
Apo-Ibuprofen[7]
Apo-Indomethacin[8]
Apo-Keto[9]
Apo-Keto-E[9]
Apo-Napro-Na[13]
Apo-Napro-Na DS[13]
Apo-Naproxen[13]
Apo-Phenylbutazone[15]
Apo-Piroxicam[16]
Apo-Sulin[17]
Butazolidin[15]
Clinoril[17]
Dolobid[2]
Feldene[16]
Froben[6]
Froben SR[6]

Idarac[5]
Indocid[8]
Indocid SR[8]
Medipren Caplets[7]
Mobiflex[18]
Motrin[7]
Motrin-IB[7]
Nalfon[4]
Naprosyn[13]
Naprosyn-E[13]
Naprosyn-SR[13]
Naxen[13]
Novo-Difenac[1]
Novo-Difenac SR[1]
Novo-Diflunisal[2]
Novo-Flurprofen[6]
Novo-Keto-EC[9]
Novo-Methacin[8]
Novo-Naprox[13]
Novo-Naprox Sodium[13]
Novo-Naprox Sodium DS[13]
Novo-Pirocam[16]
Novo-Profen[7]
Novo-Sundac[17]
Novo-Tolmetin[20]
Nu-Diclo[11]
Nu-Flurbiprofen[6]

In Canada (cont'd)—

Nu-Ibuprofen[7]
Nu-Indo[8]
Nu-Naprox[13]
Nu-Pirox[16]
Nu-Sulindac[17]
Orudis[9]
Orudis-E[9]
Orudis-SR[9]
Oruvail[9]
Ponstan[11]
Relafen[12]
Rhodis[9]

Rhodis-EC[9]
Surgam[19]
Surgam SR[19]
Synflex[13]
Synflex DS[13]
Tolectin 200[20]
Tolectin 600[20]
Tolectin DS[20]
Voltaren[1]
Voltaren Rapide[1]
Voltaren SR[1]

Other commonly used names are:

Etodolic acid[3]
Indometacin[8]

Meclofenamic acid[10]

Note: For quick reference, the following (family name) are numbered to match the corresponding brand names.

This information applies to the following medicines:

1. Diclofenac (dye-KLOE-fen-ak)
2. Diflunisal (dye-FLOO-ni-sal)‡
3. Etodolac (ee-TOE-doe-lak)†
4. Fenoprofen (fen-oh-PROE-fen)‡
5. Floctafenine (flok-ta-FEN-een)*
6. Flurbiprofen (flure-BI-proe-fen)‡§
7. Ibuprofen (eye-byoo-PROE-fen)‡§
8. Indomethacin (in-doe-METH-a-sin)‡
9. Ketoprofen (kee-toe-PROE-fen)‡
10. Meclofenamate (me-kloe-FEN-am-ate)†‡
11. Mefenamic (me-fe-NAM-ik) Acid
12. Nabumetone (na-BYOO-me-tone)
13. Naproxen (na-PROX-en)‡
14. Oxaprozin (ox-a-PROE-zin)†
15. Phenylbutazone (fen-ill-BYOO-ta-zone)‡
16. Piroxicam (peer-OX-i-kam)‡
17. Sulindac (sul-IN-dak)‡
18. Tenoxicam (ten-OX-i-kam)*
19. Tiaprofenic (tie-a-pro-FEN-ik) Acid*
20. Tolmetin (TOLE-met-in)‡

This information does *not* apply to aspirin or other salicylates or to ketorolac (e.g., Toradol).

---

*Not commercially available in the U.S.
†Not commercially available in Canada.
‡Generic name product may also be available in the U.S.
§Generic name product may also be available in the Canada.

Description

Nonsteroidal anti-inflammatory drugs (also called NSAIDs) are used to relieve some symptoms caused by arthritis (rheumatism), such as inflammation, swelling, stiffness, and joint pain. However, this medicine does not cure arthritis and will help you only as long as you continue to take it.

Some of these medicines are also used to relieve other kinds of pain or to treat other painful conditions, such as:

- gout attacks;
- bursitis;
- tendinitis;
- sprains, strains, or other injuries; or
- menstrual cramps.

Ibuprofen and naproxen are also used to reduce fever.

Meclofenamate is also used to reduce the amount of bleeding in some women who have very heavy menstrual periods.

Nonsteroidal anti-inflammatory drugs may also be used to treat other conditions as determined by your doctor.

Any nonsteroidal anti-inflammatory drug can cause side effects, especially when it is used for a long time or in large doses. Some of the side effects are painful or uncomfortable. Others can be more serious, resulting in the need for medical care and sometimes even death. If you will be taking this medicine for more than one or two months or in large amounts, you should discuss with your doctor the good that it can do as well as the risks of taking it. Also, it is a good idea to ask your doctor about other forms of treatment that might help to reduce the amount of this medicine that you take and/or the length of treatment.

One of the nonsteroidal anti-inflammatory drugs, phenylbutazone, is especially likely to cause very serious side effects. These serious side effects are more likely to occur in patients 40 years of age or older than in younger adults, and the risk becomes greater as the patient's age increases. Before you take phenylbutazone, be sure that you have discussed its use with your doctor. *Also, do not use phenyl-butazone to treat any painful condition other than the one for which it was prescribed by your doctor.*

Although ibuprofen and naproxen may be used instead of aspirin to treat many of the same medical problems, they must not be used by people who are allergic to aspirin.

The 200-mg strength of ibuprofen and the 220-mg strength of naproxen are available without a prescription. However, your health care professional may have special instructions on the proper dose of these medicines for your medical condition.

Other nonsteroidal anti-inflammatory drugs and other strengths of ibuprofen and naproxen are available only with your medical doctor's or dentist's prescription. These medicines are available in the following dosage forms:

Oral

Diclofenac
  • Tablets (U.S. and Canada)
  • Delayed-release tablets (U.S. and Canada)
  • Extended-release tablets (Canada)
Diflunisal
  • Tablets (U.S. and Canada)
Etodolac
  • Capsules (U.S.)
  • Tablets (U.S.)
Fenoprofen
  • Capsules (U.S. and Canada)
  • Tablets (U.S. and Canada)
Floctafenine
  • Tablets (Canada)
Flurbiprofen
  • Extended-release capsules (Canada)
  • Tablets (U.S. and Canada)

Ibuprofen
- Oral suspension (U.S.)
- Tablets (U.S. and Canada)

Indomethacin
- Capsules (U.S. and Canada)
- Extended-release capsules (U.S. and Canada)
- Oral suspension (U.S.)

Ketoprofen
- Capsules (U.S. and Canada)
- Extended-release capsules (U.S. and Canada)
- Delayed-release tablets (Canada)
- Extended-release tablets (Canada)

Meclofenamate
- Capsules (U.S.)

Mefenamic Acid
- Capsules (U.S. and Canada)

Nabumetone
- Tablets (U.S. and Canada)

Naproxen
- Oral suspension (U.S. and Canada)
- Tablets (U.S. and Canada)
- Delayed-release tablets (Canada)
- Extended-release tablets (Canada)

Oxaprozin
- Tablets (U.S.)

Phenylbutazone
- Capsules (U.S.)
- Tablets (U.S. and Canada)
- Buffered tablets (Canada)

Piroxicam
- Capsules (U.S. and Canada)

Sulindac
- Tablets (U.S. and Canada)

Tenoxicam
- Tablets (Canada)

Tiaprofenic Acid
- Extended-release capsules (Canada)
- Tablets (Canada)

Tolmetin
- Capsules (U.S. and Canada)
- Tablets (U.S. and Canada)

Rectal
Diclofenac
  • Suppositories (Canada)
Indomethacin
  • Suppositories (U.S. and Canada)
Ketoprofen
  • Suppositories (Canada)
Naproxen
  • Suppositories (Canada)
Piroxicam
  • Suppositories (Canada)

Before Using This Medicine

In deciding to use a medicine, the risks of taking the medicine must be weighed against the good it will do. This is a decision you and your health care professional will make. For the nonsteroidal anti-inflammatory drugs, the following should be considered:

Allergies—Tell your health care professional if you have ever had any unusual or allergic reaction to any of the nonsteroidal anti-inflammatory drugs, or to any of the following medicines:

  • Aspirin or other salicylates
  • Ketorolac (e.g., Toradol)
  • Oxyphenbutazone (e.g., Oxalid, Tandearil)
  • Suprofen (e.g., Suprol)
  • Zomepirac (e.g., Zomax)

Also tell your health care professional if you are allergic to any other substances, such as foods, preservatives, or dyes.

Diet—Make certain your health care professional knows if you are on any special diet, such as a low-sodium or low-sugar diet. Some of these medicines contain sodium or sugar.

Pregnancy—Studies on birth defects with these medicines have not been done in humans. However, there is a chance that these medicines may cause unwanted effects on the heart or blood flow of the fetus or newborn baby if they are taken regularly during the last few months of pregnancy. Also, studies in animals have shown that these medicines, if taken late in pregnancy, may increase the length of pregnancy, prolong labor, or cause other problems during delivery. If you are pregnant, do not take any of these medicines, including nonprescription (over-the-counter [OTC]) ibuprofen or naproxen, without first discussing its use with your doctor.

Studies in animals have not shown that fenoprofen, floctafenine, flurbiprofen, ibuprofen, ketoprofen, nabumetone, naproxen, phenylbutazone, piroxicam, tiaprofenic acid, or tolmetin causes birth defects. Diflunisal caused birth defects of the spine and ribs in rabbits, but not in mice or rats. Diclofenac and meclofenamate caused unwanted effects on the formation of bones in animals. Etodolac and oxaprozin caused birth defects in animals. Indomethacin caused slower development of bones and damage to nerves in animals. In some animal studies, sulindac caused unwanted effects on the development of bones and organs. Studies on birth defects with mefenamic acid have not been done in animals.

Even though most of these medicines did not cause birth defects in animals, many of them did cause other harmful or toxic effects on the fetus, usually when they were given in such large amounts that the pregnant animals became sick.

Breast-feeding—

- *For indomethacin:* Indomethacin passes into the breast milk and has been reported to cause unwanted effects in nursing babies.

- *For meclofenamate:* Use of meclofenamate by nursing mothers is not recommended because in animal studies it caused unwanted effects on the newborn's development.

- *For phenylbutazone:* Phenylbutazone passes into the breast milk and may cause unwanted effects, such as blood problems, in nursing babies.
- *For piroxicam:* Studies in animals have shown that piroxicam may decrease the amount of milk.

Although other anti-inflammatory analgesics have not been reported to cause problems in nursing babies, diclofenac, diflunisal, fenoprofen, flurbiprofen, meclofenamate, mefenamic acid, naproxen, piroxicam, and tolmetin pass into the breast milk. It is not known whether etodolac, floctafenine, ibuprofen, ketoprofen, nabumetone, oxaprozin, sulindac, or tiaprofenic acid passes into human breast milk.

Children—

- *For ibuprofen:* Ibuprofen has been tested in children 6 months of age and older. It has not been shown to cause different side effects or problems than it does in adults.
- *For indomethacin and for tolmetin:* Indomethacin and tolmetin have been tested in children 2 years of age and older and have not been shown to cause different side effects or problems than they do in adults.
- *For naproxen:* Studies with naproxen in children 2 years of age and older have shown that skin rash may be more likely to occur.
- *For oxaprozin:* Oxaprozin has been used in children with arthritis. However, there is no specific information comparing use of this medicine in children with use in other age groups.
- *For phenylbutazone:* Use of phenylbutazone in children up to 15 years of age is not recommended.
- *For other anti-inflammatory analgesics:* There is no specific information on the use of other anti-inflammatory analgesics in children.

Most of these medicines, especially indomethacin and phenylbutazone, can cause serious side effects in any patient. Therefore, it is especially important that you discuss with the child's doctor the good that this medicine may do as well as the risks of using it.

Older adults—Certain side effects, such as confusion, swelling of the face, feet, or lower legs, or sudden decrease in the amount of urine, may be especially likely to occur in elderly patients, who are usually more sensitive than younger adults to the effects of nonsteroidal anti-inflammatory drugs. Also, elderly people are more likely than younger adults to get very sick if these medicines cause stomach problems. With phenylbutazone, blood problems may also be more likely to occur in the elderly.

Other medicines—Although certain medicines should not be used together at all, in other cases two different medicines may be used together even if an interaction might occur. In these cases, your doctor may want to change the dose, or other precautions may be necessary. When you are taking a nonsteroidal anti-inflammatory drug, it is especially important that your health care professional know if you are taking any of the following:

- Anticoagulants (blood thinners) or
- Cefamandole (e.g., Mandol) or
- Cefoperazone (e.g., Cefobid) or
- Cefotetan (e.g., Cefotan) or
- Heparin or
- Plicamycin (e.g., Mithracin) or
- Valproic acid—The chance of bleeding may be increased
- Aspirin—The chance of serious side effects may be increased if aspirin is used together with a nonsteroidal anti-inflammatory drug on a regular basis
- Ciprofloxacin (e.g., Cipro) or
- Enoxacin (e.g., Penetrex) or
- Itraconazole (e.g., Sporanox) or
- Ketoconazole (e.g., Nizoral) or
- Lomefloxacin (e.g., Maxaquin) or
- Norfloxacin (e.g., Noroxin) or
- Ofloxacin (e.g., Floxin) or

- Tetracyclines, oral—The buffered form of phenylbutazone (e.g., Alka Butazolidin) may keep these medicines from working properly if the 2 medicines are taken too close together

- Cyclosporine (e.g., Sandimmune) or
- Digitalis glycosides (heart medicine) or
- Lithium (e.g., Lithane) or
- Methotrexate (e.g., Mexate) or
- Phenytoin (e.g., Dilantin)—Higher blood levels of these medicines and an increased chance of side effects may occur

- Penicillamine (e.g., Cuprimine)—The chance of serious side effects may be increased, especially with phenylbutazone (e.g., Cotylbutazone)

- Probenecid (e.g., Benemid)—Higher blood levels of the nonsteroidal anti-inflammatory drug and an increased chance of side effects may occur

- Triamterene (e.g., Dyrenium)—The chance of kidney problems may be increased, especially with indomethacin

- Zidovudine (e.g., AZT, Retrovir)—The chance of serious side effects may be increased, especially with indomethacin

Other medical problems—The presence of other medical problems may affect the use of nonsteroidal anti-inflammatory drugs. Make sure you tell your doctor if you have any other medical problems, especially:

- Alcohol abuse or
- Bleeding problems or
- Colitis, Crohn's disease, diverticulitis, stomach ulcer, or other stomach or intestinal problems or
- Diabetes mellitus (sugar diabetes) or
- Hemorrhoids or
- Hepatitis or other liver disease or
- Kidney disease (or history of) or
- Rectal irritation or bleeding, recent, or
- Systemic lupus erythematosus (SLE) or
- Tobacco use (or recent history of)—The chance of side effects may be increased

- Anemia or
- Asthma or
- Epilepsy or
- Fluid retention (swelling of feet or lower legs) or
- Heart disease or
- High blood pressure or
- Kidney stones (or history of) or
- Low platelet count or
- Low white blood cell count or
- Mental illness or
- Parkinson's disease or
- Polymyalgia rheumatica or
- Porphyria or
- Temporal arteritis—Some nonsteroidal anti-inflammatory drugs may make these conditions worse
- Ulcers, sores, or white spots in mouth—Ulcers, sores, or white spots in the mouth sometimes mean that the medicine is causing serious side effects; if these sores or spots are already present before you start taking the medicine, it will be harder for you and your doctor to recognize that these side effects might be occurring

---

Proper Use of This Medicine

For patients taking *a capsule, tablet (including caplet), or liquid form* of this medicine:

- *Take tablet or capsule forms of these medicines with a full glass (8 ounces) of water.* Also, do not lie down for about 15 to 30 minutes after taking the medicine. This helps to prevent irritation that may lead to trouble in swallowing.

- To lessen stomach upset, these medicines should be taken with food or an antacid. This is especially important when you are taking indomethacin, mefenamic acid, phenylbutazone, or piroxicam, which should always be taken with food or an antacid. Taking the extended-release tablet dosage form of flurbiprofen or naproxen and taking nabumetone with food may also help the medicine be absorbed into your body more quickly. However, your doctor may want you to take the first 1 or 2 doses of other nonsteroidal anti-inflammatory drugs 30 minutes before meals or 2 hours after meals. This helps the medicine start working a little faster when you first begin to take it. However, after the first few doses, take the medicine with food or an antacid.

- It is not necessary to take delayed-release (enteric-coated) tablets with food or an antacid, because the enteric coating helps protect your stomach from the irritating effects of the medicine. Also, it is not necessary to take ketoprofen extended-release capsules (e.g., Oruvail) with food or an antacid, because the medicine inside the capsules is enteric coated.

- If you will be taking your medicine together with an antacid, one that contains magnesium and aluminum hydroxides (e.g., Maalox) may be the best kind of antacid to use, unless your doctor has directed you to use another antacid. However, do not mix the liquid form of ibuprofen, indomethacin, or naproxen together with an antacid, or any other liquid, before taking it. To do so may cause the medicine to break down. If stomach upset (indigestion, nausea, vomiting, stomach pain, or diarrhea) continues or if you have any questions about how you should be taking this medicine, check with your health care professional.

- Some of these medicines must be swallowed whole. Tablets should not be crushed, chewed, or broken, and capsules should not be emptied out, before you take the medicine. These include delayed-release (enteric-coated) or extended-release tablets or capsules, diflunisal tablets (e.g., Dolobid), and phenylbutazone tablets (e.g., Butazolidin). If you are not sure whether you are taking a delayed-release or extended-release form of your medicine, check with your pharmacist.

For patients using *a suppository form* of this medicine:

- If the suppository is too soft to insert, chill it in the refrigerator for 30 minutes or run cold water over it before removing the foil wrapper.

- To insert the suppository: First remove the foil wrapper and moisten the suppository with cold water. Lie down on your side and use your finger to push the suppository well up into the rectum.

- Indomethacin suppositories should be kept inside the rectum for at least one hour so that all of the medicine can be absorbed by your body. This helps the medicine work better.

For patients taking *nonprescription (over-the-counter [OTC]) ibuprofen or naproxen:*

- This medicine comes with a patient information sheet. Read it carefully. If you have any questions about this information, check with your health care professional.

For safe and effective use of this medicine, do not take more of it, do not take it more often, and do not take it for a longer time than ordered by your health care professional or directed on the nonprescription (over-the-counter [OTC]) package label. Taking too much of any of these medicines may increase the chance of unwanted effects, especially in elderly patients.

When used for severe or continuing arthritis, a nonsteroidal anti-inflammatory drug must be taken regularly as ordered by your doctor in order for it to help you. These medicines usually begin to work within one week, but in severe cases up to two weeks or even longer may pass before you begin to feel better. Also, several weeks may pass before you feel the full effects of the medicine.

For patients taking *mefenamic acid:*

- *Always take mefenamic acid with food or antacids.*

- *Do not take mefenamic acid for more than 7 days at a time* unless otherwise directed by your doctor. To do so may increase the chance of side effects, especially in elderly patients.

For patients taking *phenylbutazone:*

- Phenylbutazone is intended to treat your current medical problem only. *Do not take it for any other aches or pains.* Also, phenylbutazone should be used for the shortest time possible because of the chance of serious side effects, especially in patients who are 40 years of age or older.

Dosing—The dose of these medicines will be different for different patients. *Follow your doctor's orders or the directions on the label.* The following information includes only the average doses of these medicines. *If your dose is different, do not change it* unless your doctor tells you to do so.

The number of capsules or tablets or teaspoonfuls of suspension that you take, or the number of suppositories that you use, depends on the strength of the medicine. Also, *the number of doses you take each day, the time allowed between doses, and the length of time you take the medicine depend on the medical problem for which you are taking the medicine.*

People with arthritis usually need to take more of a nonsteroidal anti-inflammatory drug during a "flare-up" than they do between "flare-ups" of arthritis symptoms. Therefore, your dose may need to be increased or decreased as your condition changes.

For diclofenac

- For *tablet* dosage form:
  - —For relieving pain or menstrual cramps:
    - Adults—50 milligrams (mg) three times a day as needed. Your doctor may direct you to take 100 mg for the first dose only.
    - Children—Use and dose must be determined by your doctor.
  - —For rheumatoid arthritis:
    - Adults—At first, 50 mg three or four times a

day. Your doctor may increase the dose, if necessary, up to a total of 225 mg a day. After your condition improves your doctor may direct you to take a lower dose.

• Children—Use and dose must be determined by your doctor.

—For osteoarthritis:

• Adults—At first, 50 mg two or three times a day. Usually, no more than a total of 150 mg a day should be taken. After your condition improves your doctor may direct you to take a lower dose.

• Children—Use and dose must be determined by your doctor.

—For spondylitis (lower back pain):

• Adults—At first, 25 mg four or five times a day. After your condition improves your doctor may direct you to take a lower dose.

• Children—Use and dose must be determined by your doctor.

• For *delayed-release tablet* dosage form:

—For rheumatoid arthritis:

• Adults—At first, 50 mg three or four times a day. Your doctor may increase the dose, if necessary, up to a total of 225 mg a day. After your condition improves your doctor may direct you to take a lower dose.

• Children—Use and dose must be determined by your doctor.

—For osteoarthritis:

• Adults—At first, 50 mg two or three times a day. Usually, no more than a total of 150 mg a day should be taken. After your condition improves your doctor may direct you to take a lower dose.

- Children—Use and dose must be determined by your doctor.

—For spondylitis (lower back pain):

- Adults—At first, 25 mg four or five times a day. After your condition improves your doctor may direct you to take a lower dose.

- Children—Use and dose must be determined by your doctor.

- For *extended-release tablet* dosage form:

—For rheumatoid arthritis, osteoarthritis, or spondylitis:

- Adults—Usually 75 or 100 mg once a day, in the morning or evening. Some people may need 75 mg twice a day, in the morning and evening. Take the medicine at the same time every day.

- Children—Use and dose must be determined by your doctor.

- For *rectal* dosage form (suppositories):

—For rheumatoid arthritis, osteoarthritis, or spondylitis:

- Adults—One 50-mg or 100-mg suppository, inserted into the rectum. The suppository is usually used only at night by people who take tablets during the day. Usually, no more than a total of 150 mg of diclofenac should be used in a day from all dosage forms combined.

- Children—Use and dose must be determined by your doctor.

For diflunisal

- For *oral* dosage form (tablets):

—For pain:

- Adults—1000 milligrams (mg) for the first dose, then 500 mg every eight to twelve hours as needed. Some people may need only 500 mg for the first dose, then 250 mg every eight to twelve hours as needed. Usually, no more than a total of 1500 mg a day should be taken.

• Children—Dose must be determined by your doctor.

—For rheumatoid arthritis or osteoarthritis:

• Adults—At first, 250 or 500 mg twice a day. Your doctor may increase the dose, if necessary, up to a total of 1500 mg a day. After your condition improves your doctor may direct you to take a lower dose.

• Children—Dose must be determined by your doctor.

For etodolac

• For *oral* dosage forms (capsules or tablets):

—For pain:

• Adults—400 milligrams (mg) for the first dose, then 200 to 400 mg every six to eight hours as needed. Usually, no more than a total of 1200 mg a day should be taken.

• Children—Use and dose must be determined by your doctor.

—For osteoarthritis:

• Adults—At first, 400 mg two or three times a day or 300 mg three or four times a day. Usually, no more than a total of 1200 mg a day should be taken. After your condition improves your doctor may direct you to take a lower dose.

• Children—Use and dose must be determined by your doctor.

For fenoprofen

• For *oral* dosage forms (capsules or tablets):

—For pain:

• Adults—200 milligrams (mg) every four to six hours as needed.

• Children—Use and dose must be determined by your doctor.

—For arthritis:

• Adults—At first, 300 to 600 mg three or four times a day. Your doctor may increase the dose, if necessary, up to a total of 3200 mg a day. After your condition improves your doctor may direct you to take a lower dose.

• Children—Use and dose must be determined by your doctor.

For floctafenine

• For *oral* dosage form (tablets):

—For pain:

• Adults—200 to 400 milligrams (mg) every six to eight hours, as needed. Usually, no more than 1200 mg a day should be taken.

• Children—Use is not recommended.

For flurbiprofen

• For *oral tablet* dosage form:

—For menstrual cramps:

• Adults—50 milligrams (mg) four times a day.

• Children—Use and dose must be determined by your doctor.

—For bursitis, tendinitis, or athletic injuries:

• Adults—50 mg every four to six hours as needed.

• Children—Use and dose must be determined by your doctor.

—For rheumatoid arthritis or osteoarthritis:

• Adults—At first, 200 to 300 mg a day, divided into smaller amounts that are taken two to four times a day. Usually, no more than a total of 300 mg a day should be taken. After your condition improves your doctor may direct you to take a lower dose.

• Children—Use and dose must be determined by your doctor.

—For spondylitis (lower back pain):

• Adults—At first, 50 mg four times a day. Your doctor may increase the dose, if necessary, up to a total of 300 mg a day. After your condition improves your doctor may direct you to take a lower dose.

• Children—Use and dose must be determined by your doctor.

• For *extended-release capsule* dosage form:

—For arthritis:

• Adults—200 mg once a day, in the evening. Take the medicine at the same time every day.

• Children—Use and dose must be determined by your doctor.

For ibuprofen

• For *oral* dosage forms (tablets or oral suspension):

—For pain or menstrual cramps:

• Adults and teenagers—200 to 400 milligrams (mg) every four to six hours as needed. If you are taking the medicine without a prescription from your health care professional, do not take more than a total of 1200 mg (six 200-mg tablets) a day.

• Children up to 12 years of age—Use and dose must be determined by your doctor.

—For fever:

• Adults and teenagers—200 to 400 mg every four to six hours as needed. If you are taking the medicine without a prescription from your health care professional, do not take more than a total of 1200 mg (six 200-mg tablets) a day.

• Children 6 months to 12 years of age—The medicine should be used only with a prescription from your doctor. The dose is based on body weight and on the body temperature. For fevers lower than 102.5°F (39.2°C) the dose is 5 mg per kilogram (kg) (about 2.2 mg per pound) of body weight. For higher fevers the dose is 10 mg per kg (about 4.5 mg per pound) of body weight.

• Infants younger than 6 months of age—Use and dose must be determined by your doctor.

—For arthritis:

• Adults and teenagers—At first, a total of 1200 to 3200 mg a day, divided into smaller amounts that are taken three or four times a day. After your condition improves your doctor may direct you to take a lower dose.

• Children 6 months to 12 years of age—The dose is based on body weight. At first, a total of 30 to 40 mg per kg (about 13.6 to 18 mg per pound) of body weight a day, divided into smaller amounts that are taken three or four times a day. Your doctor may increase the dose, if necessary, up to a total of 50 mg per kg (about 21 mg per pound) of body weight a day. After your condition improves your doctor may direct you to take a lower dose.

• Infants younger than 6 months of age—Use and dose must be determined by your doctor.

For indomethacin

• For *capsule or oral suspension* dosage forms:

—For arthritis:

• Adults—At first, 25 or 50 milligrams (mg) two to four times a day. Your doctor may increase the dose, if necessary, up to a total of 200 mg a day. After your condition improves your doctor may direct you to take a lower dose.

• Children—The dose is based on body weight. At first, 1.5 to 2.5 mg per kilogram (kg) (about 0.7 to 1.1 mg per pound) of body weight a day, divided into smaller amounts that are taken three or four times a day. Your doctor may increase the dose, if necessary, up to a total of 4 mg per kg (about 1.8 mg per pound) of body weight or 200 mg a day, whichever is less. After your condition improves your doctor may direct you to take a lower dose.

—For gout:

• Adults—100 mg for the first dose, then 50 mg three times a day. After the pain is relieved, your doctor may direct you to take a lower dose for a while before stopping treatment completely.

• Children—Use and dose must be determined by your doctor.

—For bursitis or tendinitis:

• Adults—25 mg three or four times a day or 50 mg three times a day.

• Children—Use and dose must be determined by your doctor.

• For *extended-release capsule* dosage form:

—For arthritis:

• Adults—75 mg once a day, in the morning or evening. Some people may need to take 75 mg twice a day, in the morning and evening. Take the medicine at the same time each day.

• Children—Dose must be determined by your doctor.

• For *rectal suppository* dosage form:

—For arthritis, bursitis, tendinitis, or gout:

• Adults—One 50-mg suppository, inserted into the rectum up to four times a day.

• Children—One 50-mg suppository, inserted into the rectum up to four times a day. The suppository dosage form is too strong for small children. However, the suppositories may be used for large or heavy children if they need doses as large as 50 mg.

For ketoprofen

• For *capsule or delayed-release tablet* dosage forms:
—For pain or menstrual cramps:

• Adults—25 to 50 milligrams (mg) every six to eight hours as needed. Some people may need to take as much as 75 mg every six to eight hours. Doses larger than 75 mg are not likely to give better relief.

• Children—Use and dose must be determined by your doctor.

—For arthritis:

• Adults—At first, 50 mg four times a day or 75 mg three times a day. Your doctor may increase the dose, if necessary, up to a total of 300 mg a day. After your condition improves your doctor may direct you to take a lower dose.

• Children—Use and dose must be determined by your doctor.

• For *extended-release capsule or extended-release tablet* dosage forms:
—For arthritis:

• Adults—150 or 200 mg once a day, in the morning or evening. Take the medicine at the same time every day.

• Children—Use and dose must be determined by your doctor.

• For *rectal suppository* dosage form:

—For arthritis:

• Adults—50 or 100 mg twice a day, inserted into the rectum, in the morning and evening. Sometimes, the suppository is used only at night by people who take an oral dosage form (capsules or delayed-release tablets) during the day. Usually, no more than a total of 300 mg of ketoprofen should be used in a day from all dosage forms combined.

• Children—Use and dose must be determined by your doctor.

For meclofenamate

• For *oral* dosage form (capsules):

—For arthritis:

• Adults and teenagers 14 years of age and older—At first, 50 milligrams (mg) four times a day. Your doctor may increase the dose, if necessary, up to a total of 400 mg a day. After your condition improves your doctor may direct you to take a lower dose.

• Children up to 14 years of age—Use and dose must be determined by your doctor.

—For pain:

• Adults and teenagers 14 years of age and older—50 mg every four to six hours. Some people may need as much as 100 mg every four to six hours.

• Children up to 14 years of age—Use and dose must be determined by your doctor.

—For menstrual cramps and heavy menstrual bleeding:

• Adults and teenagers 14 years of age and older—100 mg three times a day for up to six days.

• Children up to 14 years of age—Use and dose must be determined by your doctor.

For mefenamic acid
- For *oral* dosage form (capsules):
  —For pain and for menstrual cramps:
  - Adults and teenagers 14 years of age and older—500 milligrams (mg) for the first dose, then 250 mg every six hours as needed for up to seven days.
  - Children up to 14 years of age—Use and dose must be determined by your doctor.

For nabumetone
- For *oral* dosage form (tablets):
  —For arthritis:
  - Adults—At first, 1000 milligrams (mg) once a day, in the morning or evening, or 500 mg twice a day, in the morning and evening. Your doctor may increase the dose, if necessary, up to a total of 2000 mg a day. After your condition improves your doctor may direct you to take a lower dose.
  - Children—Use and dose must be determined by your doctor.

For naproxen
- For *naproxen (e.g., Naprosyn) tablet, oral suspension, and delayed-release tablet* dosage forms:
  —For arthritis:
  - Adults—At first, 250, 375, or 500 milligrams (mg) two times a day, in the morning and evening. Your doctor may increase the dose, if necessary, up to a total of 1500 mg a day. After your condition improves your doctor may direct you to take a lower dose.
  - Children—The dose is based on body weight. At first, 5 mg per kilogram (kg) (about 2.25 mg per pound) of body weight twice a day. After your condition improves your doctor may direct you to take a lower dose.

—For bursitis, tendinitis, menstrual cramps, and other kinds of pain:

- Adults—500 mg for the first dose, then 250 mg every six to eight hours as needed.
- Children—Use and dose must be determined by your doctor.

—For gout:

- Adults—750 mg for the first dose, then 250 mg every eight hours until the attack is relieved.
- Children—Use and dose must be determined by your doctor.

• For *naproxen extended-release tablet (e.g., Naprosyn-E)* dosage form:

—For arthritis:

- Adults—750 mg once a day, in the morning or evening.
- Children—The extended-release tablets are too strong for use in children.

• For *naproxen (e.g., Naprosyn) rectal suppository* dosage form:

—For arthritis:

- Adults—One 500-mg suppository, inserted into the rectum at bedtime. The suppository is usually used only at night by people who take an oral dosage form (tablets, oral suspension, or delayed-release tablets) during the day. Usually, no more than a total of 1500 mg of naproxen should be used in a day from all dosage forms combined.
- Children—The suppositories are too strong for use in children.

• For *naproxen sodium (e.g., Aleve, Anaprox) tablet* dosage form:

—For arthritis:

- Adults—At first, 275 or 550 mg two times a day, in the morning and evening, or 275 mg in the morning and 550 mg in the evening. Your doctor may increase the dose, if necessary, up to a total of 1650 mg a day. After your condition improves your doctor may direct you to take a lower dose.

• Children—Naproxen sodium tablets are too strong for most children. Naproxen (e.g., Naprosyn) tablets or oral suspension are usually used for children.

—For bursitis and tendinitis:

• Adults—550 mg for the first dose, then 275 mg every six to eight hours as needed.

• Children—Use and dose must be determined by your doctor. Naproxen sodium tablets are too strong for most children.

—For gout:

• Adults—825 mg for the first dose, then 275 mg every eight hours until the attack is relieved.

• Children—Use and dose must be determined by your doctor. Naproxen sodium tablets are too strong for most children.

—For pain, fever, and menstrual cramps:

• Adults and children 12 years of age or older—For nonprescription (over-the-counter [OTC]) use: 220 mg (one tablet) every eight to twelve hours as needed. Some people may get better relief if they take 440 mg (two tablets) for the first dose, then 220 mg twelve hours later on the first day only. If you are taking this medicine without a prescription from your health care professional, do not take more than three 220-mg tablets a day. If you are older than 65 years of age, do not take more than two 220-mg tablets a day. Your health care professional may direct you to take larger doses.

• Children up to 12 years of age—Use and dose must be determined by your doctor.

For oxaprozin

• For *oral* dosage form (tablets):

—For arthritis:

• Adults—At first, 600 milligrams (mg) once or twice a day, or 1200 mg once a day. Some people may need a larger amount for the first dose only. Your doctor may increase the dose, if necessary, up to 1800 mg a day. This large dose should always be divided into smaller amounts that are taken two or three times a day. After your condition improves your doctor may direct you to take a lower dose.

• Children—Use and dose must be determined by your doctor.

For phenylbutazone

• For *oral* dosage forms (capsules, tablets, and buffered tablets):

—For severe arthritis:

• Adults and teenagers 15 years of age and older—At first, 100 milligrams (mg) three or four times a day. Some people may need a higher dose of 200 mg three times a day. After your condition improves your doctor may direct you to take a lower dose for a while before stopping treatment completely. This medicine should not be taken for longer than a few weeks.

• Children up to 15 years of age—Use is not recommended.

—For gout:

• Adults—400 mg for the first dose, then 100 mg every four hours for one week or less.

• Children up to 15 years of age—Use is not recommended.

For piroxicam
- For *oral* dosage form (capsules):
  - —For arthritis:
    - Adults—20 milligrams (mg) once a day or 10 mg twice a day.
    - Children—Dose must be determined by your doctor.
  - —For menstrual cramps:
    - Adults—40 mg once a day for one day only, then 20 mg once a day if needed.
    - Children—Dose must be determined by your doctor.
- For *rectal* dosage form (suppositories):
  - —For arthritis:
    - Adults—20 mg once a day or 10 mg twice a day.
    - Children—Dose must be determined by your doctor.

For sulindac
- For *oral* dosage form (tablets):
  - —For arthritis:
    - Adults—At first, 150 or 200 milligrams (mg) twice a day. After your condition improves, your doctor may direct you to take a lower dose.
    - Children—Use and dose must be determined by your doctor.
  - —For gout, bursitis, or tendinitis:
    - Adults—At first, 200 mg twice a day. After the pain is relieved, your doctor may direct you to take a lower dose for a while before treatment is stopped completely.
    - Children—Use and dose must be determined by your doctor.

For tenoxicam
- For *oral* dosage form (tablets):

—For arthritis:

• Adults and teenagers 16 years of age and older—At first, 20 milligrams (mg) once a day, at the same time each day. For some people, a smaller dose of 10 mg (one-half tablet) a day may be enough.

• Children and teenagers up to 16 years of age— Dose must be determined by your doctor.

For tiaprofenic acid

• For *oral tablet* dosage form:

—For arthritis:

• Adults—At first, 200 milligrams (mg) three times a day or 300 mg twice a day. After your condition improves, your doctor may direct you to take a lower dose.

• Children—Use and dose must be determined by your doctor.

• For *extended-release capsule* dosage form:

—For arthritis:

• Adults—600 mg (two capsules) once a day, at the same time each day.

• Children—Use and dose must be determined by your doctor.

For tolmetin

• For *oral* dosage forms (capsules or tablets):

—For arthritis:

• Adults—At first, 400 milligrams (mg) three times a day. Your doctor may increase the dose, if necessary, up to a total of 1800 mg a day. After your condition improves, your doctor may direct you to take a lower dose.

• Children 2 years of age and older—The dose is based on body weight. At first, 20 mg per kilogram (kg) (about 9 mg per pound) of body weight a day, divided into smaller amounts that are taken three or four times a day. Your doctor may increase the dose, if necessary, up to 30 mg per kg (about 13.5 mg per pound) of body weight a day. After your condition improves, your doctor may direct you to take a lower dose.

• Children up to 2 years of age—Dose must be determined by your doctor.

Missed dose—If your health care professional has ordered you to take this medicine according to a regular schedule, and you miss a dose, take it as soon as you remember. However, if it is almost time for your next dose, skip the missed dose and go back to your regular dosing schedule. (For long-acting medicines or extended-release dosage forms that are only taken once or twice a day, take the missed dose only if you remember within an hour or two after the dose should have been taken. If you do not remember until later, skip the missed dose and go back to your regular dosing schedule.) Do not double doses.

Storage—To store this medicine:

• Keep out of the reach of children.

• Store away from heat and direct light.

• Do not store tablets or capsules in the bathroom, near the kitchen sink, or in other damp places. Heat or moisture may cause the medicine to break down.

• Keep liquid and suppository forms of this medicine from freezing.

• Do not keep outdated medicine or medicine no longer needed. Be sure that any discarded medicine is out of the reach of children.

Precautions While Using This Medicine

If you will be taking this medicine for a long time, as for arthritis (rheumatism), your doctor should check your progress at regular visits. Your doctor may want to do certain tests to find out if unwanted effects are occurring, especially if you are taking phenylbutazone. The tests are very important because serious side effects, including ulcers, bleeding, or blood problems, can occur without any warning.

Stomach problems may be more likely to occur if you drink alcoholic beverages while being treated with this medicine. Also, alcohol may add to the depressant side effects of phenylbutazone. Therefore, *do not regularly drink alcoholic beverages while taking this medicine,* unless otherwise directed by your doctor.

Taking two or more of the nonsteroidal anti-inflammatory drugs together on a regular basis may increase the chance of unwanted effects. Also, taking acetaminophen, aspirin or other salicylates, or ketorolac (e.g., Toradol) regularly while you are taking a nonsteroidal anti-inflammatory drug may increase the chance of unwanted effects. The risk will depend on how much of each medicine you take every day, and on how long you take the medicines together. If your health care professional directs you to take these medicines together on a regular basis, follow his or her directions carefully. However, *do not take acetaminophen or aspirin or other salicylates together with this medicine for more than a few days, and do not take any ketorolac (e.g., Toradol) while you are taking this medicine, unless your doctor has directed you to do so and is following your progress.*

Before having any kind of surgery (including dental surgery), tell the medical doctor or dentist in charge that you are taking this medicine. If possible, this should be done when your surgery is first being planned. Some of the nonsteroidal anti-inflammatory drugs can increase the chance of bleeding during and after surgery. It may be necessary for you to stop treatment for a while, or to change to a different nonsteroidal anti-inflammatory drug that is less likely to cause bleeding.

This medicine may cause some people to become confused, drowsy, dizzy, lightheaded, or less alert than they are normally. It may also cause blurred vision or other vision problems in some people. *Make sure you know how you react to this medicine before you drive, use machines, or do anything else that could be dangerous if you are confused, dizzy, or drowsy, or if you are not alert and able to see well*. If these reactions are especially bothersome, check with your doctor.

For patients taking *the buffered form of phenylbutazone (e.g., Alka-Butazolidin)*:

• This medicine contains antacids that can keep other medicines from working properly if the two medicines are taken to close together. *Always take this medicine*:

—*At least 6 hours before or 2 hours after taking ciprofloxacin (e.g., Cipro) or lomefloxacin (e.g., Maxaquin)*.

—*At least 8 hours before or 2 hours after taking enoxacin (e.g., Penetrex)*.

—*At least 2 hours after taking itraconazole (e.g., Sporanox)*.

—*At least 3 hours before or after taking ketoconazole (e.g., Nizoral)*.

—*At least 2 hours before or after taking norfloxacin (e.g., Noroxin) or ofloxacin (e.g., Floxin)*.

—*At least 1 to 3 hours before or after taking a tetracycline antibiotic by mouth*.

—*At least 1 or 2 hours before or after taking any other medicine by mouth*.

For patients taking *mefenamic acid*:

• If diarrhea occurs while you are using this medicine, *stop taking it and check with your doctor immedi-*

ately. Do not take it again without first checking with your doctor, because severe diarrhea may occur each time you take it.

Some people who take nonsteroidal anti-inflammatory drugs may become more sensitive to sunlight than they are normally. Exposure to sunlight, even for brief periods of time, may cause severe sunburn; blisters on the skin; skin rash, redness, itching, or discoloration; or vision changes. When you begin taking this medicine:

- Stay out of direct sunlight, especially between the hours of 10:00 a.m. and 3:00 p.m., if possible.
- Wear protective clothing, including a hat and sunglasses.
- Apply a sun block product that has a skin protection factor (SPF) of at least 15. Some patients may require a product with a higher SPF number, especially if they have a fair complexion. If you have any questions about this, check with your health care professional.
- Do not use a sunlamp or tanning bed or booth.

If you have a severe reaction from the sun, check with your doctor.

Serious side effects, including ulcers or bleeding, can occur during treatment with this medicine. Sometimes serious side effects can occur without any warning. However, possible warning signs often occur, including severe abdominal or stomach cramps, pain, or burning; black, tarry stools; severe, continuing nausea, heartburn, or indigestion; and/or vomiting of blood or material that looks like coffee grounds. *Stop taking this medicine and check with your doctor immediately if you notice any of these warning signs.*

Check with your doctor immediately if chills, fever, muscle aches or pains, or other influenza-like symptoms occur, especially if they occur shortly before, or together with, a skin rash. Very rarely, these effects may be the first signs of a serious reaction to this medicine.

Nonsteroidal anti-inflammatory drugs may cause a serious type of allergic reaction called anaphylaxis. Although this is rare, it may occur more often in patients who are allergic to aspirin or to any of the nonsteroidal anti-inflammatory drugs. *Anaphylaxis requires immediate medical attention.* The most serious signs of this reaction are very fast or irregular breathing, gasping for breath, wheezing, or fainting. Other signs may include changes in color of the skin of the face; very fast but irregular heartbeat or pulse; hive-like swellings on the skin; and puffiness or swellings of the eyelids or around the eyes. If these effects occur, get emergency help at once. Ask someone to drive you to the nearest hospital emergency room. If this is not possible, do not try to drive yourself. Call an ambulance, lie down, cover yourself to keep warm, and prop your feet higher than your head. Stay in that position until help arrives.

For patients taking *ibuprofen* or *naproxen* without a prescription:

- Check with your medical doctor or dentist:

    —if your symptoms do not improve or if they get worse.

    —if you are using this medicine to bring down a fever and the fever lasts more than 3 days or returns.

    —if the painful area is red or swollen.

Side Effects of This Medicine

Along with its needed effects, a medicine may cause some unwanted effects. Although not all of these side effects may occur, if they do occur they may need medical attention.

Stop taking this medicine and get emergency help right away if any of the following side effects occur:

Rare—For all nonsteroidal anti-inflammatory drugs

Fainting; fast or irregular breathing; fast, irregular heart-beat or pulse; hive-like swellings (large) on face, eyelids, mouth, lips, or tongue; puffiness or swelling of the eyelids or around the eyes; shortness of breath, troubled breathing, wheezing, or tightness in chest

Also, stop taking this medicine and check with your doctor immediately if any of the following side effects occur:

More common—for mefenamic acid only

Diarrhea

More common—for phenylbutazone only

Swelling of face, hands, feet, or lower legs; weight gain (rapid)

Symptoms of phenylbutazone overdose

Bluish color of fingernails, lips, or skin; headache (severe and continuing)

Rare—for all nonsteroidal anti-inflammatory drugs

Abdominal or stomach pain, cramping, or burning (severe); bloody or black, tarry stools; chest pain; convulsions (seizures); fever with or without chills; nausea, heartburn, and/or indigestion (severe and continuing); pinpoint red spots on skin; sores, ulcers, or white spots on lips or in mouth; spitting up blood; unexplained nosebleeds; unusual bleeding or bruising; vomiting of blood or material that looks like coffee grounds

Also, check with your doctor as soon as possible if any of the following side effects occur:

More common

Bleeding from rectum (with suppositories); headache (severe), especially in the morning (for indomethacin only); skin rash

Less common or rare

Bladder pain; bleeding from cuts or scratches that lasts longer than usual; bleeding or crusting sores on lips;

bloody or cloudy urine or any problem with urination, such as difficult, burning, or painful urination; change in urine color or odor; frequent urge to urinate; sudden, large increase or decrease in the amount of urine; or loss of bladder control; blurred vision or any change in vision; burning feeling in throat, chest, or stomach; confusion, forgetfulness, mental depression, or other mood or mental changes; cough or hoarseness; decreased hearing, any other change in hearing, or ringing or buzzing in ears; difficulty in swallowing; eye pain, irritation, dryness, redness, and/or swelling; hallucinations (seeing, hearing, or feeling things that are not there); headache (severe), throbbing, or with stiff neck or back; hives, itching of skin, or any other skin problem, such as blisters, redness or other color change, tenderness, burning, peeling, thickening, or scaliness; increased blood pressure; irritated tongue; light-colored stools; loosening or splitting of fingernails; muscle cramps, pain, or weakness; numbness, tingling, pain, or weakness in hands or feet; pain in lower back and/or side (severe); swelling and/or tenderness in upper abdominal or stomach area; swelling of face, feet, or lower legs (if taking phenylbutazone, stop taking it and check with your doctor immediately); swelling of lips or tongue; swollen and/or painful glands (especially in the neck or throat area); thirst (continuing); trouble in speaking; unexplained runny nose or sneezing; unexplained, unexpected, or unusually heavy vaginal bleeding; unusual tiredness or weakness; weight gain (rapid) (if taking phenylbutazone, stop taking it and check with your doctor immediately); yellow eyes or skin

Other side effects may occur that usually do not need medical attention. These side effects may go away during treatment as your body adjusts to the medicine. However, check with your doctor if any of the following side effects continue or are bothersome:

More common

Abdominal or stomach cramps, pain, or discomfort (mild to moderate); diarrhea (if taking mefenamic acid, stop taking it and check with your doctor immediately); dizziness, drowsiness, or lightheadedness; headache (mild to moderate); heartburn, indigestion, nausea, or vomiting

Less common or rare

Bitter taste or other taste change; bloated feeling, gas, or constipation; decreased appetite or loss of appetite; fast or pounding heartbeat; flushing or hot flashes; general feeling of discomfort or illness; increased sensitivity of eyes to light; increased sensitivity of skin to sunlight; increased sweating; irritation, dryness, or soreness of mouth; nervousness, anxiety, irritability, trembling, or twitching; rectal irritation (with suppositories); trouble in sleeping; unexplained weight loss; unusual tiredness or weakness without any other symptoms

Although not all of the side effects listed above have been reported for all of these medicines, they have been reported for at least one of them. However, since all anti-inflammatory analgesics are very similar, it is possible that any of the above side effects may occur with any of these medicines.

Some side effects may occur many days or weeks after you have stopped using phenylbutazone. During this time *check with your doctor immediately* if you notice any of the following side effects:

Sore throat and fever; ulcers, sores, or white spots in mouth; unusual bleeding or bruising; unusual tiredness or weakness

Other side effects not listed above may also occur in some patients. If you notice any other effects, check with your doctor.

OLSALAZINE   Oral

A commonly used brand name in the U.S. and Canada is Dipentum.

Other commonly used names are sodium azodisalicylate and azodisal sodium.

Description

Olsalazine (ole-SAL-a-zeen) is used in patients who have had ulcerative colitis to prevent the condition from occurring again. It works inside the bowel by helping to reduce the inflammation and other symptoms of the disease.

Olsalazine is available only with your doctor's prescription, in the following dosage form:

Oral
- Capsules (U.S. and Canada)

Before Using This Medicine

In deciding to use a medicine, the risks of taking the medicine must be weighed against the good it will do. This is a decision you and your doctor will make. For olsalazine, the following should be considered:

Allergies—Tell your doctor if you have ever had any unusual or allergic reaction to olsalazine, mesalamine, or any salicylates (for example, aspirin). Also tell your health care professional if you are allergic to any other substances, such as foods, preservatives, or dyes.

Pregnancy—Studies have not been done in humans. However, studies in rats have shown that olsalazine causes birth defects and other problems at doses 5 to 20 times the human dose. Before taking this medicine, make sure your doctor knows if you are pregnant or if you may become pregnant.

Breast-feeding—It is not known whether olsalazine passes into the breast milk.

Children—Studies on this medicine have been done only in adult patients, and there is no specific information comparing use of olsalazine in children with use in other age groups.

Older adults—Many medicines have not been studied specifically in older people. Therefore, it may not be known whether they work exactly the same way they do in younger adults. Although there is no specific information comparing use of olsalazine in the elderly with use in other age groups, this medicine is not expected to cause different side effects or problems in older people than it does in younger adults.

Other medicines—Although certain medicines should not be used together at all, in other cases two different medicines may be used together even if an interaction might occur. In these cases, your doctor may want to change the dose, or other precautions may be necessary. When you are using olsalazine, it is especially important that your health care professional know if you are taking any other medicines.

Other medical problems—The presence of other medical problems may affect the use of olsalazine. Make sure you tell your doctor if you have any other medical problems, especially:

- Kidney disease—The use of olsalazine may cause further damage to the kidneys

---

Proper Use of This Medicine

Olsalazine is best taken with food, to lessen stomach upset and diarrhea. If stomach or intestinal problems continue or are bothersome, check with your doctor.

Keep taking this medicine for the full time of treatment, even if you begin to feel better after a few days. *Do not miss any doses.*

Dosing—The dose of olsalazine will be different for different patients. *Follow your doctor's orders or the directions on the label.* The following information includes only the average doses of olsalazine. *If your dose is different, do not change it* unless your doctor tells you to do so.

- For *oral* dosage form (capsules):
  - —To prevent ulcerative colitis from occurring again:
    - Adults and teenagers—500 milligrams (mg) two times a day.
    - Children—Use and dose must be determined by your doctor.

Missed dose—If you miss a dose of this medicine, take it as soon as possible. However, if it is almost time for your next dose, skip the missed dose and go back to your regular dosing schedule. Do not double doses.

Storage—To store this medicine:

- Keep out of the reach of children.
- Store away from heat and direct light.
- Do not store this medicine in the bathroom, near the kitchen sink, or in other damp places. Heat or moisture may cause the medicine to break down.
- Do not keep outdated medicine or medicine no longer needed. Be sure that any discarded medicine is out of the reach of children.

Precautions While Using This Medicine

It is very important that your doctor check your progress at regular visits, especially if you will be taking it for a long time. Olsalazine may cause blood problems.

Side Effects of This Medicine

Along with its needed effects, a medicine may cause some unwanted effects. Although not all of these side effects

may occur, if they do occur they may need medical attention.

Check with your doctor as soon as possible if any of the following side effects occur:

> *Rare*

>> Bloody diarrhea; fever; pale skin; skin rash; sore throat; unusual bleeding or bruising; unusual tiredness or weakness; yellow eyes or skin

Other side effects may occur that usually do not need medical attention. These side effects may go away during treatment as your body adjusts to the medicine. However, check with your doctor if any of the following side effects continue or are bothersome:

> *More common*

>> Abdominal or stomach pain or upset; diarrhea; loss of appetite; nausea or vomiting

> *Less common*

>> Aching joints and muscles; acne; anxiety or depression, drowsiness or dizziness; headache; insomnia

Other side effects not listed above may also occur in some patients. If you notice any other effects, check with your doctor.

OMEPRAZOLE   Systemic

Some commonly used brand names are:
In the U.S.—
  Prilosec
In Canada—
  Losec

Description

Omeprazole (o-MEP-ra-zole) is used to treat certain conditions in which there is too much acid in the stomach. It is used to treat duodenal ulcers and gastroesophageal reflux disease, a condition in which the acid in the stomach washes back up into the esophagus. Omeprazole is also used to treat Zollinger-Ellison syndrome, a condition in which the stomach produces too much acid. It may also be used for other conditions as determined by your doctor.

Omeprazole works by decreasing the amount of acid produced by the stomach.

This medicine is available only with your doctor's prescription.

Oral

  • Delayed-release capsules (U.S. and Canada)

Before Using This Medicine

In deciding to use a medicine, the risks of taking the medicine must be weighed against the good it will do. This is a decision you and your doctor will make. For omeprazole, the following should be considered:

Allergies—Tell your doctor if you have ever had any unusual or allergic reaction to omeprazole. Also tell your health care professional if you are allergic to any other substances, such as foods, preservatives, or dyes.

Pregnancy—Studies have not been done in humans. However, studies in animals have shown that omeprazole may cause harm to the fetus.

Breast-feeding—Omeprazole may pass into the breast milk. Since this medicine has been shown to cause unwanted effects, such as tumors and cancer in animals, it may be necessary for you to take another medicine or to stop breast-feeding during treatment. Be sure you have discussed the risks and benefits of the medicine with your doctor.

Children—There is no specific information comparing the use of omeprazole in children with use in other age groups.

Older adults—Many medicines have not been studied specifically in older people. Therefore, it may not be known whether they work exactly the same way they do in younger adults or if they cause different side effects or problems in older people. There is no specific information comparing use of omeprazole in the elderly with use in other age groups.

Other medicines—Although certain medicines should not be used together at all, in other cases two different medicines may be used together even if an interaction might occur. In these cases, your doctor may want to change the dose, or other precautions may be necessary. When you are taking omeprazole, it is especially important that your health care professional know if you are taking any of the following:

- Anticoagulants (blood thinners) or
- Diazepam (e.g., Valium) or
- Phenytoin (e.g., Dilantin)—Use with omeprazole may cause high blood levels of these medicines, which may increase the chance of side effects

Other medical problems—The presence of other medical problems may affect the use of omeprazole. Make sure you tell your doctor if you have any other medical problems, especially:

- Liver disease or a history of liver disease—This condition may cause omeprazole to build up in the body

Proper Use of This Medicine

Take omeprazole immediately before a meal, preferably in the morning.

It may take several days before this medicine begins to relieve stomach pain. To help relieve this pain, antacids may be taken with omeprazole, unless your doctor has told you not to use them.

Swallow the capsule whole. Do not crush, break, chew, or open the capsule.

Take this medicine for the full time of treatment, even if you begin to feel better. Also, keep your appointments with your doctor for check-ups so that your doctor will be better able to tell you when to stop taking this medicine.

Dosing—The dose of omeprazole will be different for different patients. *Follow your doctor's orders or the directions on the label.* The following information includes only the average doses of omeprazole. *If your dose is different, do not change it* unless your doctor tells you to do so.

- For *oral* dosage form (capsules):
  - —To treat gastroesophageal reflux disease:
    - Adults—20 milligrams (mg) taken once a day for four to eight weeks. Or, your doctor may tell you to take 40 mg a day for certain conditions.
    - Children—Dose must be determined by your doctor.
  - —To treat conditions in which the stomach produces too much acid:
    - Adults—60 milligrams (mg) taken once a day. Your doctor may change the dose as needed. Your treatment may be continued for as long as it is needed.
    - Children—Dose must be determined by your doctor.
  - —To treat duodenal ulcers:
    - Adults—20 mg taken once a day. Or, your doctor may tell you to take 40 mg a day for certain conditions.
    - Children—Dose must be determined by your doctor.

Missed dose—If you miss a dose of this medicine, take it as soon as possible. However, if it is almost time for your next dose, skip the missed dose and go back to your regular dosing schedule. Do not double doses.

Storage—To store this medicine:

- Keep out of the reach of children.
- Store away from heat and direct light.
- Do not store in the bathroom, near the kitchen sink, or in other damp places. Heat or moisture may cause the medicine to break down.
- Do not keep outdated medicine or medicine no longer needed. Be sure that any discarded medicine is out of the reach of children.

Precautions While Using This Medicine

If your condition does not improve, or if it becomes worse, check with your doctor.

Side Effects of This Medicine

Along with its needed effects, a medicine may cause some unwanted effects. Although not all of these side effects may occur, if they do occur they may need medical attention.

Check with your doctor as soon as possible if any of the following side effects occur:

Rare

Bloody or cloudy urine; continuing ulcers or sores in mouth; difficult, burning, or painful urination; frequent urge to urinate; sore throat and fever; unusual bleeding or bruising; unusual tiredness or weakness

Other side effects may occur that usually do not need

medical attention. These side effects may go away during treatment as your body adjusts to the medicine. However, check with your doctor if any of the following side effects continue or are bothersome:

More common

Abdominal or stomach pain

Less common

Chest pain; constipation; diarrhea or loose stools; dizziness; gas; headache; heartburn; muscle pain; nausea and vomiting; skin rash or itching; unusual drowsiness; unusual tiredness

Other side effects not listed above may also occur in some patients. If you notice any other effects, check with your doctor.

Additional Information

Once a medicine has been approved for marketing for a certain use, experience may show that it is also useful for other medical problems. Although this use is not included in product labeling, omeprazole is used in certain patients with the following medical condition:

• Gastric ulcer

Other than the above information, there is no additional information relating to proper use, precautions, or side effects for these uses.

ORPHENADRINE AND ASPIRIN   Systemic

Some commonly used brand names are:

In the U.S.—

Norgesic	Norphadrine
Norgesic Forte	Norphadrine Forte

In the U.S. (cont'd)—
   N3 Gesic   Orphenagesic
   N3 Gesic Forte   Orphenagesic Forte
In Canada—‡
   Norgesic   Norgesic Forte

---

‡In Canada, *Aspirin* is a brand name. Acetylsalicylic acid is the generic name in Canada. ASA, a synonym for acetylsalicylic acid, is the term that commonly appears on Canadian product labels.

Description

Orphenadrine (or-FEN-a-dreen) and aspirin (AS-pir-in) combination is used to help relax certain muscles in your body and relieve the pain and discomfort caused by strains, sprains, or other injury to your muscles. However, this medicine does not take the place of rest, exercise, or other treatment that your doctor may recommend for your medical problem.

Orphenadrine acts in the central nervous system (CNS) to produce its muscle relaxant effects. Actions in the CNS may also be responsible for some of its side effects. Orphenadrine also has other actions (antimuscarinic) that may be responsible for some of its side effects.

This combination medicine also contains caffeine (kaf-EEN).

In the U.S., this combination medicine is available only with your doctor's prescription. In Canada, it is available without a prescription.

These medicines are available in the following dosage forms:

   Oral
     • Tablets (U.S. and Canada)

Before Using This Medicine

In deciding to use a medicine, the risks of taking the medicine must be weighed against the good it will do.

This is a decision you and your doctor will make. For orphenadrine and aspirin combination, the following should be considered:

Allergies—Tell your doctor if you have ever had any unusual or allergic reaction to orphenadrine, caffeine, aspirin or other salicylates including methyl salicylate (oil of wintergreen), or to any of the following medicines:

Diclofenac (e.g., Voltaren)
Diflunisal (e.g., Dolobid)
Etodolac (e.g., Lodine)
Fenoprofen (e.g., Nalfon)
Floctafenine (e.g., Idarac)
Flurbiprofen, oral (e.g., Ansaid)
Ibuprofen (e.g., Motrin)
Indomethacin (e.g., Indocin)
Ketoprofen (e.g., Orudis)
Ketorolac (e.g., Toradol)
Meclofenamate (e.g., Meclomen)
Mefenamic acid (e.g., Ponstel)
Nabumetone (e.g., Relafen)
Naproxen (e.g., Naprosyn)
Oxaprozin (e.g., Daypro)
Oxyphenbutazone (e.g., Tandearil)
Phenylbutazone (e.g., Butazolidin)
Piroxicam (e.g., Feldene)
Sulindac (e.g., Clinoril)
Suprofen (e.g., Suprol)
Tenoxicam (e.g., Mobiflex)
Tiaprofenic acid (e.g., Surgam)
Tolmetin (e.g., Tolectin)
Zomepirac (e.g., Zomax)

Also tell your health care professional if you are allergic to any other substances, such as foods, preservatives, or dyes.

Pregnancy—

- *For aspirin:* Studies in humans have not shown that aspirin causes birth defects. However, aspirin has caused birth defects in animal studies.

  Some reports have suggested that too much use of

aspirin late in pregnancy may cause a decrease in the newborn's weight and possible death of the fetus or newborn baby. However, the mothers in these reports had been taking much larger amounts of aspirin than are usually recommended. Studies of mothers taking aspirin in the doses that are usually recommended did not show these unwanted effects.

Regular use of aspirin late in pregnancy may cause unwanted effects on the heart or blood flow in the fetus or in the newborn baby. Also, use of aspirin during the last 2 weeks of pregnancy may cause bleeding problems in the fetus before or during delivery or in the newborn baby. In addition, too much use of aspirin during the last 3 months of pregnancy may increase the length of pregnancy, prolong labor, cause other problems during delivery, or cause severe bleeding in the mother before, during, or after delivery. *Do not take aspirin during the last 3 months of pregnancy unless it has been ordered by your doctor.*

- *For orphenadrine:* Orphenadrine has not been reported to cause birth defects or other problems in humans.

Breast-feeding—This medicine has not been shown to cause problems in nursing babies. However, aspirin passes into the breast milk. Also, caffeine passes into the breast milk in small amounts. It is not known whether orphenadrine passes into the breast milk.

Children—*Do not give a medicine containing aspirin to a child or a teenager with a fever or other symptoms of a virus infection, especially flu or chickenpox, without first discussing its use with your child's doctor.* This is very important because aspirin may cause a serious illness called Reye's syndrome in children with fever caused by a virus infection, especially flu or chickenpox. Children who do not have a virus infection may also be more sensitive to the effects of aspirin, especially if they have a fever or have lost large amounts of body fluid because of vomiting, diarrhea, or sweating. This may increase the chance of side effects during treatment.

There is no specific information about the use of orphenadrine in children.

Older adults—Elderly people are especially sensitive to the effects of aspirin. This may increase the chance of side effects during treatment.

There is no specific information about the use of orphenadrine in the elderly.

Other medicines—Although certain medicines should not be used together at all, in other cases two different medicines may be used together even if an interaction might occur. In these cases, your doctor may want to change the dose, or other precautions may be necessary. When you are taking orphenadrine and aspirin combination, it is especially important that your health care professional know if you are taking any of the following:

- Anticoagulants (blood thinners) or
- Carbenicillin by injection (e.g., Geopen) or
- Cefamandole (e.g., Mandol) or
- Cefoperazone (e.g., Cefobid) or
- Cefotetan (e.g., Cefotan) or
- Dipyridamole (e.g., Persantine) or
- Divalproex (e.g., Depakote) or
- Heparin or
- Medicine for inflammation or pain, except narcotics, or
- Moxalactam (e.g., Moxam) or
- Pentoxifylline (e.g., Trental) or
- Plicamycin (e.g., Mithracin) or
- Ticarcillin (e.g., Ticar) or
- Valproic acid (e.g., Depakene)—Taking these medicines together with aspirin may increase the chance of bleeding
- Anticholinergics (medicine for abdominal or stomach spasms or cramps) or
- Central nervous system (CNS) depressants or
- Methotrexate (e.g., Mexate) or

- Tricyclic antidepressants (amitriptyline [e.g., Elavil], amoxapine [e.g., Asendin], clomipramine [e.g., Anafranil], desipramine [e.g., Pertofrane], doxepin [e.g., Sinequan], imipramine [e.g., Tofranil], nortriptyline [e.g., Aventyl], protriptyline [e.g., Vivactil], trimipramine [e.g., Surmontil]) or
- Vancomycin (e.g., Vancocin)—The chance of side effects may be increased
- Antidiabetics, oral (diabetes medicine you take by mouth)—Aspirin may increase the effects of the antidiabetic medicine; a change in dose may be needed if aspirin is taken regularly
- Probenecid (e.g., Benemid) or
- Sulfinpyrazone (e.g., Anturane)—Aspirin can keep these medicines from working properly for treating gout; also, taking aspirin together with sulfinpyrazone may increase the chance of bleeding
- Urinary alkalizers (medicine that makes the urine less acid, such as acetazolamide [e.g., Diamox], dichlorphenamide [e.g., Daranide], methazolamide [e.g., Neptazane], potassium or sodium citrate and/or citric acid)—These medicines may make aspirin less effective by causing it to be removed from the body more quickly
- Zidovudine (e.g., AZT; Retrovir)—Aspirin may increase the blood levels of zidovudine, which increases the chance of serious side effects

Other medical problems—The presence of other medical problems may affect the use of orphenadrine and aspirin combination. Make sure you tell your doctor if you have any other medical problems, especially:

- Anemia or
- Overactive thyroid or
- Stomach ulcer or other stomach problems—Aspirin may make your condition worse
- Asthma, allergies, and nasal polyps, history of or
- Glucose-6-phosphate dehydrogenase (G6PD) deficiency or
- Kidney disease or
- Liver disease—The chance of side effects may be increased

- Disease of the digestive tract, especially esophagus disease or intestinal blockage, or
- Enlarged prostate or
- Fast or irregular heartbeat or
- Glaucoma or
- Myasthenia gravis or
- Urinary tract blockage—Orphenadrine has side effects that may be harmful to people with these conditions
- Gout—Aspirin can make this condition worse and can also lessen the effects of some medicines used to treat gout
- Heart disease—The chance of some side effects may be increased. Also, the caffeine present in this combination medicine can make your condition worse
- Hemophilia or other bleeding problems or
- Vitamin K deficiency—Aspirin may increase the chance of bleeding

---

Proper Use of This Medicine

Take this medicine with food or a full glass (8 ounces) of water to lessen stomach irritation.

Do not take this medicine if it has a strong vinegar-like odor. This odor means the aspirin in it is breaking down. If you have any questions about this, check with your health care professional.

Do not take more of this medicine than your doctor ordered to lessen the chance of side effects or overdose.

Dosing—The dose of orphenadrine and aspirin combination medicine will be different for different people. *Follow your doctor's orders or the directions on the label.* The following information includes only the average doses of the combination medicine. *If your dose is different, do not change it* unless your doctor tells you to do so.

- For *oral* dosage forms (tablets):
    —For muscle pain and stiffness:

- Adults and teenagers—One or two tablets containing 25 milligrams (mg) of orphenadrine and 385 mg of aspirin, or one-half or one tablet containing 50 mg of orphenadrine and 770 mg of aspirin, three or four times a day.
- Children—Dose must be determined by your doctor.

Missed dose—If you miss a dose of this medicine and remember within an hour or so of the missed dose, take it right away. But if you do not remember until later, skip the missed dose and go back to your regular dosing schedule. Do not double doses.

Storage—To store this medicine:
- Keep out of the reach of children. Overdose of aspirin is especially dangerous in young children.
- Store away from heat and direct light.
- Do not store this medicine in the bathroom, near the kitchen sink, or in other damp places. Heat or moisture may cause the medicine to break down.
- Do not keep outdated medicine or medicine no longer needed. Be sure that any discarded medicine is out of the reach of children.

Precautions While Using This Medicine

If you will be taking this medicine for a long time (for example, more than a few weeks), your doctor should check your progress at regular visits.

Check the labels of all nonprescription (over-the-counter [OTC]) and prescription medicines you now take. If any contain orphenadrine or aspirin or other salicylates be especially careful, since taking them while taking this medicine may lead to overdose. If you have any questions about this, check with your health care professional.

Too much use of acetaminophen or certain other medicines together with the aspirin in this combination medicine may increase the chance of unwanted effects. The risk depends on how much of each medicine you take every day, and on how long you take the medicines together. If your doctor directs you to take these medicines together on a regular basis, follow his or her directions carefully. However, do not take acetaminophen or any of the following medicines together with this combination medicine for more than a few days, unless your doctor has directed you to do so and is following your progress:

    Diclofenac (e.g., Voltaren)
    Diflunisal (e.g., Dolobid)
    Etodolac (e.g., Lodine)
    Fenoprofen (e.g., Nalfon)
    Floctafenine (e.g., Idarac)
    Flurbiprofen, oral (e.g., Ansaid)
    Ibuprofen (e.g., Motrin)
    Indomethacin (e.g., Indocin)
    Ketoprofen (e.g., Orudis)
    Ketorolac (e.g., Toradol)
    Meclofenamate (e.g., Meclomen)
    Mefenamic acid (e.g., Ponstel)
    Nabumetone (e.g., Relafen)
    Naproxen (e.g., Naprosyn)
    Oxaprozin (e.g., Daypro)
    Phenylbutazone (e.g., Butazolidin)
    Piroxicam (e.g., Feldene)
    Sulindac (e.g., Clinoril)
    Tenoxicam (e.g., Mobiflex)
    Tiaprofenic acid (e.g., Surgam)
    Tolmetin (e.g., Tolectin)

For *diabetic patients:*

- The aspirin in this combination medicine may cause false urine sugar test results if you are regularly taking 6 or more of the regular-strength tablets or 3 or more of the double-strength tablets of this medicine a day. Smaller doses or occasional use of aspirin usually will not affect urine sugar tests. If you have any questions about this, check with your health care professional especially if your diabetes is not well controlled.

Do not take this medicine for 5 days before any surgery, including dental surgery, unless otherwise directed by your medical doctor or dentist. Taking aspirin during this time may cause bleeding problems.

The orphenadrine in this combination medicine may add to the effects of alcohol and other CNS depressants (medicines that slow down the nervous system, possibly causing drowsiness). Some examples of CNS depressants are antihistamines or medicine for hay fever, other allergies, or colds; sedatives, tranquilizers, or sleeping medicine; prescription pain medicine or narcotics; barbiturates; medicine for seizures; other muscle relaxants; or anesthetics, including some dental anesthetics. Also, stomach problems may be more likely to occur if you drink alcoholic beverages while you are taking aspirin. *Do not drink alcoholic beverages, and check with your doctor before taking any of the medicines listed above, while you are using this medicine.*

This medicine may cause some people to have blurred vision or to become drowsy, dizzy, lightheaded, faint, or less alert than they are normally. *Make sure you know how you react to this medicine before you drive, use machines, or do anything else that could be dangerous if you are dizzy or are not alert.*

Dryness of the mouth may occur while you are taking this medicine. For temporary relief, use sugarless candy or gum, melt bits of ice in your mouth, or use a saliva substitute. However, if dry mouth continues for more than 2 weeks, check with your dentist. Continuing dryness of the mouth may increase the chance of dental disease, including tooth decay, gum disease, and fungus infections.

If you think that you or someone else may have taken an overdose of this medicine, get emergency help at once.

Taking an overdose of this medicine may cause unconsciousness or death. Signs of overdose include convulsions
(seizures), hearing loss, confusion, ringing or buzzing in
the ears, severe drowsiness or tiredness, severe excitement
or nervousness, and fast or deep breathing.

Side Effects of This Medicine

Along with its needed effects, a medicine may cause some
unwanted effects. Although not all of these side effects
may occur, if they do occur they may need medical
attention.

*Get emergency help immediately if any of the following
symptoms of overdose occur:*

> Any loss of hearing; bloody urine; confusion; convulsions
> (seizures); diarrhea; dizziness or lightheadedness (severe);
> drowsiness (severe); excitement or nervousness (severe);
> fast or deep breathing; hallucinations (seeing, hearing, or
> feeling things that are not there); headache (severe or con-
> tinuing); increased sweating; nausea or vomiting (severe
> or continuing); ringing or buzzing in the ears (continuing);
> uncontrollable flapping movements of the hands, especially
> in elderly patients; unexplained fever; unusual thirst; vi-
> sion problems

Symptoms of overdose in children

> Changes in behavior; drowsiness or tiredness (severe); fast
> or deep breathing

Also, check with your doctor as soon as possible if any
of the following side effects occur:

Less common or rare

> Abdominal or stomach pain, cramping, or burning (se-
> vere); bloody or black, tarry stools; decreased urination;
> eye pain; fainting; fast or pounding heartbeat; shortness
> of breath, troubled breathing, tightness in chest, or
> wheezing; skin rash, hives, itching, or redness; sores,
> ulcers, or white spots on lips or in mouth; swollen and/

or painful glands; unusual bleeding or bruising; unusual tiredness or weakness; vomiting of blood or material that looks like coffee grounds

Other side effects may occur that usually do not need medical attention. These side effects may go away during treatment as your body adjusts to the medicine. However, check with your doctor if any of the following side effects continue or are bothersome:

More common

Abdominal or stomach cramps, pain, or discomfort (mild to moderate); dryness of mouth; heartburn or indigestion; nausea or vomiting (mild)

Less common

Blurred or double vision or other vision problems; confusion; constipation; difficult urination; dizziness or lightheadedness; drowsiness; excitement, nervousness, or restlessness; headache; muscle weakness; trembling; unusually large pupils of eyes

Other side effects not listed above may also occur in some patients. If you notice any other effects, check with your doctor.

PAROXETINE   Systemic

A commonly used brand name in the U.S. and Canada is Paxil.

Description

Paroxetine (pa-ROX-uh-teen) is used to treat mental depression.

This medicine is available only with your doctor's prescription, in the following dosage form:

Oral

• Tablets (U.S. and Canada)

Before Using This Medicine

In deciding to use a medicine, the risks of taking the medicine must be weighed against the good it will do. This is a decision you and your doctor will make. For paroxetine, the following should be considered:

Allergies—Tell your doctor if you have ever had any unusual or allergic reaction to paroxetine. Also tell your health care professional if you are allergic to any other substances, such as foods, preservatives, or dyes.

Pregnancy—Studies have not been done in pregnant women. However, studies in animals have shown that paroxetine may cause miscarriages and decreased survival rates of offspring when given in doses many times the usual human dose. Before taking this medicine, make sure your doctor knows if you are pregnant or if you may become pregnant.

Breast-feeding—Paroxetine passes into the breast milk. However, this medicine has not been reported to cause problems in nursing babies.

Children—Studies on this medicine have been done only in adult patients, and there is no specific information comparing use of paroxetine in children with use in other age groups.

Older adults—In studies done to date that have included elderly people, paroxetine did not cause different side effects or problems in older people than it did in younger adults.

Other medicines—Although certain medicines should not be used together at all, in other cases two different medicines may be used together even if an interaction might occur. In these cases, your doctor may want to change the dose, or other precautions may be necessary. When you

are taking paroxetine, it is especially important that your health care professional know if you are taking any of the following:

- Monoamine oxidase (MAO) inhibitors (furazolidone [e.g., Furoxone], isocarboxazid [e.g., Marplan], phenelzine [e.g., Nardil], procarbazine [e.g., Matulane], selegiline [e.g., Eldepryl], tranylcypromine [e.g., Parnate])—Taking paroxetine while you are taking or within 2 weeks of taking MAO inhibitors may cause confusion, agitation, restlessness, stomach or intestinal symptoms, sudden high body temperature, extremely high blood pressure, and severe convulsions; at least 14 days should be allowed between stopping treatment with one medicine and starting treatment with the other

- Tryptophan—Taking this medicine while you are taking paroxetine may increase the risk of serious side effects

- Warfarin (e.g., Coumadin)—Taking this medicine together with paroxetine may cause bleeding problems; your doctor may need to adjust the dosage of either medicine

Other medical problems—The presence of other medical problems may affect the use of paroxetine. Make sure you tell your doctor if you have any other medical problems, especially:

- Drug abuse or dependence (or history of)—Because paroxetine is a new medicine, it is not known if it could become habit-forming, causing mental or physical dependence

- Kidney disease, severe, or
- Liver disease, severe—Higher blood levels of paroxetine may occur, increasing the chance of side effects

- Seizures, history of—The risk of seizures may be increased

Proper Use of This Medicine

Take this medicine only as directed by your doctor to benefit your condition as much as possible. Do not take more of it, do not take it more often, and do not take it for a longer time than your doctor ordered.

You may have to take paroxetine for up to 4 weeks or longer before you begin to feel better. Your doctor should check your progress at regular visits during this time.

Paroxetine may be taken with or without food or on a full or empty stomach. However, if your doctor tells you to take the medicine a certain way, take it exactly as directed.

Dosing—The dose of paroxetine will be different for different patients. *Follow your doctor's orders or the directions on the label.* The following information includes only the average doses of paroxetine. *If your dose is different, do not change it* unless your doctor tells you to do so.

- For *oral* dosage form (tablets):

  —For treatment of depression:

  - Adults—At first, 20 milligrams (mg) once a day, usually taken in the morning. Your doctor may increase your dose if needed. However, the dose is usually not more than 50 mg a day.

  - Children—Use and dose must be determined by your doctor.

  - Older adults—At first, 10 mg once a day, usually taken in the morning. Your doctor may increase your dose if needed. However, the dose is usually not more than 40 mg a day.

Missed dose—If you miss a dose of this medicine, take it as soon as possible. However, if it is almost time for your next dose, skip the missed dose and go back to your regular dosing schedule. Do not double doses.

Storage—To store this medicine:

- Keep out of the reach of children.
- Store away from heat and direct light.
- Do not store in the bathroom, near the kitchen sink,

or in other damp places. Heat or moisture may cause the medicine to break down.

- Do not keep outdated medicine or medicine no longer needed. Be sure that any discarded medicine is out of the reach of children.

Precautions While Using This Medicine

It is important that your doctor check your progress at regular visits, to allow for changes in your dose and to help reduce any side effects.

Do not stop taking this medicine without first checking with your doctor. Your doctor may want you to gradually reduce the amount you are taking before stopping completely. This is to decrease the chance of side effects.

This medicine could possibly add to the effects of alcohol and other CNS depressants (medicines that cause drowsiness). Some examples of CNS depressants are antihistamines or medicine for hay fever, other allergies, or colds; sedatives, tranquilizers, or sleeping medicine; prescription pain medicine or narcotics; barbiturates; medicine for seizures; muscle relaxants; or anesthetics, including some dental anesthetics. *Check with your doctor before taking any of the above while you are using this medicine.*

Paroxetine may cause some people to become drowsy or have blurred vision. *Make sure you know how you react to this medicine before you drive, use machines, or do anything else that could be dangerous if you are not alert or able to see clearly.*

Dizziness, lightheadedness, or fainting may occur, especially when you get up from a lying or sitting position. Getting up slowly may help. If this problem continues or gets worse, check with your doctor.

This medicine may cause dryness of the mouth. For tempo-

rary relief, use sugarless gum or candy, melt bits of ice in your mouth, or use a saliva substitute. However, if your mouth continues to feel dry for more than 2 weeks, check with your medical doctor or dentist. Continuing dryness of the mouth may increase the chance of dental disease, including tooth decay, gum disease, and fungus infections.

Side Effects of This Medicine

Along with its needed effects, a medicine may cause some unwanted effects. Although not all of these side effects may occur, if they do occur they may need medical attention.

Check with your doctor as soon as possible if any of the following side effects occur:

Less common

    Agitation; lightheadedness or fainting; muscle pain or weakness; rash

Rare

    Absence of or decrease in body movements; diarrhea; difficulty in speaking; drowsiness; dryness of mouth; fever; inability to move eyes; incomplete, sudden, or unusual body or facial movements; increased sweating; increased thirst; lack of energy; mood or behavior changes; overactive reflexes; racing heartbeat; restlessness; shivering or shaking; talking, feeling, and acting with excitement and activity you cannot control

Symptoms of overdose

    Drowsiness (severe); dryness of mouth (severe); irritability; large pupils; nausea (severe); racing heartbeat; tremor (severe); vomiting (severe)

Other side effects may occur that usually do not need medical attention. These side effects may go away during treatment as your body adjusts to the medicine. However, check with your doctor if any of the following side effects continue or are bothersome:

More common

Constipation; decreased sexual ability; dizziness; headache; nausea; problems in urinating; tremor; trouble in sleeping; unusual tiredness or weakness; vomiting

Less common

Anxiety or nervousness; blurred vision; change in your sense of taste; decreased or increased appetite; decreased sexual desire; fast or irregular heartbeat; tingling, burning, or prickly sensations; weight loss or gain

After you stop using this medicine, your body may need time to adjust. The length of time this takes depends on the amount of medicine you were using and how long you used it. During this period of time check with your doctor if you notice any of the following side effects:

Agitation, confusion, or restlessness; diarrhea; dizziness or lightheadedness; headache; increased sweating; muscle pain; nausea or vomiting; runny nose; tremor; trouble in sleeping; unusual tiredness or weakness; vision changes

Other side effects not listed above may also occur in some patients. If you notice any other effects, check with your doctor.

PENICILLINS Systemic

Some commonly used brand names are:

In the U.S.—

Amoxil[1]	Geopen[4]
Bactocill[11]	Ledercillin VK[13]
Beepen-VK[13]	Mezlin[9]
Betapen-VK[13]	Nafcil[10]
Bicillin L-A[12]	Nallpen[10]
Cloxapen[5]	Omnipen[2]
Crysticillin 300 A.S.[12]	Omnipen-N[2]
Dynapen[6]	Pathocil[6]
Dycill[6]	Pentids[12]
Geocillin[4]	Pen Vee K[13]

In the U.S. (cont'd)—

Permapen[12]
Pfizerpen[12]
Pfizerpen-AS[12]
Pipracil[14]
Polycillin[2]
Polycillin-N[2]
Polymox[1]
Principen[2]
Prostaphlin[11]
Spectrobid[3]
Staphcillin[8]

Tegopen[5]
Ticar[17]
Totacillin[2]
Totacillin-N[2]
Trimox[1]
Unipen[10]
V-Cillin K[13]
Veetids[13]
Wycillin[12]
Wymox[1]

In Canada—

Amoxil[1]
Ampicin[2]
Apo-Amoxi[1]
Apo-Ampi[2]
Apo-Cloxi[5]
Apo-Pen VK[13]
Ayercillin[12]
Bicillin L-A[12]
Fluclox[7]
Geopen Oral[4]
Ledercillin VK[13]
Megacillin[12]
Nadopen-V[13]
Nadopen-V 200[13]
Nadopen-V 400[13]
Novamoxin[1]
Novo-Ampicillin[2]
Novo-Cloxin[5]
Novo-Pen-VK[13]

Nu-Amoxi[1]
Nu-Ampi[2]
Nu-Cloxi[5]
Nu-Pen-VK[13]
Orbenin[5]
Penbritin[2]
Penglobe[3]
Pen-Vee[13]
Pipracil[14]
Pondocillin[15]
PVF[13]
PVF K[13]
Pyopen[4]
Selexid[16]
Tegopen[5]
Ticar[17]
Unipen[10]
V-Cillin K[13]
Wycillin[12]

Note: For quick reference, the following penicillins are numbered to match the corresponding brand names.

This information applies to the following medicines:

1. Amoxicillin (a-mox-i-SILL-in)‡
2. Ampicillin (am-pi-SILL-in)‡
3. Bacampicillin (ba-kam-pi-SILL-in)
4. Carbenicillin (kar-ben-i-SILL-in)
5. Cloxacillin (klox-a-SILL-in)‡
6. Dicloxacillin (dye-klox-a-SILL-in)†‡
7. Flucloxacillin (floo-klox-a-SILL-in)*
8. Methicillin (meth-i-SILL-in)†
9. Mezlocillin (mez-loe-SILL-in)†
10. Nafcillin (naf-SILL-in)‡

11. Oxacillin (ox-a-SILL-in)†‡
12. Penicillin G (pen-i-SILL-in)‡
13. Penicillin V‡
14. Piperacillin (pi-PER-a-sill-in)
15. Pivampicillin (piv-am-pi-SILL-in)*
16. Pivmecillinam (piv-me-SILL-in-am)*
17. Ticarcillin (tye-kar-SILL-in)

---

*Not commercially available in the U.S.
†Not commercially available in Canada.
‡Generic name product may also be available in the U.S.
§Generic name product may also be available in Canada.

Description

Penicillins are used to treat infections caused by bacteria. They work by killing the bacteria or preventing their growth.

There are several different kinds of penicillins. Each is used to treat different kinds of infections. One kind of penicillin usually may not be used in place of another. In addition, penicillins are used to treat bacterial infections in many different parts of the body. They are sometimes given with other antibacterial medicines (antibiotics). Some of the penicillins may also be used for other problems as determined by your doctor. However, none of the penicillins will work for colds, flu, or other virus infections.

Penicillins are available only with your doctor's prescription, in the following dosage forms:

Oral

Amoxicillin
- Capsules (U.S. and Canada)
- Oral suspension (U.S. and Canada)
- Chewable tablets (U.S. and Canada)
Ampicillin
- Capsules (U.S. and Canada)
- Oral suspension (U.S. and Canada)

Bacampicillin
- Oral suspension (U.S.)
- Tablets (U.S. and Canada)

Carbenicillin
- Tablets (U.S. and Canada)

Cloxacillin
- Capsules (U.S. and Canada)
- Oral solution (U.S. and Canada)

Dicloxacillin
- Capsules (U.S.)
- Oral suspension (U.S.)

Flucloxacillin
- Capsules (Canada)
- Oral suspension (Canada)

Nafcillin
- Capsules (U.S.)
- Tablets (U.S.)

Oxacillin
- Capsules (U.S.)
- Oral solution (U.S.)

Penicillin G Benzathine
- Oral suspension (Canada)

Penicillin G Potassium
- Oral solution (U.S.)
- Tablets (U.S. and Canada)

Penicillin V Benzathine
- Oral suspension (Canada)

Penicillin V Potassium
- Oral solution (U.S. and Canada)
- Tablets (U.S. and Canada)

Pivampicillin
- Oral suspension (Canada)
- Tablets (Canada)

Pivmecillinam
- Tablets (Canada)

Parenteral

Ampicillin
- Injection (U.S. and Canada)

Carbenicillin
- Injection (U.S. and Canada)

Cloxacillin
  • Injection (Canada)
Methicillin
  • Injection (U.S.)
Mezlocillin
  • Injection (U.S.)
Nafcillin
  • Injection (U.S. and Canada)
Oxacillin
  • Injection (U.S.)
Penicillin G Benzathine
  • Injection (U.S. and Canada)
Penicillin G Potassium
  • Injection (U.S. and Canada)
Penicillin G Procaine
  • Injection (U.S. and Canada)
Penicillin G Sodium
  • Injection (U.S. and Canada)
Piperacillin
  • Injection (U.S. and Canada)
Ticarcillin
  • Injection (U.S. and Canada)

Before Using This Medicine

In deciding to use a medicine, the risks of taking the medicine must be weighed against the good it will do. This is a decision you and your doctor will make. For penicillins, the following should be considered:

Allergies—Tell your doctor if you have ever had any unusual or allergic reaction to any of the penicillins or cephalosporins. Also tell your health care professional if you are allergic to any other substances, such as foods, preservatives, or dyes, or procaine (e.g., Novocain) or other ester-type anesthetics (medicines that cause numbing) if you are receiving penicillin G procaine.

Diet—Make certain your health care professional knows

if you are on a low-sodium (low-salt) diet. Some of these medicines contain enough sodium to cause problems in some people.

Pregnancy—Penicillins have not been studied in pregnant women. However, penicillins have been widely used in pregnant women and have not been shown to cause birth defects or other problems in animal studies.

Breast-feeding—Penicillins pass into the breast milk. Even though only small amounts may pass into breast milk, allergic reactions, diarrhea, fungus infections, and skin rash may occur in nursing babies.

Children—Many penicillins have been used in children and, in effective doses, are not expected to cause different side effects or problems in children than they do in adults.

Older adults—Penicillins have been used in the elderly and have not been shown to cause different side effects or problems in older people than they do in younger adults.

Other medicines—Although certain medicines should not be used together at all, in other cases two different medicines may be used together even if an interaction might occur. In these cases, your doctor may want to change the dose, or other precautions may be necessary. When you are taking a penicillin, it is especially important that your health care professional know if you are taking any of the following:

- Acetaminophen (e.g., Tylenol) (with long-term, high-dose use) or
- Amiodarone (e.g., Cordarone) or
- Anabolic steroids (nandrolone [e.g., Anabolin], oxandrolone [e.g., Anavar], oxymetholone [e.g., Anadrol], stanozolol [e.g., Winstrol]) or
- Androgens (male hormones) or
- Antithyroid agents (medicine for overactive thyroid) or
- Carmustine (e.g., BiCNU) or
- Chloroquine (e.g., Aralen) or
- Dantrolene (e.g., Dantrium) or

- Daunorubicin (e.g., Cerubidine) or
- Disulfiram (e.g., Antabuse) or
- Divalproex (e.g., Depakote) or
- Estrogens (female hormones) or
- Etretinate (e.g., Tegison) or
- Gold salts (medicine for arthritis) or
- Hydroxychloroquine (e.g., Plaquenil) or
- Mercaptopurine (e.g., Purinethol) or
- Methotrexate (e.g., Mexate) or
- Methyldopa (e.g., Aldomet) or
- Naltrexone (e.g., Trexan) (with long-term, high-dose use) or
- Oral contraceptives (birth control pills) containing estrogen or
- Other anti-infectives by mouth or by injection (medicine for infection) or
- Phenothiazines (acetophenazine [e.g., Tindal], chlorpromazine [e.g., Thorazine], fluphenazine [e.g., Prolixin], mesoridazine [e.g., Serentil], perphenazine [e.g., Trilafon], prochlorperazine [e.g., Compazine], promazine [e.g., Sparine], promethazine [e.g., Phenergan], thioridazine [e.g., Mellaril], trifluoperazine [e.g., Stelazine], triflupromazine [e.g., Vesprin], trimeprazine [e.g., Temaril]) or
- Plicamycin (e.g., Mithracin) or
- Valproic acid (e.g., Depakene)—These medicines may increase the chance of liver damage if taken with cloxacillin, dicloxacillin, flucloxacillin, mezlocillin, nafcillin, oxacillin, or piperacillin

- Amiloride (e.g., Midamor) or
- Benazepril (e.g., Lotensin) or
- Captopril (e.g., Capoten) or
- Enalapril (e.g., Vasotec) or
- Fosinopril (e.g., Monopril) or
- Lisinopril (e.g., Prinivil, Zestril) or
- Potassium-containing medicine or
- Quinapril (e.g., Accupril) or
- Ramipril (e.g., Altace) or
- Spironolactone (e.g., Aldactone) or
- Triamterene (e.g., Dyrenium)—Use of these medicines with penicillin G by injection may cause an increase in side effects

- Anticoagulants (blood thinners) or

- Dipyridamole (e.g., Persantine) or
- Divalproex (e.g., Depakote) or
- Heparin (e.g., Panheprin) or
- Inflammation or pain medicine (except narcotics) or
- Pentoxifylline (e.g., Trental) or
- Plicamycin (e.g., Mithracin) or
- Sulfinpyrazone (e.g., Anturane) or
- Valproic acid (e.g., Depakene)—Use of these medicines with high doses of carbenicillin, piperacillin, or ticarcillin may increase the chance of bleeding

- Cloramphenicol (e.g., Chloromycetin) or
- Erythromycins (e.g., E.E.S., E-Mycin, ERYC) or
- Sulfonamides (e.g., Gantanol, Gantrisin) or
- Tetracyclines (e.g., Achromycin, Minocin, Vibramycin)—Use of these medicines with penicillins may prevent the penicillin from working properly

- Cholestyramine (e.g., Questran) or
- Colestipol (e.g., Colestid)—Use of these medicines with oral penicillin G may prevent penicillin G from working properly

- Oral contraceptives (birth control pills) containing estrogen—Use of ampicillin, amoxicillin, or penicillin V with estrogen-containing oral contraceptives may prevent oral contraceptives from working properly, increasing the chance of pregnancy

- Methotrexate (e.g., Mexate)—Use of methotrexate with penicillins may increase the chance of side effects of methotrexate

- Probenecid (e.g., Benemid)—Probenecid causes penicillins to build up in the blood. This may increase the chance of side effects. However, your doctor may want to give you probenecid with a penicillin to treat some infections

Other medical problems—The presence of other medical problems may affect the use of penicillins. Make sure you tell your doctor if you have any other medical problems, especially:

- Allergy, general (such as asthma, eczema, hay fever, hives), history of—Patients with a history of general allergies may be more likely to have a severe reaction to penicillins

- Bleeding problems, history of—Patients with a history of bleeding problems may be more likely to have bleeding when receiving carbenicillin, piperacillin, or ticarcillin
- Congestive heart failure (CHF) or
- High blood pressure—Large doses of carbenicillin or ticarcillin may make these conditions worse, because these medicines contains a large amount of salt
- Cystic fibrosis—Patients with cystic fibrosis may have an increased chance of fever and skin rash when receiving piperacillin
- Kidney disease—Patients with kidney disease may have an increased chance of side effects
- Mononucleosis (''mono'')—Patients with mononucleosis may have an increased chance of skin rash when receiving ampicillin, bacampicillin, or pivampicillin
- Stomach or intestinal disease, history of (especially colitis, including colitis caused by antibiotics)—Patients with a history of stomach or intestinal disease may be more likely to develop colitis while taking penicillins

---

Proper Use of This Medicine

Penicillins (except bacampicillin tablets, amoxicillin, penicillin V, pivampicillin, and pivmecillinam) are best taken with a full glass (8 ounces) of water on an empty stomach (either 1 hour before or 2 hours after meals) unless otherwise directed by your doctor.

For patients taking *amoxicillin, penicillin V, pivampicillin, and pivmecillinam:*

- Amoxicillin, penicillin V, pivampicillin, and pivmecillinam may be taken on a full or empty stomach.
- The *liquid form of amoxicillin* may also be taken by itself or mixed with formulas, milk, fruit juice, water, ginger ale, or other cold drinks. If mixed with other liquids, take immediately after mixing. Be sure to drink all the liquid to get the full dose of medicine.

For patients taking *bacampicillin:*

- The liquid form of this medicine is best taken with a full glass (8 ounces) of water on an empty stomach (either 1 hour before or 2 hours after meals) unless otherwise directed by your doctor.

- The tablet form of this medicine may be taken on a full or empty stomach.

For patients taking *penicillin G by mouth:*

- Do not drink acidic fruit juices (for example, orange or grapefruit juice) or other acidic beverages within 1 hour of taking penicillin G since this may keep the medicine from working properly.

For patients taking the *oral liquid form of penicillins:*

- This medicine is to be taken by mouth even if it comes in a dropper bottle. If this medicine does not come in a dropper bottle, use a specially marked measuring spoon or other device to measure each dose accurately. The average household teaspoon may not hold the right amount of liquid.

- Do not use after the expiration date on the label. The medicine may not work properly after that date. If you have any questions about this, check with your pharmacist.

For patients taking the *chewable tablet form of amoxicillin:*

- Tablets should be chewed or crushed before they are swallowed.

To help clear up your infection completely, *keep taking this medicine for the full time of treatment*, even if you begin to feel better after a few days. *If you have a "strep" infection, you should keep taking this medicine for at least 10 days. This is especially important in "strep" infections. Serious heart problems could develop later if your infec-*

tion is not cleared up completely. Also, if you stop taking this medicine too soon, your symptoms may return.

This medicine works best when there is a constant amount in the blood or urine. *To help keep the amount constant, do not miss any doses. Also, it is best to take the doses at evenly spaced times, day and night.* For example, if you are to take 4 doses a day, the doses should be spaced about 6 hours apart. If this interferes with your sleep or other daily activities, or if you need help in planning the best times to take your medicine, check with your health care professional.

Dosing—The dose of these medicines will be different for different patients. *Follow your doctor's orders or the directions on the label.* The following information includes only the average doses of these medicines. *If your dose is different, do not change it* unless your doctor tells you to do so.

The number of tablets or teaspoonfuls of suspension that you take depends on the strength of the medicine. Also, *the number of doses you take each day, the time allowed between doses, and the length of time you take the medicine depend on the medical problem for which you are taking a penicillin.*

For amoxicillin

- For bacterial infections:

    —For *oral* dosage forms (capsules, chewable tablets, and oral suspension):

    • Adults, teenagers, and children weighing more than 20 kilograms (kg) (44 pounds)—250 to 500 milligrams (mg) every eight hours.

    • Infants and children weighing 8 to 20 kg (17 to 44 pounds): Dose is based on body weight and must be determined by your doctor. The usual dose is 6.7 to 13.3 mg per kg (3 to 6 mg per pound) of body weight every eight hours.

• Infants weighing 6 to 8 kg (13 to 17 pounds):
50 to 100 mg every eight hours.

• Infants weighing up to 6 kg (13 pounds): 25 to
50 mg every eight hours.

For ampicillin

• For bacterial infections:

—For *oral* dosage forms (capsules and oral
suspension):

• Adults, teenagers, and children weighing more
than 20 kilograms (kg) (44 pounds)—250 to
500 milligrams (mg) every six hours.

• Infants and children weighing up to 20 kg (44
pounds)—Dose is based on body weight and must
be determined by your doctor. The usual dose is
12.5 to 25 mg per kg (5.7 to 11.4 mg per pound)
of body weight every six hours; or 16.7 to
33.3 mg per kg (7.6 to 15 mg per pound) of body
weight every eight hours.

—For *injection* dosage form:

• Adults, teenagers, and children weighing more
than 20 kg (44 pounds)—250 to 500 mg, injected
into a vein or muscle every three to six hours.

• Infants and children weighing up to 20 kg (44
pounds)—Dose is based on body weight and must
be determined by your doctor. The usual dose is
12.5 mg per kg (5.7 mg per pound) of body
weight, injected into a vein or muscle every six
hours.

For bacampicillin

• For bacterial infections:

—For *oral* dosage forms (oral suspension and
tablets):

• Adults, teenagers, and children weighing more
than 25 kilograms (kg) (55 pounds)—400 to
800 milligrams (mg) every twelve hours.

• Children weighing up to 25 kg (55 pounds)—Bacampicillin tablets are not recommended for use in children weighing up to 25 kg (55 pounds). The dose of the oral suspension is based on body weight and must be determined by your doctor. The usual dose is 12.5 to 25 mg per kg (5.7 to 11.4 mg per pound) of body weight every twelve hours.

For carbenicillin

• For bacterial infections:

—For *oral* dosage form (tablets):

• Adults and teenagers—500 milligrams (mg) to 1 gram every six hours.

• Children—Dose must be determined by your doctor.

—For *injection* dosage form:

• Adults and teenagers—Dose is based on body weight and must be determined by your doctor. The usual dose is 50 to 83.3 mg per kilogram (kg) (22.8 to 37.9 mg per pound) of body weight, injected into a vein or muscle every four hours.

• Older infants and children—Dose is based on body weight and must be determined by your doctor. The usual dose is 16.7 to 75 mg per kg (7.6 to 34 mg per pound) of body weight, injected into a vein or muscle every four to six hours.

For cloxacillin

• For bacterial infections:

—For *oral* dosage form (capsules and oral solution):

• Adults, teenagers, and children weighing more than 20 kilograms (kg) (44 pounds)—250 to 500 milligrams (mg) every six hours.

• Infants and children weighing up to 20 kg (44 pounds)—Dose is based on body weight and must be determined by your doctor. The usual dose is

6.25 to 12.5 mg per kg (2.8 to 5.7 mg per pound) of body weight every six hours.

—For *injection* dosage form:

• Adults, teenagers, and children weighing more than 20 kg—250 to 500 mg, injected into a vein every six hours.

• Infants and children weighing up to 20 kg (44 pounds)—Dose is based on body weight and must be determined by your doctor. The usual dose is 6.25 to 12.5 mg per kg (2.8 to 5.7 mg per pound) of body weight, injected into a vein every six hours.

For dicloxacillin

• For bacterial infections:

—For *oral* dosage form (capsules and oral suspension):

• Adults, teenagers, and children weighing more than 40 kilograms (kg) (88 pounds)—125 to 250 milligrams (mg) every six hours.

• Infants and children weighing up to 40 kg (88 pounds)—Dose is based on body weight and must be determined by your doctor. The usual dose is 3.1 to 6.2 mg per kg (1.4 to 2.8 mg per pound) of body weight every six hours.

For flucloxacillin

• For bacterial infections:

—For *oral* dosage form (capsules and oral suspension):

• Adults, teenagers, and children more than 12 years of age and weighing more than 40 kilograms (kg) (88 pounds)—250 to 500 milligrams (mg) every six hours.

• Children less than 12 years of age and weighing up to 40 kg (88 pounds)—125 to 250 mg every six hours; or 6.25 to 12.5 mg per kg (2.8 to 5.7 mg per pound) of body weight every six hours.

• Infants up to 6 months of age—Dose is based on body weight and must be determined by your doctor. The usual dose is 6.25 mg per kg (2.8 mg per pound) of body weight every six hours.

For methicillin

• For bacterial infections:

—For *injection* dosage form:

• Adults, teenagers, and children weighing more than 40 kilograms (kg) (88 pounds)—1 gram injected into a muscle every four to six hours; or 1 gram injected into a vein every six hours.

• Children weighing up to 40 kg (88 pounds)—Dose is based on body weight and must be determined by your doctor. The usual dose is 25 milligrams (mg) per kg (11.4 mg per pound) of body weight, injected into a vein or muscle every six hours.

For mezlocillin

• For bacterial infections:

—For *injection* dosage form:

• Adults and teenagers—Dose is based on body weight and must be determined by your doctor. The usual dose is 33.3 to 87.5 milligrams (mg) per kilogram (kg) (15.1 to 39.8 mg per pound) of body weight, injected into a vein or muscle every four to six hours; or 3 to 4 grams every four to six hours.

• Infants over 1 month of age and children up to 12 years of age—Dose is based on body weight and must be determined by your doctor. The usual dose is 50 mg per kg (22.7 mg per pound) of body weight, injected into a vein or muscle every four hours.

For nafcillin

- For bacterial infections:

    —For *oral* dosage form (capsules and tablets):

    - Adults and teenagers—250 milligrams (mg) to 1 gram every four to six hours.

    - Older infants and children—Dose is based on body weight and must be determined by your doctor. The usual dose is 6.25 to 12.5 mg per kilogram (kg) (2.8 to 5.7 mg per pound) of body weight every six hours.

    - Newborns—Dose is based on body weight and must be determined by your doctor. The usual dose is 10 mg per kg (4.5 mg per pound) of body weight every six to eight hours.

    —For *injection* dosage form:

    - Adults and teenagers—500 mg to 2 grams injected into a vein or muscle every four to six hours.

    - Infants and children—Dose is based on body weight and must be determined by your doctor. The usual dose is 10 to 25 mg per kg (4.5 to 11.4 mg per pound) of body weight, injected into a muscle every twelve hours; or 10 to 40 mg per kg (4.5 to 18.2 mg per pound) of body weight, injected into a vein every four to eight hours.

For oxacillin

- For bacterial infections:

    —For *oral* dosage form (capsules and oral solution):

    - Adults, teenagers, and children weighing more than 40 kilograms (kg) (88 pounds)—500 milligrams (mg) to 1 gram every four to six hours.

    - Children weighing up to 40 kg (88 pounds)—Dose is based on body weight and must be determined by your doctor. The usual dose is 12.5 to

25 mg per kg (5.7 to 11.4 mg per pound) of body weight every six hours.

—For *injection* dosage form:

• Adults, teenagers, and children weighing more than 40 kg (88 pounds)—250 mg to 1 gram injected into a vein or muscle every four to six hours.

• Children weighing up to 40 kg (88 pounds)—Dose is based on body weight and must be determined by your doctor. The usual dose is 12.5 to 25 mg per kg (5.7 to 11.4 mg per pound) of body weight, injected into a vein or muscle every four to six hours.

• Premature infants and newborns—Dose is based on body weight and must be determined by your doctor. The usual dose is 6.25 mg per kg (2.8 mg per pound) of body weight, injected into a vein or muscle every six hours.

For penicillin G

• For bacterial infections:

—For *oral* dosage form (oral solution, oral suspension, and tablets):

• Adults and teenagers—200,000 to 500,000 Units (125 to 312 milligrams [mg]) every four to six hours.

• Infants and children less than 12 years of age—Dose is based on body weight and must be determined by your doctor. The usual dose is 4167 to 30,000 Units per kilogram (kg) (189 to 13,636 Units per pound) of body weight every four to eight hours.

—For *benzathine injection* dosage form:

• Adults and teenagers—1,200,000 to 2,400,000 Units injected into a muscle as a single dose.

• Infants and children—300,000 to 1,200,000

Units injected into a muscle as a single dose; or 50,000 Units per kg (22,727 Units per pound) of body weight injected into a muscle as a single dose.

—For *injection* dosage forms (potassium and sodium salts):

• Adults and teenagers—1,000,000 to 5,000,000 Units, injected into a vein or muscle every four to six hours.

• Older infants and children—Dose is based on body weight and must be determined by your doctor. The usual dose is 8,333 to 25,000 Units per kg (3,788 to 11,363 Units per pound) of body weight, injected into a vein or muscle every four to six hours.

• Premature infants and newborns—Dose is based on body weight and must be determined by your doctor. The usual dose is 30,000 Units per kg (13,636 Units per pound) of body weight, injected into a vein or muscle every twelve hours.

—For *procaine injection* dosage form:

• Adults and teenagers—600,000 to 1,200,000 Units injected into a muscle once a day.

• Children—Dose is based on body weight and must be determined by your doctor. The usual dose is 50,000 Units per kg (22,727 Units per pound) of body weight, injected into a muscle once a day.

For penicillin V

• For bacterial infections:

—For the *benzathine salt oral* dosage form (oral solution):

• Adults and teenagers—200,000 to 500,000 Units every six to eight hours.

• Children—100,000 to 250,000 Units every six to eight hours.

—For the *potassium salt oral* dosage forms (oral solution, oral suspension, and tablets):

• Adults and teenagers—125 to 500 milligrams (mg) every six to eight hours.

• Children—Dose is based on body weight and must be determined by your doctor. The usual dose is 2.5 to 16.7 mg per kilogram (kg) (1.1 to 7.6 mg per pound) of body weight every four to eight hours.

For piperacillin

• For bacterial infections:

—For *injection* dosage form:

• Adults and teenagers—3 to 4 grams, injected into a vein or muscle every four to six hours.

• Infants and children—Dose must be determined by your doctor.

For pivampicillin

• For bacterial infections:

—For *oral* dosage form (oral suspension):

• Adults, teenagers, and children 10 years of age and older—525 to 1050 milligrams (mg) two times a day.

• Children 7 to 10 years of age—350 mg two times a day.

• Children 4 to 6 years of age—262.5 mg two times a day.

• Children 1 to 3 years of age—175 mg two times a day.

• Infants 3 to 12 months of age—Dose is based on body weight and must be determined by your doctor. The usual dose is 20 to 30 mg per kilogram (kg) (9.1 to 13.6 mg per pound) of body weight two times a day.

—For *oral* dosage form (tablets):

• Adults, teenagers, and children 10 years of age and older—500 mg to 1 gram two times a day.

• Children up to 10 years of age—Dose must be determined by your doctor.

For pivmecillinam
• For bacterial infections:
—For *oral* dosage form (tablets):
• Adults, teenagers, and children weighing more than 40 kilograms (kg) (88 pounds)—200 milligrams (mg) two to four times a day for three days.
• Children up to 40 kg (88 pounds)—Dose must be determined by your doctor.

For ticarcillin
• For bacterial infections:
—For *injection* dosage form:
• Adults, teenagers, and children weighing more than 40 kilograms (kg) (88 pounds)—3 grams injected into a vein every four hours; or 4 grams injected into a vein every six hours.
• Children up to 40 kg (88 pounds)—Dose is based on body weight and must be determined by your doctor. The usual dose is 33.3 to 75 milligrams (mg) per kg (15 to 34 mg per pound) of body weight, injected into a vein every four to six hours.

Missed dose—If you miss a dose of this medicine, take it as soon as possible. This will help to keep a constant amount of medicine in the blood or urine. However, if it is almost time for your next dose, skip the missed dose and go back to your regular dosing schedule. Do not double doses.

Storage—To store this medicine:
• Keep out of the reach of children.

- Store away from heat and direct light.
- Do not store the capsule or tablet form of penicillins in the bathroom, near the kitchen sink, or in other damp places. Heat or moisture may cause the medicine to break down.
- Store the oral liquid form of penicillins in the refrigerator because heat will cause this medicine to break down. However, keep the medicine from freezing. Follow the directions on the label.
- Do not keep outdated medicine or medicine no longer needed. Be sure that any discarded medicine is out of the reach of children.

Precautions While Using This Medicine

If your symptoms do not improve within a few days, or if they become worse, check with your doctor.

Penicillins may cause diarrhea in some patients.

- *Check with your doctor if severe diarrhea occurs. Severe diarrhea may be a sign of a serious side effect. Do not take any diarrhea medicine without first checking with your doctor.* Diarrhea medicines may make your diarrhea worse or make it last longer.
- For mild diarrhea, diarrhea medicine containing kaolin or attapulgite (e.g., Kaopectate tablets, Diasorb) may be taken. However, other kinds of diarrhea medicine should not be taken. They may make your diarrhea worse or make it last longer.
- If you have any questions about this or if mild diarrhea continues or gets worse, check with your health care professional.

Oral contraceptives (birth control pills) containing estrogen may not work properly if you take them while you are taking ampicillin, amoxicillin, or penicillin V. Unplanned pregnancies may occur. You should use a different or additional means of birth control while you are taking any of these penicillins. If you have any questions about this, check with your health care professional.

For *diabetic patients:*

* *Penicillins may cause false test results with some urine sugar tests.* Check with your doctor before changing your diet or the dosage of your diabetes medicine.

Before you have any medical tests, tell the doctor in charge that you are taking this medicine. The results of some tests may be affected by this medicine.

Side Effects of This Medicine

Along with its needed effects, a medicine may cause some unwanted effects. Although not all of these side effects may occur, if they do occur they may need medical attention.

Stop taking this medicine and get emergency help immediately if any of the following side effects occur:

Less common

Fast or irregular breathing; fever; joint pain; lightheadedness or fainting (sudden); puffiness or swelling around the face; red, scaly skin; shortness of breath; skin rash, hives, itching

In addition to the side effects mentioned above, *check with your doctor immediately* if any of the following side effects occur:

Rare

Abdominal or stomach cramps and pain (severe); abdominal tenderness; convulsions (seizures); decreased amount of urine; diarrhea (watery and severe), which may also be bloody; mental depression; nausea and vomiting;

pain at place of injection; sore throat and fever; unusual bleeding or bruising; yellow eyes or skin

Note: Some of the above side effects (severe abdominal or stomach cramps and pain, and watery and severe diarrhea, which may also be bloody) may also occur up to several weeks after you stop taking any of these medicines.

Rare—For penicillin G procaine only

Agitation or combativeness; anxiety; confusion; fear of impending death; feeling, hearing, or seeing things that are not real

Other side effects may occur that usually do not need medical attention. These side effects may go away during treatment as your body adjusts to the medicine. However, check with your doctor if any of the following side effects continue or are bothersome:

More common

Diarrhea (mild); headache; sore mouth or tongue; vaginal itching and discharge; white patches in the mouth and/ or on the tongue

Other side effects not listed above may also occur in some patients. If you notice any other effects, check with your doctor.

Additional Information

Once a medicine has been approved for marketing for a certain use, experience may show that it is also useful for other medical problems. Although these uses are not included in product labeling, penicillins are used in certain patients with the following medical conditions:

- Chlamydia infections in pregnant women—Amoxicillin and ampicillin
- Gas gangrene—Penicillin G
- *Helicobacter pylori*-associated gastritis or peptic ulcer disease—Amoxicillin

- Leptospirosis—Ampicillin and penicillin G
- Lyme disease—Amoxicillin and penicillin V
- Typhoid fever—Amoxicillin and ampicillin

Other than the above information, there is no additional information relating to proper use, precautions, or side effects for these uses.

PENICILLINS AND BETA-LACTAMASE INHIBITORS   Systemic

Some commonly used brand names are:

In the U.S.—

Augmentin[1]	Unasyn[2]
Timentin[4]	Zosyn[3]

In Canada—

Clavulin-250[1]	Clavulin-500F[1]
Clavulin-125F[1]	Tazocin[3]
Clavulin-250F[1]	Timentin[4]

Note: For quick reference, the following penicillins and beta-lactamase inhibitors are numbered to match the corresponding brand names.

This information applies to the following medicines:

1. Amoxicillin and Clavulanate (a-mox-i-SILL-in and klav-yoo-LAN-ate)
2. Ampicillin and Sulbactam (am-pi-SILL-in and sul-BAK-tam)†
3. Piperacillin and Tazobactam (pi-PER-a-sill-in and ta-zoe-BAK-tam)
4. Ticarcillin and Clavulanate (tye-kar-SILL-in and klav-yoo-LAN-ate)

---

†Not commercially available in Canada.

Description

Penicillins and beta-lactamase inhibitors are used to treat infections caused by bacteria. They work by killing the bacteria or preventing their growth. The beta-lactamase inhibitor is added to the pencillin to protect the penicillin from certain substances (enzymes) that will destroy the penicillin before it can kill the bacteria.

There are several different kinds of penicillins. Each is used to treat different kinds of infections. One kind of penicillin usually may not be used in place of another. In addition, penicillins are used to treat bacterial infections in many different parts of the body. They are sometimes given with other antibacterial medicines. Some of the penicillins may also be used for other problems as determined by your doctor. However, none of the penicillins will work for colds, flu, or other virus infections.

Penicillins are available only with your doctor's prescription, in the following dosage forms:

Oral

Amoxicillin and Clavulanate
- Oral suspension (U.S. and Canada)
- Tablets (U.S. and Canada)
- Chewable tablets (U.S.)

Parenteral

Ampicillin and Sulbactam
- Injection (U.S.)

Piperacillin and Tazobactam
- Injection (U.S.)

Ticarcillin and Clavulanate
- Injection (U.S. and Canada)

Before Using This Medicine

In deciding to use a medicine, the risks of taking the medicine must be weighed against the good it will do. This is a decision you and your doctor will make. For penicillins, the following should be considered:

Allergies—Tell your doctor if you have ever had any unusual or allergic reaction to any of the penicillins, cephalosporins, or beta-lactamase inhibitors. Also tell your health care professional if you are allergic to any other substances, such as foods, preservatives, or dyes.

Diet—Tell your doctor if you are on a low-sodium (low-salt) diet. Some of these medicines contain enough sodium to cause problems in some people.

Pregnancy—Penicillins and beta-lactamase inhibitors have not been studied in pregnant women. However, penicillins have not been shown to cause birth defects or other problems in animal studies.

Breast-feeding—Penicillins and sulbactam, a beta-lactamase inhibitor, pass into the breast milk. Even though only small amounts may pass into breast milk, allergic reactions, diarrhea, fungus infections, and skin rash may occur in nursing babies.

Children—Penicillins and beta-lactamase inhibitors have been used in children and, in effective doses, are not expected to cause different side effects or problems in children than they do in adults.

Older adults—Penicillins and beta-lactamase inhibitors have been used in the elderly and have not been shown to cause different side effects or problems in older people than they do in younger adults.

Other medicines—Although certain medicines should not be used together at all, in other cases two different medicines may be used together even if an interaction might occur. In these cases, your doctor may want to change the dose, or other precautions may be necessary. When you are taking a penicillin and beta-lactamase inhibitor combination, it is especially important that your health care professional know if you are taking any of the following:

- Anticoagulants (blood thinners) or
- Dipyridamole (e.g., Persantine) or
- Divalproex (e.g., Depakote) or
- Heparin (e.g., Panheprin) or
- Inflammation or pain medicine (except narcotics) or
- Pentoxifylline (e.g., Trental) or
- Plicamycin (e.g., Mithracin) or

- Sulfinpyrazone (e.g., Anturane) or
- Valproic acid (e.g., Depakene)—Use of these medicines with piperacillin and tazobactam combination or with ticarcillin and clavulanate combination may increase the chance of bleeding
- Probenecid (e.g., Benemid)—Probenecid causes penicillins, sulbactam, and tazobactam to build up in the blood. This may increase the chance of side effects. However, your doctor may want to give you probenecid with a penicillin and beta-lactamase inhibitor combination to treat some infections

Other medical problems—The presence of other medical problems may affect the use of penicillin and beta-lactamase inhibitor combinations. Make sure you tell your doctor if you have any other medical problems, especially:

- Allergies or a history of allergies, such as asthma, eczema, hay fever, or hives—Patients with a history of allergies may be more likely to have a severe allergic reaction to a penicillin and beta-lactamase inhibitor combination
- Bleeding problems, history of—Patients with a history of bleeding problems may be more likely to have bleeding when receiving piperacillin and tazobactam combination or ticarcillin and clavulanate combination
- Congestive heart failure (CHF) or
- High blood pressure—Large doses of ticarcillin and clavulanate combination may make these conditions worse, because this medicine contains a large amount of salt
- Cystic fibrosis—Patients with cystic fibrosis may have an increased chance of fever and skin rash when receiving piperacillin and tazobactam combination
- Kidney disease—Patients with kidney disease may have an increased chance of side effects
- Mononucleosis (''mono'')—Patients with mononucleosis may have an increased chance of skin rash when receiving ampicillin and sulbactam combination
- Stomach or intestinal disease, history of (especially colitis, including colitis caused by antibiotics)—Patients with a history of stomach or intestinal disease may be more likely

to develop colitis while taking penicillins and beta-lactamase inhibitors

---

Proper Use of This Medicine

Amoxicillin and clavulanate combination may be taken on
a full or empty stomach. Taking amoxicillin and clavulanate combination with food may decrease the chance of
diarrhea, nausea, and vomiting.

For patients taking the *oral liquid form of amoxicillin and
clavulanate combination:*

- Use a specially marked measuring spoon or other device to measure each dose accurately. The average
  household teaspoon may not hold the right amount
  of liquid.
- Do not use after the expiration date on the label. The
  medicine may not work properly after that date. If
  you have any questions about this, check with your
  pharmacist.

For patients taking the *chewable tablet form of amoxicillin
and clavulanate combination:*

- Tablets should be chewed or crushed before they
  are swallowed.

To help clear up your infection completely, *keep taking
this medicine for the full time of treatment*, even if you
begin to feel better after a few days.

This medicine works best when there is a constant amount
in the blood or urine. *To help keep the amount constant,
do not miss any doses. Also, it is best to take the doses
at evenly spaced times, day and night.* For example, if you
are to take 4 doses a day, the doses should be spaced
about 6 hours apart. If this interferes with your sleep or
other daily activities, or if you need help in planning the

best times to take your medicine, check with your health care professional.

Dosing—The dose of these medicines will be different for different patients. *Follow your doctor's orders or the directions on the label.* The following information includes only the average doses of these medicines. *If your dose is different, do not change it* unless your doctor tells you to do so.

The number of tablets or teaspoonfuls of suspension that you take depends on the strength of the medicine. Also, *the number of doses you take each day, the time allowed between doses, and the length of time you take the medicine depend on the medical problem for which you are taking a penicillin and beta-lactamase inhibitor combination.*

For amoxicillin and clavulanate combination

- For bacterial infections:

  —For *oral* dosage forms (chewable tablets and suspension):

  - Adults, teenagers, and children weighing more than 40 kilograms (kg) (88 pounds)—250 to 500 milligrams (mg) of amoxicillin, in combination with 62.5 to 125 mg of clavulanate, every eight hours for seven to ten days.

  - Infants and children weighing up to 40 kg (88 pounds)—6.7 to 13.3 mg of amoxicillin per kg (3 to 6 mg per pound) of body weight, in combination with 1.7 to 3.3 mg of clavulanate per kg (0.8 to 1.5 mg per pound) of body weight, every eight hours for seven to ten days.

  —For *oral* dosage form (tablets):

  - Adults, teenagers, and children weighing more than 40 kg (88 pounds)—250 to 500 mg of amoxicillin, in combination with 125 mg of clavulanate, every eight hours for seven to ten days.

• Infants and children weighing up to 40 kg (88 pounds)—6.7 to 13.3 mg of amoxicillin per kg (3 to 6 mg per pound) of body weight, in combination with 1.7 to 3.3 mg of clavulanate per kg (0.8 to 1.5 mg per pound) of body weight, every eight hours for seven to ten days.

For ampicillin and sulbactam combination

• For bacterial infections:

—For *injection* dosage form:

• Adults and teenagers—1 to 2 grams of ampicillin, in combination with 500 milligrams (mg) to 1 gram of sulbactam, injected into a vein or a muscle every six hours.

• Children up to 12 years of age—Use and dose must be determined by your doctor.

For piperacillin and tazobactam combination

• For bacterial infections:

—For *injection* dosage form:

• Adults and teenagers—3 to 4 grams of piperacillin, in combination with 0.375 to 0.5 grams of tazobactam, injected into a vein every six to eight hours for seven to ten days.

• Children up to 12 years of age—Use and dose must be determined by your doctor.

For ticarcillin and clavulanate combination

• For bacterial infections:

—For *injection* dosage form:

• Adults and teenagers weighing 60 kilograms (kg) (132 pounds) or more—3 grams of ticarcillin, in combination with 100 milligrams (mg) of clavulanate, injected into a vein every four to six hours.

• Adults and teenagers weighing less than 60 kg (132 pounds)—33.3 to 75 mg of ticarcillin per kg (15 to 34.1 mg per pound) of body weight, in combination with 1.1 to 2.5 mg of clavulanate per kg (0.5 to 1.1 mg per pound) of body weight, injected into a vein every four to six hours.

• Infants and children 1 month to 12 years of age—50 mg of ticarcillin per kg (22.7 mg per pound) of body weight, in combination with 1.7 mg of clavulanate per kg (0.8 mg per pound) of body weight, injected into a vein every four to six hours.

Missed dose—If you miss a dose of this medicine, take it as soon as possible. This will help to keep a constant amount of medicine in the blood or urine. However, if it is almost time for your next dose, skip the missed dose and go back to your regular dosing schedule. Do not double doses.

Storage—To store this medicine:

• Keep out of the reach of children.

• Store away from heat and direct light.

• Do not store capsules or tablets in the bathroom, near the kitchen sink, or in other damp places. Heat or moisture may cause the medicine to break down.

• Store the oral liquid form of penicillins in the refrigerator because heat will cause this medicine to break down. However, keep the medicine from freezing. Follow the directions on the label.

• Do not keep outdated medicine or medicine no longer needed. Be sure that any discarded medicine is out of the reach of children.

Precautions While Using This Medicine

If your symptoms do not improve within a few days, or if they become worse, check with your doctor.

Penicillins may cause diarrhea in some patients.

- *Check with your doctor if severe diarrhea occurs.* Severe diarrhea may be a sign of a serious side effect. *Do not take any diarrhea medicine.* Diarrhea medicines may make your diarrhea worse or make it last longer.

- For mild diarrhea, diarrhea medicine containing kaolin or attapulgite (e.g., Kaopectate tablets, Diasorb) may be taken. However, other kinds of diarrhea medicine should not be taken. They may make your diarrhea worse or make it last longer.

- If you have any questions about this or if mild diarrhea continues or gets worse, check with your health care professional.

For *diabetic patients:*

- *Penicillin and beta-lactamase inhibitor combinations may cause false test results with some urine sugar tests.* Check with your doctor before changing your diet or the dosage of your diabetes medicine.

Before you have any medical tests, tell the doctor in charge that you are taking this medicine. The results of some tests may be affected by this medicine.

Side Effects of This Medicine

Along with its needed effects, a medicine may cause some unwanted effects. Although not all of these side effects may occur, if they do occur they may need medical attention.

Stop taking this medicine and get emergency help immediately if any of the following side effects occur:

  Less common

    Fast or irregular breathing; fever; joint pain; lightheadedness or fainting (sudden); puffiness or swelling around the face; shortness of breath; skin rash, hives, itching

In addition to the side effects mentioned above, *check with your doctor immediately* if any of the following side effects occur:

> *Rare*
>> Abdominal or stomach cramps and pain (severe); convulsions (seizures); diarrhea (watery and severe), which may also be bloody; pain at place of injection; sore throat and fever; unusual bleeding or bruising
>>
>> Note: Some of the above side effects (severe abdominal or stomach cramps and pain, and watery and severe diarrhea, which may also be bloody) may also occur up to several weeks after you stop taking any of these medicines.

Other side effects may occur that usually do not need medical attention. These side effects may go away during treatment as your body adjusts to the medicine. However, check with your doctor if any of the following side effects continue or are bothersome:

> *More common*
>> Diarrhea (mild); headache; nausea or vomiting; sore mouth or tongue; stomach pain; vaginal itching and discharge; white patches in the mouth and/or on the tongue

Other side effects not listed above may also occur in some patients. If you notice any other effects, check with your doctor.

PENTOXIFYLLINE Systemic

A commonly used brand name in the U.S. and Canada is Trental. Another commonly used name is oxypentifylline.

Description

Pentoxifylline (pen-tox-IF-i-lin) improves the flow of blood through blood vessels. It is used to reduce leg pain caused by poor blood circulation. Pentoxifylline makes it possible to walk farther before having to rest because of leg cramps.

Pentoxifylline is available only with your doctor's prescription, in the following dosage form:

Oral

• Extended-release tablets (U.S. and Canada)

Before Using This Medicine

In deciding to use a medicine, the risks of taking the medicine must be weighed against the good it will do. This is a decision you and your doctor will make. For pentoxifylline, the following should be considered:

Allergies—Tell your doctor if you have ever had any unusual or allergic reaction to pentoxifylline or to other xanthines such as aminophylline, caffeine, dyphylline, ethylenediamine (contained in aminophylline), oxtriphylline, theobromine, or theophylline. Also tell your health care professional if you are allergic to any other substances, such as foods, preservatives, or dyes.

Pregnancy—Pentoxifylline has not been studied in pregnant women. Studies in animals have not shown that it causes birth defects. However, at very high doses it has caused other harmful effects. Before taking this medicine, make sure your doctor knows if you are pregnant or if you may become pregnant.

Breast-feeding—Pentoxifylline passes into breast milk. The medicine has not been reported to cause problems in nursing babies. However, pentoxifylline has caused noncancerous tumors in animals when given for a long time in doses much larger than those used in humans. Therefore, your doctor may not want you to breast-feed while taking it. Be sure that you discuss the risks and benefits of this medicine with your doctor.

Children—Studies on this medicine have been done only in adult patients, and there is no specific information comparing use of pentoxifylline in children with use in other age groups.

Older adults—Side effects may be more likely to occur in the elderly, who are usually more sensitive than younger adults to the effects of pentoxifylline.

Other medicines—Although certain medicines should not be used together at all, in other cases two different medicines may be used together even if an interaction might occur. In these cases, your doctor may want to change the dose, or other precautions may be necessary. When you are taking pentoxifylline, it is important that your health care professional know if you are taking any other prescription or nonprescription (over-the-counter [OTC]) medicine, or if you smoke tobacco.

Other medical problems—The presence of other medical problems may affect the use of pentoxifylline. Make sure you tell your doctor if you have any other medical problems, especially:

- Any condition in which there is a risk of bleeding (e.g., recent stroke)—Pentoxifylline may make the condition worse
- Kidney disease or
- Liver disease—The chance of side effects may be increased

Proper Use of This Medicine

Swallow the tablet whole. Do not crush, break, or chew it before swallowing.

Pentoxifylline should be taken with meals to lessen the chance of stomach upset. Taking an antacid with the medicine may also help.

Dosing—The dose of pentoxifylline will be different for different patients. *Follow your doctor's orders or the directions on the label.* The following information includes only the average doses of pentoxifylline. *If your dose is different, do not change it* unless your doctor tells you to do so.

- For *oral* dosage form (extended-release tablets):
    - —For peripheral vascular disease (circulation problems):
        - Adults—400 milligrams (mg) two to three times a day, taken with meals.
        - Children—Use must be determined by your doctor.

Missed dose—If you miss a dose of this medicine, take it as soon as possible. However, if it is almost time for your next dose, skip the missed dose and go back to your regular dosing schedule. Do not double doses.

Storage—To store this medicine:

- Keep out of the reach of children.
- Store away from heat and direct light.
- Do not store in the bathroom, near the kitchen sink, or in other damp places. Heat or moisture may cause the medicine to break down.
- Do not keep outdated medicine or medicine no longer needed. Be sure that any discarded medicine is out of the reach of children.

Precautions While Using This Medicine

It may take several weeks for this medicine to work. If you feel that pentoxifylline is not working, do not stop taking it on your own. Instead, check with your doctor.

Smoking tobacco may worsen your condition since nicotine may further narrow your blood vessels. Therefore, it is best to avoid smoking.

Side Effects of This Medicine

Along with its needed effects, a medicine may cause some unwanted effects. Although not all of these side effects may occur, if they do occur they may need medical attention.

Check with your doctor as soon as possible if any of the following side effects occur:

Rare

Chest pain; irregular heartbeat

Signs and symptoms of overdose (in the order in which they may occur)

Drowsiness; flushing; faintness; unusual excitement; convulsions (seizures)

Other side effects may occur that usually do not need medical attention. These side effects may go away during treatment as your body adjusts to the medicine. However, check with your doctor if any of the following side effects continue or are bothersome:

Less common

Dizziness; headache; nausea or vomiting; stomach discomfort

Other side effects not listed above may also occur in some patients. If you notice any other effects, check with your doctor.

PHENOTHIAZINES Systemic

Some commonly used brand names are:

In the U.S.—

Compa-Z[9]	Cotranzine[9]
Compazine[9]	Levoprome[5]
Compazine Spansule[9]	Mellaril[13]

In the U.S. (cont'd)—

Mellaril Concentrate[13]

Mellaril-S[13]

Ormazine[2]

Permitil[3]

Permitil Concentrate[3]

Primazine[10]

Prolixin[3]

Prolixin Concentrate[3]

Prolixin Decanoate[3]

Prolixin Enanthate[3]

Prozine-50[10]

Serentil[4]

Serentil Concentrate[4]

Sparine[10]

Stelazine[14]

Stelazine Concentrate[14]

Thorazine[2]

Thorazine Concentrate[2]

Thorazine Spansule[2]

Thor-Prom[2]

Tindal[1]

Trilafon[7]

Trilafon Concentrate[7]

Ultrazine-10[9]

Vesprin[15]

In Canada—

Apo-Fluphenazine[3]

Apo-Perphenazine[7]

Apo-Thioridazine[13]

Apo-Trifluoperazine[14]

Chlorpromanyl-5[2]

Chlorpromanyl-20[2]

Chlorpromanyl-40[2]

Dartal[11]

Largactil[2]

Largactil Liquid[2]

Largactil Oral Drops[2]

Majeptil[12]

Mellaril[13]

Modecate[3]

Modecate Concentrate[3]

Moditen Enanthate[3]

Moditen HCl[3]

Moditen HCl-H.P.[3]

Neuleptil[6]

Novo-Chlorpromazine[2]

Novo-Flurazine[14]

Novo-Ridazine[13]

Nozinan[5]

Nozinan Liquid[5]

Nozinan Oral Drops[5]

PMS Perphenazine[7]

PMS Prochlorperazine[9]

PMS Thioridazine[13]

PMS Trifluoperazine[14]

Prorazin[9]

Solazine[14]

Stelazine[14]

Stelazine Concentrate[14]

Stemetil[9]

Stemetil Liquid[9]

Permitil[3]

Piportil L[4][8]

Serentil[4]

Terfluzine[14]

Terfluzine Concentrate[14]

Trilafon[7]

Trilafon Concentrate[7]

Note: For quick reference, the following phenothiazines are numbered to match the corresponding brand names.

This information applies to the following medicines:

1. Acetophenazine (a-set-oh-FEN-a-zeen)†
2. Chlorpromazine (klor-PROE-ma-zeen)‡§
3. Fluphenazine (floo-FEN-a-zeen)‡
4. Mesoridazine (mez-oh-RID-a-zeen)
5. Methotrimeprazine (meth-oh-trim-EP-ra-zeen)
6. Pericyazine (pair-ee-SYE-a-zeen)*
7. Perphenazine (per-FEN-a-zeen)‡§

8. Pipotiazine (pip-oh-TYE-a-zeen)*
9. Prochlorperazine (proe-klor-PAIR-a-zeen)‡§
10. Promazine (PROE-ma-zeen)‡§
11. Thiopropazate (thye-oh-PROE-pa-zayt)*
12. Thioproperazine (thye-oh-proe-PAIR-a-zeen)*
13. Thioridazine (thye-oh-RID-a-zeen)‡
14. Trifluoperazine (trye-floo-oh-PAIR-a-zeen)‡
15. Triflupromazine (trye-floo-PROE-ma-zeen)†

Note: This information does *not* apply to Ethopropazine, Promethazine, Propiomazine, and Trimeprazine.

---

*Not commercially available in the U.S.
†Not commercially available in Canada.
‡Generic name product may also be available in the U.S.
§Generic name product may also be available in Canada.

Description

Phenothiazines (FEE-noe-THYE-a-zeens) are used to treat nervous, mental, and emotional disorders. Some are used also to control anxiety or agitation in certain patients, severe nausea and vomiting, severe hiccups, and moderate to severe pain in some hospitalized patients. Chlorpromazine is also used in the treatment of certain types of porphyria, and with other medicines in the treatment of tetanus. Phenothiazines may also be used for other conditions as determined by your doctor.

Phenothiazines are available only with your doctor's prescription in the following dosage forms:

Oral

Acetophenazine
• Tablets (U.S.)
Chlorpromazine
• Extended-release capsules (U.S.)
• Oral concentrate (U.S. and Canada)
• Syrup (U.S. and Canada)
• Tablets (U.S. and Canada)
Fluphenazine
• Elixir (U.S. and Canada)
• Oral solution (U.S.)

- Tablets (U.S. and Canada)

Mesoridazine
- Oral solution (U.S.)
- Tablets (U.S. and Canada)

Methotrimeprazine
- Oral solution (Canada)
- Syrup (Canada)
- Tablets (Canada)

Pericyazine
- Capsules (Canada)
- Oral solution (Canada)

Perphenazine
- Oral solution (U.S. and Canada)
- Syrup (Canada)
- Tablets (U.S. and Canada)

Prochlorperazine
- Extended-release capsules (U.S.)
- Syrup (U.S. and Canada)
- Tablets (U.S. and Canada)

Promazine
- Tablets (U.S.)

Thiopropazate
- Tablets (Canada)

Thioproperazine
- Tablets (Canada)

Thioridazine
- Oral solution (U.S. and Canada)
- Oral suspension (U.S. and Canada)
- Tablets (U.S. and Canada)

Trifluoperazine
- Oral solution (U.S. and Canada)
- Syrup (Canada)
- Tablets (U.S. and Canada)

Parenteral

Chlorpromazine
- Injection (U.S. and Canada)

Fluphenazine
- Injection (U.S. and Canada)

Mesoridazine
- Injection (U.S.)

Methotrimeprazine

- Injection (U.S. and Canada)

Perphenazine
- Injection (U.S. and Canada)

Pipotiazine
- Injection (Canada)

Prochlorperazine
- Injection (U.S. and Canada)

Promazine
- Injection (U.S. and Canada)

Trifluoperazine
- Injection (U.S. and Canada)

Triflupromazine
- Injection (U.S.)

Rectal

Chlorpromazine
- Suppositories (U.S. and Canada)

Prochlorperazine
- Suppositories (U.S. and Canada)

Before Using This Medicine

In deciding to use a medicine, the risks of taking the medicine must be weighed against the good it will do. This is a decision you and your doctor will make. For phenothiazines, the following should be considered:

Allergies—Tell your doctor if you have ever had any unusual or allergic reaction to phenothiazines. Also tell your health care professional if you are allergic to any other substances, such as foods, preservatives, or dyes.

Pregnancy—Although studies have not been done in pregnant women, some side effects, such as jaundice and muscle tremors and other movement disorders, have occurred in a few newborns whose mothers received phenothiazines close to the time of delivery. Studies in animals have shown that chlorpromazine and trifluoperazine, given in doses many times the usual human dose, may cause birth defects.

Breast-feeding—Phenothiazines pass into the breast milk and may cause drowsiness and a greater chance of unusual muscle movement in the nursing baby.

Children—Certain side effects, such as muscle spasms of the face, neck, and back, tic-like or twitching movements, inability to move the eyes, twisting of the body, or weakness of the arms and legs, are more likely to occur in children, especially those with severe illness or dehydration. Children are usually more sensitive than adults to some of the side effects of phenothiazines.

Older adults—Constipation, dizziness or fainting, drowsiness, dryness of mouth, trembling of the hands and fingers, and symptoms of tardive dyskinesia (such as rapid, worm-like movements of the tongue or any other uncontrolled movements of the mouth, tongue, or jaw, and/or arms and legs) are especially likely to occur in elderly patients, who are usually more sensitive than younger adults to the effects of phenothiazines.

Other medicines—Although certain medicines should not be used together at all, in other cases two different medicines may be used together even if an interaction might occur. In these cases, your doctor may want to change the dose, or other precautions may be necessary. When you are taking phenothiazines, it is especially important that your health care professional know if you are taking any of the following:

- Amantadine (e.g., Symmetrel) or
- Antihypertensives (high blood pressure medicine) or
- Bromocriptine (e.g., Parlodel) or
- Deferoxamine (e.g., Desferal) or
- Diuretics (water pills) or
- Levobunolol (e.g., Betagan) or
- Medicine for heart disease or
- Metipranolol (e.g., OptiPranolol)
- Nabilone (e.g., Cesamet) (with high doses) or
- Narcotic pain medicine or
- Nimodipine (e.g., Nimotop) or

- Other antipsychotics (medicine for mental illness) or
- Pentamidine (e.g., Pentam) or
- Pimozide (e.g., Orap) or
- Promethazine (e.g., Phenergan) or
- Trimeprazine (e.g., Temaril)—Severe low blood pressure may occur
- Antidepressants (medicine for depression)—The risk of serious side effects may be increased
- Antithyroid agents (medicine for overactive thyroid) or
- Central nervous system (CNS) depressants (medicines that cause drowsiness)—There may be an increased chance of blood problems
- Epinephrine (e.g., Adrenalin)—Severe low blood pressure and fast heartbeat may occur
- Levodopa (e.g., Dopar)—Phenothiazines may prevent levodopa from working properly in the treatment of Parkinson's disease
- Lithium (e.g., Lithane, Lithizine)—The amount of medicine you need to take may change
- Methyldopa (e.g., Aldomet) or
- Metoclopramide (e.g., Reglan) or
- Metyrosine (e.g. Demser) or
- Pemoline (e.g., Cylert) or
- Rauwolfia alkaloids (alseroxylon [e.g., Rauwiloid], deserpidine [e.g., Harmonyl], rauwolfia serpentina [e.g., Raudixin], reserpine [e.g., Serpasil])—Taking these medicines with phenothiazines may increase the chance and severity of certain side effects
- Metrizamide—When this dye is used for myelograms, the risk of seizures may be increased

Other medical problems—The presence of other medical problems may affect the use of phenothiazines. Make sure you tell your doctor if you have any other medical problems, especially:

- Alcohol abuse—Certain side effects such as heat stroke may be more likely to occur
- Blood disease or
- Breast cancer or
- Difficult urination or

- Enlarged prostate or
- Glaucoma or
- Heart or blood vessel disease or
- Lung disease or
- Parkinson's disease or
- Seizure disorders or
- Stomach ulcers—Phenothiazines may make the condition worse
- Liver disease—Higher blood levels of phenothiazines may occur, increasing the chance of side effects
- Reye's syndrome—There may be an increased chance of unwanted effects on the liver

---

Proper Use of This Medicine

For patients taking this medicine *by mouth:*

- This medicine may be taken with food or a full glass (8 ounces) of water or milk to reduce stomach irritation.

- *If your medicine comes in a dropper bottle,* measure each dose with the special dropper provided with your prescription and dilute it in ½ a glass (4 ounces) of orange or grapefruit juice or water.

- If you are taking the *extended-release capsule form* of this medicine, each dose should be swallowed whole. Do not break, crush, or chew before swallowing.

For patients using the *suppository form* of this medicine:

- If the suppository is too soft to insert, chill it in the refrigerator for 30 minutes or run cold water over it before removing the foil wrapper.

- To insert the suppository: First remove the foil wrapper and moisten the suppository with cold water. Lie down on your side and use your finger to push the suppository well up into the rectum.

Do not take more of this medicine and do not take it more often than your doctor ordered. This is particularly important for children or elderly patients, since they may react very strongly to this medicine.

Sometimes this medicine must be taken for several weeks before its full effect is reached when it is used to treat mental and emotional conditions.

Dosing—The dose of phenothiazines will be different for different patients. *Follow your doctor's orders or the directions on the label.* The following information includes only the average doses of phenothiazines. *If your dose is different, do not change it* unless your doctor tells you to do so.

The number of capsules, tablets, or teaspoonfuls of elixir, solution, suspension, or syrup that you take, or the number of injections you receive or suppositories that you use, depends on the strength of the medicine. Also, *the number of doses you use each day, the time allowed between doses, and the length of time you take the medicine depend on the medical problem for which you are taking phenothiazines.*

For acetophenazine

- For *oral* dosage form (tablets):
  - —For nervous, mental, or emotional disorders:
    - Adults and teenagers—20 milligrams (mg) three times a day. Your doctor may change your dose if needed.
    - Children up to 12 years of age—Dose must be determined by your doctor.

For chlorpromazine

- For *oral extended-release capsule* dosage form:
  - —For nervous, mental, or emotional disorders:
    - Adults—30 to 300 milligrams (mg) one to three times a day. Your doctor may increase your dose

if needed. However, the dose is usually not more than 1000 mg a day.

• Children—This dosage form is not recommended for use in children.

• For *oral concentrate, syrup, or tablet* dosage forms:

—For nervous, mental, or emotional disorders:

• Adults and teenagers—At first, 10 to 25 mg two to four times a day. Your doctor may increase your dose if needed. However, the dose is usually not more than 1000 mg a day.

• Children up to 6 months of age—Dose must be determined by your doctor.

• Children 6 months of age and older—Dose is based on body weight or size, and must be determined by your doctor. The usual dose is 0.55 mg per kilogram (kg) (0.25 mg per pound) of body weight, every four to six hours.

—For nausea and vomiting:

• Adults and teenagers—10 to 25 mg every four hours as needed.

• Children up to 6 months of age—Dose must be determined by your doctor.

• Children 6 months of age and older—Dose is based on body weight or size, and must be determined by your doctor. The usual dose is 0.55 mg per kg (0.25 mg per pound) of body weight, every four to six hours.

—For sedation before surgery:

• Adults and teenagers—25 to 50 mg two to three hours before surgery.

• Children—Dose is based on body weight or size, and must be determined by your doctor. The usual dose is 0.55 mg per kg (0.25 mg per pound) of body weight, two or three hours before surgery.

—For treatment of hiccups:

• Adults and teenagers—25 to 50 mg three or four times a day.

• Children—Dose must be determined by your doctor.

—For porphyria:

• Adults and teenagers—25 to 50 mg three or four times a day.

• Children—Use and dose must be determined by your doctor.

• For *injection* dosage form:

—For severe nervous, mental, or emotional disorders:

• Adults—At first, 25 to 50 mg, injected into a muscle. The dose may be repeated in one hour, and every three to twelve hours thereafter. Your doctor may increase your dose if needed.

• Children up to 6 months of age—Dose must be determined by your doctor.

• Children 6 months of age and over—Dose is based on body weight or size and must be determined by your doctor. The usual dose is 0.55 mg per kg (0.25 mg per pound) of body weight, injected into a muscle every six to eight hours as needed.

—For nausea and vomiting:

• Adults—At first, 25 mg injected into a muscle. The dose may be increased to 25 to 50 mg every three to four hours if needed.

• Children up to 6 months of age—Dose must be determined by your doctor.

• Children 6 months of age and over—Dose is based on body weight or size and must be determined by your doctor. The usual dose is 0.55 mg per kg (0.25 mg per pound) of body weight, in-

jected into a muscle every six to eight hours as
needed.

—For nausea and vomiting during surgery:

• Adults—At first, 12.5 mg injected into a muscle. The dose may be repeated if needed. Or, up
to 25 mg, diluted and injected slowly into a vein.

• Children—Dose is based on body weight or
size and must be determined by your doctor. The
usual dose is 0.275 mg per kg (0.125 mg per
pound) of body weight, injected into a muscle, or
diluted and injected slowly into a vein.

—For sedation before surgery:

• Adults—12.5 to 25 mg, injected into a muscle
one or two hours before surgery.

• Children—Dose is based on body weight and
must be determined by your doctor. The usual
dose is 0.55 mg per kg (0.25 mg per pound) of
body weight, injected into a muscle one to two
hours before surgery.

—For treatment of hiccups:

• Adults—25 to 50 mg, injected into a muscle
three or four times a day. Or, 25 to 50 mg diluted
and injected slowly into a vein.

• Children—Dose must be determined by your
doctor.

—For porphyria:

• Adults—25 mg injected into a muscle every six
or eight hours.

• Children—Dose must be determined by your
doctor.

—For tetanus:

• Adults—25 to 50 mg, injected into a muscle
three or four times a day. Or, 25 to 50 mg, diluted
and injected slowly into a vein. Your doctor may
increase your dose if needed.

• Children—Dose is based on body weight and must be determined by your doctor. The usual dose is 0.55 mg per kg (0.25 mg per pound) of body weight, injected into a muscle every six to eight hours. Or, 0.55 mg per kg (0.25 mg per pound) of body weight, diluted and injected slowly into a vein.

• For *rectal* dosage form (suppositories):

—For nausea and vomiting:

• Adults and teenagers—50 to 100 mg, inserted into the rectum every six to eight hours as needed.

• Children up to 6 months of age—Dose must be determined by your doctor.

• Children 6 months of age and over—Dose is based on body weight and must be determined by your doctor. The usual dose is 1 mg per kg (0.45 mg per pound) of body weight, inserted into the rectum every six to eight hours as needed.

For fluphenazine

• For *oral* dosage form (elixir, solution, or tablets):

—For nervous, mental, or emotional disorders:

• Adults—At first, 2.5 to 10 milligrams (mg) a day, taken in smaller doses every six to eight hours during the day. Your doctor may increase your dose if needed. However, the dose is usually not more than 20 mg a day.

• Children—0.25 to 0.75 mg one to four times a day.

• Older adults—1 to 2.5 mg a day. Your doctor may increase your dose if needed.

• For *long-acting decanoate injection* dosage form:

—For nervous, mental, or emotional disorders:

• Adults—At first, 12.5 to 25 mg, injected into a muscle or under the skin every one to three weeks. Your doctor may increase your dose if needed. However, the dose is usually not more than 100 mg.

• Children 5 to 12 years of age—3.125 to 12.5 mg, injected into a muscle or under the skin every one to three weeks.

• Children 12 years of age and over—At first, 6.25 to 18.75 mg a week, injected into a muscle or under the skin. Your doctor may increase your dose if needed. However, the dose is usually not more than 25 mg every one to three weeks.

• For *long-acting enanthate injection* dosage form:

—For nervous, mental, or emotional disorders:

• Adults and teenagers—25 mg, injected into a muscle or under the skin every one to three weeks. Your doctor may increase your dose if needed. However, the dose is usually not more than 100 mg.

• Children up to 12 years of age—Dose must be determined by your doctor.

• For *short-acting hydrochloride injection* dosage form:

—For nervous, mental, or emotional disorders:

• Adults and teenagers—1.25 to 2.5 mg, injected into a muscle every six to eight hours. Your doctor may increase your dose if needed. However, the dose is usually not more than 10 mg a day.

• Children up to 12 years of age—Dose must be determined by your doctor.

• Older adults—1 to 2.5 mg a day, injected into a muscle. Your doctor may increase your dose if needed.

For mesoridazine

• For *oral* dosage form (solution or tablets):

—For nervous, mental, or emotional disorders:

• Adults and teenagers—30 to 150 milligrams

(mg), taken in smaller doses two or three times during the day.

• Children up to 12 years of age—Dose must be determined by your doctor.

• For *injection* dosage form:

—For nervous, mental, or emotional disorders:

• Adults and teenagers—25 mg injected into a muscle. The dose may be repeated in thirty to sixty minutes if needed.

• Children up to 12 years of age—Dose must be determined by your doctor.

For methotrimeprazine

• For *oral* dosage form (solution, syrup, or tablets):

—For nervous, mental, or emotional disorders:

• Adults and teenagers—At first, 6 to 75 milligrams (mg) a day, taken in smaller doses two or three times a day with meals. Your doctor may increase your dose if needed.

• Children—Dose is based on body weight and must be determined by your doctor. At first, the usual dose is 0.25 mg per kilogram (kg) (0.11 mg per pound) of body weight a day, taken in smaller doses two or three times a day with meals. Your doctor may increase your dose if needed.

—For pain:

• Adults and teenagers—At first, 6 to 25 mg a day, taken in smaller doses three times a day with meals. For more severe pain, 50 to 75 mg a day, taken in smaller doses two or three times a day with meals. Your doctor may increase your dose if needed.

• Children—Dose is based on body weight and must be determined by your doctor. At first, the usual dose is 0.25 mg per kg (0.11 mg per pound) of body weight a day, taken in smaller doses two or three times a day with meals. Your doctor may increase your dose if needed. However, the dose is usually not more than 40 mg a day.

—For sedation before surgery:

• Adults and teenagers—At first, 6 to 25 mg a day, taken in smaller doses three times a day with meals. Your doctor may increase your dose if needed.

• Children—Dose is based on body weight and must be determined by your doctor. At first, the usual dose is 0.25 mg per kg (0.11 mg per pound) of body weight a day, taken in smaller doses two or three times a day with meals. Your doctor may increase your dose if needed. However, the dose is usually not more than 40 mg a day.

• For *injection* dosage form:

—For nervous, mental, or emotional disorders:

• Adults and teenagers—At first, 10 to 20 mg, injected into a muscle every four to six hours. Your doctor may increase your dose if needed.

• Children—Dose must be determined by your doctor.

—For pain:

• Adults and teenagers—At first, 2.5 to 20 mg, injected into a muscle. Your doctor may increase your dose if needed.

• Children—Dose is based on body weight and must be determined by your doctor. The usual dose is 0.062 to 0.125 mg per kg (0.028 to 0.057 mg per pound) of body weight, injected into a muscle.

• Older adults—At first, 5 to 10 mg injected into a muscle every four to six hours. Your doctor may increase your dose if needed.

—For sedation before surgery:

- Adults and teenagers—2 to 20 mg, injected into a muscle forty-five minutes to three hours before surgery.
- Children—Dose must be determined by your doctor.

For pericyazine

- For *oral* dosage form (capsules or solution):

  —For nervous, mental, or emotional disorders:

  - Adults—At first, 5 to 20 milligrams (mg) taken in the morning, and 10 to 40 mg taken in the evening. Your doctor may change your dose if needed.
  - Children 5 years of age and over—2.5 to 10 mg taken in the morning, and 5 to 30 mg taken in the evening.
  - Older adults—At first, 5 mg a day. Your doctor may increase your dose if needed. However, the dose is usually not more than 30 mg a day.

For perphenazine

- For *oral solution* dosage form:

  —For nervous, mental, or emotional disorders in hospitalized patients:

  - Adults and teenagers—8 to 16 milligrams (mg) two to four times a day.
  - Children up to 12 years of age—Dose must be determined by your doctor.

- For *oral syrup* dosage form:

  —For nervous, mental, or emotional disorders:

  - Adults and teenagers—2 to 16 mg two to four times a day.
  - Children up to 12 years of age—Dose must be determined by your doctor.

  —For nausea and vomiting:

  - Adults and teenagers—2 to 4 mg two to four times a day.

      • Children up to 12 years of age—Dose must be determined by your doctor.

• For *oral tablet* dosage form:

      —For nervous, mental, or emotional disorders:

           • Adults and teenagers—4 to 16 mg two to four times a day.

           • Children up to 12 years of age—Dose must be determined by your doctor.

      —For nausea and vomiting:

           • Adults and teenagers—8 to 16 mg a day, taken in smaller doses during the day. Your doctor will lower your dose as soon as possible.

           • Children up to 12 years of age—Dose must be determined by your doctor.

• For *injection* dosage form:

      —For nervous, mental, or emotional disorders:

           • Adults and teenagers—5 to 10 mg injected into a muscle every six hours. Hospitalized patients may need higher doses.

           • Children up to 12 years of age—Dose must be determined by your doctor.

      —For nausea and vomiting:

           • Adults and teenagers—At first, 5 mg injected into a muscle, or diluted and injected slowly into a vein. Your doctor may increase your dose if needed.

           • Children up to 12 years of age—Dose must be determined by your doctor.

For pipotiazine

• For *injection* dosage form:

      —For nervous, mental, or emotional disorders:

           • Adults and teenagers—At first, 50 to 100 milligrams (mg) injected into a muscle.Your doctor may increase your dose if needed. However, the dose is usually not more than 150 mg every four weeks.

• Children up to 12 years of age—Dose must be determined by your doctor.

For prochlorperazine

• For *oral syrup* dosage form:

—For nervous, mental, or emotional disorders:

• Adults and teenagers—At first, 5 to 10 milligrams (mg) three or four times a day. Your doctor may increase your dose if needed. However, the dose is usually not more than 150 mg a day.

• Children up to 2 years of age—Dose must be determined by your doctor.

• Children 2 to 12 years of age—2.5 mg two or three times a day.

—For nausea and vomiting:

• Adults and teenagers—5 to 10 mg three or four times a day.

• Children—Dose is based on body weight and must be determined by your doctor. The usual dose is 2.5 mg taken one to three times a day. For children 2 to 5 years of age, the dose is usually not more than 20 mg a day. For children 6 to 12 years of age, the dose is usually not more than 25 mg a day.

—For anxiety:

• Adults and teenagers—5 mg three or four times a day. This dose is usually not taken for longer than twelve weeks.

• Children—Dose must be determined by your doctor.

• For *oral extended-release capsule* dosage form:

—For nervous, mental, or emotional disorders:

• Adults and teenagers—At first, 5 to 10 mg every three or four hours. Your doctor may increase your dose if needed. However, the dose is usually not more than 150 mg a day.

• Children—This dosage form is not recommended for use in children.

—For nausea and vomiting:

• Adults and teenagers—15 to 30 mg once a day in the morning, or 10 mg taken every twelve hours. Your doctor may increase your dose if needed. However, the dose is usually not more than 40 mg a day.

• Children—This dosage form is not recommended for use in children.

—For anxiety:

• Adults and teenagers—15 mg once a day in the morning, or 10 mg taken every twelve hours. This dose is usually not taken for longer than twelve weeks.

• Children—This dosage form is not recommended for use in children.

• For *oral tablet* dosage form:

—For nervous, mental, or emotional disorders:

• Adults and teenagers—5 to 10 mg three or four times a day. Your doctor may increase your dose if needed. However, the dose is usually not more than 150 mg a day.

• Children—The tablet dosage form is often not suitable for use in children. The syrup dosage form is usually recommended.

—For nausea and vomiting:

• Adults and teenagers—5 to 10 mg three or four times a day.

• Children—The tablet dosage form is often not suitable for use in children. The syrup dosage form is usually recommended.

—For anxiety:

- Adults and teenagers—5 mg three or four times a day. This dose is usually not taken for longer than twelve weeks.

- Children—The tablet dosage form is often not suitable for use in children. The syrup dosage form is usually recommended.

- For *injection* dosage form:

  —For nervous, mental, or emotional disorders:

  - Adults and teenagers—At first, 10 to 20 mg injected into a muscle. The dose may be repeated every two to four hours if needed for up to four doses. Later, the dose is usually 10 to 20 mg every four to six hours. However, the dose is usually not more than 200 mg a day.

  - Children up to 2 years of age—Dose must be determined by your doctor.

  - Children 2 to 12 years of age—Dose is based on body weight and must be determined by your doctor. The usual dose is 0.132 mg per kilogram (kg) (0.06 mg per pound) of body weight, injected into a muscle. However, the dose for children 2 to 5 years of age is usually not more than 20 mg a day. The dose for children 6 to 12 years of age is usually not more than 25 mg a day.

  —For nausea and vomiting:

  - Adults and teenagers—5 to 10 mg, injected into a muscle every three to four hours as needed. Or, 2.5 to 10 mg injected slowly into a vein. The dose is usually not more than 40 mg a day.

  - Children up to 2 years of age—Dose must be determined by your doctor.

  - Children 2 to 12 years of age—Dose is based on body weight and must be determined by your doctor. The usual dose is 0.132 mg per kg (0.06 mg per pound) of body weight, injected into a muscle. However, the dose for children 2 to 5

years of age is usually not more than 20 mg a
day. The dose for children 6 to 12 years of age
is usually not more than 25 mg a day.

—For nausea and vomiting in surgery:

• Adults and teenagers—5 to 10 mg, injected into
a muscle. Or, up to 20 mg injected slowly into a
vein. The dose is usually not more than 40 mg
a day.

• Children—Dose must be determined by your
doctor.

—For anxiety:

• Adults and teenagers—5 to 10 mg injected into
a muscle every three to four hours. Or, 2.5 to 10
mg injected slowly into a vein. The dose is usually not more than 40 mg a day.

• Children up to 2 years of age—Dose must be
determined by your doctor.

• Children 2 to 12 years of age—Dose is based
on body weight and must be determined by your
doctor. The usual dose is 0.132 mg per kg (0.06
mg per pound) of body weight, injected into a
muscle. However, the dose for children 2 to 5
years of age is usually not more than 20 mg a
day. The dose for children 6 to 12 years of age
is usually not more than 25 mg a day.

• For *rectal* dosage form (suppositories):

—For nervous, mental, or emotional disorders:

• Adults and teenagers—10 mg inserted into the
rectum three or four times a day. Your doctor
may increase your dose if needed.

• Children—Dose must be determined by your
doctor.

—For nausea and vomiting:

• Adults and teenagers—25 mg inserted into the
rectum two times a day.

• Children up to 2 years of age—Dose must be determined by your doctor.

• Children 2 to 12 years of age—Dose is based on body weight and must be determined by your doctor. The usual dose is 2.5 mg inserted into the rectum one to three times a day. The dose in children 2 to 5 years of age is usually not more than 20 mg a day. The dose for children 6 to 12 years of age is usually not more than 25 mg a day.

For promazine

• For *oral* dosage form (tablets):

—For nervous, mental, or emotional disorders:

• Adults—10 to 200 milligrams (mg) every four to six hours.

• Children up to 12 years of age—Dose must be determined by your doctor.

• Children 12 years of age and over—10 to 25 mg every four to six hours.

• For *injection* dosage form:

—For nervous, mental, or emotional disorders:

• Adults—At first, 50 to 150 mg injected into a muscle, or diluted and injected into a vein. Later, 10 to 200 mg, injected into a muscle or vein, every four to six hours.

• Children up to 12 years of age—Dose must be determined by your doctor.

• Children 12 years of age and over—10 to 25 mg, injected into a muscle, every four to six hours.

For thiopropazate

• For *oral* dosage form (tablets):

—For nervous, mental, or emotional disorders:

• Adults and teenagers—At first, 10 milligrams (mg) three times a day. Your doctor may increase your dose if needed. However, the dose is usually not more than 100 mg a day.

• Children—Dose must be determined by your doctor.

For thioproperazine

• For *oral* dosage form (tablets):

—For nervous, mental, or emotional disorders:

• Adults and teenagers—At first, 5 milligrams (mg) a day. Your doctor may increase your dose if needed.

• Children—Dose must be determined by your doctor.

For thioridazine

• For *oral* dosage form (suspension, solution, or tablets):

—For nervous, mental, or emotional disorders:

• Adults and teenagers—At first, 25 to 100 milligrams (mg) three times a day. Your doctor may increase your dose if needed. However, the dose is usually not more than 800 mg a day.

• Children up to 2 years of age—Dose must be determined by your doctor.

• Children 2 to 12 years of age—Dose is based on body weight or size and must be determined by your doctor. The usual dose is 10 to 25 mg two or three times a day.

For trifluoperazine

• For *oral* dosage form (solution, syrup, or tablets):

—For nervous, mental, or emotional disorders:

• Adults and teenagers—At first, 2 to 5 milligrams (mg) two times a day. Your doctor may increase your dose if needed. However, the dose is usually not more than 40 mg a day.

• Children up to 6 years of age—Dose must be determined by your doctor.

• Children 6 years of age and over—1 mg one or two times a day.

—For anxiety:

• Adults and teenagers—1 to 2 mg a day. Your doctor may increase your dose if needed. However, the dose is usually not more than 6 mg a day, and is usually not taken for longer than twelve weeks.

• Children—Dose must be determined by your doctor.

• For *injection* dosage form:

—For nervous, mental, or emotional disorders:

• Adults and teenagers—1 to 2 mg, injected into a muscle every four to six hours as needed. However, the dose is usually not more than 10 mg a day.

• Children up to 6 years of age—Dose must be determined by your doctor.

• Children 6 years of age and over—1 mg injected into a muscle one or two times a day.

For triflupromazine

• For *injection* dosage form:

—For nervous, mental, or emotional disorders:

• Adults and teenagers—60 milligrams (mg) injected into a muscle as needed. However, the dose is usually not more than 150 mg a day.

• Children up to 2½ years of age—Dose must be determined by your doctor.

• Children 2½ years of age and over—Dose is based on body weight and must be determined by your doctor. The usual dose is 0.2 to 0.25 mg per kilogram (kg) (0.09 to 0.11 mg per pound) of body weight, injected into a muscle. However, the dose is usually not more than 10 mg a day.

—For nausea and vomiting:

- Adults and teenagers—5 to 15 mg injected into a muscle every four hours, or 1 mg injected into a vein as needed. Your doctor may increase your dose if needed. However, the dose is usually not more than 60 mg a day injected into a muscle, or 3 mg a day injected into a vein.

- Children up to 2½ years of age—Dose must be determined by your doctor.

- Children 2½ years of age and over—Dose is based on body weight and must be determined by your doctor. The usual dose is 0.2 to 0.25 mg per kg (0.09 to 0.11 mg per pound) of body weight, injected into a muscle. However, the dose is usually not more than 10 mg a day.

Missed dose—If you miss a dose of this medicine and your dosing schedule is:

- One dose a day: Take the missed dose as soon as possible. Then go back to your regular dosing schedule. However, if you do not remember the missed dose until the next day, skip it and go back to your regular dosing schedule. Do not double doses.

- More than one dose a day: If you remember within an hour or so of the missed dose, take it right away. However, if you do not remember until later, skip the missed dose and go back to your regular dosing schedule. Do not double doses.

If you have any questions about this, check with your doctor.

Storage—To store this medicine:

- Keep out of the reach of children.

- Store away from heat and direct light.

- Do not store the capsule or tablet form of this medicine in the bathroom, near the kitchen sink, or in other damp places. Heat or moisture may cause the medicine to break down.

- Keep the liquid form of this medicine from freezing.
- Do not keep outdated medicine or medicine no longer needed. Be sure that any discarded medicine is out of the reach of children.

Precautions While Using This Medicine

Your doctor should check your progress at regular visits, especially during the first few months of treatment with this medicine. This will allow your dosage to be changed if necessary to meet your needs.

Do not stop taking this medicine without first checking with your doctor. Your doctor may want you to reduce gradually the amount you are taking before stopping completely. This is to prevent side effects and to keep your condition from becoming worse.

Do not take this medicine within two hours of taking antacids or medicine for diarrhea. Taking these products too close together may make this medicine less effective.

This medicine will add to the effects of alcohol and other CNS depressants (medicines that slow down the nervous system, possibly causing drowsiness). Some examples of CNS depressants are antihistamines or medicine for hay fever, other allergies, or colds; sedatives, tranquilizers, or sleeping medicine; prescription pain medicine or narcotics; barbiturates; medicine for seizures; muscle relaxants; or anesthetics, including some dental anesthetics. *Check with your doctor before taking any of the above while you are using this medicine.*

Before using any prescription or over-the-counter (OTC) medicine for colds or allergies, check with your doctor. These medicines may increase the chance of heat stroke or other unwanted effects, such as dizziness, dry mouth, blurred vision, and constipation, while you are taking a phenothiazine.

Before you have any medical tests, tell the medical doctor in charge that you are taking this medicine. The results of some tests (such as electrocardiogram [ECG] readings, certain pregnancy tests, the metyrapone test, and urine bilirubin tests) may be affected by this medicine.

Before having any kind of surgery, dental treatment, or emergency treatment, tell the medical doctor or dentist in charge that you are using this medicine.

This medicine may cause some people to become drowsy or less alert than they are normally. Even if this medicine is taken only at bedtime, it may cause some people to feel drowsy or less alert on arising. *Make sure you know how you react to this medicine before you drive, use machines, or do anything else that could be dangerous if you are not alert.*

Phenothiazines may cause blurred vision, difficulty in reading, or other changes in vision, especially during the first few weeks of treatment. Do not drive, use machines, or do anything else that could be dangerous if you are not able to see well. *If the problem continues or gets worse, check with your doctor.*

Dizziness, lightheadedness, or fainting may occur, especially when you get up from a lying or sitting position. Getting up slowly may help. If the problem continues or gets worse, check with your doctor.

This medicine may make you sweat less, causing your body temperature to increase. *Use extra care not to become overheated during exercise or hot weather while you are taking this medicine,* since overheating may result in heat stroke. Also, hot baths or saunas may make you feel dizzy or faint while you are taking this medicine.

This medicine may also make you more sensitive to cold temperatures. Dress warmly during cold weather. Be careful during prolonged exposure to cold, such as in winter sports or swimming in cold water.

Phenothiazines may cause dryness of the mouth. For temporary relief, use sugarless candy or gum, melt bits of ice in your mouth, or use a saliva substitute. However, if your mouth continues to feel dry for more than 2 weeks, check with your medical doctor or dentist. Continuing dryness of the mouth may increase the chance of dental disease, including tooth decay, gum disease, and fungus infections.

Phenothiazines may cause your skin to be more sensitive to sunlight than it is normally. Exposure to sunlight, even for brief periods of time, may cause a skin rash, itching, redness or other discoloration of the skin, or a severe sunburn. When you begin taking this medicine:

- Stay out of direct sunlight, especially between the hours of 10:00 a.m. and 3:00 p.m., if possible.
- Wear protective clothing, including a hat. Also, wear sunglasses.
- Apply a sun block product that has a skin protection factor (SPF) of at least 15. Some patients may require a product with a higher SPF number, especially if they have a fair complexion. If you have any questions about this, check with your health care professional.
- Apply a sun block lipstick that has an SPF of at least 15 to protect your lips.
- Do not use a sunlamp or tanning bed or booth.

If you have a severe reaction from the sun, check with your doctor.

Phenothiazines may cause your eyes to be more sensitive to sunlight than they are normally. Exposure to sunlight over a period of time (several months to years) may cause blurred vision, change in color vision, or difficulty in seeing at night. When you go out during the daylight hours, even on cloudy days, wear sunglasses that block ultraviolet (UV) light. Ordinary sunglasses may not protect your eyes. If you have any questions about the kind of sunglasses to wear, check with your medical doctor or eye doctor.

If you are taking a liquid form of this medicine, avoid getting it on your skin or clothing because it may cause a skin rash or other irritation.

If you are receiving this medicine by injection:

- The effects of the long-acting injection form of this medicine may last for up to 12 weeks. *The precautions and side effects information for this medicine applies during this time.*

Side Effects of This Medicine

Along with their needed effects, phenothiazines can sometimes cause serious side effects. Tardive dyskinesia (a movement disorder) may occur and may not go away after you stop using the medicine. Signs of tardive dyskinesia include fine, worm-like movements of the tongue, or other uncontrolled movements of the mouth, tongue, cheeks, jaw, or arms and legs. Other serious but rare side effects may also occur. These include severe muscle stiffness, fever, unusual tiredness or weakness, fast heartbeat, difficult breathing, increased sweating, loss of bladder control, and seizures (neuroleptic malignant syndrome). *You and your doctor should discuss the good this medicine will do as well as the risks of taking it.*

Stop taking this medicine and check with your doctor immediately if any of the following side effects occur:

Rare

Convulsions (seizures); difficult or fast breathing; fast

heartbeat or irregular pulse; fever; high or low blood pressure; increased sweating; loss of bladder control; muscle stiffness (severe); unusually pale skin; unusual tiredness or weakness

Check with your doctor immediately if any of the following side effects occur:

More common

Lip smacking or puckering; puffing of cheeks; rapid or fine, worm-like movements of tongue; uncontrolled chewing movements; uncontrolled movements of arms or legs

Also, check with your doctor as soon as possible if any of the following side effects occur:

More common

Blurred vision, change in color vision, or difficulty in seeing at night; difficulty in speaking or swallowing; fainting; inability to move eyes; loss of balance control; mask-like face; muscle spasms (especially of face, neck, and back); restlessness or need to keep moving; shuffling walk; stiffness of arms or legs; tic-like or twitching movements; trembling and shaking of hands and fingers; twisting movements of body; weakness of arms and legs

Less common

Difficulty in urinating; skin rash; sunburn (severe)

Rare

Abdominal or stomach pains; aching muscles and joints; confusion; fever and chills; hot, dry skin or lack of sweating; muscle weakness; nausea, vomiting, or diarrhea; painful, inappropriate penile erection (continuing); skin discoloration (tan or blue-gray); skin itching (severe); sore throat and fever; unusual bleeding or bruising; yellow eyes or skin

Other side effects may occur that usually do not need medical attention. These side effects may go away during treatment as your body adjusts to the medicine. However,

check with your doctor if any of the following side effects continue or are bothersome:

More common

   Constipation; decreased sweating; dizziness; drowsiness; dryness of mouth; nasal congestion

Less common

   Changes in menstrual period; decreased sexual ability; increased sensitivity of skin to sunlight (skin rash, itching, redness or other discoloration of skin, or severe sunburn); swelling or pain in breasts; unusual secretion of milk; weight gain (unusual)

After you stop using this medicine, your body may need time to adjust. The length of time this takes depends on the amount of medicine you are using and how long you used it. During this time, check with your doctor if you notice dizziness, nausea and vomiting, stomach pain, trembling of the fingers and hands, or any of the following symptoms of tardive dyskinesia:

   Lip smacking or puckering; puffing of cheeks; rapid or fine, worm-like movements of tongue; uncontrolled chewing movements; uncontrolled movements of arms or legs

Although not all of the side effects listed above have been reported for all of these medicines, they have been reported for at least one of them. However, since all of the phenothiazines are very similar, any of the above side effects may occur with any of these medicines.

Other side effects not listed above may also occur in some patients. If you notice any other effects, check with your doctor.

Additional Information

Once a medicine has been approved for marketing for a certain use, experience may show that it is also useful for other medical problems. Although these uses are not in-

cluded in product labeling, phenothiazines are used in certain patients with the following medical conditions:

- Chronic neurogenic pain (certain continuing pain conditions)
- Huntington's chorea (hereditary movement disorder)

Other than the above information, there is no additional information relating to proper use, precautions, or side effects for these uses.

PILOCARPINE   Systemic†

A commonly used brand name in the U.S. is Salagen.

†Not commercially available in Canada.

Description

Pilocarpine (pye-loe-KAR-peen) tablets are used to treat dryness of the mouth and throat caused by a decrease in the amount of saliva that may occur after radiation treatment for cancer of the head and neck. This medicine may help you speak without having to sip liquids. It may also help with chewing, tasting, and swallowing. This medicine may reduce your need for other oral comfort agents, such as hard candy, sugarless gum, or artificial saliva agents.

This medicine is available only with your doctor's prescription, in the following dosage form:

Oral
- Tablets (U.S.)

Before Using This Medicine

In deciding to use a medicine, the risks of using the medicine must be weighed against the good it will do. This is

a decision you and your doctor will make. For pilocarpine, the following should be considered:

Allergies—Tell your doctor if you have ever had any unusual or allergic reaction to pilocarpine taken by mouth or used in the eye. Also tell your health care professional if you are allergic to any other substances, such as foods, preservatives, or dyes.

Pregnancy—Pilocarpine has not been studied in pregnant women. However, studies in animals have shown that pilocarpine, when given in very high doses, may cause birth defects. Before using this medicine, make sure your doctor knows if you are pregnant or if you may become pregnant.

Breast-feeding—It is not known whether pilocarpine passes into the breast milk. However, this medicine has not been reported to cause problems in nursing babies.

Children—Studies on this medicine have been done only in adult patients and there is no specific information comparing use of pilocarpine in children with use in other age groups.

Older adults—This medicine has been tested and has not been shown to cause different side effects or problems in older people than it does in younger adults.

Other medicines—Although certain medicines should not be used together at all, in other cases two different medicines may be used together even if an interaction might occur. In these cases, your doctor may want to change the dose, or other precautions may be necessary. When you are using pilocarpine, it is especially important that your health care professional know if you are taking any of the following:

- Amantadine (e.g., Symmetrel) or
- Anticholinergics (medicine for abdominal or stomach spasms or cramps) or
- Antidepressants (medicine for depression) or

- Antidyskinetics (medicine for Parkinson's disease or other conditions affecting control of muscles) or
- Antihistamines or
- Antipsychotics (medicine for mental illness) or
- Buclizine (e.g., Bucladin) or
- Carbamazepine (e.g., Tegretol) or
- Cyclizine (e.g., Marezine) or
- Cyclobenzaprine (e.g., Flexeril) or
- Disopyramide (e.g., Norpace) or
- Flavoxate (e.g., Urispas) or
- Ipratropium (e.g., Atrovent) or
- Meclizine (e.g., Antivert) or
- Methylphenidate (e.g., Ritalin) or
- Orphenadrine (e.g., Norflex) or
- Oxybutynin (e.g., Ditropen) or
- Procainamide (e.g., Pronestyl) or
- Promethazine (e.g., Phenergan) or
- Quinidine (e.g., Quinidex) or
- Trimeprazine (e.g., Temaril)—Pilocarpine may reduce the effect of these medicines or these medicines may reduce the effects of pilocarpine
- Antimyasthenics (ambenonium [e.g., Mytelase], neostigmine [e.g., Prostigmin], pyridostigmine [Mestinon]) or
- Beta-adrenergic blocking agents (acebutolol [e.g., Sectral], atenolol [e.g., Tenormin], betaxolol [e.g., Kerlone], carteolol [e.g., Cartrol], labetalol [e.g., Normodyne], metoprolol [e.g., Lopressor], nadolol [e.g., Corgard], oxprenolol [e.g., Trasicor], penbutolol [e.g., Levatol], pindolol [e.g., Visken], propranolol [e.g., Inderal], sotalol [e.g., Sotacor], timolol [e.g., Blocadren]) or
- Bethanechol (e.g., Urecholine) or
- Ophthalmic beta-adrenergic blocking agents (betaxolol [e.g., Betoptic], carteolol [e.g., Ocupress], levobunolol [e.g., Betagan], metipranolol [e.g., OptiPranolol], timolol [e.g., Timoptic])—Pilocarpine may increase the side effects of these medicines

- Carbachol (e.g., Isopto Carbachol) or
- Demecarium (e.g., Humorsol) or
- Echothiophate (e.g., Phospholine Iodide) or
- Isoflurophate (e.g., Floropryl) or
- Physostigmine (e.g., Isopto Eserine) or

- Pilocarpine (ophthalmic) (e.g., Isopto Carpine)—Pilocarpine may increase the effects of these ophthalmic glaucoma medicines

Other medical problems—The presence of other medical problems may affect the use of pilocarpine. Make sure you tell your doctor if you have any other medical problems, especially:

- Asthma, bronchitis, or other breathing problems, or
- Gallbladder problems or
- Glaucoma, angle closure, or
- Heart or blood vessel disease or
- Iritis (inflammation of the iris [colored part] of the eye) or
- Kidney problems or
- Mental problems—Pilocarpine may make the condition worse
- Retinal detachment, tendency for, or
- Retinal disease—Pilocarpine may increase the risk of a detached retina

---

Proper Use of This Medicine

Take this medicine only as directed. Do not take it more often and do not take a larger dose than directed. To do so may increase the chance of side effects.

It is important that you visit your dentist regularly even though this medicine may make your dry mouth feel better. Having a dry mouth condition makes you more likely to have dental and other mouth problems.

Dosing—The dose of pilocarpine will be different for different patients. *Follow your doctor's orders or the directions on the label.* The following information includes only the average dose of pilocarpine. *If your dose is different, do not change it* unless your doctor tells you to do so.

- For *oral* dosage form (tablets):
    - —For dryness of mouth and throat:

• Adults—5 milligrams (mg) three times a day.

• Children—Use and dose must be determined by your doctor.

Missed dose—If you miss a dose of this medicine, take it as soon as possible. However, if it is almost time for your next dose, skip the missed dose and go back to your regular dosing schedule. Do not double doses.

Storage—To store this medicine:

• *Keep out of the reach of children.*

• Store away from heat and direct light.

• Do not store in the bathroom, near the kitchen sink, or in other damp places. Heat or moisture may cause the medicine to break down.

• Do not keep outdated medicine or medicine no longer needed. Be sure that any discarded medicine is out of the reach of children.

Precautions While Using This Medicine

This medicine may cause difficulty in reading or other vision problems, especially at night. It may also cause some people to become dizzy or lightheaded. *Make sure you know how you react to this medicine before you drive, use machines, or do anything else that could be dangerous if you are not alert or able to see well.* If these reactions are especially bothersome, check with your doctor.

This medicine may cause you to sweat more than is usual. *If you do, it is important that you drink extra liquids to offset this sweating so you do not lose too much fluid and become dehydrated.* Check with your doctor if you are not sure how much extra liquid to drink or if you cannot drink as much liquid as you should.

Side Effects of This Medicine

Along with its needed effects, a medicine may cause some unwanted effects. Although not all of these side effects may occur, if they do occur they may need medical attention.

Check with your doctor as soon as possible if any of the following side effects occur:

Symptoms of overdose

> Chest pain; confusion; diarrhea (continuing or severe); fainting; fast, slow, or irregular heartbeat (continuing or severe); headache (continuing or severe); nausea or vomiting (continuing or severe); shortness of breath or troubled breathing; stomach cramps or pain; tiredness or weakness (continuing or severe); trembling or shaking (continuing or severe); trouble seeing (continuing or severe)

Other side effects may occur that usually do not need medical attention. These side effects may go away during treatment as your body adjusts to the medicine. However, check with your doctor if any of the following side effects continue or are bothersome:

More common

> Sweating

Less common or rare

> Chills; diarrhea; dizziness; fast heartbeat; headache; holding more body water; indigestion; nausea; nosebleeds; passing urine more often; redness of face or feeling of warmth; runny nose; swelling of face, fingers, ankles, or feet; trembling or shaking; trouble swallowing; trouble seeing; unusual weak feeling; voice change; vomiting

Other side effects not listed above may also occur in some patients. If you notice any other effects, check with your doctor.

POTASSIUM SUPPLEMENTS Systemic

Some commonly used brand names are:

In the U.S.—

Cena-K[5]
Effer-K[4]
Gen-K[5]
K+ 10[5]
Kaochlor 10%[5]
Kaochlor-Eff[6]
Kaochlor S-F 10%[5]
Kaon[7]
Kaon-Cl[5]
Kaon-Cl-10[5]
Kaon-Cl 20% Liquid[5]
Kato[5]
Kay Ciel[5]
Kaylixir[7]
K+ Care[5]
K+ Care ET[2]
K-Dur[5]
K-G Elixir[7]
K-Ide[2,5]
K-Lease[5]
K-Lor[5]
Klor-Con 8[5]
Klor-Con 10[5]
Klor-Con/EF[2]
Klor-Con Powder[5]

Klor-Con/25 Powder[5]
Klorvess[3]
Klorvess Effervescent
  Granules[3]
Klorvess 10% Liquid[5]
Klotrix[5]
K-Lyte[2]
K-Lyte/Cl[3]
K-Lyte/Cl 50[3]
K-Lyte/Cl Powder[5]
K-Lyte DS[4]
K-Norm[5]
Kolyum[8]
K-Tab[5]
Micro-K[5]
Micro-K 10[5]
Micro-K LS[5]
Potage[5]
Potasalan[5]
Rum-K[5]
Slow-K[5]
Ten-K[5]
Tri-K[10]
Twin-K[9]

In Canada—

Apo-K[5]
K-10[5]
Kalium Durules[5]
Kaochlor-10[5]
Kaochlor-20[5]
Kaon[7]
KCL 5%[5]
K-Dur[5]
K-Long[5]
K-Lor[5]
Klor-Con/EF[2]

K-Lyte[2]
K-Lyte/Cl[5]
Micro-K[5]
Micro-K 10[5]
Neo-K[3]
Novolente-K[5]
Potassium-Rougier[7]
Potassium-Sandoz[3]
Roychlor-10%[5]
Slow-K[5]

Note: For quick reference, the following potassium supplements are numbered to match the corresponding brand names.

This information applies to the following medicines:

1. Potassium Acetate (poe-TAS-ee-um AS-a-tate)‡§
2. Potassium Bicarbonate (bi-KAR-bo-nate)
3. Potassium Bicarbonate and Potassium Chloride (KLOR-ide)
4. Potassium Bicarbonate and Potassium Citrate (SIH-trayt)†
5. Potassium Chloride‡§
6. Potassium Chloride, Potassium Bicarbonate, and Potassium Citrate†
7. Potassium Gluconate (GLOO-ko-nate)‡
8. Potassium Gluconate and Potassium Chloride†
9. Potassium Gluconate and Potassium Citrate†
10. Trikates (TRI-kates)‡

---

†Not commercially available in Canada.
‡Generic name product may be available in the U.S.
§Generic name product may be available in Canada.

Description

Potassium is needed to maintain good health. Although a balanced diet usually supplies all the potassium a person needs, potassium supplements may be needed by patients who do not have enough potassium in their regular diet or have lost too much potassium because of illness or treatment with certain medicines.

There is no evidence that potassium supplements are useful in the treatment of high blood pressure.

Lack of potassium may cause muscle weakness, irregular heartbeat, mood changes, or nausea and vomiting.

Some forms of potassium may be available in stores without a prescription. Since too much potassium may cause health problems, you should take potassium supplements only if directed by your doctor. Potassium supplements are available with your doctor's prescription in the following dosage forms:

Oral

Potassium Bicarbonate
• Tablets for solution (U.S. and Canada)

Potassium Bicarbonate and Potassium Chloride
- Powder for solution (U.S. and Canada)
- Tablets for solution (U.S. and Canada)

Potassium Bicarbonate and Potassium Citrate
- Tablets for solution (U.S.)

Potassium Chloride
- Extended-release capsules (U.S. and Canada)
- Solution (U.S. and Canada)
- Powder for solution (U.S. and Canada)
- Powder for suspension (U.S.)
- Extended-release tablets (U.S. and Canada)

Potassium Chloride, Potassium Bicarbonate, and Potassium Citrate
- Tablets for solution (U.S.)

Potassium Gluconate
- Elixir (U.S. and Canada)
- Tablets (U.S.)

Potassium Gluconate and Potassium Chloride
- Solution (U.S.)
- Powder for solution (U.S.)

Potassium Gluconate and Potassium Citrate
- Solution (U.S.)

Trikates
- Solution (U.S.)

Parenteral

Potassium Acetate
- Injection (U.S. and Canada)

Potassium Chloride
- Concentrate for injection (U.S. and Canada)

Importance of Diet

Many nutritionists recommend that, if possible, people get the potassium they need from the foods they eat. However, many people do not get enough potassium from their diets. For example, people on weight-loss diets may consume too little food to get enough potassium. Others may lose potassium from the body because of illness or treatment with certain medicines. For such people, a potassium supplement, given under a doctor's supervision, is important.

In order to get enough vitamins and minerals in your diet, it is important that you eat a balanced and varied diet. Follow carefully any diet program your doctor may recommend. For your specific vitamin and/or mineral needs, ask your doctor for a list of appropriate foods.

The following table includes some potassium-rich foods.

Food (amount)	Milligrams of potassium	Milli-equivalents of potassium
Acorn squash, cooked (1 cup)	896	23
Potato with skin, baked (1 long)	844	22
Spinach, cooked (1 cup)	838	21
Lentils, cooked (1 cup)	731	19
Kidney beans, cooked (1 cup)	713	18
Split peas, cooked (1 cup)	710	18
White navy beans, cooked (1 cup)	669	17
Butternut squash, cooked (1 cup)	583	15
Watermelon (1/16)	560	14
Raisins (1/2 cup)	553	14
Yogurt, low-fat, plain (1 cup)	531	14
Orange juice, frozen (1 cup)	503	13
Brussel sprouts, cooked (1 cup)	494	13
Zucchini, cooked, sliced (1 cup)	456	12
Banana (medium)	451	12
Collards, frozen, cooked (1 cup)	427	11
Cantaloupe (1/4)	412	11
Milk, low-fat 1% (1 cup)	348	9
Broccoli, frozen, cooked (1 cup)	332	9

Experts have developed a list of recommended dietary allowances (RDA) for most of the vitamins and some minerals. The RDA are not an exact number but a general idea of how much you need. They do not cover amounts needed for problems caused by a serious lack of vitamins or minerals. Because lack of potassium is rare, there are no RDA for this mineral. However, it is thought that 1600 to 2000 mg (40 to 50 mEq) per day for adults is adequate.

Remember:

- The total amount of potassium that you get every day includes what you get from food *and* what you may take as a supplement. Read the labels of processed foods. Many foods now have added potassium.

- Your total intake of potassium should not be greater than the recommended amounts, unless ordered by your doctor. In some cases, too much potassium may cause muscle weakness, confusion, irregular heartbeat, or difficult breathing.

Before Using This Medicine

In deciding to use a medicine, the risks of taking the medicine must be weighed against the good it will do. This is a decision you and your doctor will make. For potassium supplements, the following should be considered:

Allergies—Tell your doctor if you have ever had any unusual or allergic reaction to potassium preparations. Also tell your health care professional if you are allergic to any other substances, such as foods, preservatives, or dyes.

Pregnancy—Potassium supplements have not been shown to cause problems in humans.

Breast-feeding—Potassium supplements pass into breast milk. However, this medicine has not been reported to cause problems in nursing babies.

Children—Although there is no specific information comparing use of potassium supplements in children with use in other age groups, they are not expected to cause different side effects or problems in children than they do in adults.

Older adults—Many medicines have not been studied specifically in older people. Therefore, it may not be known whether they work exactly the same way they do in younger adults. Although there is no specific information comparing use of potassium supplements in the elderly with use in other age groups, they are not expected to cause different side effects or problems in older people than they do in younger adults.

Older adults may be at a greater risk of developing high blood levels of potassium (hyperkalemia).

Other medicines—Although certain medicines should not be used together at all, in other cases two different medicines may be used together even if an interaction might occur. In these cases, your doctor may want to change the dose, or other precautions may be necessary. When you are taking potassium supplements, it is especially important that your health care professional know if you are taking any of the following:

- Amantadine (e.g., Symmetrel) or
- Anticholinergics (medicine for abdominal or stomach spasms or cramps) or
- Antidepressants (medicine for depression) or
- Antidyskinetics (medicine for Parkinson's disease or other conditions affecting control of muscles) or
- Antihistamines or
- Antipsychotic medicine (medicine for mental illness) or
- Buclizine (e.g., Bucladin) or
- Carbamazepine (e.g., Tegretol) or
- Cyclizine (e.g., Marezine) or
- Cyclobenzaprine (e.g., Flexeril) or
- Disopyramide (e.g., Norpace) or
- Flavoxate (e.g., Urispas) or
- Ipratropium (e.g., Atrovent) or
- Meclizine (e.g., Antivert) or
- Methylphenidate (e.g., Ritalin) or
- Orphenadrine (e.g., Norflex) or
- Oxybutynin (e.g., Ditropan) or
- Procainamide (e.g., Pronestyl) or
- Promethazine (e.g., Phenergan) or
- Quinidine (e.g., Quinidex) or

- Trimeprazine (e.g., Temaril)—Use with potassium supplements may cause or worsen certain stomach or intestine problems
- Angiotensin-converting enzyme (ACE) inhibitors (benazepril [e.g., Lotensin], captopril [e.g., Capoten], enalapril [e.g., Vasotec], fosinopril [e.g., Monotril], lisinopril [e.g., Prinivil, Zestril], quinapril [e.g., Accupril], ramipril [e.g., Altace]) or
- Amiloride (e.g., Midamor) or
- Beta-adrenergic blocking agents (acebutolol [e.g., Sectral], atenolol [e.g., Tenormin], betaxolol [e.g., Kerlone], carteolol [e.g., Cartrol], labetalol [e.g., Normodyne], metoprolol [e.g., Lopressor], nadolol [e.g., Corgard], oxprenolol [e.g., Trasicor], penbutolol [e.g., Levatol], pindolol [e.g., Visken], propranolol [e.g., Inderal], sotalol [e.g., Sotacor], timolol [e.g., Blocadren]) or
- Heparin (e.g., Panheprin) or
- Inflammation or pain medicine (except narcotics) or
- Potassium-containing medicines (other) or
- Salt substitutes, low-salt foods, or milk or
- Spironolactone (e.g., Aldactone) or
- Triamterene (e.g., Dyrenium)—Use with potassium supplements may further increase potassium blood levels, which may cause or worsen heart problems
- Digitalis glycosides (heart medicine)—Use with potassium supplements may make heart problems worse
- Thiazide diuretics (water pills)—If you have been taking a potassium supplement and a thiazide diuretic together, stopping the thiazide diuretic may cause hyperkalemia (high blood levels of potassium)

Other medical problems—The presence of other medical problems may affect the use of potassium supplements. Make sure you tell your doctor if you have any other medical problems, especially:

- Addison's disease (underactive adrenal glands) or
- Dehydration (excessive loss of body water, continuing or severe)
- Diabetes mellitus or
- Kidney disease—Potassium supplements may increase the

risk of hyperkalemia (high blood levels of potassium), which may worsen or cause heart problems in patients with these conditions

- Diarrhea (continuing or severe)—The loss of fluid in combination with potassium supplements may cause kidney problems, which may increase the risk of hyperkalemia (high blood levels of potassium)

- Heart disease—Potassium supplements may make this condition worse

- Intestinal or esophageal blockage—Potassium supplements may damage the intestines

- Stomach ulcer—Potassium supplements may make this condition worse

---

Proper Use of This Medicine

For patients taking the *liquid form* of this medicine:

- This medicine *must be diluted* in at least one-half glass (4 ounces) of cold water or juice to reduce its possible stomach-irritating or laxative effect.

- If you are on a salt (sodium)-restricted diet, check with your doctor before using tomato juice to dilute your medicine. Tomato juice has a high salt content.

For patients taking the *soluble granule, soluble powder, or soluble tablet form* of this medicine:

- This medicine must be completely dissolved in at least one-half glass (4 ounces) of cold water or juice to reduce its possible stomach-irritating or laxative effect.

- Allow any "fizzing" to stop before taking the dissolved medicine.

- If you are on a salt (sodium)-restricted diet, check with your doctor before using tomato juice to dilute your medicine. Tomato juice has a high salt content.

For patients taking the *extended-release tablet form* of this medicine:

- Swallow the tablets whole with a full (8-ounce) glass of water. Do not chew or suck on the tablet.

- Some tablets may be broken or crushed and sprinkled on applesauce or other soft food. However, check with your health care professional first, since this should not be done for most tablets.

- If you have trouble swallowing tablets or if they seem to stick in your throat, check with your doctor. When this medicine is not properly released, it can cause irritation that may lead to ulcers.

For patients taking the *extended-release capsule form* of this medicine:

- Do not crush or chew the capsule. Swallow the capsule whole with a full (8-ounce) glass of water.

- Some capsules may be opened and the contents sprinkled on applesauce or other soft food. However, check with your health care professional first, since this should not be done for most capsules.

Take this medicine immediately after meals or with food to lessen possible stomach upset or laxative action.

Take this medicine only as directed by your doctor. Do not take more of it, do not take it more often, and do not take it for a longer time than your doctor ordered. *This is especially important if you are also taking both diuretics (water pills) and digitalis medicines for your heart.*

Dosing—The dose of these single or combination medicines will be different for different patients. *Follow your doctor's orders or the directions on the label.* The following information includes only the average dose of these medicines. *If your dose is different, do not change it* unless your doctor tells you to do so.

The number of ounces of solution that you drink, or the number of tablets or capsules you take, depends on the strength of the medicine. Also, *the number of doses you take each day, the time allowed between doses, and the length of time you take the medicine depend on the medical problem for which you are taking the single or combination medicine.*

For potassium bicarbonate

- For *oral* dosage form (tablets for solution):

  —To replace potassium lost by the body:

    • Adults and teenagers—25 to 50 milliequivalents (mEq) dissolved in one-half to one glass of cold water, taken one or two times a day. Your doctor may change the dose if needed. However, most people will not take more than 100 mEq a day.

    • Children—Dose must be determined by your doctor.

For potassium bicarbonate and potassium chloride

- For *oral* dosage form (granules for solution):

  —To replace potassium lost by the body:

    • Adults and teenagers—20 milliequivalents (mEq) dissolved in one-half to one glass of cold water, taken one or two times a day. Your doctor may change the dose if needed. However, most people will not take more than 100 mEq a day.

    • Children—Dose must be determined by your doctor.

- For *oral* dosage form (tablets for solution):

  —To replace potassium lost by the body:

    • Adults and teenagers—20, 25, or 50 mEq dissolved in one-half to one glass of cold water, taken one or two times a day. Your doctor may change the dose if needed. However, most people will not take more than 100 mEq a day.

    • Children—Dose must be determined by your doctor.

For potassium bicarbonate and potassium citrate

- For *oral* dosage form (tablets for solution):

—To replace potassium lost by the body:

• Adults and teenagers—25 or 50 milliequivalents (mEq) dissolved in one-half to one glass of cold water, taken one or two times a day. Your doctor may change the dose if needed. However, most people will not take more than 100 mEq a day.

• Children—Dose must be determined by your doctor.

For potassium chloride

• For *oral* dosage form (extended-release capsules):

—To replace potassium lost by the body:

• Adults and teenagers—40 to 100 milliequivalents (mEq) a day, divided into two or three smaller doses during the day. Your doctor may change the dose if needed. However, most people will not take more than 100 mEq a day.

—To prevent potassium loss:

• Adults and teenagers—16 to 24 mEq a day, divided into two or three smaller doses during the day. Your doctor may change the dose if needed. However, most people will not take more than 100 mEq a day.

• Children—Dose must be determined by your doctor.

• For *oral* dosage form (liquid for solution):

—To replace potassium lost by the body:

• Adults and teenagers—20 mEq mixed into one-half glass of cold water or juice, taken one to four times a day. Your doctor may change the dose if needed. However, most people will not take more than 100 mEq a day.

• Children—Dose is based on body weight and must be determined by your doctor. The usual dose is 1 to 3 mEq of potassium per kilogram (kg) (0.45 to 1.36 mEq per pound) of body weight taken in smaller doses during the day. The solution should be well mixed in water or juice.

• For *oral* dosage form (powder for solution):

—To replace potassium lost by the body:

• Adults and teenagers—15 to 25 mEq dissolved in four to six ounces of cold water, taken two or four times a day. Your doctor may change the dose if needed. However, most people will not take more than 100 mEq a day.

• Children—Dose is based on body weight and must be determined by your doctor. The usual dose is 1 to 3 mEq per kg (0.45 to 1.36 mEq per pound) of body weight taken in smaller doses during the day. The solution should be mixed into water or juice.

• For *oral* dosage form (powder for suspension):

—To replace potassium lost by the body:

• Adults and teenagers—20 mEq dissolved in two to six ounces of cold water, taken one to five times a day. Your doctor may change the dose if needed. However, most people will not take more than 100 mEq a day.

• Children—Dose must be determined by your doctor.

• For *oral* dosage form (extended-release tablets):

—To replace potassium lost by the body:

• Adults and teenagers—6.7 to 20 mEq taken three times a day. However, most people will not take more than 100 mEq a day.

• Children—Dose must be determined by your doctor.

For potassium chloride, potassium bicarbonate and potassium citrate

• For *oral* dosage form (tablets for solution):

—To replace potassium lost by the body:

• Adults and teenagers—20 milliequivalents (mEq) dissolved in one-half to one glass of cold water, taken one to four times a day. Your doctor may change the dose if needed. However, most people will not take more than 100 mEq a day.

• Children—Dose must be determined by your doctor.

For potassium gluconate

• For *oral* dosage form (liquid for solution):

—To replace potassium lost by the body:

• Adults and teenagers—20 milliequivalents (mEq) mixed into one-half glass of cold water or juice, taken two to four times a day. Your doctor may change the dose if needed. However, most people will not take more than 100 mEq a day.

• Children—Dose is based on body weight and must be determined by your doctor. The usual dose is 2 to 3 mEq per kilogram (kg) (0.9 to 1.36 mEq per pound) of body weight a day, taken in smaller doses during the day. The solution should be completely mixed into water or juice.

• For *oral* dosage form (tablets):

—To replace potassium lost by the body:

• Adults and teenagers—5 to 10 mEq taken two to four times a day. However, most people will not take more than 100 mEq a day.

• Children—Dose must be determined by your doctor.

For potassium gluconate and potassium chloride

• For *oral* dosage form (liquid for solution):

—To replace potassium lost by the body:

• Adults and teenagers—20 milliequivalents (mEq) diluted in 2 tablespoonfuls or more of cold water or juice, taken two to four times a day. Your doctor may change the dose if needed.

However, most people will not take more than 100 mEq a day.

• Children—Dose is based on body weight and must be determined by your doctor. The usual dose is 2 to 3 mEq per kilogram (kg) (0.9 to 1.36 mEq per pound) of body weight taken in smaller doses during the day. The solution should be well mixed into water or juice.

• For *oral* dosage form (powder for solution):

  —To replace potassium lost by the body:

• Adults and teenagers—20 mEq mixed in 2 tablespoonfuls or more of cold water or juice taken two to four times a day. Your doctor may change the dose if needed. However, most people will not take more than 100 mEq a day.

• Children—Dose is base on body weight and must be determined by your doctor. The usual dose is 2 to 3 mEq per kg (0.9 to 1.36 mEq per pound) of body weight taken in smaller doses during the day. The solution should be well mixed into water or juice.

For potassium gluconate and potassium citrate

• For *oral* dosage form (liquid for solution):

  —To replace potassium lost by the body:

• Adults and teenagers—20 milliequivalents (mEq) mixed into one-half glass of cold water or juice, taken two to four times a day. Your doctor may change the dose if needed. However, most people will not take more than 100 mEq a day.

• Children—Dose is based on body weight and must be determined by your doctor. The usual dose is 2 to 3 mEq per kg (0.9 to 1.36 mEq per pound) of body weight taken in smaller doses during the day. The solution should be well mixed into water or juice.

For trikates
- For *oral* dosage form (liquid for solution):
  —To replace potassium lost by the body:
    - Adults and teenagers—15 milliequivalents (mEq) mixed into one-half glass of cold water or juice, taken three or four times a day. Your doctor may change the dose if needed. However, most people will not take more than 100 mEq a day.
    - Children—Dose is based on body weight and must be determined by your doctor. The usual dose is 2 to 3 mEq per kilogram (kg) (0.9 to 1.36 mEq per pound) of body weight taken in smaller doses during the day. The solution should be well mixed into water or juice.

Missed dose—If you miss a dose of this medicine and remember within 2 hours, take the missed dose right away with food or liquids. Then go back to your regular dosing schedule. However, if you do not remember until later, skip the missed dose and go back to your regular dosing schedule. Do not double doses.

Storage—To store this medicine:
- Keep out of the reach of children.
- Store away from heat and direct light.
- Do not store in the bathroom, near the kitchen sink, or in other damp places. Heat or moisture may cause the medicine to break down.
- Keep the liquid form of this medicine from freezing.
- Do not keep outdated medicine or medicine no longer needed. Be sure that any discarded medicine is out of the reach of children.

Precautions While Using This Medicine

Your doctor should check your progress at regular visits to make sure the medicine is working properly and that possible side effects are avoided. Laboratory tests may be necessary.

Do not use salt substitutes, eat low-sodium foods, especially some breads and canned foods, or drink low-sodium milk unless you are told to do so by your doctor, since these products may contain potassium. It is important to read the labels carefully on all low-sodium food products.

Check with your doctor before starting any physical exercise program, especially if you are out of condition and are taking any other medicine. Exercise and certain medicines may increase the amount of potassium in the blood.

Check with your doctor at once if you notice blackish stools or other signs of stomach or intestinal bleeding. This medicine may cause such a condition to become worse, especially when taken in tablet form.

Side Effects of This Medicine

Along with its needed effects, a medicine may cause some unwanted effects. Although not all of these side effects may occur, if they do occur they may need medical attention.

Stop taking this medicine and check with your doctor immediately if any of the following side effects occur:

Less common

> Confusion; irregular or slow heartbeat; numbness or tingling in hands, feet, or lips; shortness of breath or difficult breathing; unexplained anxiety; unusual tiredness or weakness; weakness or heaviness of legs

Also, check with your doctor if any of the following side effects occur:

Rare

> Abdominal or stomach pain, cramping, or soreness (continuing); chest or throat pain, especially when swallowing; stools with signs of blood (red or black color)

Other side effects may occur that usually do not need medical attention. These side effects may go away during treatment as your body adjusts to the medicine. However, check with your doctor if any of the following side effects continue or are bothersome:

More common

Diarrhea; nausea; stomach pain, discomfort, or gas (mild); vomiting

Sometimes you may see what appears to be a whole tablet in the stool after taking certain extended-release potassium chloride tablets. This is to be expected. Your body has absorbed the potassium from the tablet and the shell is then expelled.

Other side effects not listed above may also occur in some patients. If you notice any other effects, check with your doctor.

PRAZOSIN Systemic

A commonly used brand name in the U.S. and Canada is Minipress. Generic name product may also be available.

Description

Prazosin (PRA-zoe-sin) belongs to the general class of medicines called antihypertensives. It is used to treat high blood pressure (hypertension).

High blood pressure adds to the work load of the heart and arteries. If it continues for a long time, the heart and arteries may not function properly. This can damage the blood vessels of the brain, heart, and kidneys, resulting in a stroke, heart failure, or kidney failure. High blood pressure may also increase the risk of heart attacks. These problems may be less likely to occur if blood pressure is controlled.

Prazosin works by relaxing blood vessels so that blood passes through them more easily. This helps to lower blood pressure.

Prazosin may also be used for other conditions as determined by your doctor.

Prazosin is available only with your doctor's prescription, in the following dosage forms:

Oral
- Capsules (U.S.)
- Tablets (Canada)

Before Using This Medicine

In deciding to use a medicine, the risks of taking the medicine must be weighed against the good it will do. This is a decision you and your doctor will make. For prazosin, the following should be considered:

Allergies—Tell your doctor if you have ever had any unusual or allergic reaction to prazosin, doxazosin, or terazosin. Also tell your health care professional if you are allergic to any other substance, such as foods, preservatives, or dyes.

Pregnancy—Limited use of prazosin to control high blood pressure in pregnant women has not shown that prazosin causes birth defects or other problems. Studies in animals given many times the highest recommended human dose of prazosin also have not shown that prazosin causes birth defects. However, in rats given many times the highest recommended human dose, lower birth weights were seen.

Breast-feeding—Prazosin passes into breast milk in small amounts. However, it has not been reported to cause problems in nursing babies.

Children—Studies on this medicine have been done only

in adult patients, and there is no specific information comparing use of prazosin in children with use in other age groups.

Older adults—Dizziness, lightheadedness, or fainting (especially when getting up from a lying or sitting position) may be more likely to occur in the elderly, who are more sensitive to the effects of prazosin. In addition, prazosin may reduce tolerance to cold temperatures in elderly patients.

Other medicines—Although certain medicines should not be used together at all, in other cases two different medicines may be used together even if an interaction might occur. In these cases, your doctor may want to change the dose, or other precautions may be necessary. Tell your health care professional if you are taking any other prescription or nonprescription (over-the-counter [OTC]) medicine.

Other medical problems—The presence of other medical problems may affect the use of prazosin. Make sure you tell your doctor if you have any other medical problems, especially:

- Angina (chest pain) or
- Heart disease (severe)—Prazosin may make these conditions worse
- Kidney disease—Possible increased sensitivity to the effects of prazosin

Proper Use of This Medicine

For patients *taking this medicine for high blood pressure:*

- In addition to the use of the medicine your doctor has prescribed, treatment for your high blood pressure may include weight control and care in the types of foods you eat, especially foods high in sodium. Your doctor will tell you which of these are most important for you. You should check with your doctor before changing your diet.

- Many patients who have high blood pressure will not notice any signs of the problem. In fact, many may feel normal. It is very important that you *take your medicine exactly as directed* and that you keep your appointments with your doctor even if you feel well.

- Remember that prazosin will not cure your high blood pressure but it does help control it. Therefore, you must continue to take it as directed if you expect to lower your blood pressure and keep it down. *You may have to take high blood pressure medicine for the rest of your life.* If high blood pressure is not treated, it can cause serious problems such as heart failure, blood vessel disease, stroke, or kidney disease.

To help you remember to take your medicine, try to get into the habit of taking it at the same time each day.

Dosing—The dose of prazosin will be different for different patients. *Follow your doctor's orders or the directions on the label.* The following information includes only the average doses of prazosin. *If your dose is different, do not change it* unless your doctor tells you to do so.

The number of capsules or tablets that you take depends on the strength of the medicine.

- For *oral* dosage form (capsules or tablets):
  —For high blood pressure:
  - Adults—At first, 0.5 or 1 milligram (mg) two or three times a day. Then, your doctor will slowly increase your dose to 6 to 15 mg a day. This is divided into two or three doses.
  - Children—Dose is based on body weight and must be determined by your doctor. The usual dose is 50 to 400 micrograms (mcg) (0.05 to 0.4 mg) per kilogram of body weight (22.73 to

181.2 mcg per pound [0.023 to 0.18 mg per pound]) a day. This is divided into two or three doses.

Missed dose—If you miss a dose of this medicine, take it as soon as possible. However, if it is almost time for your next dose, skip the missed dose and go back to your regular dosing schedule. Do not double doses.

Storage—To store this medicine:

• Keep out of the reach of children.

• Store away from heat and direct light.

• Do not store in the bathroom, near the kitchen sink, or in other damp places. Heat or moisture may cause the medicine to break down.

• Do not keep outdated medicine or medicine no longer needed. Be sure that any discarded medicine is out of the reach of children.

Precautions While Using This Medicine

It is important that your doctor check your progress at regular visits to make sure that this medicine is working properly.

For patients *taking this medicine for high blood pressure:*

• *Do not take other medicines unless they have been discussed with your doctor.* This especially includes over-the-counter (nonprescription) medicines for appetite control, asthma, colds, cough, hay fever, or sinus problems, since they may tend to make prazosin less effective.

Dizziness, lightheadedness, or sudden fainting may occur after you take this medicine, especially when you get up from a lying or sitting position. These effects are more likely to occur when you take the first dose of this medicine. Taking the first dose at bedtime may prevent problems. However, *be especially careful if you need to get up during the night.* These effects may also occur with any doses you take after the first dose. Getting up slowly may help lessen this problem. *If you feel dizzy, lie down so that you do not faint.* Then sit for a few moments before standing to prevent the dizziness from returning.

The dizziness, lightheadedness, or fainting is more likely to occur if you drink alcohol, stand for a long time, exercise, or if the weather is hot. *While you are taking this medicine, be careful to limit the amount of alcohol you drink. Also, use extra care during exercise or hot weather or if you must stand for a long time.*

Prazosin may cause some people to become drowsy or less alert than they are normally. *Make sure you know how you react to this medicine before you drive, use machines, or do anything else that could be dangerous if you are dizzy, drowsy, or are not alert.* After you have taken several doses of this medicine, these effects should lessen.

Side Effects of This Medicine

Along with its needed effects, a medicine may cause some unwanted effects. Although not all of these side effects may occur, if they do occur they may need medical attention.

Check with your doctor as soon as possible if any of the following side effects occur:

> *More common*
>> Dizziness or lightheadedness, especially when getting up from a lying or sitting position; fainting (sudden)
>
> *Less common*
>> Loss of bladder control; pounding heartbeat; swelling of feet or lower legs

Rare

Chest pain; painful inappropriate erection of penis (continuing); shortness of breath

Other side effects may occur that usually do not need medical attention. These side effects may go away during treatment as your body adjusts to the medicine. However, check with your doctor if any of the following side effects continue or are bothersome:

More common

Drowsiness; headache; lack of energy

Less common

Dryness of mouth; nervousness; unusual tiredness or weakness

Rare

Frequent urge to urinate; nausea

Other side effects not listed above may also occur in some patients. If you notice any other effects, check with your doctor.

Additional Information

Once a medicine has been approved for marketing for a certain use, experience may show that it is also useful for other medical problems. Although these uses are not included in product labeling, prazosin is used in certain patients with the following medical conditions:

- Congestive heart failure
- Ergot alkaloid poisoning
- Pheochromocytoma
- Raynaud's disease
- Benign enlargement of the prostate

For patients taking this medicine for *benign enlargement of the prostate*:

- Prazosin will not shrink the size of your prostate, but it does help to relieve the symptoms.

Other than the above information, there is no additional information relating to proper use, precautions, or side effects for these uses.

PROBENECID   Systemic

Some commonly used brand names are:

In the U.S.—

Benemid   Probalan

Generic name product may also be available.

In Canada—

Benemid   Benuryl

Description

Probenecid (proe-BEN-e-sid) is used in the treatment of chronic gout or gouty arthritis. These conditions are caused by too much uric acid in the blood. The medicine works by removing the extra uric acid from the body. Probenecid does not cure gout, but after you have been taking it for a few months it will help prevent gout attacks. This medicine will help prevent gout attacks only as long as you continue to take it.

Probenecid is also used to prevent or treat other medical problems that may occur if too much uric acid is present in the body.

Probenecid is sometimes used with certain kinds of antibiotics to make them more effective in the treatment of infections.

Probenecid is available only with your doctor's prescription, in the following dosage form:

Oral

- Tablets (U.S. and Canada)

Before Using This Medicine

In deciding to use a medicine, the risks of taking the medicine must be weighed against the good it will do. This is a decision you and your doctor will make. For probenecid, the following should be considered:

Allergies—Tell your doctor if you have ever had any unusual or allergic reaction to probenecid. Also tell your health care professional if you are allergic to any other substances, such as foods, preservatives, or dyes.

Pregnancy—Probenecid has not been shown to cause birth defects or other problems in humans.

Breast-feeding—Probenecid has not been reported to cause problems in nursing babies.

Children—Probenecid has been tested in children 2 to 14 years of age for use together with antibiotics. It has not been shown to cause different side effects or problems than it does in adults. Studies on the effects of probenecid in patients with gout have been done only in adults. Gout is very rare in children.

Older adults—Many medicines have not been studied specifically in older people. Therefore, it may not be known whether they work exactly the same way they do in younger adults. There is no specific information comparing use of probenecid in the elderly with use in other age groups.

Other medicines—Although certain medicines should not be used together at all, in other cases two different medicines may be used together even if an interaction might occur. In these cases, your doctor may want to change the dose, or other precautions may be necessary. When you are taking probenecid, it is especially important that your health care professional know if you are taking any of the following:

- Antineoplastics (cancer medicine)—The chance of serious side effects may be increased
- Aspirin or other salicylates—These medicines may keep probenecid from working properly for treating gout, depending on the amount of aspirin or other salicylate that you take and how often you take it
- Heparin—Probenecid may increase the effects of heparin, which increases the chance of side effects
- Indomethacin (e.g., Indocin) or
- Ketoprofen (e.g., Orudis) or
- Methotrexate (e.g., Mexate)—Probenecid may increase the blood levels of these medicines, which increases the chance of side effects
- Medicine for infection, including tuberculosis or virus infection—Probenecid may increase the blood levels of many of these medicines. In some cases, this is a desired effect and probenecid may be used to help the other medicine work better. However, the chance of side effects is sometimes also increased
- Nitrofurantoin (e.g., Furadantin)—Probenecid may keep nitrofurantoin from working properly
- Zidovudine (e.g., AZT, Retrovir)—Probenecid increases the blood level of zidovudine and may allow lower doses of zidovudine to be used. However, the chance of side effects is also increased

Other medical problems—The presence of other medical problems may affect the use of probenecid. Make sure you tell your doctor if you have any other medical problems, especially:

- Blood disease or
- Cancer being treated by antineoplastics (cancer medicine) or radiation (x-rays) or
- Kidney disease or stones (or history of) or
- Stomach ulcer (history of)—The chance of side effects may be increased

Proper Use of This Medicine

If probenecid upsets your stomach, it may be taken with food. If this does not work, an antacid may be taken. If stomach upset (nausea, vomiting, or loss of appetite) continues, check with your doctor.

For patients taking probenecid *for gout:*

- After you begin to take probenecid, gout attacks may continue to occur for a while. However, if you take this medicine regularly as directed by your doctor, the attacks will gradually become less frequent and less painful than before. After you have been taking probenecid for several months, they may stop completely.

- This medicine will help prevent gout attacks, but it will not relieve an attack that has already started. *Even if you take another medicine for gout attacks, continue to take this medicine also.* If you have any questions about this, check with your doctor.

For patients taking probenecid *for gout or to help remove uric acid from the body:*

- When you first begin taking probenecid, the amount of uric acid in the kidneys is greatly increased. This may cause kidney stones or other kidney problems in some people. To help prevent this, your doctor may want you to drink at least 10 to 12 full glasses (8 ounces each) of fluids each day, or to take another medicine to make your urine less acid. It is important that you follow your doctor's instructions very carefully.

Dosing—The dose of probenecid will be different for different patients. *Follow your doctor's orders or the directions on the label.* The following information includes only the average doses of probenecid. *If your dose is different, do not change it* unless your doctor tells you to do so.

- *For treating gout or removing uric acid from the body:*

    —Adults: 250 mg (one-half of a 500-mg tablet) two times a day for about one week, then 500 mg (one tablet) two times a day for a few weeks. After this, the dose will depend on the amount of uric acid in your blood or urine. Most people need 2, 3, or 4 tablets a day, but some people may need higher doses.

    —Children: It is not likely that probenecid will be needed to treat gout or to remove uric acid from the body in children. If a child needs this medicine, however, the dose would have to be determined by the doctor.

- *For helping antibiotics work better:*

    —Adults: The amount of probenecid will depend on the condition being treated. Sometimes, only one dose of 2 tablets is needed. Other times, the dose will be 1 tablet four times a day.

    —Children: The dose will have to be determined by the doctor. It depends on the child's weight, as well as on the condition being treated. Older children and teenagers may need the same amount as adults.

Missed dose—If you are taking probenecid regularly and you miss a dose, take the missed dose as soon as possible. However, if you do not remember until it is almost time for the next dose, skip the missed dose and go back to your regular dosing schedule. Do not double doses.

Storage—To store this medicine:

- Keep out of the reach of children.
- Store away from heat and direct light.
- Do not store this medicine in the bathroom, near the kitchen sink, or in other damp places. Heat or moisture may cause the medicine to break down.
- Do not keep outdated medicine or medicine no longer

needed. Be sure that any discarded medicine is out of the reach of children.

Precautions While Using This Medicine

If you will be taking probenecid for more than a few weeks, your doctor should check your progress at regular visits.

Before you have any medical tests, tell the person in charge that you are taking this medicine. The results of some tests may be affected by probenecid.

For *diabetic patients:*

• Probenecid may cause false test results with copper sulfate urine sugar tests (Clinitest®), but not with glucose enzymatic urine sugar tests (Clinistix®). If you have any questions about this, check with your health care professional.

For patients taking probenecid *for gout or to help remove uric acid from the body:*

• Taking aspirin or other salicylates may lessen the effects of probenecid. This will depend on the dose of aspirin or other salicylate that you take, and on how often you take it. Also, drinking too much alcohol may increase the amount of uric acid in the blood and lessen the effects of this medicine. Therefore, *do not take aspirin or other salicylates or drink alcoholic beverages while taking this medicine*, unless you have first checked with your doctor.

Side Effects of This Medicine

Along with its needed effects, a medicine may cause some unwanted effects. Although not all of these side effects

may occur, if they do occur they may need medical
attention.

The following side effects may mean that you are having
an allergic reaction to this medicine. *Check with your doctor immediately* if any of the following side effects occur:

Rare

Fast or irregular breathing; puffiness or swellings of the
eyelids or around the eyes; shortness of breath, troubled
breathing, tightness in chest, or wheezing; changes in
the skin color of the face occurring together with any
of the other side effects listed here; or skin rash, hives,
or itching occurring together with any of the other side
effects listed here

Also, check with your doctor as soon as possible if any
of the following side effects occur:

Less common

Bloody urine; difficult or painful urination; lower back or
side pain (especially if severe or sharp); skin rash,
hives, or itching (occurring without other signs of an
allergic reaction)

Rare

Cloudy urine; cough or hoarseness; fast or irregular breathing; fever; pain in back and/or ribs; sores, ulcers, or
white spots on lips or in mouth; sore throat and fever
with or without chills; sudden decrease in the amount
of urine; swelling of face, fingers, feet, and/or lower
legs; swollen and/or painful glands; unusual bleeding
or bruising; unusual tiredness or weakness; yellow eyes
or skin; weight gain

Other side effects may occur that usually do not need
medical attention. These side effects may go away during
treatment as your body adjusts to the medicine. However,
check with your doctor if any of the following side effects
continue or are bothersome:

More common

Headache; joint pain, redness, or swelling; loss of appetite;
nausea or vomiting (mild)

Less common

> Dizziness; flushing or redness of face (occurring without any signs of an allergic reaction); frequent urge to urinate; sore gums

Other side effects not listed above may also occur in some patients. If you notice any other effects, check with your doctor.

PROBUCOL Systemic

Some commonly used brand names are:

In the U.S.—
Lorelco

In Canada—
Lorelco

Other—
Bifenabid
Lesterol
Lurselle

Panesclerina
Superlipid

Description

Probucol (PROE-byoo-kole) is used to lower levels of cholesterol (a fat-like substance) in the blood. This may help prevent medical problems caused by cholesterol clogging the blood vessels.

Probucol is available only with your doctor's prescription, in the following dosage form:

Oral

- Tablets (U.S. and Canada)

Before Using This Medicine

In deciding to use a medicine, the risks of taking the medicine must be weighed against the good it will do.

This is a decision you and your doctor will make. For probucol, the following should be considered:

Allergies—Tell your doctor if you have ever had any unusual or allergic reaction to probucol. Also tell your health care professional if you are allergic to any other substances, such as foods, preservatives, or dyes.

Diet—Before prescribing medicine for your condition, your doctor will probably try to control your condition by prescribing a personal diet for you. Such a diet may be low in fats, sugars, and/or cholesterol. Many people are able to control their condition by carefully following their doctor's orders for proper diet and exercise. Medicine is prescribed only when additional help is needed and is effective only when a schedule of diet and exercise is properly followed.

Also, this medicine is less effective if you are greatly overweight. It may be very important for you to go on a reducing diet. However, check with your doctor before going on any diet.

Make certain your health care professional knows if you are on a low-sodium, low-sugar, or any other special diet.

Pregnancy—Probucol has not been studied in pregnant women. However, it has not been shown to cause birth defects or other problems in rats or rabbits.

Breast-feeding—It is not known whether probucol passes into the breast milk. However, this medicine is not recommended for use during breast-feeding because it may cause unwanted effects in nursing babies.

Children—There is no specific information about the use of probucol in children. However, use is not recommended in children under 2 years of age since cholesterol is needed for normal development.

Older adults—Many medicines have not been studied specifically in older people. Therefore, it may not be known whether they work exactly the same way they do in younger adults or if they cause different side effects or problems in older people. There is no specific information comparing use of probucol in the elderly with use in other age groups.

Other medicines—Although certain medicines should not be used together at all, in other cases two different medicines may be used together even if an interaction might occur. In these cases, your doctor may want to change the dose, or other precautions may be necessary. Tell your health care professional if you are taking any other prescription or nonprescription (over-the-counter [OTC]) medicine.

Other medical problems—The presence of other medical problems may affect the use of probucol. Make sure you tell your doctor if you have any other medical problems, especially:

- Gallbladder disease or gallstones or
- Heart disease—Probucol may make these conditions worse
- Liver disease—Higher blood levels of probucol may result, which may increase the chance of side effects

---

Proper Use of This Medicine

Many patients who have high cholesterol levels will not notice any signs of the problem. In fact, many may feel normal. *Take this medicine exactly as directed by your doctor, even though you may feel well.* Try not to miss any doses and do not take more medicine than your doctor ordered.

Remember that this medicine will not cure your condition but it does help control it. Therefore, you must continue to take it as directed if you expect to keep your cholesterol levels down.

Follow carefully the special diet your doctor gave you. This is the most important part of controlling your condition, and is necessary if the medicine is to work properly.

This medicine works better when taken with meals.

Dosing—The dose of probucol will be different for different patients. *Follow your doctor's orders or the directions on the label.* The following information includes only the average doses of probucol. *If your dose is different, do not change it* unless your doctor tells you to do so:

- The number of tablets that you take depends on the strength of the medicine.
- For *oral* dosage form (tablets):

  —Adults: 500 milligrams two times a day taken with the morning and evening meals.

  —Children:
    - Up to 2 years of age—Use is not recommended.
    - 2 years of age and over—Dose must be determined by your doctor.

Missed dose—If you miss a dose of this medicine, take it as soon as possible. However, if it is almost time for your next dose, skip the missed dose and go back to your regular dosing schedule. Do not double doses.

Storage—To store this medicine:

- Keep out of the reach of children.
- Store away from heat and direct light.
- Do not store in the bathroom, near the kitchen sink, or in other damp places. Heat or moisture may cause the medicine to break down.
- Do not keep outdated medicine or medicine no longer needed. Be sure that any discarded medicine is out of the reach of children.

Precautions While Using This Medicine

It is very important that your doctor check your progress at regular visits. This will allow your doctor to see if the medicine is working properly to lower your cholesterol levels and to decide if you should continue to take it.

Do not stop taking this medicine without first checking with your doctor. When you stop taking this medicine, your blood fat levels may increase again. Your doctor may want you to follow a special diet to help prevent this.

Side Effects of This Medicine

Along with its needed effects, a medicine may cause some unwanted effects. Although not all of these side effects may occur, if they do occur they may need medical attention.

Check with your doctor as soon as possible if any of the following side effects occur:

More common

Dizziness or fainting; fast or irregular heartbeat

Rare

Swellings on face, hands, or feet, or in mouth; unusual bleeding or bruising; unusual tiredness or weakness

Other side effects may occur that usually do not need medical attention. These side effects may go away during treatment as your body adjusts to the medicine. However, check with your doctor if any of the following side effects continue or are bothersome:

More common

Bloating; diarrhea; nausea and vomiting; stomach pain

Less common

Headache; numbness or tingling of fingers, toes, or face

Other side effects not listed above may also occur in some patients. If you notice any other effects, check with your doctor.

PROCAINAMIDE   Systemic

Some commonly used brand names are:

In the U.S.—

Procan SR	Pronestyl
Promine	Pronestyl-SR

Generic name product may also be available.

In Canada—

Procan SR	Pronestyl-SR
Pronestyl	

Generic name product may also be available.

Description

Procainamide (proe-KANE-a-mide) is used to correct ir-regular heartbeats to a normal rhythm and to slow an over-active heart. This allows the heart to work more efficiently. Procainamide produces its beneficial effects by slowing nerve impulses in the heart and reducing sensitivity of heart tissues.

Procainamide is available only with your doctor's prescription, in the following dosage forms:

Oral

- Capsules (U.S. and Canada)
- Tablets (U.S.)
- Extended-release tablets (U.S. and Canada)

Parenteral

- Injection (U.S. and Canada)

Before Using This Medicine

In deciding to use a medicine, the risks of taking the medicine must be weighed against the good it will do. This is a decision you and your doctor will make. For procainamide, the following should be considered:

Allergies—Tell your doctor if you have ever had any unusual or allergic reaction to procainamide, procaine, or any other "caine-type" medicine. Also tell your health care professional if you are allergic to any other substance, such as foods, preservatives, or dyes.

Pregnancy—Procainamide has not been studied in pregnant women. However, it has been used in some pregnant women and has not been shown to cause problems. Before taking this medicine, make sure your doctor knows if you are pregnant or if you may become pregnant.

Breast-feeding—Procainamide passes into breast milk.

Children—Procainamide has been used in a limited number of children. In effective doses, the medicine has not been shown to cause different side effects or problems than it does in adults.

Older adults—Dizziness or lightheadedness is more likely to occur in the elderly, who are usually more sensitive to the effects of this medicine.

Other medicines—Although certain medicines should not be used together at all, in other cases two different medicines may be used together even if an interaction might occur. In these cases, your doctor may want to change the dose, or other precautions may be necessary. When you are taking procainamide, it is especially important that your health care professional know if you are taking any of the following:

- Antiarrhythmics (medicines for heart rhythm problems), other—Effects on the heart may be increased
- Antihypertensives (high blood pressure medicine)—Effects on blood pressure may be increased
- Antimyasthenics (ambenonium [e.g., Mytelase], neostigmine [e.g., Prostigmin], pyridostigmine [e.g., Mestinon])—Effects may be blocked by procainamide
- Pimozide (e.g., Orap)—May increase the risk of heart rhythm problems

Other medical problems—The presence of other medical problems may affect the use of procainamide. Make sure you tell your doctor if you have any other medical problems, especially:

- Asthma—Possible allergic reaction
- Kidney disease or
- Liver disease—Effects may be increased because of slower removal of procainamide from the body
- Lupus erythematosus (history of)—Procainamide may cause the condition to become active
- Myasthenia gravis—Procainamide may increase muscle weakness

---

Proper Use of This Medicine

Take procainamide exactly as directed by your doctor, even though you may feel well. Do not take more medicine than ordered.

Procainamide should be taken with a glass of water on an empty stomach 1 hour before or 2 hours after meals so that it will be absorbed more quickly. However, to lessen stomach upset, your doctor may want you to take the medicine with food or milk.

For patients taking the *extended-release tablets:*

- Swallow the tablet whole without breaking, crushing, or chewing it.

This medicine works best when there is a constant amount in the blood. *To help keep the amount constant, do not miss any doses. Also, it is best to take the doses at evenly spaced times day and night.* For example, if you are to take 6 doses a day, the doses should be spaced about 4 hours apart. If this interferes with your sleep or other daily activities, or if you need help in planning the best times to take your medicine, check with your health care professional.

Dosing—The dose of procainamide will be different for different patients. *Follow your doctor's orders or the directions on the label.* The following information includes only the average doses of procainamide. *If your dose is different, do not change it* unless your doctor tells you to do so.

The number of capsules or tablets that you take depends on the strength of the medicine.

- For *regular (short-acting) oral* dosage forms (capsules or tablets):

  —For atrial arrhythmias (fast or irregular heartbeat):

  - Adults—500 milligrams (mg) to 1000 mg (1 gram) every four to six hours.

  - Children—12.5 mg per kilogram (5.68 mg per pound) of body weight four times a day.

  —For ventricular arrhythmias (fast or irregular heartbeat):

  - Adults—50 mg per kilogram (22.73 mg per pound) of body weight per day divided into eight doses taken every three hours.

  - Children—12.5 mg per kilogram (5.68 mg per pound) of body weight four times a day.

- For *long-acting oral* dosage form (extended-release tablets):

  —For atrial arrhythmias (fast or irregular heartbeat):

  - Adults—1000 mg (1 gram) every six hours.

  - Children—Use is not recommended.

  —For ventricular arrhythmias (fast or irregular heartbeat):

  - Adults—50 mg per kilogram (22.73 mg per pound) of body weight per day divided into four doses taken every six hours.

- For *injection* dosage form:

  —For arrhythmias (fast or irregular heartbeat):

- Adults—

—*First few doses:* May be given intramuscularly (into the muscle) at 50 mg per kilogram (22.73 mg per pound) of body weight per day in divided doses every three hours; or may be given intravenously (into the vein) by slowly injecting 100 mg (mixed in fluid) every five minutes or infusing 500 to 600 mg (mixed in fluid) over a twenty-five- to thirty-minute period.

—*Doses after the first few doses:* 2 to 6 mg (mixed in fluid) per minute infused into the vein.

- Children—Dose must be determined by your doctor.

Missed dose—If you miss a dose of this medicine and remember within 2 hours (4 hours if you are taking the long-acting tablets), take it as soon as possible. However, if you do not remember until later, skip the missed dose and go back to your regular dosing schedule. Do not double doses.

Storage—To store this medicine:

- Keep out of the reach of children.
- Store away from heat and direct light.
- Do not store in the bathroom, refrigerator, near the kitchen sink, or in other damp places. Moisture usually present in these areas may cause the medicine to break down. Keep the container tightly closed and store in a dry place.
- Do not keep outdated medicine or medicine no longer needed. Be sure that any discarded medicine is out of the reach of children.

Precautions While Using This Medicine

It is important that your doctor check your progress at regular visits to make sure the medicine is working properly.

This will allow necessary changes in the amount of medicine you are taking, which also may help reduce side effects.

Do not stop taking this medicine without first checking with your doctor. Stopping it suddenly may cause a serious change in the activity of your heart. Your doctor may want you to reduce gradually the amount you are taking before stopping completely.

Before having any kind of surgery (including dental surgery) or emergency treatment, tell the medical doctor or dentist in charge that you are taking this medicine.

Your doctor may want you to carry a medical identification card or bracelet stating that you are taking this medicine.

Dizziness or lightheadedness may occur, especially in elderly patients and when large doses are used. *Elderly patients should use extra care to avoid falling. Make sure you know how you react to this medicine before you drive, use machines, or do anything else that could be dangerous if you are dizzy or are not alert.*

Tell the doctor in charge that you are taking this medicine before you have any medical tests. The results of some tests may be affected by this medicine.

Side Effects of This Medicine

Along with its needed effects, a medicine may cause some unwanted effects. Although not all of these side effects may occur, if they do occur they may need medical attention.

Check with your doctor as soon as possible if any of the following side effects occur:

Less common
>Fever and chills; joint pain or swelling; pains with breathing; skin rash or itching

Rare

Confusion; fever or sore mouth, gums, or throat; hallucinations (seeing, hearing, or feeling things that are not there); mental depression; unusual bleeding or bruising; unusual tiredness or weakness

Signs and symptoms of overdose

Confusion; decrease in urination; dizziness (severe) or fainting; drowsiness; fast or irregular heartbeat; nausea and vomiting

Other side effects may occur that usually do not need medical attention. These side effects may go away during treatment as your body adjusts to the medicine. However, check with your doctor if any of the following side effects continue or are bothersome:

More common

Diarrhea; loss of appetite

Less common

Dizziness or lightheadedness

The medicine in the extended-release tablets is contained in a special wax form (matrix). The medicine is slowly released, after which the wax matrix passes out of the body. Sometimes it may be seen in the stool. This is normal and is no cause for concern.

Other side effects not listed above may also occur in some patients. If you notice any other effects, check with your doctor.

PROGESTINS   Systemic

Some commonly used brand names are:

In the U.S.—

Amen[2]	Cycrin[2]
Aygestin[4]	Depo-Provera[2]
Curretab[2]	Gesterol 50[6]

In the U.S. (cont'd)—

Hy/Gestrone[1]

Hylutin[1]

Megace[3]

Micronor[4]

Norlutate[4]

Norlutin[4]

Nor-QD[4]

Ovrette[5]

Pro-Depo[1]

Prodrox[1]

Pro-Span[1]

Provera[2]

In Canada—

Depo-Provera[2]

Megace[3]

Micronor[4]

Norlutate[4]

PMS-Progesterone[6]

Provera[2]

Another commonly used name is norethisterone.

Note: For quick reference, the following progestins are numbered to match the corresponding brand names.

This information applies to the following medicines:

1. Hydroxyprogesterone (hye-drox-ee-proe-JESS-te-rone)†‡
2. Medroxyprogesterone (me-DROX-ee-proe-JESS-te-rone)‡
3. Megestrol (me-JESS-trole)‡
4. Norethindrone (nor-eth-IN-drone)
5. Norgestrel (nor-JESS-trel)†
6. Progesterone (proe-JESS-ter-one)‡

---

†Not commercially available in Canada.

‡Generic name product may also be available in the U.S.

Description

Progestins (proe-JESS-tins) are sometimes called female hormones. They are produced by the body and are necessary during the childbearing years for the development of the milk-producing glands, and for the proper regulation of the menstrual cycle.

Progestins are prescribed for several reasons:

- for the proper regulation of the menstrual cycle.
- to treat a certain type of disorder of the uterus known as endometriosis.
- to prevent pregnancy, when used in birth-control pills.
- to help treat selected cases of cancer of the breast, kidney, or uterus.

- for testing the body's production of certain hormones.

Progestins may also be used for other conditions as determined by your doctor.

Progestins should not be used in pregnancy tests or in most cases of threatened miscarriage, since there have been some reports that these medications may cause harmful effects on the fetus. However, progesterone is sometimes used in a few patients to treat a certain type of infertility. These patients are given progesterone because their bodies do not produce enough natural progesterone to support a pregnancy. Progesterone is used if this problem has not responded well to other types of treatment.

To make the use of a progestin as safe and reliable as possible, you should understand how and when to take it and what effects may be expected. A paper with information for the patient may be given to you with your filled prescription, and will provide many details concerning most uses of this medicine. Read this paper carefully and ask your health care professional if you need additional information or explanation.

Progestins are available only with your doctor's prescription, in the following dosage forms:

Oral

Medroxyprogesterone
- Tablets (U.S. and Canada)

Megestrol
- Tablets (U.S. and Canada)

Norethindrone
- Tablets (U.S. and Canada)

Norgestrel
- Tablets (U.S.)

Parenteral

Hydroxyprogesterone
- Injection (U.S.)

Medroxyprogesterone
- Injection (U.S. and Canada)

Progesterone
- Injection (U.S. and Canada)

Rectal

Progesterone
- Suppositories

Vaginal

Progesterone
- Suppositories

Before Using This Medicine

In deciding to use a medicine, the risks of taking the medicine must be weighed against the good it will do. This is a decision you and your doctor will make. For progestins, the following should be considered:

Allergies—Tell your doctor if you have ever had any unusual or allergic reaction to progestins. Also tell your health care professional if you are allergic to any other substances, such as foods, preservatives, or dyes.

Pregnancy—Progestins are not recommended for use during pregnancy since there have been some reports that these medications may cause harmful effects on the fetus. However, progesterone is sometimes used in a few patients to treat a certain type of infertility. These patients are given progesterone because their bodies do not produce enough natural progesterone to support a pregnancy. Progesterone is used if this problem has not responded well to other types of treatment.

Breast-feeding—Progestins pass into the breast milk and may cause unwanted effects in the nursing baby. It may be necessary for you to take another medicine or to stop breast-feeding during treatment.

Children—Studies on this medicine have been done only

in adults, and there is no specific information about its use in children.

Older adults—This medicine has been tested and has not been shown to cause different side effects or problems in older people than it does in younger adults.

Other medicines—Although certain medicines should not be used together at all, in other cases two different medicines may be used together even if an interaction might occur. In these cases, your doctor may want to change the dose, or other precautions may be necessary. When you are taking a progestin, it is especially important that your health care professional know if you are taking any of the following:

- Bromocriptine (e.g., Parlodel)

Other medical problems—The presence of other medical problems may affect the use of progestins. Make sure you tell your doctor if you have any other medical problems, especially:

- Asthma
- Blood clots (or history of)
- Cancer (or history of)
- Changes in vaginal bleeding
- Diabetes mellitus (sugar diabetes)
- Epilepsy
- Heart or circulation disease
- High blood cholesterol
- Kidney disease
- Liver or gallbladder disease
- Mental depression (or history of)
- Migraine headaches
- Stroke (or history of)

Proper Use of This Medicine

Take this medicine only as directed by your doctor. Do not take more of it and do not take it for a longer time than your doctor ordered. To do so may increase the chance of side effects. Try to take the medicine at the same time each day to reduce the possibility of side effects and to allow it to work better. When used for birth control, this medicine should be taken every day of the year, with doses taken 24 hours apart without interruption.

For patients using the rectal suppository form of this medicine:

- If the suppository is too soft to insert, chill it in the refrigerator for 30 minutes.
- To insert the suppository: Moisten the suppository with cold water. Lie down on your side and use your finger to push the suppository well up into the rectum.

For patients using the vaginal suppository form of this medicine:

- Use as directed by your doctor.

Dosing—The dose of these medicines will be different for different patients. *Follow your doctor's orders or the directions on the label.* The following information includes only the average doses of these medicines. *If your dose is different, do not change it* unless your doctor tells you to do so.

The number of tablets, injections, or suppositories that you take, receive, or use depends on the strength of the medicine. Also, *the number of doses you take or use each day, the time allowed between doses, and the length of time you take or use the medicine depend on the medical problem for which you are taking progestins.*

For hydroxyprogesterone

- For *injection* dosage form:

    —For starting the menstrual cycle (amenorrhea) or controlling unusual and heavy bleeding of the uterus (dysfunctional uterine bleeding):

    - Adults and teenagers—At first, 375 milligrams

(mg) injected into a muscle as a single dose. Depending on your response, your doctor may want you to receive another dose in four or twenty-one days. Then, you will receive another dose every twenty-eight days for four more months.

—For testing the amount of estrogen produced:

• Adults and teenagers—250 mg injected into a muscle as a single dose once a month for two months.

—For treating cancer of the uterus:

• Adults and teenagers—1 gram injected into a muscle one to seven times a week for up to twelve weeks.

—For treating unusual menstrual cycles:

• Adults and teenagers—250 or 375 mg injected into a muscle as a single dose. Your doctor may also want you to use another hormone called estrogen. Depending on your response, your doctor may want you to receive an additional dose in four or twenty-one days. Then, you will receive another dose every twenty-eight days if needed.

For medroxyprogesterone

• For *oral* dosage form (tablets):

—For starting the menstrual cycle (amenorrhea) or controlling unusual and heavy bleeding of the uterus (dysfunctional uterine bleeding):

• Adults or teenagers—5 to 10 milligrams (mg) a day for five to ten days. Your treatment will probably begin on Day 16 or Day 21 (counting from the beginning of your last period).

—For treating unusual menstrual cycles:

• Adults or teenagers—10 mg daily for ten or thirteen days. Your treatment will probably begin on Day 13 through Day 16 (counting from the beginning of your last period). Your doctor may also want you to use another hormone called estrogen.

- For *injection* dosage form:

  —For treating cancer of the uterus or kidneys:

  - Adults and teenagers—At first, 400 to 1000 milligrams (mg) injected into a muscle as a single dose once a week. Then, your doctor may lower your dose to 400 mg once a month.

  —For preventing pregnancy:

  - Adults and teenagers—150 mg injected into a muscle every three months.

For megestrol

- For *oral* dosage form (tablets):

  —For treating cancer of the breast:

  - Adults and teenagers—40 milligrams (mg) four times a day for two or more months.

  —For treating cancer of the uterus:

  - Adults and teenagers—10 to 80 mg four times a day for two or more months.

For norethindrone (base)

- For *oral* dosage form (tablets):

  —For starting the menstrual cycle (amenorrhea) or controlling unusual and heavy bleeding of the uterus (dysfunctional uterine bleeding):

  - Adults or teenagers—5 to 20 milligrams (mg) a day from Day 5 through Day 25 (counting from the first day of the last menstrual cycle).

  —For treating endometriosis:

  - Adults or teenagers—At first, 10 mg a day for two weeks. Then, your doctor may increase your dose slowly to 30 mg a day for six to nine months. Let your doctor know if your menstrual period starts. Your doctor may want you to stop taking the medicine for a short period of time.

—For preventing pregnancy:

• Adults or teenagers—0.35 mg every day without interruption beginning on Day 1 of your menstrual cycle.

For norethindrone acetate

• For *oral* dosage form (tablets):

—For starting the menstrual cycle (amenorrhea) or controlling unusual and heavy bleeding of the uterus (dysfunctional uterine bleeding):

• Adults or teenagers—2.5 to 10 milligrams (mg) a day from Day 5 through Day 25 (counting from the first day of the last menstrual cycle).

—For treating endometriosis:

• Adults or teenagers—At first, 5 mg a day for two weeks. Then, your doctor may increase your dose slowly to 15 mg a day for six to nine months. Let your doctor know if your menstrual period starts. Your doctor may want you to stop taking the medicine for a short period of time.

For norgestrel

—For preventing pregnancy:

• Adults or teenagers—75 micrograms (mcg) every day without interruption beginning on Day 1 of your menstrual cycle.

For progesterone

• For *injection* dosage form:

—For starting the menstrual cycle (amenorrhea) or controlling unusual and heavy bleeding of the uterus (dysfunctional uterine bleeding):

• Adults or teenagers—50 to 100 milligrams (mg) injected into a muscle as a single dose. Or, your doctor may want you to receive 5 to 10 mg injected into a muscle a day for six to eight days. Your doctor may want you to take another hormone called estrogen first. If your menstrual period starts, your doctor will want you to stop taking the medicine.

—For maintaining a pregnancy (at ovulation and at the beginning of pregnancy)

• Adults or teenagers—12.5 mg injected into a muscle a day at the time of ovulation for up to two weeks. If needed, your doctor may want you to receive the medicine for up to eleven weeks.

• For *suppositories* dosage form (rectal or vaginal):

—For maintaining a pregnancy (at ovulation and at the beginning of pregnancy):

• Adults or teenagers—25 mg (one suppository) inserted into the rectum or the vagina two times a day at the time of ovulation for up to two weeks. If needed, your doctor may want you to receive the medicine for up to eleven weeks.

Missed dose—If you miss a dose of this medicine:

• If you are *not* taking this medicine for birth control, take the missed dose as soon as possible. However, if it is almost time for your next dose, skip the missed dose and go back to your regular dosing schedule. Do not double doses.

• *If you are taking this medicine for birth control,* the safest thing to do when you miss 1 day's dose is to stop taking the medicine immediately and use another method of birth control until your period begins or until your doctor determines that you are not pregnant. This procedure is different from the one used after missed doses of birth control tablets that contain more than one hormone.

Storage—To store this medicine:

• Keep out of the reach of children.

• Store away from heat and direct light.

• Do not store in the bathroom medicine cabinet because the heat or moisture may cause the medicine to break down.

- Keep the injectable form of this medicine from freezing.
- Do not keep outdated medicine or medicine no longer needed. Be sure that any discarded medicine is out of the reach of children.

Precautions While Using This Medicine

It is very important that your doctor check your progress at regular visits. This will allow your dosage to be adjusted to your changing needs, and will allow any unwanted effects to be detected. These visits will usually be every 6 to 12 months, but some doctors require them more often.

Check with your doctor right away:

- if vaginal bleeding continues for an unusually long time.
- if your menstrual period has not started within 45 days of your last period.
- *if you suspect that you may have become pregnant. You should stop taking this medicine immediately*, since there have been some reports that these medications may cause harmful effects on the fetus when used during pregnancy. However, progesterone is sometimes used during early pregnancy to treat a certain type of infertility.

If you are scheduled for any laboratory tests, tell your doctor that you are taking a progestin.

In some patients, tenderness, swelling, or bleeding of the gums may occur. Brushing and flossing your teeth carefully and regularly and massaging your gums may help prevent this. See your dentist regularly to have your teeth cleaned. Check with your medical doctor or dentist if you have any questions about how to take care of your teeth and gums, or if you notice any tenderness, swelling, or bleeding of your gums.

If you are taking this medicine for birth control:

- *When you begin to use birth control tablets,* your body will require time to adjust before pregnancy will be prevented; therefore, you should *use a second method of birth control for at least the first 3 weeks to ensure full protection.*

- Since one of the most important factors in the proper use of birth control tablets is taking every dose exactly on schedule, you should make sure you never run out of tablets. Therefore, always keep 1 extra month's supply of tablets on hand. To keep the extra month's supply from becoming too old, use it next, after the pills now being used, and replace the extra supply each month on a regular schedule. The tablets will keep well when kept dry and at room temperature (light will fade some tablet colors but will not change the tablets' effect).

- Keep the tablets in the container in which you received them. Most containers aid you in keeping track of dosage schedule.

- Your doctor has prescribed this medicine only for you after studying your health record and the results of your physical examination. Use of the tablets by other persons may be dangerous because of differences in health and body make-up. Therefore, do not give your birth control tablets to anyone else, and do not take tablets prescribed for someone else. Also, check with your doctor before taking any leftover birth control tablets from an old prescription, especially after a pregnancy. This medicine may be dangerous if your health has changed since your last physical examination.

Side Effects of This Medicine

Along with their needed effects, progestins sometimes cause some unwanted effects such as blood clots, heart attacks, and strokes, and problems of the liver and eyes. Although these effects are rare, they can be very serious and may cause death.

The following side effects may be caused by blood clots. Although not all of these side effects may occur, if they do occur they need immediate medical attention. *Get emergency help immediately* if any of the following side effects occur:

Headache (severe or sudden); loss of coordination (sudden); loss of vision or change in vision (sudden); pains in chest, groin, or leg (especially in calf of leg); shortness of breath (sudden); slurred speech (sudden); weakness, numbness, or pain in arm or leg

Also, check with your doctor as soon as possible if any of the following side effects occur:

More common

Changes in vaginal bleeding (spotting, breakthrough bleeding, prolonged or complete stoppage of bleeding)

Less common or rare

Bulging eyes; discharge from breasts; double vision; loss of vision (gradual, partial, or complete); mental depression; pains in stomach, side, or abdomen; skin rash or itching; yellow eyes or skin

Other side effects may occur that usually do not need medical attention. These side effects may go away during treatment as your body adjusts to the medicine. However, check with your doctor if any of the following side effects continue or are bothersome:

More common

Changes in appetite; changes in weight; pain or irritation

at injection site (with progesterone); swelling of ankles and feet; unusual tiredness or weakness

Less common or rare

Acne; brown, blotchy spots on exposed skin; fever; increased body and facial hair; increased breast tenderness; nausea; some loss of scalp hair; trouble in sleeping

Other side effects not listed above may also occur in some patients. If you notice any other effects, check with your doctor.

QUINIDINE Systemic

Some commonly used brand names are:

In the U.S.—

Cardioquin	Quinalan
Cin-Quin	Quinidex Extentabs
Duraquin	Quinora
Quinaglute Dura-tabs	

Generic name product may also be available.

In Canada—

Apo-Quinidine	Quinaglute Dura-tabs
Cardioquin	Quinate
Novoquinidin	Quinidex Extentabs

Generic name product may also be available.

Description

Quinidine (KWIN-i-deen) is used to correct certain irregular heartbeats to a normal rhythm and to slow an overactive heart. The injection dosage form is also used to treat malaria.

Quinidine acts directly on the heart tissues to make them less responsive. It also slows impulses along special nerve networks to the heart. This allows the heart to work more efficiently.

Do not confuse this medicine with *quinine*, which, although related, has different medical uses.

Quinidine is available only with your doctor's prescription, in the following dosage forms:

Oral
- Capsules (U.S.)
- Tablets (U.S. and Canada)
- Extended-release tablets (U.S. and Canada)

Parenteral
- Injection (U.S. and Canada)

Before Using This Medicine

In deciding to use a medicine, the risks of taking the medicine must be weighed against the good it will do. This is a decision you and your doctor will make. For quinidine, the following should be considered:

Allergies—Tell your doctor if you have ever had any unusual or allergic reaction to quinidine or quinine. Also tell your health care professional if you are allergic to any other substance, such as foods, preservatives, or dyes.

Pregnancy—Studies on effects in pregnancy have not been done in either humans or animals. However, a closely related medicine, quinine, has been shown to cause birth defects of the nervous system, fingers, and toes, and decreased hearing in the infant. Quinine also may cause contractions of the uterus.

Breast-feeding—Quinidine passes into breast milk. However, it has not been reported to cause problems in nursing babies.

Children—Studies on this medicine have been done only in adult patients, and there is no specific information comparing use of quinidine in children with use in other age groups. Use of the extended-release tablets in children is not recommended.

Older adults—Many medicines have not been studied specifically in older people. Therefore, it may not be known whether they work exactly the same way they do in younger adults. Although there is no specific information comparing use of quinidine in the elderly with use in other age groups, this medicine is not expected to cause different side effects or problems in older people than it does in younger adults.

Other medicines—Although certain medicines should not be used together at all, in other cases two different medicines may be used together even if an interaction might occur. In these cases, your doctor may want to change the dose, or other precautions may be necessary. When you are taking quinidine, it is especially important that your health care professional knows if you are taking any of the following:

- Anticoagulants (blood thinners)—Risk of bleeding may be increased
- Other heart medicine (especially digoxin)—Effects on the heart may be increased
- Pimozide (e.g., Orap)—Risk of heart rhythm problems may be increased
- Urinary alkalizers (medicine that makes the urine less acid, such as acetazolamide [e.g., Diamox], calcium- and/or magnesium-containing antacids, dichlorphenamide [e.g., Daranide], methazolamide [e.g., Neptazane], potassium or sodium citrate and/or citric acid, sodium bicarbonate [baking soda])—Effects may be increased because levels of quinidine in the body may be increased

Other medical problems—The presence of other medical problems may affect the use of quinidine. Make sure you tell your doctor if you have any other medical problems, especially:

- Asthma or emphysema—Possible allergic reaction

- Blood disease
- Infection
- Kidney disease or
- Liver disease—Effects may be increased because of slower removal of quinidine from the body
- Myasthenia gravis—Muscle weakness may be increased
- Overactive thyroid
- Psoriasis

Proper Use of This Medicine

Take quinidine with a full glass (8 ounces) of water on an empty stomach 1 hour before or 2 hours after meals so that it will be absorbed more quickly. However, to lessen stomach upset, your doctor may want you to take the medicine with food or milk.

For patients taking the *extended-release tablet* form of this medicine:

- Swallow the tablets whole.
- Do not break, crush, or chew before swallowing.

Take quinidine exactly as directed by your doctor even though you may feel well. Do not take more medicine than ordered and do not miss any doses.

Dosing—The dose of quinidine will be different for different patients. *Follow your doctor's orders or the directions on the label.* The following information includes only the average doses of quinidine. *If your dose is different, do not change it* unless your doctor tells you to do so.

The number of capsules or tablets that you take depends on the strength of the medicine. Also, *the number of doses you take each day, the time allowed between doses, and the length of time you take the medicine depend on the medical problem for which you are taking quinidine.* When you first begin to take quinidine for irregular heartbeat, you may need to take a higher number of doses each day. This depends on what type of irregular heartbeat you have and will be determined by your doctor.

- For *regular (short-acting) oral* dosage forms (capsules and tablets):

    —For irregular heartbeat:

    - Adults—200 to 650 milligrams (mg) two to four times a day.

    - Children—6 to 8.25 mg per kilogram (kg) (2.73 to 3.75 mg per pound) of body weight five times a day.

- For *long-acting oral* dosage forms (tablets):

    —For irregular heartbeat:

    - Adults—300 to 660 mg every six to twelve hours.

    - Children—Use is not recommended.

- For *injection* dosage form:

    —For irregular heartbeat:

    - Adults—400 to 600 mg injected into the muscle every two hours. Or, 600 to 800 mg in a solution and injected into a vein.

    - Children—Dose must be determined by your doctor.

    —For malaria:

    - Adults—10 mg per kg (4.54 mg per pound) of body weight in a solution and injected slowly into a vein over one to two hours. Then, 0.02 mg per kg (0.009 mg per pound) of body weight per minute is given. Or, 12 to 24 mg per kg (5.45 to 10.91 mg per pound) of body weight in a solution and injected slowly into a vein over a four hour period every eight hours.

    - Children—Dose must be determined by your doctor.

Missed dose—If you miss a dose of this medicine and remember within 2 hours of the missed dose, take it as soon as possible. However, if you do not remember until later, skip the missed dose and go back to your regular dosing schedule. Do not double doses.

Storage—To store this medicine:

- Keep out of the reach of children.
- Store away from heat and direct light.
- Do not store in the bathroom, near the kitchen sink, or in other damp places. Heat or moisture may cause the medicine to break down.
- Do not keep outdated medicine or medicine no longer needed. Be sure that any discarded medicine is out of the reach of children.

Precautions While Using This Medicine

It is very important that your doctor check your progress at regular visits to make sure that the quinidine is working properly and does not cause unwanted effects.

Do not stop taking this medicine without first checking with your doctor, to avoid possible worsening of your condition.

Before having any kind of surgery (including dental surgery) or emergency treatment, tell the medical doctor or dentist in charge that you are taking this medicine.

Your doctor may want you to carry a medical identification card or bracelet stating that you are using this medicine.

Some people who are unusually sensitive to this medicine may have side effects after the first dose or first few doses. Check with your doctor right away if the following side effects occur: breathing difficulty, changes in vision, dizziness, fever, headache, ringing in ears, or skin rash.

Side Effects of This Medicine

Along with its needed effects, a medicine may cause some unwanted effects. Although not all of these side effects may occur, if they do occur they may need medical attention.

Check with your doctor immediately if any of the following side effects occur:

> *Less common*
>> Blurred vision or any change in vision; dizziness, light-headedness, or fainting; fever; headache (severe); ringing or buzzing in the ears or any loss of hearing; skin rash, hives, or itching; wheezing, shortness of breath, or troubled breathing

> *Rare*
>> Fast heartbeat; unusual bleeding or bruising; unusual tiredness or weakness

Other side effects may occur that usually do not need medical attention. These side effects may go away during treatment as your body adjusts to the medicine. However, check with your doctor if any of the following side effects continue or are bothersome:

> *More common*
>> Bitter taste; diarrhea; flushing of skin with itching; loss of appetite; nausea or vomiting; stomach pain or cramping

> *Less common*
>> Confusion

Other side effects not listed above may also occur in some patients. If you notice any other effects, check with your doctor.

RIMANTADINE   Systemic†

A commonly used brand name in the U.S. is Flumadine.

———————————————————————————————————
†Not commercially available in Canada.
———————————————————————————————————

Description

Rimantadine (ri-MAN-ta-deen) is an antiviral. It is used to prevent or treat certain influenza (flu) infections (type A). It may be given alone or along with flu shots. Rimantadine will not work for colds, other types of flu, or other virus infections.

Rimantadine is available only with your doctor's prescription, in the following dosage forms:

Oral

- Syrup (U.S.)
- Tablets (U.S.)

Before Using This Medicine

In deciding to use a medicine, the risks of taking the medicine must be weighed against the good it will do. This is a decision you and your doctor will make. For rimantadine, the following should be considered:

Allergies—Tell your doctor if you have ever had any unusual or allergic reaction to rimantadine or amantadine. Also tell your health care professional if you are allergic to any other substances, such as foods, preservatives, or dyes.

Pregnancy—Studies have not been done in humans. However, studies in some animals have shown that rimantadine is harmful to the fetus and causes birth defects.

Breast-feeding—It is not known if rimantadine passes into breast milk. Although most medicines pass into breast milk in small amounts, many of them may be used safely while breast-feeding. Mothers who are taking this medicine and who wish to breast-feed should discuss this with their doctor.

Children—This medicine has been tested in children over one year of age and has not been shown to cause different side effects or problems in these children than it does in adults. There is no specific information comparing the use of rimantadine in children under one year of age with use in other age groups.

Older adults—Elderly people are especially sensitive to the effects of rimantadine. Difficulty in sleeping, difficulty in concentrating, dizziness, headache, nervousness, and weakness may be especially likely to occur. Stomach pain, nausea, vomiting, and loss of appetite may also occur.

Other medicines—Although certain medicines should not be used together at all, in other cases two different medicines may be used together even if an interaction might occur. In these cases, your doctor may want to change the dose, or other precautions may be necessary. Tell your health care professional if you are taking any other prescription or nonprescription (over-the-counter [OTC]) medicine.

Other medical problems—The presence of other medical problems may affect the use of rimantadine. Make sure you tell your doctor if you have any other medical problems, especially:

- Epilepsy or other seizures (history of)—Rimantadine may increase the frequency of convulsions (seizures) in patients with a seizure disorder
- Kidney disease—Rimantadine is removed from the body by the kidneys; patients with severe kidney disease will need to receive a lower dose of rimantadine
- Liver disease—Patients with severe liver disease may need to receive a lower dose of rimantadine

Proper Use of This Medicine

Talk to your doctor about the *possibility of getting a flu shot* if you have not had one yet.

This medicine is *best taken before exposure, or as soon as possible after exposure,* to people who have the flu.

To help keep yourself from getting the flu, *keep taking this medicine for the full time of treatment.*

If you already have the flu, *continue taking this medicine for the full time of treatment even if you begin to feel better after a few days.* This will help to clear up your infection completely. If you stop taking this medicine too soon, your symptoms may return. This medicine should be taken for at least 5 to 7 days.

This medicine works best when there is a constant amount in the blood. *To help keep the amount constant, do not miss any doses. Also, it is best to take the doses at evenly spaced times day and night.*

If you are using the oral liquid form of rimantadine, use a specially marked measuring spoon or other device to measure each dose accurately. The average household teaspoon may not hold the right amount of liquid.

Dosing—The dose of rimantadine will be different for different patients. *Follow your doctor's orders or the directions on the label.* The following information includes only the average doses of rimantadine. Your dose may be different if you have kidney disease or liver disease. *If your dose is different, do not change it* unless your doctor tells you to do so.

- For *oral* dosage forms (syrup, tablets):
  - For the prevention or treatment of flu:
    - Elderly adults—100 milligrams (mg) once a day.

- Adults and children 10 years of age and older—100 mg two times a day.
- Children up to 10 years of age—5 mg per kilogram (2.3 mg per pound) of body weight once a day. Children in this age group should not receive more than 150 mg a day.

Missed dose—If you do miss a dose of this medicine, take it as soon as possible. This will help to keep a constant amount of medicine in the blood. However, if it is almost time for your next dose, skip the missed dose and go back to your regular dosing schedule. Do not double doses.

Storage—To store this medicine:
- Keep out of the reach of children.
- Store away from heat and direct light.
- Keep the syrup form of this medicine from freezing.
- Do not keep outdated medicine or medicine no longer needed. Be sure that any discarded medicine is out of the reach of children.

Precautions While Using This Medicine

This medicine may cause some people to become dizzy or confused, or to have trouble concentrating. *Make sure you know how you react to this medicine before you drive, use machines, or do anything else that could be dangerous if you are dizzy or confused.* If these reactions are especially bothersome, check with your doctor.

If your symptoms do not improve within a few days, or if they become worse, check with your doctor.

Side Effects of This Medicine

Along with its needed effects, a medicine may cause some unwanted effects. Although not all of these side effects

may occur, if they do occur they may need medical attention.

Side effects may occur that usually do not need medical attention. These side effects may go away during treatment as your body adjusts to the medicine. However, check with your doctor if any of the following side effects continue or are bothersome:

Less common

Difficulty in concentrating; dizziness; dryness of mouth; headache; loss of appetite; nausea; nervousness; stomach pain; trouble in sleeping; unusual tiredness; vomiting

Other side effects not listed above may also occur in some patients. If you notice any other effects, check with your doctor.

SALMETEROL   Inhalation

A commonly used brand name in the U.S. and Canada is Serevent.

Description

Salmeterol (sal-ME-te-role) is used with anti-inflammatory medication to prevent asthma attacks. It is used by oral inhalation (breathed in through the mouth) to open up the bronchial tubes (air passages) of the lungs. Salmeterol should not be used to relieve an asthma attack that has already started because it does not act quickly enough.

Salmeterol is also used before exercise to prevent bronchospasm (wheezing or difficulty in breathing).

Salmeterol is available only with your doctor's prescription, in the following dosage forms:

Inhalation
- Inhalation aerosol (U.S. and Canada)
- Powder for inhalation (Canada)

Before Using This Medicine

In deciding to use a medicine, the risks of taking the medicine must be weighed against the good it will do. This is a decision you and your doctor will make. For salmeterol, the following should be considered:

Allergies—Tell your doctor if you have ever had any unusual or allergic reaction to salmeterol or to other inhalation aerosol medicines.

Pregnancy—Salmeterol has not been studied in pregnant women. However, studies in rabbits have shown that this medicine causes birth defects when given in doses many times higher than the usual human inhalation dose.

Breast-feeding—It is not known whether salmeterol passes into the breast milk. Although most medicines pass into breast milk in small amounts, many of them may be used safely while breast-feeding. Mothers who are using salmeterol and who wish to breast-feed should discuss this with their doctor.

Children—Although there is no specific information about the use of salmeterol in children younger than 12 years of age, this medicine is not expected to cause different side effects or problems in children than it does in adults.

Older adults—This medicine has been tested in a limited number of patients 65 years of age or older. It has not been shown to cause different side effects or problems in older people than it does in younger adults.

Other medicines—Although certain medicines should not be used together at all, in other cases two different medi-

cines may be used together even if an interaction might occur. In these cases, your doctor may want to change the dose, or other precautions may be necessary. When you are using salmeterol, it is especially important that your health care professional know if you are taking any of the following:

- Beta-blockers (acebutolol [e.g., Sectral], atenolol [e.g., Tenormin], betaxolol [e.g., Betoptic, Kerlone], bisoprolol [e.g., Zebeta], carteolol [e.g., Cartrol], labetalol [e.g., Normodyne], levobunolol [e.g., Betagan], metipranolol [e.g., Optipranolol], metoprolol [e.g., Lopressor], nadolol [e.g., Corgard], oxprenolol [e.g., Trasicor], penbutolol [e.g., Levatol], pindolol [e.g., Visken], propranolol [e.g., Inderal], sotalol [e.g., Sotacor], timolol [e.g., Blocadren, Timoptic])—These medicines may make your condition worse and prevent salmeterol from working properly

Other medical problems—The presence of other medical problems may affect the use of salmeterol. Make sure you tell your doctor if you have any other medical problems, especially:

- Heart or blood vessel disease—Salmeterol may make this condition worse
- Overactive thyroid—The chance of side effects may be increased in patients with this condition

---

Proper Use of This Medicine

Salmeterol is used to prevent asthma attacks. It is not used to relieve an attack that has already started. For relief of an asthma attack that has already started, you should use a medicine that starts working faster than salmeterol does. *If you do not have another medicine to use for an attack or if you have any questions about this, check with your doctor.*

Salmeterol comes with patient directions. Read them carefully before using the medicine. If you do not understand the directions or if you are not sure how to use the inhaler, ask your health care professional to show you what to do. Also, ask your health care professional to check regularly how you use the inhaler to make sure you are using it properly.

Use this medicine only as directed. Do not use more of it and do not use it more often than recommended on the label, unless otherwise directed by your doctor. Because the effects of salmeterol usually last about 12 hours, doses should never be taken more than two times a day or less than 12 hours apart. Using the medicine more often may increase the chance of serious unwanted effects. Deaths have occurred when too much inhalation bronchodilator medicine was used.

For patients using *salmeterol inhalation aerosol:*

- Keep the spray away from your eyes because it may cause irritation.
- The salmeterol aerosol canister provides 60 or 120 inhalations, depending on the size of the canister your doctor ordered. You should keep a record of the number of inhalations you use so you will know when the canister is almost empty. This canister, unlike other aerosol canisters, cannot be floated in water to test its fullness.
- When you use the inhaler for the first time, or if you have not used it for more than 4 weeks, the inhaler may not deliver the right amount of medicine with the first puff. Therefore, before using the inhaler, test or prime it.
- *To test or prime the inhaler:*

  —Insert the medicine container (canister) firmly into the clean mouthpiece according to the manufacturer's directions. Check to make sure it is placed properly into the mouthpiece.

  —Take the cap off the mouthpiece and shake the inhaler 3 or 4 times.

—Hold the inhaler well away from you at arm's length and press the top of the canister, spraying the medicine into the air *two* times. The inhaler will now be ready to provide the right amount of medicine when you use it.

• *To use the inhaler:*

—Using your thumb and 1 or 2 fingers, hold the inhaler upright, with the mouthpiece end down and pointing toward you.

—Take the cap off the mouthpiece. Check the mouthpiece for any foreign object. Then, gently shake the inhaler and canister 3 or 4 times.

—Hold the mouthpiece away from your mouth and breathe out slowly and completely.

—Use the inhalation method recommended by your doctor.

• Open-mouth method—Place the mouthpiece about 1 or 2 inches (2 fingerwidths) in front of your widely opened mouth. Make sure the inhaler is aimed into your mouth so the spray does not hit the roof of your mouth or your tongue.

• Closed-mouth method—Place the mouthpiece in your mouth between your teeth and over your tongue with your lips closed tightly around it. Make sure your tongue or teeth are not blocking the opening.

—Start to breathe in slowly through your mouth. At the same time, press the top of the canister 1 time to get one puff of medicine. Continue to breathe in slowly until you have taken a full breath. Try to inhale for 3 to 4 seconds. It is important to press down on the top of the canister and breathe in slowly at the same time so the medicine is pulled into your lungs. This step may be difficult at first. If you are using the closed-mouth method and you see a fine mist coming from your mouth or nose, the inhaler is not being used correctly.

—After inhaling the spray into your lungs, hold your breath as long as you can up to 10 seconds. This gives the medicine time to settle into your airways and lungs.

—Take the mouthpiece away from your mouth and breathe out slowly.

—If your doctor has told you to inhale more than 1 puff of medicine at each dose, wait about 30 seconds between puffs. Then, gently shake the inhaler again and take the next puff, following exactly the same steps you used for the first puff. Press the canister 1 time for each breath in.

—When you are finished, wipe off the mouthpiece and replace the cap to keep the mouthpiece clean and free of foreign objects.

• Clean the inhaler and mouthpiece at least once a week.

To clean the inhaler:

• Remove the metal canister from the inhaler and set the canister aside.
• Wash the mouthpiece and cap with soap and hot water. Rinse well with warm, running water.
• Shake off the excess water and let the inhaler parts air dry completely before replacing the metal canister and cap.
• The metal canister stem may get dirty or blocked. While the canister is out of the mouthpiece, check the small hole in the stem of the canister.
• If the hole seems blocked, rinse it with clear, lukewarm water.
• Let the canister dry completely before you put it back into the dry mouthpiece.
• Replace the cap to keep the mouthpiece clean.

• Save your inhaler. Refill units may be available.

For patients using *salmeterol powder for inhalation:*

- *To load the inhaler:*

—Take the cap off the mouthpiece. Check the mouthpiece for any foreign object and make sure the mouthpiece is clean.

—Hold the white tray by the corners and pull it out gently until you can see all of the plastic ridges on the sides of the tray.

—Squeeze the ridged sides and gently pull the tray out of the body of the inhaler.

—Place the disk containing the medication onto the white wheel with the numbers facing up. Allow the underside of the disk to fit into the holes of the wheel.

—Slide the tray with the wheel and disk back into the body of the inhaler.

—Gently push the tray in and pull it out again. The disk will turn.

—Continue to turn the disk in this way until the number 4 appears in the top indicator window. Each disk has 4 blisters containing medicine. The window will display how many doses you have left after you use it each time.

- *To use the inhaler:*

—Hold the inhaler flat in your hand. Lift the lid until it is fully upright.

—The plastic needle on the front of the lid will break the blister containing one inhalation of medicine. When the lid is raised as far as it will go, both the upper and lower surfaces of the blister will be pierced. Some resistance will be felt as both sides of the blister are pierced. Do not try to lift the lid unless the tray is fully within the body of the inhaler or is completely removed, as it would be for cleaning. Lifting the lid when the tray is not completely pushed into the inhaler will break the needle and you will need a new inhaler.

—After the blister is broken open, close the lid. Keeping the inhaler flat and well away from your mouth, breathe out to the end of a normal breath.

—Raise the inhaler to your mouth, and place the mouthpiece in your mouth.

—Close your lips around the mouthpiece and tilt your head slightly back. Do not block the mouthpiece with your teeth or tongue. Do not cover the air holes on the side of the mouthpiece.

—Breathe in slowly and deeply through your mouth until you have taken a full breath.

—Hold your breath and remove the mouthpiece from your mouth. Continue holding your breath as long as you can up to 10 seconds before breathing out. This gives the medicine time to settle into your airways and lungs.

—Hold the inhaler well away from your mouth and breathe out to the end of a normal breath.

—Prepare the disk for your next inhalation. Pull the disk out once and push it in once. The disk will turn to the next numbered dose as seen in the indicator window. Do not pierce the blister until just before your next inhalation.

—Replace the mouthpiece cover.

- When the indicator window shows the number 4 again, the disk is empty and should be replaced with a new disk. Do not throw the inhaler wheel away with the empty disk.

- *To clean the inhaler:* A brush is provided at the rear of the inhaler body to clean any remaining powder from the inhaler device. This should be done after the tray and wheel have been removed from the inhaler body and before a new disk is inserted.

- The inhaler may need to be replaced after about 6 months of use.

Dosing   The dose of salmeterol will be different for different patients. *Follow your doctor's orders or the directions on the label.* The following information includes only the average doses of salmeterol. *If your dose is different, do not change it* unless your doctor tells you to do so.

- For the *inhalation aerosol dosage form:*
  - —For preventing attacks of bronchial asthma:
    - Adults and children 12 years of age and older—Two inhalations (puffs) two times a day, in the morning and evening. Doses should be taken about twelve hours apart.
    - Children younger than 12 years of age—Use and dose must be determined by your doctor.
  - —For preventing bronchospasm caused by exercise:
    - Adults and children 12 years of age and older—Two inhalations (puffs) taken at least thirty to sixty minutes before you start to exercise.
    - Children younger than 12 years of age—Use and dose must be determined by your doctor.
- For the *powder for inhalation dosage form:*
  - —For preventing attacks of bronchial asthma:
    - Adults and children 12 years of age and older—One inhalation (the contents of one blister) two times a day, in the morning and evening. Doses should be taken about twelve hours apart.
    - Children younger than 12 years of age—Use and dose must be determined by your doctor.

Missed dose—If you use salmeterol inhalation regularly and you miss a dose of this medicine, use it as soon as possible. Then go back to your regular schedule. Do not double doses. If you have wheezing or breathlessness before the next dose is due, you should use another inhaled bronchodilator that starts to work faster than salmeterol does to relieve the attack.

Storage—To store this medicine:

- Keep out of the reach of children.
- Store away from heat and direct light.
- Keep the medicine from freezing. Do not refrigerate.
- Do not keep outdated medicine or medicine no longer needed. Be sure that any discarded medicine is out of the reach of children.
- Store canister with the nozzle end down.
- Do not puncture, break, or burn the aerosol container, even if it is empty.
- Do not store the powder form of this medicine in the bathroom, near the kitchen sink, or in other damp places. Moisture may cause the medicine to break down.

Precautions While Using This Medicine

It is important that your doctor check your progress at regular intervals to make sure that this medicine is working properly.

If you still have trouble breathing after using this medicine, or if your condition becomes worse, check with your doctor at once.

Check with your doctor:

- If you need to use 4 or more inhalations (puffs) a day of a fast-acting inhaled bronchodilator for 2 or more days in a row to relieve asthma attacks.
- If you need to use more than 1 canister (a total of 200 inhalations per canister) of a fast-acting inhaled bronchodilator in a 2-month period to relieve asthma attacks.

You may also be taking an anti-inflammatory medicine for asthma along with this medicine. *Do not stop taking the anti-inflammatory medicine even if your asthma seems better, unless you are told to do so by your doctor.*

Side Effects of This Medicine

Along with its needed effects, a medicine may cause some unwanted effects. Although not all of these side effects may occur, if they do occur they may need medical attention.

Check with your doctor immediately if any of the following side effects occur:

Rare

Increased shortness of breath, troubled breathing, tightness in chest or wheezing; hives, skin rash, or swelling of face, lips, or eyelids

Symptoms of overdose

Chest discomfort or pain; convulsions (seizures); dizziness or lightheadedness; fast heartbeat, continuing; irregular heartbeat; nervousness or restlessness, continuing; trembling, continuing; vomiting

Other side effects may occur that usually do not need medical attention. These side effects may go away during treatment as your body adjusts to the medicine. However, check with your doctor if any of the following side effects continue or are bothersome:

More common

Headache

Less common

Abdominal pain; cough; diarrhea; fast heartbeat; muscle cramps or soreness; nausea; nervousness; unusual pounding heartbeat; trembling

SERTRALINE　Systemic

A commonly used brand name in the U.S. and Canada is Zoloft.

Description

Sertraline (SER-tral-leen) is used to treat mental depression.

This medicine is available only with your doctor's prescription, in the following dosage form:

Oral

- Capsules (Canada)
- Tablets (U.S.)

Before Using This Medicine

In deciding to use a medicine, the risks of taking the medicine must be weighed against the good it will do. This is a decision you and your doctor will make. For sertraline, the following should be considered:

Allergies—Tell your doctor if you have ever had any unusual or allergic reaction to sertraline. Also tell your health care professional if you are allergic to any other substances, such as foods, preservatives, or dyes.

Pregnancy—Studies have not been done in pregnant women. However, studies in animals have shown that sertraline may cause delayed development and decreased survival rates of offspring when given in doses many times the usual human dose. Before taking this medicine, make sure your doctor knows if you are pregnant or if you may become pregnant.

Breast-feeding—It is not known whether sertraline is excreted in breast milk.

Children—Studies on this medicine have been done only in adult patients, and there is no specific information comparing use of sertraline in children with use in other age groups.

Older adults—In studies done to date that have included elderly people, sertraline did not cause different side effects or problems in older people than it did in younger adults.

Other medicines—Although certain medicines should not be used together at all, in other cases two different medicines may be used together even if an interaction might occur. In these cases, your doctor may want to change the dose, or other precautions may be necessary. When you are taking sertraline, it is especially important that your health care professional know if you are taking any of the following:

- Digitoxin (e.g., Crystodigin) or
- Warfarin (e.g., Coumadin)—Higher or lower blood levels of these medicines or sertraline may occur, which may increase the chance of unwanted effects; your doctor may need to change the dose of either these medicines or sertraline
- Monoamine oxidase (MAO) inhibitors (furazolidone [e.g., Furoxone], isocarboxazid [e.g., Marplan], phenelzine [e.g., Nardil], procarbazine [e.g., Matulane], selegiline [e.g., Eldepryl], tranylcypromine [e.g., Parnate])—Taking sertraline while you are taking or within 2 weeks of taking MAO inhibitors may cause confusion, agitation, restlessness, stomach or intestinal symptoms, sudden high body temperature, extremely high blood pressure, and severe convulsions; at least 14 days should be allowed between stopping treatment with one medicine and starting treatment with the other

Other medical problems—The presence of other medical problems may affect the use of sertraline. Make sure you tell your doctor if you have any other medical problems, especially:

- Drug abuse or dependence (or history of)—Because sertraline is a new drug, it is not known if it could become habit-forming, causing mental or physical dependence
- Kidney disease, severe, or
- Liver disease—Higher blood levels of sertraline may occur, increasing the chance of side effects

---

Proper Use of This Medicine

Take this medicine only as directed by your doctor, to benefit your condition as much as possible. Do not take more of it, do not take it more often, and do not take it for a longer time than your doctor ordered.

You may have to take sertraline for up to 4 weeks or longer before you begin to feel better. Your doctor should check your progress at regular visits during this time.

This medicine should always be taken at the same time in relation to meals and snacks to make sure that it is absorbed in the same way.

Dosing—The dose of sertraline will be different for different patients. *Follow your doctor's orders or the directions on the label.* The following information includes only the average doses of sertraline. *If your dose is different, do not change it* unless your doctor tells you to do so.

- The number of capsules or tablets that you take depends on the strength of the medicine and the medical problem for which you are taking sertraline.
- For *oral* dosage forms (capsules or tablets):

  —Adults: To start, usually 50 milligrams once a day, taken either in the morning or evening. Your doctor may gradually increase your dose if needed.

  —Children: Dose must be determined by the doctor.

  —Older adults: To start, usually 12.5 to 25 milligrams once a day, taken either in the morning or evening. Your doctor may gradually increase your dose if needed.

Missed dose—Because sertraline may be given to different patients at different times of the day, you and your doctor should discuss what to do about any missed doses.

Storage—To store this medicine:

- Keep out of the reach of children.
- Store away from heat and direct light.
- Do not store in the bathroom, near the kitchen sink, or in other damp places. Heat or moisture may cause the medicine to break down.
- Do not keep outdated medicine or medicine no longer needed. Be sure that any discarded medicine is out of the reach of children.

Precautions While Using This Medicine

It is important that your doctor check your progress at regular visits, to allow for changes in your dose and to help reduce any side effects.

This medicine could possibly add to the effects of alcohol and other CNS depressants (medicines that slow down the nervous system, possibly causing drowsiness). Some examples of CNS depressants are antihistamines or medicine for hay fever, other allergies, or colds; sedatives, tranquilizers, or sleeping medicine; prescription pain medicine or narcotics; barbiturates; medicine for seizures; muscle relaxants; or anesthetics, including some dental anesthetics. *Check with your doctor before taking any of the above while you are using this medicine.*

This medicine may cause some people to become drowsy. *Make sure you know how you react to sertraline before you drive, use machines, or do anything else that could be dangerous if you are not alert.*

This medicine may cause dryness of the mouth. For temporary relief, use sugarless gum or candy, melt bits of ice in your mouth, or use a saliva substitute. However, if your mouth continues to feel dry for more than 2 weeks, check with your medical doctor or dentist. Continuing dryness of the mouth may increase the chance of dental disease, including tooth decay, gum disease, and fungus infections.

Side Effects of This Medicine

Along with its needed effects, a medicine may cause some unwanted effects. Although not all of these side effects may occur, if they do occur they may need medical attention.

Check with your doctor as soon as possible if any of the following side effects occur:

Less common or rare

> Fast talking and excited feelings or actions that are out of control; fever; skin rash, hives, or itching

Other side effects may occur that usually do not need medical attention. These side effects may go away during treatment as your body adjusts to the medicine. However, check with your doctor if any of the following side effects continue or are bothersome:

More common

> Decreased appetite or weight loss; decreased sexual drive or ability; diarrhea; drowsiness; dryness of mouth; headache; nausea; stomach or abdominal cramps, gas, or pain; tiredness or weakness; tremor; trouble in sleeping

Less common

> Anxiety, agitation, nervousness or restlessness; changes in vision, including blurred vision; constipation; fast or irregular heartbeat; flushing or redness of skin, with feeling of warmth or heat; increased appetite; vomiting

Other side effects not listed above may also occur in some patients. If you notice any other effects, check with your doctor.

SKELETAL MUSCLE RELAXANTS   Systemic

Some commonly used brand names are:

In the U.S.—

Carbacot[5]   Robaxin[5]
Delaxin[5]   Robomol[5]
Maolate[2]   Skelaxin[4]
Marbaxin[5]   Skelex[5]
Paraflex[3]   Sodol[1]
Parafon Forte DSC[3]   Soma[1]
Rela[1]   Soprodol[1]
Robamol[5]   Soridol[1]

In Canada—

Robaxin[5]
Soma[1]

Note: For quick reference, the following skeletal muscle relaxants are numbered to match the corresponding brand names.

This information applies to the following medicines:

1. Carisoprodol (kar-eye-soe-PROE-dole)‡
2. Chlorphenesin (klor-FEN-e-sin)
3. Chlorzoxazone (klor-ZOX-a-zone)‡
4. Metaxalone (me-TAX-a-lone)
5. Methocarbamol (meth-oh-KAR-ba-mole)‡

This information does *not* apply to Baclofen, Cyclobenzaprine, Dantrolene, Diazepam, or Orphenadrine.

‡Generic name product may also be available in the U.S.

Description

Skeletal muscle relaxants are used to relax certain muscles in your body and relieve the pain and discomfort caused by strains, sprains, or other injury to your muscles. However, these medicines do not take the place of rest, exercise or physical therapy, or other treatment that your doctor may recommend for your medical problem. Methocarbamol also has been used to relieve some of the muscle problems caused by tetanus.

Skeletal muscle relaxants act in the central nervous system (CNS) to produce their muscle relaxant effects. Their actions in the CNS may also produce some of their side effects.

In the U.S., these medicines are available only with your doctor's prescription. In Canada, some of these medicines are available without a prescription.

These medicines are available in the following dosage forms:

Oral

Carisoprodol
  • Tablets (U.S. and Canada)
Chlorphenesin
  • Tablets (U.S.)
Chlorzoxazone
  • Tablets (U.S.)
Metaxalone
  • Tablets (U.S.)
Methocarbamol
  • Tablets (U.S. and Canada)

Parenteral

Methocarbamol
  • Injection (U.S. and Canada)

Before Using This Medicine

In deciding to use a medicine, the risks of taking the medicine must be weighed against the good it will do. This is a decision you and your doctor will make. For the skeletal muscle relaxants, the following should be considered:

Allergies—Tell your doctor if you have ever had any unusual or allergic reaction to any of the skeletal muscle relaxants or to carbromal, mebutamate, meprobamate (e.g., Equanil), or tybamate. Also tell your health care professional if you are allergic to any other substances, such as foods, preservatives, or dyes.

Pregnancy—Although skeletal muscle relaxants have not been shown to cause birth defects or other problems, studies on birth defects have not been done in pregnant women. Studies in animals with metaxalone have not shown that it causes birth defects.

Breast-feeding—Carisoprodol passes into the breast milk and may cause drowsiness or stomach upset in nursing babies. Chlorphenesin, chlorzoxazone, metaxalone, and methocarbamol have not been shown to cause problems in nursing babies. However, methocarbamol passes into the breast milk in small amounts. It is not known whether chlorphenesin, chlorzoxazone, or metaxalone passes into the breast milk.

Children—Chlorzoxazone has been tested in children and has not been shown to cause different side effects or problems than it does in adults.

Although there is no specific information about the use of carisoprodol in children, it is not expected to cause different side effects or problems in children than it does in adults.

There is no specific information about the use of other skeletal muscle relaxants in children.

Older adults—Many medicines have not been tested in older people. Therefore, it may not be known whether they work exactly the same way they do in younger adults or if they cause different side effects or problems in older people. There is no specific information about the use of skeletal muscle relaxants in the elderly.

Other medicines—Although certain medicines should not be used together at all, in other cases two different medicines may be used together even if an interaction might occur. In these cases, your doctor may want to change the dose, or other precautions may be necessary. When you are taking a skeletal muscle relaxant, it is especially important that your health care professional know if you are taking any of the following:

- Central nervous system (CNS) depressants or
- Tricyclic antidepressants (amitriptyline [e.g., Elavil], amoxapine [e.g., Asendin], clomipramine [e.g., Anafranil], desipramine [e.g., Pertofrane], doxepin [e.g., Sinequan], imipramine [e.g., Tofranil], nortriptyline [e.g., Aventyl], protriptyline [e.g., Vivactil], trimipramine [e.g., Surmontil])—The chance of side effects may be increased

Other medical problems—The presence of other medical problems may affect the use of a skeletal muscle relaxant. Make sure you tell your doctor if you have any other medical problems, especially:

- Allergies, history of, or
- Blood disease caused by an allergy or reaction to any other medicine, history of, or
- Drug abuse or dependence, or history of, or
- Kidney disease or
- Liver disease or
- Porphyria—Depending on which of the skeletal muscle relaxants you take, the chance of side effects may be increased; your doctor can choose a muscle relaxant that is less likely to cause problems
- Epilepsy—Convulsions may be more likely to occur if methocarbamol is given by injection

Proper Use of This Medicine

Chlorzoxazone, metaxalone, or methocarbamol tablets may be crushed and mixed with a little food or liquid if needed to make the tablets easier to swallow.

Missed dose—If you miss a dose of this medicine and remember within an hour or so of the missed dose, take it right away. But if you do not remember until later, skip the missed dose and go back to your regular dosing schedule. Do not double doses.

Storage—To store this medicine:

- Keep out of the reach of children.
- Store away from heat and direct light.
- Do not store this medicine in the bathroom, near the kitchen sink, or in other damp places. Heat or moisture may cause the medicine to break down.
- Do not keep outdated medicine or medicine no longer needed. Be sure that any discarded medicine is out of the reach of children.

Precautions While Using This Medicine

If you will be taking this medicine for a long time (for example, more than a few weeks), your doctor should check your progress at regular visits.

This medicine will add to the effects of alcohol and other CNS depressants (medicines that slow down the nervous system, possibly causing drowsiness). Some examples of CNS depressants are antihistamines or medicine for hay fever, other allergies, or colds; sedatives, tranquilizers, or sleeping medicine; prescription pain medicine or narcotics; barbiturates; medicine for seizures; other muscle relaxants; or anesthetics, including some dental anesthetics. *Do not drink alcoholic beverages, and check with your doctor before taking any of the medicines listed above, while you are using this medicine.*

Skeletal muscle relaxants may cause blurred vision or clumsiness or unsteadiness in some people. They may also cause some people to feel drowsy, dizzy, lightheaded, faint, or less alert than they are normally. *Make sure you know how you react to this medicine before you drive, use machines, or do anything else that could be dangerous if you are dizzy or are not alert, well-coordinated, and able to see well.*

For *diabetic patients:*

- Metaxalone (e.g., Skelaxin) may cause false test results with one type of test for sugar in your urine. If your urine sugar test shows an unusually large amount of sugar, or if you have any questions about this, check with your health care professional. This is especially important if your diabetes is not well controlled.

Side Effects of This Medicine

Along with its needed effects, a medicine may cause some unwanted effects. Although not all of these side effects may occur, if they do occur they may need medical attention.

Check with your doctor as soon as possible if any of the following side effects occur:

Less common

Fainting; fast heartbeat; fever; hive-like swellings (large) on face, eyelids, mouth, lips, and/or tongue; mental depression; shortness of breath, troubled breathing, tightness in chest, and/or wheezing; skin rash, hives, itching, or redness; slow heartbeat (methocarbamol injection only); stinging or burning of eyes; stuffy nose and red or bloodshot eyes

Rare

Blood in urine; bloody or black, tarry stools; convulsions (seizures) (methocarbamol injection only); cough or hoarseness; fast or irregular breathing; lower back or side pain; muscle cramps or pain (not present before treatment or more painful than before treatment); painful or difficult urination; pain, tenderness, heat, redness, or swelling over a blood vessel (vein) in arm or leg (methocarbamol injection only); pinpoint red spots on skin; puffiness or swelling of the eyelids or around the eyes; sores, ulcers, or white spots on lips or in mouth; sore throat and fever with or without chills; swollen and/or painful glands; unusual bruising or bleeding; unusual tiredness or weakness; vomiting of blood or material that looks like coffee grounds; yellow eyes or skin

Other side effects may occur that usually do not need medical attention. These side effects may go away during treatment as your body adjusts to the medicine. However, check with your doctor if any of the following side effects continue or are bothersome:

More common

Blurred or double vision or any change in vision; dizziness or lightheadedness; drowsiness

Less common or rare

Abdominal or stomach cramps or pain; clumsiness or unsteadiness; confusion; constipation; diarrhea; excitement, nervousness, restlessness, or irritability; flushing or redness of face; headache; heartburn; hiccups; muscle weakness; nausea or vomiting; pain or peeling of skin at place of injection (methocarbamol only); trembling; trouble in sleeping; uncontrolled movements of eyes (methocarbamol injection only)

Although not all of the side effects listed above have been reported for all of these medicines, they have been reported for at least one of them. However, since all of these skeletal muscle relaxants have similar effects, it is possible that any of the above side effects may occur with any of these medicines.

In addition to the other side effects listed above, chlorzoxazone may cause your urine to turn orange or reddish purple. Methocarbamol may cause your urine to turn black, brown, or green. This effect is harmless and will go away when you stop taking the medicine. However, if you have any questions about this, check with your doctor.

Other side effects not listed above may also occur in some patients. If you notice any other effects, check with your doctor.

STAVUDINE   Systemic†

A commonly used brand name in the U.S. is Zerit.
Another commonly used name is d4T.

> †Not commercially available in Canada.

Description

Stavudine (STAV-yoo-deen) (also known as d4T) is used in the treatment of the infection caused by the human immunodeficiency virus (HIV). HIV is the virus responsible for acquired immune deficiency syndrome (AIDS).

Stavudine (d4T) will not cure or prevent HIV infection or AIDS; however, it helps to keep HIV from reproducing and appears to slow down the destruction of the immune system. This may help delay the development of problems usually related to AIDS or HIV disease. Stavudine will not keep you from spreading HIV to other people. People who receive this medicine may continue to have the problems usually related to AIDS or HIV disease.

Stavudine may cause some serious side effects, including peripheral neuropathy. Symptoms of peripheral neuropathy include tingling, burning, numbness, and pain in the hands or feet. *Check with your doctor if any new health problems or symptoms occur while you are taking stavudine.*

Stavudine is available only with your doctor's prescription, in the following dosage form:

Oral
  • Capsules (U.S.)

Before Using This Medicine

In deciding to use a medicine, the risks of taking the medicine must be weighed against the good it will do. This is a decision you and your doctor will make. For stavudine, the following should be considered:

Allergies—Tell your doctor if you have ever had any unusual or allergic reaction to stavudine. Also tell your health care professional if you are allergic to any other substances, such as foods, preservatives, or dyes.

Pregnancy—Stavudine has not been studied in pregnant women. However, studies in animals have shown that stavudine causes birth defects when given in very high doses. Before taking this medicine, make sure your doctor knows if you are pregnant or if you may become pregnant.

Breast-feeding—It is not known whether stavudine passes into the breast milk. However, if your baby does not already have the AIDS virus, there is a chance that you could pass it to your baby by breast-feeding. Talk to your doctor first if you are thinking about breast-feeding your baby.

Children—Studies on this medicine have been done only in adult patients, and there is no specific information comparing use of stavudine in children with use in other age groups.

Older adults—Stavudine has not been studied specifically in older people. Therefore, it is not known whether it causes different side effects or problems in the elderly than it does in younger adults.

Other medicines—Although certain medicines should not be used together at all, in other cases two different medicines may be used together even if an interaction might

occur. In these cases, your doctor may want to change the dose, or other precautions may be necessary. When you are taking stavudine, it is especially important that your health care professional know if you are taking any of the following:

- Chloramphenicol (e.g., Chloromycetin) or
- Cisplatin (e.g., Platinol) or
- Dapsone (e.g., Avlosulfon) or
- Didanosine (e.g. ddI, Videx) or
- Ethambutol (e.g., Myambutol) or
- Ethionamide (e.g., Trecator-SC) or
- Hydralazine (e.g., Apresoline) or
- Isoniazid (e.g., Nydrazid) or
- Lithium (e.g., Eskalith, Lithobid) or
- Metronidazole (e.g., Flagyl) or
- Nitrofurantoin (e.g., Macrodantin) or
- Phenytoin (e.g., Dilantin) or
- Vincristine (e.g., Oncovin) or
- Zalcitabine (e.g. ddC, HIVID)—Use of these medicines with stavudine may increase the chance of peripheral neuropathy (tingling, burning, numbness, or pain in your hands or feet)

Other medical problems—The presence of other medical problems may affect the use of stavudine. Make sure you tell your doctor if you have any other medical problems, especially:

- Alcohol abuse, active or a history of, or
- Liver disease—Stavudine may make liver disease worse in patients with liver disease, active alcohol abuse, or a history of alcohol abuse
- Kidney disease—Patients with kidney disease may have an increased chance of side effects
- Peripheral neuropathy—Stavudine may make this condition worse

---

Proper Use of This Medicine

Take this medicine exactly as directed by your doctor. Do not take more of it, do not take it more often, and do not take it for a longer time than your doctor ordered. Also, do not stop taking this medicine without checking with your doctor first.

Keep taking stavudine for the full time of treatment, even if you begin to feel better.

This medicine works best when there is a constant amount in the blood. *To help keep the amount constant, do not miss any doses.* If you need help in planning the best times to take your medicine, check with your health care professional.

Only take medicine that your doctor has prescribed specifically for you. Do not share your medicine with others.

Dosing—The dose of stavudine will be different for different patients. *Follow your doctor's orders or the directions on the label.* The following information includes only the average doses of stavudine. Your dose may be different if you have kidney disease. *If your dose is different, do not change it* unless your doctor tells you to do so:

- For *oral* dosage form (capsules):
  —For treatment of HIV infection:
    - Adults and teenagers weighing 60 kilograms (kg) (132 pounds) or more—40 milligrams (mg) two times a day.
    - Adults and teenagers weighing up to 60 kg (132 pounds)—30 mg two times a day.
    - Children—Use and dose must be determined by your doctor.

Missed dose—If you miss a dose of this medicine, take it as soon as possible. However, if it is almost time for your next dose, skip the missed dose and go back to your regular dosing schedule. Do not double doses.

Storage—To store this medicine:
- Keep out of the reach of children.

- Store away from heat and direct light.
- Do not store in the bathroom, near the kitchen sink, or in other damp places. Heat or moisture may cause the medicine to break down.
- Do not keep outdated medicine or medicine no longer needed. Be sure that any discarded medicine is out of the reach of children.

Precautions While Using This Medicine

It is very important that your doctor check your progress at regular visits.

Do not take any other medicines without checking with your doctor first. To do so may increase the chance of side effects from stavudine.

HIV may be acquired from or spread to other people through infected body fluids, including blood, vaginal fluid, or semen. *If you are infected, it is best to avoid any sexual activity involving an exchange of body fluids with other people. If you do have sex, always wear (or have your partner wear) a condom ("rubber").* Only use condoms made of latex, and *use them every time you have vaginal, anal, or oral sex.* The use of a spermicide (such as nonoxynol-9) may also help prevent transmission of HIV if it is not irritating to the vagina, rectum, or mouth. Spermicides have been shown to kill HIV in lab tests. Do not use oil-based jelly, cold cream, baby oil, or shortening as a lubricant—these products can cause the condom to break. Lubricants without oil, such as *K-Y Jelly*, are recommended. Women may wish to carry their own condoms. Birth control pills and diaphragms will help protect against pregnancy, but they will not prevent someone from giving or getting the AIDS virus. *If you inject drugs*, get help to stop. *Do not share needles or equipment with anyone.* In some cities, more than half of the drug users are infected, and sharing even one needle or syringe can spread the virus. If you have any questions about this, check with your health care professional.

Side Effects of This Medicine

Along with its needed effects, a medicine may cause some unwanted effects. Although not all of these side effects may occur, if they do occur they may need medical attention.

Check with your doctor immediately if any of the following side effects occur:

  More common

   Tingling, burning, numbness, or pain in the hands or feet

  Less common

   Fever; joint pain; muscle pain; skin rash

  Rare

   Nausea and vomiting; stomach pain (severe); unusual tiredness or weakness

Other side effects may occur that usually do not need medical attention. These side effects may go away during treatment as your body adjusts to the medicine. However, check with your doctor if any of the following side effects continue or are bothersome:

  Less common

   Diarrhea; difficulty in sleeping; headache; lack of strength or energy; loss of appetite

Other side effects not listed above may also occur in some patients. If you notice any other effects, check with your doctor.

SULFAMETHOXAZOLE AND TRIMETHOPRIM Systemic

Some commonly used brand names are:

In the U.S.—

Bactrim	Sulfatrim
Bactrim DS	Sulfatrim DS
Cotrim	Sulfoxaprim
Cotrim DS	Sulfoxaprim DS
Septra	Triazole
Septra DS	Triazole DS
Sulfamethoprim	Trimeth-Sulfa
Sulfamethoprim DS	Trisulfam
Sulfaprim	Uroplus DS
Sulfaprim DS	Uroplus SS

Generic name product may also be available.

In Canada—

Apo-Sulfatrim	Nu-Cotrimox
Apo-Sulfatrim DS	Nu-Cotrimox DS
Bactrim	Roubac
Bactrim DS	Septra
Novotrimel	Septra DS
Novotrimel DS	

Some other commonly used names are cotrimoxazole and SMZ-TMP.

Description

Sulfamethoxazole and trimethoprim (sul-fa-meth-OX-a-zole and trye-METH-oh-prim) combination is used to treat infections, such as bronchitis, middle ear infection, urinary tract infection, and traveler's diarrhea. It is also used for the prevention and treatment of *Pneumocystis carinii* pneumonia (PCP). It will not work for colds, flu, or other virus infections. It may also be used for other conditions as determined by your doctor.

Sulfamethoxazole and trimethoprim combination is available only with your doctor's prescription, in the following dosage forms:

Oral
- Oral suspension (U.S. and Canada)
- Tablets (U.S. and Canada)

Parenteral
- Injection (U.S. and Canada)

Before Using This Medicine

In deciding to use a medicine, the risks of taking the medicine must be weighed against the good it will do. This is a decision you and your doctor will make. For sulfamethoxazole and trimethoprim combination, the following should be considered:

Allergies—Tell your doctor if you have ever had any unusual or allergic reaction to sulfa medicines, furosemide (e.g., Lasix) or thiazide diuretics (water pills), oral antidiabetics (diabetes medicine you take by mouth), glaucoma medicine you take by mouth (for example, acetazolamide [e.g., Diamox], dichlorphenamide [e.g., Daranide], methazolamide [e.g., Neptazane]), or trimethoprim (e.g., Trimpex). Also tell your health care professional if you are allergic to any other substances, such as foods, preservatives, or dyes.

Pregnancy—Sulfamethoxazole and trimethoprim combination has not been reported to cause birth defects or other problems in humans. However, studies in mice, rats, and rabbits have shown that some sulfonamides cause birth defects, including cleft palate and bone problems. Studies in rabbits have also shown that trimethoprim causes birth defects, as well as a decrease in the number of successful pregnancies.

Breast-feeding—Sulfamethoxazole and trimethoprim pass into the breast milk. This medicine is not recommended for use during breast-feeding. It may cause liver problems, anemia, and other unwanted effects in nursing babies, especially those with glucose-6-phosphate dehydrogenase (G6PD) deficiency.

Children—This medicine should not be given to infants under 2 months of age unless directed by the child's doctor, because it may cause brain problems.

Older adults—Elderly people are especially sensitive to the effects of sulfamethoxazole and trimethoprim combination. Severe skin problems and blood problems may be more likely to occur in the elderly. These problems may also be more likely to occur in patients who are taking diuretics (water pills) along with this medicine.

Other medicines—Although certain medicines should not be used together at all, in other cases two different medicines may be used together even if an interaction might occur. In these cases, your doctor may want to change the dose, or other precautions may be necessary. When you are taking sulfamethoxazole and trimethoprim combination, it is especially important that your health care professional knows if you are taking any of the following:

- Acetaminophen (e.g., Tylenol) (with long-term, high-dose use) or
- Amiodarone (e.g., Cordarone) or
- Anabolic steroids (nandrolone [e.g., Anabolin], oxandrolone [e.g., Anavar], oxymetholone [e.g., Anadrol], stanozolol [e.g., Winstrol]) or
- Androgens (male hormones) or
- Antithyroid agents (medicine for overactive thyroid) or
- Carbamazepine (e.g., Tegretol) or
- Carmustine (e.g., BiCNU) or
- Chloroquine (e.g., Aralen) or
- Dantrolene (e.g., Dantrium) or
- Daunorubicin (e.g., Cerubidine) or
- Disulfiram (e.g., Antabuse) or
- Divalproex (e.g., Depakote) or
- Estrogens (female hormones) or
- Etretinate (e.g., Tegison) or
- Gold salts (medicine for arthritis) or

- Hydroxychloroquine (e.g., Plaquenil) or
- Mercaptopurine (e.g., Purinethol) or
- Naltrexone (e.g., Trexan) (with long-term, high-dose use) or
- Oral contraceptives (birth control pills) containing estrogens or
- Other anti-infectives by mouth or by injection (medicine for infection) or
- Phenothiazines (acetophenazine [e.g., Tindal], chlorpromazine [e.g., Thorazine], fluphenazine [e.g., Prolixin], mesoridazine [e.g., Serentil], perphenazine [e.g., Trilafon], prochlorperazine [e.g., Compazine], promazine [e.g., Sparine], promethazine [e.g., Phenergan], thioridazine [e.g., Mellaril], trifluoperazine [e.g., Stelazine], triflupromazine [e.g., Vesprin], trimeprazine [e.g., Temaril]) or
- Plicamycin (e.g., Mithracin) or
- Valproic acid (e.g., Depakene)—Use of sulfamethoxazole and trimethoprim combination with these medicines may increase the chance of side effects affecting the liver
- Acetohydroxamic acid (e.g., Lithostat) or
- Dapsone or
- Furazolidone (e.g., Furoxone) or
- Nitrofurantoin (e.g., Furadantin) or
- Primaquine or
- Procainamide (e.g., Pronestyl) or
- Quinidine (e.g., Quinidex) or
- Quinine (e.g., Quinamm)—Use of sulfamethoxazole and trimethoprim combination with these medicines may increase the chance of side effects affecting the blood
- Anticoagulants (blood thinners) or
- Ethotoin (e.g., Peganone) or
- Mephenytoin (e.g., Mesantoin)—Use of sulfamethoxazole and trimethoprim combination with these medicines may increase the chance of side effects of these medicines
- Antidiabetics, oral (diabetes medicine you take by mouth)—Use of oral antidiabetics with sulfamethoxazole and trimethoprim combination may increase the chance of side effects affecting the blood and/or the side effects of the oral antidiabetics
- Methenamine (e.g., Mandelamine)—Use of methenamine with sulfamethoxazole and trimethoprim combination may increase the chance of side effects of the sulfamethoxazole

- Methotrexate (e.g., Mexate) or
- Phenytoin (e.g., Dilantin)—Use of these medicines with sulfamethoxazole and trimethoprim combination may increase the chance of side effects affecting the liver and/or the side effects of these medicines
- Methyldopa (e.g., Aldomet)—Use of methyldopa with sulfamethoxazole and trimethoprim combination may increase the chance of side effects affecting the liver and/or the blood

Other medical problems—The presence of other medical problems may affect the use of sulfamethoxazole and trimethoprim combination. Make sure you tell your doctor if you have any other medical problems, especially:

- Anemia or other blood problems or
- Glucose-6-phosphate dehydrogenase (G6PD) deficiency—Patients with these problems may have an increase in side effects affecting the blood
- Kidney disease or
- Liver disease—Patients with kidney and/or liver disease may have an increased chance of side effects
- Porphyria—This medicine may bring on an attack of porphyria

---

Proper Use of This Medicine

Sulfamethoxazole and trimethoprim combination is best taken with a full glass (8 ounces) of water. Several additional glasses of water should be taken every day, unless otherwise directed by your doctor. Drinking extra water will help to prevent some unwanted effects of sulfonamides.

For patients taking the *oral liquid form* of this medicine:

- Use a specially marked measuring spoon or other device to measure each dose accurately. The average household teaspoon may not hold the right amount of liquid.

To help clear up your infection completely, *keep taking this medicine for the full time of treatment*, even if you begin to feel better after a few days. If you stop taking this medicine too soon, your symptoms may return.

This medicine works best when there is a constant amount in the blood or urine. *To help keep the amount constant, do not miss any doses. Also, it is best to take the doses at evenly spaced times day and night.* For example, if you are to take 4 doses a day, the doses should be spaced about 6 hours apart. If this interferes with your sleep or other daily activities, or if you need help in planning the best times to take your medicine, check with your health care professional.

Dosing—The dose of sulfamethoxazole and trimethoprim combination will be different for different patients. *Follow your doctor's orders or the directions on the label.* The following information includes only the average doses of sulfamethoxazole and trimethoprim combination. *If your dose is different, do not change it* unless your doctor tells you to do so.

The number of tablets or teaspoonfuls of suspension that you take depends on the strength of the medicine. Also, *the number of doses you take each day, the time allowed between doses, and the length of time you take the medicine depend on the medical problem for which you are taking sulfamethoxazole and trimethoprim combination.*

- For *oral* dosage forms (suspension, tablets):

    —For bacterial infections:

    - Adults and children over 40 kilograms (kg) of body weight (88 pounds)—160 milligrams (mg) of trimethoprim and 800 mg of sulfamethoxazole every twelve hours.

    - Infants younger than 2 months of age—Use and dose must be determined by your doctor.

    - Infants 2 months of age and older and children

up to 40 kg of weight (88 pounds)—Dose is based on body weight. The usual dose is 4 to 6 mg of trimethoprim and 20 to 30 mg of sulfamethoxazole per kg (1.8 to 2.7 mg of trimethoprim and 9.1 to 13.6 mg of sulfamethoxazole per pound) of body weight every twelve hours.

—For the treatment of *Pneumocystis carinii* pneumonia (PCP):

• Adults and children older than 2 months—Dose is based on body weight. The usual dose is 3.75 to 5 mg of trimethoprim and 18.75 to 25 mg of sulfamethoxazole per kg (1.7 to 2.3 mg of trimethoprim and 8.5 to 11.4 mg of sulfamethoxazole per pound) of body weight every six hours.

—For the prevention of *Pneumocystis carinii* pneumonia (PCP):

• Adults and teenagers—160 mg of trimethoprim and 800 mg of sulfamethoxazole one or two times a day.

• Infants and children 1 month of age and older—Dose is based on body size and must be determined by your doctor. There are several dosing regimens available that your doctor may choose from. One dosing regimen is 75 mg of trimethoprim and 375 mg of sulfamethoxazole per square meter of body surface (m^2) three times a week on consecutive days (e.g., Monday, Tuesday, Wednesday).

• For *injection* dosage form:

—For bacterial infections:

• Adults and children older than 2 months—The usual total daily dose is 8 to 10 mg of trimethoprim and 40 to 50 mg of sulfamethoxazole per kg (3.6 to 4.5 mg of trimethoprim and 18.2 to 22.7 mg of sulfamethoxazole per pound) of body weight. This total daily dose may be divided up and injected into a vein every six, eight, or twelve hours.

• Infants younger than 2 months of age—Use and dose must be determined by your doctor.

—For the treatment of *Pneumocystis carinii* pneumonia (PCP):

• Adults and children older than 2 months—The usual dose is 3.75 to 5 mg of trimethoprim and 18.75 to 25 mg of sulfamethoxazole per kg (1.7 to 2.3 mg of trimethoprim and 8.5 to 11.4 mg of sulfamethoxazole per pound) of body weight. This is injected into a vein every six hours.

• Infants younger than 2 months of age—Use and dose must be determined by your doctor.

Missed dose—If you miss a dose of this medicine, take it as soon as possible. This will help to keep a constant amount of medicine in the blood or urine. However, if it is almost time for your next dose, skip the missed dose and go back to your regular dosing schedule. Do not double doses.

Storage—To store this medicine:
• Keep out of the reach of children.
• Store away from heat and direct light.
• Do not store the tablet form of this medicine in the bathroom, near the kitchen sink, or in other damp places. Heat or moisture may cause the medicine to break down.
• Keep the oral liquid form of this medicine from freezing.
• Do not keep outdated medicine or medicine no longer needed. Be sure that any discarded medicine is out of the reach of children.

Precautions While Using This Medicine

It is very important that your doctor check your progress at regular visits. This medicine may cause blood problems, especially if it is taken for a long time.

If your symptoms do not improve within a few days, or if they become worse, check with your doctor.

Sulfamethoxazole and trimethoprim combination may cause blood problems. These problems may result in a greater chance of certain infections, slow healing, and bleeding of the gums. Therefore, you should be careful when using regular toothbrushes, dental floss, and toothpicks. Dental work should be delayed until your blood counts have returned to normal. Check with your medical doctor or dentist if you have any questions about proper oral hygiene (mouth care) during treatment.

Sulfamethoxazole and trimethoprim combination may cause your skin to be more sensitive to sunlight than it is normally. Exposure to sunlight, even for brief periods of time, may cause a skin rash, itching, redness or other discoloration of the skin, or a severe sunburn. When you begin taking this medicine:

- Stay out of direct sunlight, especially between the hours of 10:00 a.m. and 3:00 p.m., if possible.
- Wear protective clothing, including a hat. Also, wear sunglasses.
- Apply a sun block product that has a skin protection factor (SPF) of at least 15. Some patients may require a product with a higher SPF number, especially if they have a fair complexion. If you have any questions about this, check with your health care professional.
- Apply a sun block lipstick that has an SPF of at least 15 to protect your lips.
- Do not use a sunlamp or tanning bed or booth.

If you have a severe reaction from the sun, check with your doctor.

This medicine may also cause some people to become dizzy. *Make sure you know how you react to this medicine before you drive, use machines, or do anything else that could be dangerous if you are dizzy or are not alert.* If this reaction is especially bothersome, check with your doctor.

Side Effects of This Medicine

Along with its needed effects, a medicine may cause some unwanted effects. Although not all of these side effects may occur, if they do occur they may need medical attention.

Check with your doctor immediately if any of the following side effects occur:

More common

Itching; skin rash

Less common

Aching of joints and muscles; difficulty in swallowing; pale skin; redness, blistering, peeling, or loosening of skin; sore throat and fever; unusual bleeding or bruising; unusual tiredness or weakness; yellow eyes or skin

Rare

Blood in urine; bluish fingernails, lips, or skin; difficult breathing; greatly increased or decreased frequency of urination or amount of urine; increased thirst; lower back pain; pain or burning while urinating; swelling of front part of neck

Also, check with your doctor as soon as possible if the following side effect occurs:

More common

Increased sensitivity of skin to sunlight

Other side effects may occur that usually do not need medical attention. These side effects may go away during treatment as your body adjusts to the medicine. However, check with your doctor if any of the following side effects continue or are bothersome:

More common

Diarrhea; dizziness; headache; loss of appetite; nausea or vomiting

Other side effects not listed above may also occur in some patients. If you notice any other effects, check with your doctor.

Additional Information

Once a medicine has been approved for marketing for a certain use, experience may show that it is also useful for other medical problems. Although these uses are not included in product labeling, sulfamethoxazole and trimethoprim combination is used in certain patients with the following medical conditions:

- Bile infections
- Bone and joint infections
- Sexually transmitted diseases, such as gonorrhea
- Sinus infections
- Urinary tract infections (for prevention)

Other than the above information, there is no additional information relating to proper use, precautions, or side effects for these uses.

SULFASALAZINE Systemic

Some commonly used brand names are:

In the U.S.—

Azulfidine   Azulfidine EN-Tabs

Generic name product may also be available.

In Canada—

PMS Sulfasalazine   Salazopyrin EN-Tabs
PMS Sulfasalazine E.C.   S.A.S.-500
Salazopyrin   S.A.S. Enteric-500

Generic name product may also be available.

Other commonly used names are salazosulfapyridine and salicylazosulfa-
pyridine.

Description

Sulfasalazine (sul-fa-SAL-a-zeen), a sulfa medicine, is
used to prevent and treat inflammatory bowel disease, such
as ulcerative colitis. It works inside the bowel by helping
to reduce the inflammation and other symptoms of the
disease. Sulfasalazine is sometimes given with other medicines to treat inflammatory bowel disease. However, this
medicine will not work for all kinds of infection the way
other sulfa medicines do.

Sulfasalazine is available only with your doctor's prescription, in the following dosage forms:

Oral

- Enteric-coated tablets (U.S. and Canada)
- Oral suspension (U.S.)
- Tablets (U.S. and Canada)

Before Using This Medicine

In deciding to use a medicine, the risks of taking the
medicine must be weighed against the good it will do.
This is a decision you and your doctor will make. For
sulfasalazine, the following should be considered:

Allergies—Tell your doctor if you have ever had any unusual or allergic reaction to any of the sulfa medicines,
furosemide (e.g., Lasix) or thiazide diuretics (water pills),
oral antidiabetics (diabetes medicine you take by mouth),
glaucoma medicine you take by mouth (for example, acetazolamide [e.g., Diamox], dichlorphenamide [e.g., Dara-
nide], methazolamide [e.g., Neptazane]), or salicylates (for
example, aspirin). Also tell your health care professional
if you are allergic to any other substances, such as foods,
preservatives, or dyes.

Pregnancy—Studies have not been done in humans. However, reports on women who took sulfasalazine during pregnancy have not shown that it causes birth defects or other problems. In addition, sulfasalazine has not been shown to cause birth defects in studies in rats and rabbits given doses of up to 6 times the human dose.

Breast-feeding—Sulfa medicines pass into the breast milk in small amounts. They may cause unwanted effects in nursing babies with glucose-6-phosphate dehydrogenase (G6PD) deficiency.

Children—Sulfasalazine should not be used in children up to 2 years of age because it may cause brain problems. However, sulfasalazine has not been shown to cause different side effects or problems in children over the age of 2 than it does in adults.

Older adults—Many medicines have not been studied specifically in older people. Therefore, it may not be known whether they work exactly the same way they do in younger adults or if they cause different side effects or problems in older people. There is no specific information comparing use of sulfasalazine in the elderly with use in other age groups.

Other medicines—Although certain medicines should not be used together at all, in other cases two different medicines may be used together even if an interaction might occur. In these cases, your doctor may want to change the dose, or other precautions may be necessary. When you are taking sulfasalazine, it is especially important that your health care professional know if you are taking any of the following:

- Acetaminophen (e.g., Tylenol) (with long-term, high-dose use) or
- Amiodarone (e.g., Cordarone) or
- Anabolic steroids (nandrolone [e.g., Anabolin], oxandrolone [e.g., Anavar], oxymetholone [e.g., Anadrol], stanozolol [e.g., Winstrol]) or

- Androgens (male hormones) or
- Antithyroid agents (medicine for overactive thyroid) or
- Carbamazepine (e.g., Tegretol) or
- Carmustine (e.g., BiCNU) or
- Chloroquine (e.g., Aralen) or
- Dantrolene (e.g., Dantrium) or
- Daunorubicin (e.g., Cerubidine) or
- Disulfiram (e.g., Antabuse) or
- Divalproex (e.g., Depakote) or
- Estrogens (female hormones) or
- Etretinate (e.g., Tegison) or
- Gold salts (medicine for arthritis) or
- Hydroxychloroquine (e.g., Plaquenil) or
- Mercaptopurine (e.g., Purinethol) or
- Naltrexone (e.g., Trexan) (with long-term, high-dose use) or
- Oral contraceptives (birth control pills) containing estrogen or
- Other anti-infectives by mouth or by injection (medicine for infection) or
- Phenothiazines (acetophenazine [e.g., Tindal], chlorpromazine [e.g., Thorazine], fluphenazine [e.g., Prolixin], mesoridazine [e.g., Serentil], perphenazine [e.g., Trilafon], prochlorperazine [e.g., Compazine], promazine [e.g., Sparine], promethazine [e.g., Phenergan], thioridazine [e.g., Mellaril], trifluoperazine [e.g., Stelazine], triflupromazine [e.g., Vesprin], trimeprazine [e.g., Temaril]) or
- Plicamycin (e.g., Mithracin) or
- Valproic acid (e.g., Depakene)—Use of sulfasalazine with these medicines may increase the chance of side effects affecting the liver
- Acetohydroxamic acid (e.g., Lithostat) or
- Dapsone or
- Furazolidone (e.g., Furoxone) or
- Nitrofurantoin (e.g., Furadantin) or
- Primaquine or
- Procainamide (e.g., Pronestyl) or
- Quinidine (e.g., Quinidex) or
- Quinine (e.g., Quinamm) or
- Sulfoxone (e.g., Diasone) or
- Vitamin K (e.g., AquaMEPHYTON, Synkayvite)—Use of sulfasalazine with these medicines may increase the chance of side effects affecting the blood

- Anticoagulants (blood thinners) or
- Ethotoin (e.g., Peganone) or
- Mephenytoin (e.g., Mesantoin)—Use of sulfasalazine with these medicines may increase the chance of side effects of these medicines
- Antidiabetics, oral (diabetes medicine you take by mouth)— Use of oral antidiabetics with sulfasalazine may increase the chance of side effects affecting the blood and/or the side effects or oral antidiabetics
- Methotrexate (e.g., Mexate)—Use of methotrexate with sulfasalazine may increase the chance of side effects affecting the liver and/or the side effects of methotrexate
- Methyldopa (e.g., Aldomet)—Use of methyldopa with sulfasalazine may increase the chance of side effects affecting the liver and/or the blood
- Phenytoin (e.g., Dilantin)—Use of phenytoin with sulfasalazine may increase the chance of side effects affecting the liver and/or the side effects of phenytoin

Other medical problems—The presence of other medical problems may affect the use of sulfasalazine. Make sure you tell your doctor if you have any other medical problems, especially:

- Blood problems or
- Glucose-6-phosphate dehydrogenase deficiency (lack of G6PD enzyme)—Patients with these problems may have an increase in side effects affecting the blood
- Kidney disease or
- Liver disease—Patients with kidney disease or liver disease may have an increased chance of side effects
- Porphyria—Use of sulfasalazine may cause an attack of porphyria

Proper Use of This Medicine

Do not give sulfasalazine to infants up to 2 years of age, unless otherwise directed by your doctor. It may cause brain problems.

Sulfasalazine is best taken after meals or with food to lessen stomach upset. If stomach upset continues or is bothersome, check with your doctor.

Each dose of sulfasalazine should also be taken with a full glass (8 ounces) of water. Several additional glasses of water should be taken every day, unless otherwise directed by your doctor. Drinking extra water will help to prevent some unwanted effects (e.g., kidney stones) of the sulfa medicine.

For patients taking the *enteric-coated tablet form* of this medicine:

- Swallow tablets whole. Do not break or crush.

Keep taking this medicine for the full time of treatment, even if you begin to feel better after a few days. *Do not miss any doses.*

Dosing—The dose of sulfasalazine will be different for different patients. *Follow your doctor's orders or the directions on the label.* The following information includes only the average doses of sulfasalazine. *If your dose is different, do not change it* unless your doctor tells you to do so.

The number of tablets or teaspoonfuls of oral suspension that you take depends on the strength of the medicine. Also, *the number of doses you take each day, the time allowed between doses, and the length of time you take the medicine depend on the medical problem for which you are taking sulfasalazine.*

- For *oral* dosage forms (oral suspension, tablets, enteric-coated tablets):

    —For prevention or treatment of inflammatory bowel disease:

    - Adults—To start, 500 milligrams (mg) to 1000 mg (1 gram) every six to eight hours. Your doctor may then decrease the dose to 500 mg every six hours. After a time, your doctor may change your dose as needed.

• Children 2 years of age and over—Dose is based on body weight and must be determined by your doctor.

—To start, the dose is usually:

• 6.7 to 10 mg per kilogram (kg) (3.05 to 4.55 mg per pound) of body weight every four hours or

• 10 to 15 mg per kg (4.55 to 6.82 mg per pound) of body weight every six hours or

• 13.3 to 20 mg per kg (6.05 to 9.09 mg per pound) of body weight every eight hours.

—Then, the dose is usually 7.5 mg per kg (3.41 mg per pound) of body weight every six hours.

• Infants and children less than 2 years of age— Use is not recommended.

Missed dose—If you do miss a dose of this medicine, take it as soon as possible. However, if it is almost time for your next dose, skip the missed dose and go back to your regular dosing schedule. Do not double doses.

Storage—To store this medicine:

• Keep out of the reach of children.

• Store away from heat and direct light.

• Do not store the tablet form of this medicine in the bathroom, near the kitchen sink, or in other damp places. Heat or moisture may cause the medicine to break down.

• Keep the oral liquid form of this medicine from freezing.

• Do not keep outdated medicine or medicine no longer needed. Be sure that any discarded medicine is out of the reach of children.

Precautions While Using This Medicine

It is very important that your doctor check your progress at regular visits. This medicine may cause blood problems, especially if it is taken for a long time.

If your symptoms (including diarrhea) do not improve within a month or 2, or if they become worse, check with your doctor.

Sulfasalazine may cause blood problems. These problems may result in a greater chance of certain infections, slow healing, and bleeding of the gums. Therefore, you should be careful when using regular toothbrushes, dental floss, and toothpicks. Dental work should be delayed until your blood counts have returned to normal. Check with your medical doctor or dentist if you have any questions about proper oral hygiene (mouth care) during treatment.

Sulfasalazine may cause your skin to be more sensitive to sunlight than it is normally. Exposure to sunlight, even for brief periods of time, may cause a skin rash, itching, redness or other discoloration of the skin, or a severe sunburn. When you begin taking this medicine:

- Stay out of direct sunlight, especially between the hours of 10:00 a.m. and 3:00 p.m., if possible.
- Wear protective clothing, including a hat. Also, wear sunglasses.
- Apply a sun block product that has a skin protection factor (SPF) of at least 15. Some patients may require a product with a higher SPF number, especially if they have a fair complexion. If you have any questions about this, check with your health care professional.
- Apply a sun block lipstick that has an SPF of at least 15 to protect your lips.
- Do not use a sunlamp or tanning bed or booth.

If you have a severe reaction from the sun, check with your doctor.

This medicine may also cause some people to become dizzy. *Make sure you know how you react to this medicine before you drive, use machines, or do anything else that could be dangerous if you are dizzy.* If this reaction is especially bothersome, check with your doctor.

Before you have any medical tests, tell the doctor in charge that you are taking this medicine. The results of the bentiromide (e.g., Chymex) test for pancreas function are affected by this medicine.

Side Effects of This Medicine

Along with its needed effects, a medicine may cause some unwanted effects. Although not all of these side effects may occur, if they do occur, they may need medical attention.

Check with your doctor immediately if any of the following side effects occur:

> *More common*
>> Aching of joints and muscles; headache (continuing); itching; skin rash
>
> *Less common*
>> Back, leg, or stomach pains; difficulty in swallowing; fever and sore throat; pale skin; redness, blistering, peeling, or loosening of skin; unusual bleeding or bruising; unusual tiredness or weakness; yellow eyes or skin
>
> *Rare*
>> Bloody diarrhea, fever, and rash; cough; difficult breathing

Also, check with your doctor as soon as possible if the following side effect occurs:

More common
    Increased sensitivity of skin to sunlight

Other side effects may occur that usually do not need medical attention. These side effects may go away during treatment as your body adjusts to the medicine. However, check with your doctor if any of the following side effects continue or are bothersome:

More common
    Abdominal or stomach pain or upset; diarrhea; dizziness; loss of appetite; nausea or vomiting

In some patients this medicine may also cause the urine or skin to become orange-yellow. This side effect does not need medical attention.

Other side effects not listed above may also occur in some patients. If you notice any other effects, check with your doctor.

Additional Information

Once a medicine has been approved for marketing for a certain use, experience may show that it is also useful for other medical problems. Although these uses are not included in product labeling, sulfasalazine is used in certain patients with the following medical conditions:

* Ankylosing spondylitis
* Rheumatoid arthritis

Other than the above information, there is no additional information relating to proper use, precautions, or side effects for these uses.

SULFONAMIDES   Systemic

Some commonly used brand names are:

In the U.S.—

Gantanol[4]

Gantrisin[5]

Renoquid[1]

Thiosulfil Forte[3]

In Canada—

Apo-Sulfamethoxazole[4]

Gantanol[4]

Novosoxazole[5]

Another commonly used name for sulfisoxazole is sulfafurazole.

Note: For quick reference, the following sulfonamides are numbered to match the corresponding brand names.

This information applies to the following medicines:

1. Sulfacytine (sul-fa-SYE-teen)[†]
2. Sulfadiazine (sul-fa-DYE-a-zeen)[†‡]
3. Sulfamethizole (sul-fa-METH-a-zole)[†]
4. Sulfamethoxazole (sul-fa-meth-OX-a-zole)[‡]
5. Sulfisoxazole (sul-fi-SOX-a-zole)[‡§]

[†]Not commercially available in Canada.
[‡]Generic name product may also be available in the U.S.
[§]Generic name product may also be available in Canada.

Description

Sulfonamides (sul-FON-a-mides), or sulfa medicines, are used to treat infections. They will not work for colds, flu, or other virus infections.

Sulfonamides are available only with your doctor's prescription, in the following dosage forms:

Oral

Sulfacytine
- Tablets (U.S.)

Sulfadiazine
- Tablets (U.S.)

Sulfamethizole
- Tablets (U.S.)

Sulfamethoxazole
- Oral suspension (U.S.)
- Tablets (U.S. and Canada)

Sulfisoxazole
- Oral suspension (U.S.)
- Syrup (U.S.)
- Tablets (U.S. and Canada)

Before Using This Medicine

In deciding to use a medicine, the risks of taking the medicine must be weighed against the good it will do. This is a decision you and your doctor will make. For sulfonamides, the following should be considered:

Allergies—Tell your doctor if you have ever had any unusual or allergic reaction to sulfa medicines, furosemide (e.g., Lasix) or thiazide diuretics (water pills), oral antidiabetics (diabetes medicine you take by mouth), glaucoma medicine you take by mouth (for example, acetazolamide [e.g., Diamox], dichlorphenamide [e.g., Daranide], or methazolamide [e.g., Neptazane]). Also tell your health care professional if you are allergic to any other substances, such as foods, preservatives, or dyes.

Pregnancy—Studies have not been done in pregnant women. However, studies in mice, rats, and rabbits have shown that some sulfonamides cause birth defects, including cleft palate and bone problems.

Breast-feeding—Sulfonamides pass into the breast milk. This medicine is not recommended for use during breast-feeding. It may cause liver problems, anemia, and other unwanted effects in nursing babies, especially those with glucose-6-phosphate dehydrogenase (G6PD) deficiency.

Children—Sulfonamides should not be given to infants under 2 months of age unless directed by the child's doctor, because they may cause brain problems. Sulfacytine should not be given to children up to the age of 14.

Older adults—Elderly people are especially sensitive to the effects of sulfonamides. Severe skin problems and blood problems may be more likely to occur in the elderly. These problems may also be more likely to occur in patients who are taking diuretics (water pills) along with this medicine.

Other medicines—Although certain medicines should not be used together at all, in other cases two different medicines may be used together even if an interaction might occur. In these cases, your doctor may want to change the dose, or other precautions may be necessary. When you are taking sulfonamides, it is especially important that your health care professional knows if you are taking any of the following:

- Acetaminophen (e.g., Tylenol) (with long-term, high-dose use) or
- Amiodarone (e.g., Cordarone) or
- Anabolic steroids (nandrolone [e.g., Anabolin], oxandrolone [e.g., Anavar], oxymetholone [e.g., Anadrol], stanozolol [e.g., Winstrol]) or
- Androgens (male hormones) or
- Antithyroid agents (medicine for overactive thyroid) or
- Carbamazepine (e.g., Tegretol) or
- Carmustine (e.g., BiCNU) or
- Chloroquine (e.g., Aralen) or
- Dantrolene (e.g., Dantrium) or
- Daunorubicin (e.g., Cerubidine) or
- Disulfiram (e.g., Antabuse) or
- Divalproex (e.g., Depakote) or
- Estrogens (female hormones) or
- Etretinate (e.g., Tegison) or
- Gold salts (medicine for arthritis) or
- Hydroxychloroquine (e.g., Plaquenil) or
- Mercaptopurine (e.g., Purinethol) or
- Naltrexone (e.g., Trexan) (with long-term, high-dose use) or
- Oral contraceptives (birth control pills) containing estrogens or

- Other anti-infectives by mouth or by injection (medicine for infection) or
- Phenothiazines (acetophenazine [e.g., Tindal], chlorpromazine [e.g., Thorazine], fluphenazine [e.g., Prolixin], mesoridazine [e.g., Serentil], perphenazine [e.g., Trilafon], prochlorperazine [e.g., Compazine], promazine [e.g., Sparine], promethazine [e.g., Phenergan], thioridazine [e.g., Mellaril], trifluoperazine [e.g., Stelazine], triflupromazine [e.g., Vesprin], trimeprazine [e.g., Temaril]) or
- Plicamycin (e.g., Mithracin) or
- Valproic acid (e.g., Depakene)—Use of sulfonamides with these medicines may increase the chance of side effects affecting the liver

- Acetohydroxamic acid (e.g., Lithostat) or
- Dapsone or
- Furazolidone (e.g., Furoxone) or
- Nitrofurantoin (e.g., Furadantin) or
- Primaquine or
- Procainamide (e.g., Pronestyl) or
- Quinidine (e.g., Quinidex) or
- Quinine (e.g., Quinamm) or
- Sulfoxone (e.g., Diasone)—Use of sulfonamides with these medicines may increase the chance of side effects affecting the blood

- Anticoagulants (blood thinners) or
- Ethotoin (e.g., Peganone) or
- Mephenytoin (e.g., Mesantoin)—Use of sulfonamides with these medicines may increase the chance of side effects of these medicines

- Antidiabetics, oral (diabetes medicine you take by mouth)—Use of oral antidiabetics with sulfonamides may increase the chance of side effects affecting the blood and/or the side effects of oral antidiabetics

- Methenamine (e.g., Mandelamine)—Use of this medicine with sulfonamides may increase the chance of side effects of sulfonamides

- Methotrexate (e.g., Mexate) or
- Phenytoin (e.g., Dilantin)—Use of these medicines with sulfonamides may increase the chance of side effects affecting the liver and/or the side effects of these medicines

- Methyldopa (e.g., Aldomet)—Use of methyldopa with sulfonamides may increase the chance of side effects affecting the liver and/or the blood

Other medical problems—The presence of other medical problems may affect the use of sulfonamides. Make sure you tell your doctor if you have any other medical problems, especially:

- Anemia or other blood problems or
- Glucose-6-phosphate dehydrogenase (G6PD) deficiency—Patients with these problems may have an increase in side effects affecting the blood
- Kidney disease or
- Liver disease—Patients with kidney and/or liver disease may have an increased chance of side effects
- Porphyria—This medicine may bring on an attack of porphyria

---

Proper Use of This Medicine

Sulfonamides are best taken with a full glass (8 ounces) of water. Several additional glasses of water should be taken every day, unless otherwise directed by your doctor. Drinking extra water will help to prevent some unwanted effects (e.g., kidney stones) of sulfonamides.

For patients taking the *oral liquid form* of this medicine:

- Use a specially marked measuring spoon or other device to measure each dose accurately. The average household teaspoon may not hold the right amount of liquid.

To help clear up your infection completely, *keep taking this medicine for the full time of treatment,* even if you begin to feel better after a few days. If you stop taking this medicine too soon, your symptoms may return.

This medicine works best when there is a constant amount in the blood or urine. *To help keep the amount constant, do not miss any doses. Also, it is best to take the doses at evenly spaced times day and night.* For example, if you are to take 4 doses a day, the doses should be spaced about 6 hours apart. If this interferes with your sleep or other daily activities, or if you need help in planning the best times to take your medicine, check with your health care professional.

Dosing—The dose of these medicines will be different for different patients. *Follow your doctor's orders or the directions on the label.* The following information includes only the average doses of these medicines. *If your dose is different, do not change it* unless your doctor tells you to do so.

For sulfacytine

- For *tablet* dosage form:

    —For bacterial infections:

        • Adults and children 14 years of age and older—500 milligrams (mg) for the first dose, then 250 mg every six hours.

        • Children up to age 14—Use and dose must be determined by your doctor.

For sulfadiazine

- For *tablet* dosage form:

    —For bacterial infections:

        • Adults and teenagers—2 to 4 grams for the first dose, then 1 gram every four to six hours.

        • Children up to 2 months of age—Use and dose must be determined by your doctor.

        • Children 2 months of age and older—Dose is based on body weight. The usual dose is 75 milligrams (mg) per kilogram (kg) (34 mg per pound) of body weight for the first dose, then 37.5 mg per kg (17 mg per pound) of body weight every six hours, or 25 mg per kg (11.4 mg per pound) of body weight every four hours.

For sulfamethizole

- For *tablet* dosage form:

    —For bacterial infections:

    - Adults and teenagers—500 milligrams (mg) to 1 gram every six to eight hours.

    - Children up to 2 months of age—Use and dose must be determined by your doctor.

    - Children 2 months of age and older—Dose is based on body weight. The usual dose is 7.5 to 11.25 mg per kilogram (kg) (3.4 to 5.1 mg per pound) of body weight every six hours.

For sulfamethoxazole

- For *suspension or tablet* dosage forms:

    —For bacterial or protozoal infections:

    - Adults and teenagers—2 grams for the first dose, then 1 gram every eight to twelve hours.

    - Children up to 2 months of age—Use and dose must be determined by your doctor.

    - Children 2 months of age and older—Dose is based on body weight. The usual dose is 50 to 60 milligrams (mg) per kilogram (kg) (22.7 to 27.3 mg per pound) of body weight for the first dose, then 25 to 30 mg per kg (11.4 to 13.6 mg per pound) of body weight every twelve hours.

For sulfisoxazole

- For *suspension, syrup, or tablet* dosage forms:

    —For bacterial or protozoal infections:

    - Adults and teenagers—2 to 4 grams for the first dose, then 750 milligrams (mg) to 1.5 grams every four hours; or 1 to 2 grams every six hours.

    - Children up to 2 months of age—Use and dose must be determined by your doctor.

    - Children 2 months of age and older—Dose is based on body weight. The usual dose is 75 mg per kilogram (kg) (34 mg per pound) of body weight for the first dose, then 25 mg every per kg (11.4 mg per pound) of body weight every four hours, or 37.5 mg per kg (17 mg per pound) of body weight every six hours.

Missed dose—If you miss a dose of this medicine, take it as soon as possible. This will help to keep a constant amount of medicine in the blood or urine. However, if it is almost time for your next dose, skip the missed dose and go back to your regular dosing schedule. Do not double doses.

Storage—To store this medicine:

- Keep out of the reach of children.
- Store away from heat and direct light.
- Do not store the tablet form of this medicine in the bathroom, near the kitchen sink, or in other damp places. Heat or moisture may cause the medicine to break down.
- Keep the oral liquid forms of this medicine from freezing.
- Do not keep outdated medicine or medicine no longer needed. Be sure that any discarded medicine is out of the reach of children.

Precautions While Using This Medicine

It is very important that your doctor check your progress at regular visits. This medicine may cause blood problems, especially if it is taken for a long time.

If your symptoms do not improve within a few days, or if they become worse, check with your doctor.

Sulfonamides may cause blood problems. These problems may result in a greater chance of certain infections, slow healing, and bleeding of the gums. Therefore, you should be careful when using regular toothbrushes, dental floss, and toothpicks. Dental work should be delayed until your blood counts have returned to normal. Check with your medical doctor or dentist if you have any questions about proper oral hygiene (mouth care) during treatment.

Sulfonamides may cause your skin to be more sensitive to sunlight than it is normally. Exposure to sunlight, even for brief periods of time, may cause a skin rash, itching, redness or other discoloration of the skin, or a severe sunburn. When you begin taking this medicine:

- Stay out of direct sunlight, especially between the hours of 10:00 a.m. and 3:00 p.m., if possible.
- Wear protective clothing, including a hat. Also, wear sunglasses.
- Apply a sun block product that has a skin protection factor (SPF) of at least 15. Some patients may require a product with a higher SPF number, especially if they have a fair complexion. If you have any questions about this, check with your health care professional.
- Apply a sun block lipstick that has an SPF of at least 15 to protect your lips.
- Do not use a sunlamp or tanning bed or booth.

If you have a severe reaction from the sun, check with your doctor.

This medicine may also cause some people to become dizzy. *Make sure you know how you react to this medicine before you drive, use machines, or do anything else that could be dangerous if you are dizzy or are not alert.* If this reaction is especially bothersome, check with your doctor.

Side Effects of This Medicine

Along with its needed effects, a medicine may cause some unwanted effects. Although not all of these side effects

may occur, if they do occur they may need medical attention.

Check with your doctor immediately if any of the following side effects occur:

More common

Itching; skin rash

Less common

Aching of joints and muscles; difficulty in swallowing; pale skin; redness, blistering, peeling, or loosening of skin; sore throat and fever; unusual bleeding or bruising; unusual tiredness or weakness; yellow eyes or skin

Rare

Blood in urine; greatly increased or decreased frequency of urination or amount of urine; increased thirst; lower back pain; pain or burning while urinating; swelling of front part of neck

Also, check with your doctor as soon as possible if the following side effect occurs:

More common

Increased sensitivity of skin to sunlight

Other side effects may occur that usually do not need medical attention. These side effects may go away during treatment as your body adjusts to the medicine. However, check with your doctor if any of the following side effects continue or are bothersome:

More common

Diarrhea; dizziness; headache; loss of appetite; nausea or vomiting; tiredness

Other side effects not listed above may also occur in some patients. If you notice any other effects, check with your doctor.

SUMATRIPTAN   Systemic

A commonly used brand name in the U.S. and Canada is Imitrex.

Description

Sumatriptan (soo-ma-TRIP-tan) is used to treat severe migraine headaches. Many people find that their headaches go away completely after they take sumatriptan. Other people find that their headaches are much less painful, and that they are able to go back to their normal activities even though their headaches are not completely gone. Sumatriptan often relieves other symptoms that occur together with a migraine headache, such as nausea, vomiting, sensitivity to light, and sensitivity to sound.

Sumatriptan is not an ordinary pain reliever. It will not relieve any kind of pain other than migraine headaches. This medicine is usually used for people whose headaches are not relieved by acetaminophen, aspirin, or other pain relievers.

Sumatriptan is available only with your doctor's prescription, in the following dosage forms:

Oral
- Tablets (Canada)

Parenteral
- Injection (U.S. and Canada)

Before Using This Medicine

In deciding to use a medicine, the risks of using the medicine must be weighed against the good it will do. This is a decision you and your doctor will make. For sumatriptan, the following should be considered:

Allergies—Tell your doctor if you have ever had any unusual or allergic reaction to sumatriptan. Also tell your health care professional if you are allergic to any other substances, such as foods, preservatives, or dyes.

Pregnancy—Sumatriptan has not been studied in pregnant women. However, in some animal studies, sumatriptan caused harmful effects on the fetus. These unwanted effects usually occurred when sumatriptan was given in amounts that were large enough to cause harmful effects in the mother.

Breast-feeding—It is not known whether sumatriptan passes into human breast milk. However, it has been found in the breast milk of animals. Breast-feeding mothers should discuss the risks and benefits of this medicine with their doctors.

Children—Studies on this medicine have been done only in adult patients, and there is no specific information comparing use of sumatriptan in children with use in other age groups.

Teenagers—Studies on this medicine have been done only in patients 18 years of age or older, and there is no specific information comparing use of sumatriptan in younger teenagers with use in other age groups.

Older adults—This medicine has been tested in a limited number of patients between 60 and 65 years of age. It did not cause different side effects or problems in these patients than it did in younger adults. However, there is no specific information comparing use of sumatriptan in patients older than 65 years of age with use in younger adults.

Other medicines—Although certain medicines should not be used together at all, in other cases two different medicines may be used together even if an interaction might occur. In these cases, your doctor may want to change the dose, or other precautions may be necessary. Tell your health care professional if you are taking any other prescription or nonprescription (over-the-counter [OTC]) medicine, especially other prescription medicine for migraine headaches, or if you smoke tobacco.

Other medical problems—The presence of other medical problems may affect the use of sumatriptan. Make sure you tell your doctor if you have any other medical problems, especially:

- Angina (chest pain) or
- Fast or irregular heartbeat or
- Heart or blood vessel disease or
- High blood pressure or
- Kidney disease or
- Liver disease or
- Stroke (history of)—The chance of side effects may be increased

---

Proper Use of This Medicine

To relieve your migraine as soon as possible, use sumatriptan at the first sign that the headache is coming. If you get warning signals of a coming migraine (an aura), you may use the medicine before the headache pain actually starts. However, even if you do not use sumatriptan until your migraine has been present for several hours, the medicine will still work.

Lying down in a quiet, dark room for a while after you use this medicine may help relieve your migraine.

If you are not much better in 1 or 2 hours after an injection of sumatriptan, or in 2 to 4 hours after a tablet is taken, *do not use any more of this medicine for the same migraine*. A migraine that is not relieved by the first dose of sumatriptan probably will not be relieved by a second dose, either. Ask your doctor ahead of time about other medicine to be taken if sumatriptan does not work. However, even if sumatriptan does not relieve one migraine, it may still relieve the next one.

If you feel much better after a dose of sumatriptan, but your headache comes back or gets worse after a while, you may use more sumatriptan. However, *use this medicine only as directed by your doctor. Do not use more of it, and do not use it more often, than directed.* Using too much sumatriptan may increase the chance of side effects.

Your doctor may direct you to take another medicine to help prevent headaches. *It is important that you follow your doctor's directions, even if your headaches continue to occur.* Headache-preventing medicines may take several weeks to start working. Even after they do start working, your headaches may not go away completely. However, your headaches should occur less often, and they should be less severe and easier to relieve. This can reduce the amount of sumatriptan or pain relievers that you need. If you do not notice any improvement after several weeks of headache-preventing treatment, check with your doctor.

For patients taking *sumatriptan tablets*:

- Sumatriptan tablets are to be swallowed whole. *Do not break, crush, or chew the tablets before swallowing them.*

For patients using *sumatriptan injection*:

- This medicine comes with patient directions. *Read them carefully before using the medicine,* and check with your health care professional if you have any questions.

- Your health care professional will teach you how to inject yourself with the medicine. *Be sure to follow the directions carefully. Check with your health care professional if you have any problems using the medicine.*

- After you have finished injecting the medicine, be

sure to follow the precautions in the patient directions about safely discarding the empty cartridge and the needle. Always return the empty cartridge and needle to their container before discarding them. Do not throw away the autoinjector unit, because refills are available.

Dosing—The dose of sumatriptan will be different for different patients. *Follow your doctor's orders or the directions on the label.* The following information includes only the average doses of sumatriptan. *If your dose is different, do not change it* unless your doctor tells you to do so.

- For *oral* dosage form (tablets):
  - —For migraine headaches:
    - Adults—One 100-milligram (mg) tablet. Another 100-mg tablet may be taken one or two times more, if necessary, if the migraine comes back after being relieved. *Do not take more than three 100-mg tablets in any twenty-four-hour period.*
    - Children—Use and dose must be determined by your doctor.
- For *parenteral* dosage form (injection):
  - —For migraine headaches:
    - Adults—6 mg. One more 6-mg dose may be injected, if necessary, if the migraine comes back after being relieved. However, the second injection should not be given any sooner than one hour after the first one. *Do not use more than two 6-mg injections in forty-eight hours (two days).*
    - Children—Use and dose must be determined by your doctor.

Storage—To store this medicine:

- Keep out of the reach of children since overdose is especially dangerous in children.
- Store away from heat and direct light.

- Do not store tablets in the bathroom, near the kitchen sink, or in other damp places. Heat or moisture may cause the medicine to break down.
- Keep the injection form of sumatriptan from freezing.
- Do not keep outdated medicine or medicine no longer needed. Be sure that any discarded medicine is out of the reach of children.

Precautions While Using This Medicine

Check with your doctor if you have used sumatriptan for 3 headaches, and have not had good relief. Also, check with your doctor if your migraine headaches are worse, or if they are occurring more often, than before you started using sumatriptan.

Drinking alcoholic beverages can make headaches worse or cause new headaches to occur. People who suffer from severe headaches should probably avoid alcoholic beverages, especially during a headache.

Some people feel drowsy or dizzy during or after a migraine, or after taking sumatriptan to relieve a migraine. As long as you are feeling drowsy or dizzy, *do not drive, use machines, or do anything else that could be dangerous if you are dizzy or are not alert.*

Side Effects of This Medicine

Along with its needed effects, a medicine may cause some unwanted effects. Most side effects of sumatriptan are milder and occur less often with the tablets than with the injection. Although not all of these side effects may occur, if they do occur they may need medical attention.

Stop using this medicine and check with your doctor immediately if any of the following side effects occur:

Rare

Chest pain (severe); swelling of eyelids, face, or lips; wheezing

Check with your doctor right away if any of the following side effects continue for more than 1 hour. Even if they go away in less than 1 hour, *check with your doctor before using any more sumatriptan if any of the following side effects occur*:

Less common

Chest pain (mild); heaviness, tightness, or pressure in chest and/or neck

Also check with your doctor as soon as possible if any of the following side effects occur:

Less common

Difficulty in swallowing; pounding heartbeat; skin rash or bumps on skin

Other side effects may occur that usually do not need medical attention. Some of the following effects, such as nausea, vomiting, drowsiness, dizziness, and general feeling of illness or tiredness often occur during or after a migraine, even when sumatriptan has not been used. Most of the side effects caused by sumatriptan go away within a short time (less than 1 hour after an injection or 2 hours after a tablet). However, check with your doctor if any of the following side effects continue or are bothersome:

More common

Burning, pain, or redness at place of injection; feeling of burning, warmth, heat, numbness, tightness, or tingling; discomfort in jaw, mouth, tongue, throat, nose, or sinuses; dizziness; drowsiness; feeling cold, "strange," or weak; flushing; lightheadedness; muscle aches, cramps, or stiffness; nausea or vomiting

Less common or rare

Anxiety; general feeling of illness or tiredness; vision changes

Other side effects not listed above may also occur in some patients. If you notice any other effects, check with your doctor.

TACRINE   Systemic†

A commonly used brand name in the U.S. is Cognex.

Other commonly used names are THA and tetrahydroaminoacridine.

---

†Not commercially available in Canada.

Description

Tacrine (TA-crin) is used to treat the symptoms of mild to moderate Alzheimer's disease. Tacrine will not cure Alzheimer's disease, and it will not stop the disease from getting worse. However, tacrine can improve thinking ability in some patients with Alzheimer's disease.

In Alzheimer's disease, many chemical changes take place in the brain. One of the earliest and biggest changes is that there is less of a chemical messenger called acetylcholine (ACh). ACh helps the brain to work properly. Tacrine slows the breakdown of ACh, so it can build up and have a greater effect. However, as Alzheimer's disease gets worse, there will be less and less ACh, so tacrine may not work as well.

Tacrine may cause liver problems. You must have blood tests regularly while taking this medicine to see if the medicine is affecting your liver.

This medicine is available only with your doctor's prescription, in the following dosage form:

Oral

- Capsules (U.S.)

Before Using This Medicine

In deciding to use a medicine, the risks of taking the medicine must be weighed against the good it will do. This is a decision you and your doctor will make. For tacrine the following should be considered:

Allergies—Tell your doctor if you have ever had any unusual or allergic reaction to tacrine or to wound antiseptics (e.g., Akrinol, Panflavin, Monacrin). Also tell your health care professional if you are allergic to any other substances, such as foods, preservatives, or dyes.

Pregnancy—Studies on effects in pregnancy have not been done in either humans or animals.

Breast-feeding—It is not known whether tacrine passes into breast milk. However, use of tacrine is not recommended in nursing mothers.

Older adults—Studies on tacrine have been done only in middle-aged and older patients. Information on the effects of tacrine is based on these patients.

Other medicines—Although certain medicines should not be used together at all, in other cases two different medicines may be used together even if an interaction might occur. In these cases, your doctor may want to change the dose, or other precautions may be necessary. When you are taking tacrine, it is especially important that your health care professional know if you are taking any of the following:

- Cimetidine (e.g., Tagamet)—Cimetidine may cause higher blood levels of tacrine, which may increase the chance of side effects
- Inflammation or pain medicine, except narcotics—Stomach irritation may be increased
- Neuromuscular blocking agents (medicines used in surgery to relax muscles)—Tacrine may increase the effects of

these medicines; your doctor may change the dose of tacrine before you have surgery.

- Smoking tobacco—Smoking may cause lower blood levels
  of tacrine, which may decrease the effects of tacrine; if
  you smoke, your doctor may need to change the dose
  of tacrine
- Theophylline (e.g., Theo-Dur, Uniphyl)—Tacrine may
  cause higher blood levels of theophylline, which may increase the chance of side effects; your doctor may need
  to change the dose of theophylline

Other medical problems—The presence of other medical
problems may affect the use of tacrine. Make sure you
tell your doctor if you have any other medical problems,
especially:

- Asthma (or history of) or
- Heart problems, including slow heartbeat or hypotension
  (low blood pressure), or
- Intestinal blockage or
- Liver disease (or history of) or
- Parkinson's disease or
- Stomach ulcer (or history of) or
- Urinary tract blockage or difficult urination—Tacrine may
  make these conditions worse

- Brain disease, other, or
- Epilepsy or history of seizures or
- Head injury with loss of consciousness—Tacrine may
  cause seizures

Proper Use of This Medicine

Take this medicine only as directed by your doctor. Do
not take more or less of it, and do not take it more or less
often than your doctor ordered. Taking too much may
increase the chance of side effects, while taking too little
may not improve your condition.

Tacrine is best taken on an empty stomach (1 hour before
or 2 hours after meals). However, if this medicine upsets

your stomach, your doctor may want you to take it with food.

Tacrine seems to work best when it is taken at regularly spaced times, usually four times a day.

Dosing—The dose of tacrine will be different for different patients. *Follow your doctor's orders or the directions on the label.* The following information includes only the average doses of tacrine. *If your dose is different, do not change it* unless your doctor tells you to do so.

- For *oral* dosage form (capsules):
  - —For treatment of Alzheimer's disease:
    - Adults—To start, 10 milligrams (mg) four times a day. Your doctor may increase your dose gradually if you are doing well on this medicine and your liver tests are normal. However, the dose is usually not more than 40 mg four times a day.

Missed dose—If you miss a dose of this medicine, take it as soon as possible. However, if it is within 2 hours of your next dose, skip the missed dose and go back to your regular dosing schedule. Do not double doses.

Storage—To store this medicine:

- Keep out of the reach of children.
- Store away from heat and direct light.
- Do not store in the bathroom, near the kitchen sink, or in other damp places. Heat or moisture may cause the medicine to break down.
- Do not keep outdated medicine or medicine no longer needed. Be sure that any discarded medicine is out of the reach of children.

Precautions While Using This Medicine

It is important that your doctor check your progress at regular visits. Also, you must have your blood tested every week for at least 18 weeks when you first start using tacrine, and every week for at least 6 weeks every time your dose is increased to see if this medicine is affecting your liver. If all of these blood tests are normal, you will still need regular testing, but then your doctor may decide to do the tests less often.

Tell your doctor if your symptoms get worse, or if you notice any new symptoms.

Before you have any kind of surgery, dental treatment, or emergency treatment, tell the medical doctor or dentist in charge that you are taking this medicine. Taking tacrine together with medicines that are sometimes used during surgery or dental or emergency treatments may increase the effects of these medicines.

Tacrine may cause some people to become dizzy, clumsy, or unsteady. Make sure you know how you react to this medicine before you do anything that could be dangerous if you are dizzy, clumsy, or unsteady.

Do not stop taking this medicine or decrease your dose without first checking with your doctor. Stopping this medicine suddenly or decreasing the dose by a large amount may cause mental or behavior changes.

If you think you or someone else may have taken an overdose of tacrine, get emergency help at once. Taking an overdose of tacrine may lead to seizures or shock. Some signs of shock are large pupils, irregular breathing, and fast, weak pulse. Other signs of an overdose are severe nausea and vomiting, increasing muscle weakness, greatly increased sweating, and greatly increased watering of the mouth.

Side Effects of This Medicine

Along with its needed effects, a medicine may cause some unwanted effects. Some side effects will have signs or symptoms that you can see or feel. Your doctor may watch for others by doing certain tests

Tacrine may cause some serious side effects, including liver problems. You and your doctor should discuss the good this medicine will do as well as the risks of receiving it.

Check with your doctor as soon as possible if any of the following side effects occur:

>*More common*

>>Clumsiness or unsteadiness; diarrhea; loss of appetite; nausea; vomiting

>*Less common*

>>Fainting; fast or pounding heartbeat; fever; high or low blood pressure; skin rash; slow heartbeat

>*Rare*

>>Aggression, irritability, or nervousness; change in stool color; convulsions (seizures); cough, tightness in chest, troubled breathing, or wheezing; stiffness of arms or legs, slow movement, or trembling and shaking of hands and fingers; trouble in urinating; yellow eyes or skin

>*Symptoms of overdose*

>>Convulsions (seizures); greatly increased sweating; greatly increased watering of mouth; increasing muscle weakness; low blood pressure; nausea (severe); shock (fast weak pulse, irregular breathing, large pupils); slow heartbeat; vomiting (severe)

This medicine may also cause the following side effect that your doctor will watch for:

>*More common*

>>Liver problems

Other side effects may occur that usually do not need medical attention. These side effects may go away during treatment as your body adjusts to the medicine. However,

check with your doctor if any of the following side effects continue or are bothersome:

More common

Abdominal or stomach pain or cramping; dizziness; headache; indigestion; muscle aches or pain

Less common

Belching; fast breathing; flushing of skin; general feeling of discomfort or illness; increased sweating; increased urination; increased watering of eyes; increased watering of mouth; runny nose; swelling of feet or lower legs; trouble in sleeping

Other side effects not listed above may also occur in some patients. If you notice any other effects, check with your doctor.

TERAZOSIN Systemic

A commonly used brand name in the U.S. and Canada is Hytrin.

Description

Terazosin (ter-AY-zoe-sin) is used to treat high blood pressure (hypertension).

High blood pressure adds to the work load of the heart and arteries. If it continues for a long time, the heart and arteries may not function properly. This can damage the blood vessels of the brain, heart, and kidneys, resulting in a stroke, heart failure, or kidney failure. High blood pressure may also increase the risk of heart attacks. These problems may be less likely to occur if blood pressure is controlled.

Terazosin helps to lower blood pressure by relaxing blood vessels so that blood passes through them more easily.

Terazosin is also used to treat benign enlargement of the

prostate (benign prostatic hyperplasia [BPH]). Benign enlargement of the prostate is a problem that can occur in men as they get older. The prostate gland is located below the bladder. As the prostate gland enlarges, certain muscles in the gland may become tight and get in the way of the tube that drains urine from the bladder. This can cause problems in urinating, such as a need to urinate often, a weak stream when urinating, or a feeling of not being able to empty the bladder completely.

Terazosin helps relax the muscles in the prostate and the opening of the bladder. This may help increase the flow of urine and/or decrease the symptoms. However, terazosin will not help shrink the prostate. The prostate may continue to grow. This may cause the symptoms to become worse over time. Therefore, even though terazosin may lessen the problems caused by enlarged prostate now, surgery still may be needed in the future.

Terazosin is available only with your doctor's prescription, in the following dosage form:

Oral
- Tablets (U.S. and Canada)

Before Using This Medicine

In deciding to use a medicine, the risks of taking the medicine must be weighed against the good it will do. This is a decision you and your doctor will make. For terazosin, the following should be considered:

Allergies—Tell your doctor if you have ever had any unusual or allergic reaction to terazosin, prazosin, or doxazosin. Also tell your health care professional if you are allergic to any other substances, such as foods, preservatives, or dyes.

Pregnancy—Studies have not been done in humans. Studies in animals given many times the highest recommended human dose have not shown that terazosin causes birth defects. However, these studies have shown a decrease in successful pregnancies.

Breast-feeding—It is not known whether terazosin passes into breast milk. Although most medicines pass into breast milk in small amounts, many of them may be used safely while breast-feeding. Mothers who are taking this medicine and who wish to breast-feed should discuss this with their doctor.

Children—Studies on this medicine have been done only in adult patients, and there is no specific information comparing use of terazosin in children with use in other age groups.

Older adults—Dizziness, lightheadedness, or fainting (especially when getting up from a lying or sitting position) may be more likely to occur in the elderly, who are more sensitive to the effects of terazosin.

Other medicines—Although certain medicines should not be used together at all, in other cases two different medicines may be used together even if an interaction might occur. In these cases, your doctor may want to change the dose, or other precautions may be necessary. Tell your health care professional if you are taking any other prescription or nonprescription (over-the-counter [OTC]) medicine.

Other medical problems—The presence of other medical problems may affect the use of terazosin. Make sure you tell your doctor if you have any other medical problems, especially:

- Angina (chest pain)—Terazosin may make this condition worse
- Heart disease (severe)—Terazosin may make this condition worse

- Kidney disease—Possible increased sensitivity to the effects of terazosin

---

Proper Use of This Medicine

For patients *taking this medicine for high blood pressure:*

- In addition to the use of the medicine your doctor has prescribed, treatment for your high blood pressure may include weight control and care in the types of foods you eat, especially foods high in sodium. Your doctor will tell you which of these are most important for you. You should check with your doctor before changing your diet.

- Many patients who have high blood pressure will not notice any signs of the problem. In fact, many may feel normal. It is very important that you *take your medicine exactly as directed* and that you keep your appointments with your doctor even if you feel well.

- Remember that terazosin will not cure your high blood pressure but it does help control it. Therefore, you must continue to take it as directed if you expect to lower your blood pressure and keep it down. *You may have to take high blood pressure medicine for the rest of your life.* If high blood pressure is not treated, it can cause serious problems such as heart failure, blood vessel disease, stroke, or kidney disease.

For patients *taking this medicine for benign enlargement of the prostate:*

- Remember that terazosin will not shrink the size of your prostate, but it does help to relieve the symptoms.

- It may take up to 6 weeks before your symptoms get better.

To help you remember to take your medicine, try to get into the habit of taking it at the same time each day.

Dosing—The dose of terazosin will be different for different patients. *Follow your doctor's orders or the directions on the label.* The following information includes only the average doses of terazosin. *If your dose is different, do not change it* unless your doctor tells you to do so.

The number of tablets that you take depends on the strength of the medicine.

- For *oral* dosage form (tablets):
  —For benign enlargement of the prostate:
    - Adults—At first, 1 milligram (mg) taken at bedtime. Then, 5 to 10 mg once a day.
  —For high blood pressure:
    - Adults—At first, 1 mg taken at bedtime. Then, 1 to 5 mg once a day.
    - Children—Use and dose must be determined by your doctor.

Missed dose—If you miss a dose of this medicine, take it as soon as possible the same day. However, if you do not remember the missed dose until the next day, skip the missed dose and go back to your regular dosing schedule. Do not double doses.

Storage—To store this medicine:
- Keep out of the reach of children.
- Store away from heat and direct light.
- Do not store in the bathroom, near the kitchen sink, or in other damp places. Heat or moisture may cause the medicine to break down.
- Do not keep outdated medicine or medicine no longer needed. Be sure that any discarded medicine is out of the reach of children.

Precautions While Using This Medicine

It is important that your doctor check your progress at regular visits to make sure that this medicine is working properly.

For patients *taking this medicine for high blood pressure:*

- *Do not take other medicines unless they have been discussed with your doctor.* This especially includes over-the-counter (nonprescription) medicines for appetite control, asthma, colds, cough, hay fever, or sinus problems, since they may tend to increase your blood pressure.

Dizziness, lightheadedness, or sudden fainting may occur after you take this medicine, especially when you get up from a lying or sitting position. These effects are more likely to occur when you take the first dose of this medicine. Taking the first dose at bedtime may prevent problems. However, *be especially careful if you need to get up during the night*. These effects may also occur with any doses you take after the first dose. Getting up slowly may help lessen this problem. *If you feel dizzy, lie down so that you do not faint*. Then sit for a few moments before standing to prevent the dizziness from returning.

The dizziness, lightheadedness, or fainting is more likely to occur if you drink alcohol, stand for long periods of time, exercise, or if the weather is hot. *While you are taking this medicine, be careful to limit the amount of alcohol you drink. Also, use extra care during exercise or hot weather or if you must stand for long periods of time.*

Terazosin may cause some people to become drowsy or less alert than they are normally. *Make sure you know how you react to this medicine before you drive, use machines, or do anything else that could be dangerous if you are dizzy, drowsy, or are not alert.* After you have taken several doses of this medicine, these effects should lessen.

Side Effects of This Medicine

Along with its needed effects, a medicine may cause some unwanted effects. Although not all of these side effects may occur, if they do occur they may need medical attention.

Check with your doctor as soon as possible if any of the following side effects occur:

More common

Dizziness

Less common

Chest pain; dizziness or lightheadedness when getting up from a lying or sitting position; fainting (sudden); fast or irregular heartbeat; pounding heartbeat; shortness of breath; swelling of feet or lower legs

Rare

Weight gain

Other side effects may occur that usually do not need medical attention. These side effects may go away during treatment as your body adjusts to the medicine. However, check with your doctor if any of the following side effects continue or are bothersome:

More common

Headache; unusual tiredness or weakness

Less common

Back or joint pain; blurred vision; drowsiness; nausea and vomiting; stuffy nose

Other side effects not listed above may also occur in some patients. If you notice any other effects, check with your doctor.

TETRACYCLINES　Systemic

Some commonly used brand names are:

In the U.S.—

Achromycin[5]	Panmycin[5]
Achromycin V[5]	Robitet[5]
Declomycin[1]	Sumycin[5]
Doryx[2]	Terramycin[4]
Doxy[2]	Tetracyn[5]
Doxy-Caps[2]	Tija[4]
Minocin[3]	Vibramycin[2]
Monodox[2]	Vibra-Tabs[2]

In Canada—

Achromycin[5]	
Achromycin V[5]	Minocin[3]
Apo-Doxy[2]	Novodoxylin[2]
Apo-Tetra[5]	Novotetra[5]
Declomycin[1]	Nu-Tetra[5]
Doryx[2]	Tetracyn[5]
Doxycin[2]	Vibramycin[2]
	Vibra-Tabs[2]

Note: For quick reference, the following tetracyclines are numbered to match the corresponding brand names.

This information applies to the following medicines:

1. Demeclocycline (dem-e-kloe-SYE-kleen)
2. Doxycycline (dox-i-SYE-kleen)‡
3. Minocycline (mi-noe-SYE-kleen)‡
4. Oxytetracycline (ox-i-te-tra-SYE-kleen)‡
5. Tetracycline (te-tra-SYE-kleen)‡

‡Generic name product may also be available in the U.S.

Description

Tetracyclines are used to treat infections and to help control acne. Demeclocycline and doxycycline may also be used for other problems as determined by your doctor. Tetracyclines will not work for colds, flu, or other virus infections.

Tetracyclines are available only with your doctor's prescription, in the following dosage forms:

Oral

Demeclocycline
- Capsules (U.S.)
- Tablets (U.S. and Canada)

Doxycycline
- Capsules (U.S. and Canada)
- Delayed-release capsules (U.S. and Canada)
- Oral suspension (U.S.)
- Tablets (U.S. and Canada)

Minocycline
- Capsules (U.S. and Canada)
- Oral suspension (U.S.)
- Tablets (U.S.)

Oxytetracycline
- Capsules (U.S.)

Tetracycline
- Capsules (U.S. and Canada)
- Oral suspension (U.S. and Canada)
- Tablets (U.S. and Canada)

Parenteral

Doxycycline
- Injection (U.S. and Canada)

Minocycline
- Injection (U.S.)

Oxytetracycline
- Injection (U.S.)

Tetracycline
- Injection (U.S. and Canada)

Before Using This Medicine

In deciding to use a medicine, the risks of taking the medicine must be weighed against the good it will do. This is a decision you and your doctor will make. For tetracyclines, the following should be considered:

Allergies—Tell your doctor if you have ever had any unusual or allergic reaction to any of the tetracyclines or combination medicines containing a tetracycline. Also tell your health care professional if you are allergic to any other substances, such as foods, preservatives, or dyes. In addition, if you are going to be given oxytetracycline or tetracycline by injection, tell your doctor if you have ever had an unusual or allergic reaction to "caine-type" anesthetics.

Pregnancy—Use is not recommended during the last half of pregnancy. Tetracyclines may cause the unborn infant's teeth to become discolored and may slow down the growth of the infant's teeth and bones if they are taken during that time. In addition, liver problems may occur in pregnant women, especially those receiving high doses by injection into a vein.

Breast-feeding—Use is not recommended since tetracyclines pass into the breast milk. They may cause the nursing baby's teeth to become discolored and may slow down the growth of the baby's teeth and bones. They may also cause increased sensitivity of nursing babies' skin to sunlight and fungus infections of the mouth and vagina. In addition, minocycline may cause dizziness, lightheadedness, or unsteadiness in nursing babies.

Children—Tetracyclines may cause permanent discoloration of teeth and slow down the growth of bones. These medicines should not be given to children up to 8 years of age unless directed by the child's doctor.

Older adults—Many medicines have not been studied specifically in older people. Therefore, it may not be known whether they work exactly the same way they do in younger adults or if they cause different side effects or problems in older people. There is no specific information comparing use of tetracyclines in the elderly with use in other age groups.

Other medicines—Although certain medicines should not be used together at all, in other cases two different medicines may be used together even if an interaction might

occur. In these cases, your doctor may want to change the dose, or other precautions may be necessary. When you are taking tetracyclines, it is especially important that your health care professional know if you are taking any of the following:

- Antacids or
- Calcium supplements such as calcium carbonate or
- Cholestyramine (e.g., Questran) or
- Choline and magnesium salicylates (e.g., Trilisate) or
- Colestipol (e.g., Colestid) or
- Iron-containing medicine or
- Laxatives (magnesium-containing) or
- Magnesium salicylate (e.g., Magan)—Use of these medicines with tetracyclines may decrease the effect of tetracyclines
- Oral contraceptives (birth control pills) containing estrogen—Use of birth control pills with tetracyclines may decrease the effect of the birth control pills and increase the chance of unwanted pregnancy

Other medical problems—The presence of other medical problems may affect the use of tetracyclines. Make sure you tell your doctor if you have any other medical problems, especially:

- Diabetes insipidus (water diabetes)—Demeclocycline may make the condition worse
- Kidney disease (does not apply to doxycycline or minocycline)—Patients with kidney disease may have an increased chance of side effects
- Liver disease—Patients with liver disease may have an increased chance of side effects if they use doxycycline or minocycline

Proper Use of This Medicine

Do not give tetracyclines to infants or children up to 8 years of age unless directed by your doctor. Tetracyclines may cause permanently discolored teeth and other problems in this age group.

Do not take milk, milk formulas, or other dairy products within 1 to 2 hours of the time you take tetracyclines (except doxycycline and minocycline) by mouth. They may keep this medicine from working properly.

If this medicine has changed color or tastes or looks different, has become outdated (old), has been stored incorrectly (too warm or too damp area or place), do not use it. To do so may cause *serious side effects*. Discard the medicine. If you have any questions about this, check with your health care professional.

Tetracyclines should be taken with a full glass (8 ounces) of water to prevent irritation of the esophagus (tube between the throat and stomach) or stomach. In addition, most tetracyclines (except doxycycline and minocycline) are best taken on an empty stomach (either 1 hour before or 2 hours after meals). However, if this medicine upsets your stomach, your doctor may want you to take it with food.

For patients taking the *oral liquid form* of this medicine:

- Use a specially marked measuring spoon or other device to measure each dose accurately. The average household teaspoon may not hold the right amount of liquid.
- Do not use after the expiration date on the label since the medicine may not work properly after that date. Check with your pharmacist if you have any questions about this.

For patients taking *doxycycline or minocycline:*

- These medicines may be taken with food or milk if they upset your stomach.
- Swallow the capsule (with enteric-coated pellets) form of doxycycline whole. Do not break or crush.

To help clear up your infection completely, *keep taking this medicine for the full time of treatment*, even if you begin to feel better after a few days. If you stop taking this medicine too soon, your symptoms may return.

This medicine works best when there is a constant amount in the blood or urine. *To help keep the amount constant, do not miss any doses. Also, it is best to take the doses at evenly spaced times day and night.* For example, if you are to take 4 doses a day, the doses should be spaced about 6 hours apart. If this interferes with your sleep or other daily activities, or if you need help in planning the best times to take your medicine, check with your health care professional.

Dosing—The dose of these medicines will be different for different patients. *Follow your doctor's orders or the directions on the label.* The following information includes only the average doses of these medicines. *If your dose is different, do not change it* unless your doctor tells you to do so.

The number of capsules, tablets or teaspoonfuls of suspension that you take depends on the strength of the medicine. Also, *the number of doses you take each day, the time allowed between doses, and the length of time you take the medicine depend on the medical problem for which you are taking a tetracycline.*

For demeclocycline

• For *oral* dosage forms (capsules, tablets):

—For bacterial or protozoal infections:

• Adults and teenagers—150 milligrams (mg) every six hours; or 300 mg every twelve hours.

• Infants and children up to 8 years of age—Tetracyclines are usually not used in young children because tetracyclines can permanently stain teeth.

• Children 8 years of age and older—Dose is

based on body weight. The usual dose is 1.65 to 3.3 mg per kilogram (kg) (0.8 to 1.5 mg per pound) of body weight every six hours; or 3.3 to 6.6 mg per kg (1.5 to 3 mg per pound) of body weight every twelve hours.

For doxycycline

- For *oral* dosage forms (capsules, suspension, and tablets):

  —For bacterial or protozoal infections:

  - Adults and children over 45 kilograms (kg) of body weight (99 pounds)—100 milligrams (mg) every twelve hours the first day, then 100 to 200 mg once a day or 50 to 100 mg every twelve hours.

  - Infants and children up to 8 years of age—Tetracyclines are usually not used in young children because tetracyclines can permanently stain teeth.

  - Children 45 kg of body weight (99 pounds) and less—Dose is based on body weight. The usual dose is 2.2 mg per kg (1 mg per pound) of body weight the first day, then 2.2 to 4.4 mg per kg (1 to 2 mg per pound) of body weight once a day; or 1.1 to 2.2 mg per kg (0.5 to 1 mg per pound) of body weight every twelve hours.

  —For the prevention of malaria:

  - Adults and teenagers—100 mg once a day. You should take the first dose one or two days before travel to an area where malaria may occur, continue taking the medicine every day throughout travel, and for four weeks after you leave the malarious area.

  - Children over 8 years of age—Dose is based on body weight. The usual dose is 2 mg per kg (0.9 mg per pound) of body weight once a day. You should take the first dose one or two days before travel to an area where malaria may occur, continue taking the medicine every day throughout travel, and for four weeks after you leave the malarious area.

• Infants and children up to 8 years of age—Tetracyclines are usually not used in young children because tetracyclines can permanently stain teeth.

• For *injection* dosage form:

—For bacterial or protozoal infections:

• Adults and children over 45 kg of body weight (99 pounds)—200 mg injected into a vein once a day; or 100 mg injected into a vein every twelve hours the first day, then 100 to 200 mg injected into a vein once a day. Another dose is 50 to 100 mg every twelve hours.

• Infants and children up to 8 years of age—Tetracyclines are usually not used in young children because tetracyclines can permanently stain teeth.

• Children 45 kg of body weight (99 pounds) and less—Dose is based on body weight. The usual dose is 4.4 mg per kg (2 mg per pound) of body weight injected into a vein once a day; or 2.2 mg per kg (1 mg per pound) of body weight injected into a vein every twelve hours the first day, then 2.2 to 4.4 mg per kg (1 to 2 mg per pound) of body weight once a day, or 1.1 to 2.2 mg per kg (0.5 to 1 mg per pound) of body weight every twelve hours.

For minocycline

• For *oral* dosage forms (capsules, suspension, and tablets):

—For bacterial or protozoal infections:

• Adults and teenagers—200 milligrams (mg) at

first, then 100 mg every twelve hours; or 100 to 200 mg at first, then 50 mg every six hours.

• Infants and children up to 8 years of age— Tetracyclines are usually not used in young children because tetracyclines can permanently stain teeth.

• Children 8 years of age and over—Dose is based on body weight. The usual dose is 4 mg per kilogram (kg) (1.8 mg per pound) of body weight at first, then 2 mg per kg (0.9 mg per pound) of body weight every twelve hours.

• For *injection* dosage form:

—For bacterial or protozoal infections:

• Adults and teenagers—200 mg at first, then 100 mg every twelve hours, injected into a vein.

• Infants and children up to 8 years of age— Tetracyclines are usually not used in young children because tetracyclines can permanently stain teeth.

• Children 8 years of age and over—Dose is based on body weight. The usual dose is 4 mg per kg (1.8 mg per pound) of body weight at first, then 2 mg per kg (0.9 mg per pound) of body weight every twelve hours, injected into a vein.

For oxytetracycline

• For *oral* dosage form (capsules):

—For bacterial or protozoal infections:

• Adults and teenagers—250 to 500 milligrams (mg) every six hours.

• Infants and children up to 8 years of age— Tetracyclines are usually not used in young children because tetracyclines can permanently stain teeth.

• Children 8 years of age and over—Dose is based on body weight. The usual dose is 6.25 to

12.5 mg per kilogram (kg) (2.8 to 5.7 mg per pound) of body weight every six hours.

- For *injection* dosage form (muscle injection):

  —For bacterial or protozoal infections:

    • Adults and teenagers—100 mg every eight hours; or 150 mg every twelve hours; or 250 mg once a day, injected into a muscle.

    • Infants and children up to 8 years of age—Tetracyclines are usually not used in young children because tetracyclines can permanently stain teeth.

    • Children 8 years of age and over—Dose is based on body weight. The usual dose is 5 to 8.3 mg per kg (2.3 to 3.8 mg per pound) of body weight every eight hours; or 7.5 to 12.5 mg per kg (3.4 to 5.7 mg per pound) of body weight every twelve hours, injected into a muscle.

- For *injection* dosage form (vein injection):

  —For bacterial or protozoal infections:

    • Adults and teenagers—250 to 500 mg injected into a vein every twelve hours.

    • Infants and children up to 8 years of age—Tetracyclines are usually not used in young children because tetracyclines can permanently stain teeth.

    • Children 8 years of age and over—Dose is based on body weight. The usual dose is 5 to 10 mg per kg (2.3 to 4.5 mg per pound) of body weight, injected into a vein, every twelve hours.

For tetracycline

- For *oral* dosage forms (capsules, suspension, and tablets):

  —For bacterial or protozoal infections:

    • Adults and teenagers—250 to 500 milligrams

(mg) every six hours; or 500 mg to 1 gram every twelve hours.

• Infants and children up to 8 years of age— Tetracyclines are usually not used in young children because tetracyclines can permanently stain teeth.

• Children 8 years of age and over—Dose is based on body weight. The usual dose is 6.25 to 12.5 mg per kilogram (kg) (2.8 to 5.7 mg per pound) of body weight every six hours; or 12.5 to 25 mg per kg (5.7 to 11.4 mg per pound) of body weight every twelve hours.

• For *injection* dosage form:

—For bacterial or protozoal infections:

• Adults and teenagers—100 mg every eight hours; or 150 mg every twelve hours; or 250 mg once a day, injected into a muscle.

• Infants and children up to 8 years of age— Tetracyclines are usually not used in young children because tetracyclines can permanently stain teeth.

• Children 8 years of age and over—Dose is based on body weight. The usual dose is 5 to 8.3 mg per kg (2.3 to 3.8 mg per pound) of body weight every eight hours; or 7.5 to 12.5 mg per kg (3.4 to 5.7 mg per pound) of body weight every twelve hours, injected into a muscle.

Missed dose—If you miss a dose of this medicine, take it as soon as possible. This will help to keep a constant amount of medicine in the blood or urine. However, if it is almost time for your next dose, skip the missed dose and go back to your regular dosing schedule. Do not double doses.

Storage—To store this medicine:

• Keep out of the reach of children.

- Store away from heat and direct light.
- Do not store the capsule or tablet form of this medicine in the bathroom, near the kitchen sink, or in other damp places. Heat or moisture may cause the medicine to break down.
- Keep the oral liquid forms of this medicine from freezing.
- Do not keep outdated medicine or medicine no longer needed. Be sure that any discarded medicine is out of the reach of children.

Precautions While Using This Medicine

If your symptoms do not improve within a few days (or a few weeks or months for acne patients), or if they become worse, check with your doctor.

Do not take antacids; calcium supplements such as calcium carbonate; *choline and magnesium salicylates combination (e.g., Trilisate); magnesium salicylate (e.g., Magan); magnesium-containing laxatives* such as Epsom salt; *or sodium bicarbonate* (baking soda) within 1 to 2 hours of the time you take any of the tetracyclines by mouth. In addition, *do not take iron preparations* (including vitamin preparations that contain iron) within 2 to 3 hours of the time you take tetracyclines by mouth. To do so may keep this medicine from working properly.

Oral contraceptives (birth control pills) containing estrogen may not work properly if you take them while you are taking tetracyclines. Unplanned pregnancies may occur. You should use a different or additional means of birth control while you are taking tetracyclines. If you have any questions about this, check with your health care professional.

Before having surgery (including dental surgery) with a general anesthetic, tell the medical doctor or dentist in charge that you are taking a tetracycline. This does not apply to doxycycline, however.

Tetracyclines may cause your skin to be more sensitive to sunlight than it is normally. Exposure to sunlight, even for brief periods of time, may cause a skin rash, itching, redness or other discoloration of the skin, or a severe sunburn. When you begin taking this medicine:

- Stay out of direct sunlight, especially between the hours of 10:00 a.m. and 3:00 p.m., if possible.
- Wear protective clothing, including a hat. Also, wear sunglasses.
- Apply a sun block product that has a skin protection factor (SPF) of at least 15. Some patients may require a product with a higher SPF number, especially if they have a fair complexion. If you have any questions about this, check with your health care professional.
- Apply a sun block lipstick that has an SPF of at least 15 to protect your lips.
- Do not use a sunlamp or tanning bed or booth.

You may still be more sensitive to sunlight or sunlamps for 2 weeks to several months or more after stopping this medicine. *If you have a severe reaction, check with your doctor.*

For patients taking *minocycline:*

- Minocycline may also cause some people to become dizzy, lightheaded, or unsteady. *Make sure you know how you react to this medicine before you drive, use machines, or do anything else that could be dangerous if you are dizzy or are not alert.* If these reactions are especially bothersome, check with your doctor.

Side Effects of This Medicine

Along with its needed effects, a medicine may cause some unwanted effects. In some infants and children, tetracyclines may cause the teeth to become discolored. Even though this may not happen right away, check with your doctor as soon as possible if you notice this effect or if you have any questions about it.

For all tetracyclines
  More common
> Increased sensitivity of skin to sunlight (rare with minocycline)

  Rare
> Abdominal pain; bulging fontanel (soft spot on head) of infants; headache; loss of appetite; nausea and vomiting; yellowing skin; visual changes

For demeclocycline only
  Less common
> Greatly increased frequency of urination or amount of urine; increased thirst; unusual tiredness or weakness

For minocycline only
  Less common
> Pigmentation (darker color or discoloration) of skin and mucous membranes

Other side effects may occur that usually do not need medical attention. These side effects may go away during treatment as your body adjusts to the medicine. However, check with your doctor if any of the following side effects continue or are bothersome:

For all tetracyclines
  More common
> Cramps or burning of the stomach; diarrhea; nausea or vomiting

  Less common
> Itching of the rectal or genital (sex organ) areas; sore mouth or tongue

For minocycline only
  More common
> Dizziness, lightheadedness, or unsteadiness

In some patients tetracyclines may cause the tongue to become darkened or discolored. This effect is only temporary and will go away when you stop taking this medicine.

Other side effects not listed above may also occur in some patients. If you notice any other effects, check with your doctor.

Additional Information

Once a medicine has been approved for marketing for a certain use, experience may show that it is also useful for other medical problems. Although these uses are not included in product labeling, tetracyclines are used in certain patients with the following medical conditions:

- Syndrome of inappropriate antidiuretic hormone (SIADH) (for demeclocycline)
- Traveler's diarrhea (for doxycyline)

For patients taking this medicine for *SIADH:*

- Some doctors may prescribe demeclocycline for certain patients who retain (keep) more body water than usual. Although demeclocycline works like a diuretic (water pill) in these patients, it will not work that way in other patients who may need a diuretic.

For patients taking this medicine for *traveler's diarrhea:*

- Some doctors may prescribe doxycycline by mouth to help prevent or treat traveler's diarrhea. It is usually given daily for three weeks to prevent traveler's diarrhea. If you have any questions about this, check with your doctor.

Other than the above information, there is no additional information relating to proper use, precautions, or side effects for these uses.

THYROID HORMONES   Systemic

Some commonly used brand names are:

In the U.S.—

Armour Thyroid[5]	Synthroid[1]
Cytomel[2]	Thyrar[5]
Levo-T[1]	Thyroid Strong[5]
Levothroid[1]	Thyrolar[3]
Levoxine[1]	Westhroid[5]

In Canada—

Cytomel[2]	PMS-Levothyroxine Sodium[1]
Eltroxin[1]	Synthroid[1]

Note: For quick reference, the following thyroid hormones are numbered
       to match the corresponding brand names.

This information applies to the following medicines:

  1. Levothyroxine (lee-voe-thye-ROX-een)‡
  2. Liothyronine (lye-oh-THYE-roe-neen)‡
  3. Liotrix (LYE-oh-trix)†
  4. Thyroglobulin (thye-roe-GLOB-yoo-lin)*†
  5. Thyroid (THYE-roid)‡§

Note: This information does *not* apply to Thyrotropin.

---

   *Not commercially available in the U.S.
   †Not commercially available in Canada.
   ‡Generic name product may also be available in the U.S.
   §Generic name product may also be available in Canada.

Description

Thyroid medicines belong to the general group of medicines called hormones. They are used when the thyroid
gland does not produce enough hormone. They are also
used to help decrease the size of enlarged thyroid glands
(known as goiter) and to treat thyroid cancer.

These medicines are available only with your doctor's prescription, in the following dosage forms:

Oral

  Levothyroxine
    • Tablets (U.S. and Canada)

Liothyronine
- Tablets (U.S. and Canada)

Liotrix
- Tablets (U.S.)

Thyroglobulin
- Tablets

Thyroid
- Tablets (U.S. and Canada)
- Enteric-coated tablets (U.S.)

Parenteral

Levothyroxine
- Injection (U.S. and Canada)

Before Using This Medicine

In deciding to use a medicine, the risks of taking the medicine must be weighed against the good it will do. This is a decision you and your doctor will make. For thyroid hormones, the following should be considered:

Allergies—Tell your doctor if you have ever had any unusual or allergic reaction to thyroid hormones. Also tell your health care professional if you are allergic to any other substances, such as foods, preservatives, or dyes.

Pregnancy—It is essential that your baby receive the right amount of thyroid for normal development. You may need to take different amounts while you are pregnant. In addition, you may respond differently than usual to some tests. Your doctor should check your progress at regular visits while you are pregnant.

Breast-feeding—Use of proper amounts of thyroid hormones by mothers has not been shown to cause problems in nursing babies.

Children—Thyroid hormones have been tested in children and have not been shown to cause different side effects or problems in children than they do in adults.

Older adults—This medicine has been tested and has not been shown to cause different side effects or problems in older people than it does in younger adults. However, a different dose may be needed in the elderly. Therefore, it is important to take the medicine only as directed by the doctor.

Other medicines—Although certain medicines should not be used together at all, in other cases two different medicines may be used together even if an interaction might occur. In these cases, your doctor may want to change the dose, or other precautions may be necessary. When you are taking thyroid hormones, it is especially important that your health care professional know if you are taking any of the following:

- Amphetamines
- Anticoagulants (blood thinners)
- Appetite suppressants (diet pills)
- Cholestyramine (e.g., Questran)
- Colestipol (e.g., Colestid)
- Medicine for asthma or other breathing problems
- Medicine for colds, sinus problems, or hay fever or other allergies (including nose drops or sprays)

Other medical problems—The presence of other medical problems may affect the use of thyroid hormones. Make sure you tell your doctor if you have any other medical problems especially:

- Diabetes mellitus (sugar diabetes)
- Hardening of the arteries
- Heart disease
- High blood pressure
- Overactive thyroid (history of)
- Underactive adrenal gland
- Underactive pituitary gland

Proper Use of This Medicine

Use this medicine only as directed by your doctor. Do not use more or less of it, and do not use it more often than your doctor ordered. Your doctor has prescribed the exact amount your body needs, and if you take different amounts, you may experience symptoms of an overactive or underactive thyroid. Take it at the same time each day to make sure it always has the same effect.

If your condition is due to a lack of thyroid hormone, you may have to take this medicine for the rest of your life. It is very important that you *do not stop taking this medicine without first checking with your doctor.*

Dosing—The dose of these medicines will be different for different patients. *Follow your doctor's orders or the directions on the label.* The following information includes only the average doses of these medicines. *If your dose is different, do not change it* unless your doctor tells you to do so.

The number of tablets that you take depends on the strength of the medicine. The amount of thyroid hormone that you need to take every day depends on the results of your thyroid tests. However, treatment is usually started with lower doses that are increased a little at a time until you are taking the full amount. This helps prevent side effects.

For levothyroxine

- For *oral* dosage form (tablets):

    —For replacing the thyroid hormone:

    - Adults and teenagers—At first, 0.0125 to 0.05 milligrams (mg) once a day. Then, your doctor may increase your dose a little at a time to 0.075 to 0.125 mg a day. The dose is usually no higher than 0.15 mg once a day.

• Children less than 6 months of age—The dose is based on body weight and must be determined by your doctor. The usual dose is 0.025 to 0.05 mg once a day.

• Children 6 months to 12 months of age—The dose is based on body weight and must be determined by your doctor. The usual dose is 0.05 to 0.075 mg once a day.

• Children 1 to 5 years of age—The dose is based on body weight and must be determined by your doctor. The usual dose is 0.075 to 0.1 mg once a day.

• Children 6 to 10 years of age—The dose is based on body weight and must be determined by your doctor. The usual dose is 0.1 to 0.15 mg once a day.

• Children over 10 years of age—The dose is based on body weight and must be determined by your doctor. The usual dose is 0.15 to 0.2 mg once a day.

• For *injection* dosage form:

—For replacing the thyroid hormone:

• Adults and teenagers—50 to 100 micrograms (mcg) injected into a muscle or into a vein once a day. People with very serious conditions caused by too little thyroid hormone may need higher doses.

• Children less than 6 months of age—The dose is based on body weight and must be determined by your doctor. The usual dose is 0.019 to 0.038 mg once a day.

• Children 6 months to 12 months of age—The dose is based on body weight and must be determined by your doctor. The usual dose is 0.038 to 0.056 mg once a day.

• Children 1 to 5 years of age—The dose is based

on body weight and must be determined by your doctor. The usual dose is 0.056 to 0.075 mg once a day.

• Children 6 to 10 years of age—The dose is based on body weight and must be determined by your doctor. The usual dose is 0.075 to 0.113 mg once a day.

• Children over 10 years of age—The dose is based on body weight and must be determined by your doctor. The usual dose is 0.113 to 0.15 mg once a day.

For liothyronine sodium

• For *oral* dosage form (tablets):

—For replacing the thyroid hormone:

• Adults and teenagers—At first, 25 micrograms (mcg) a day. Some patients with very serious conditions caused by too little thyroid hormone may need to take only 2.5 to 5 mcg a day at first. Also, some patients with heart disease or the elderly may need lower doses at first. Then, your doctor may increase your dose a little at a time to up to 50 mcg a day if needed. Your doctor may want you to divide your dose into smaller amounts that are taken two or more times a day.

—For treating a large thyroid gland (goiter):

• Adults—At first, 5 mcg a day. Some patients with heart disease or the elderly may need lower doses at first. Then, your doctor may increase your dose a little at a time to 50 to 100 mcg a day.

For liotrix (levothyroxine and liothyronine combination)

• For *oral* dosage form (tablets):

—For replacing the thyroid hormone:

• Adults, teenagers, and children—At first, 50 micrograms (mcg) of levothyroxine and 12.5 mcg of liothyronine once a day. Some people with very serious conditions caused by too little thyroid hormone may need only 12.5 mcg of levothyroxine and 3.1 mcg of liothyronine once a day. Also, some elderly patients may need lower doses at first. Then, your doctor may want to increase your dose a little at a time to up to 100 mcg of levothyroxine and 25 mcg of liothyronine.

For thyroglobulin

• For *oral* dosage form (tablets):

—For replacing the thyroid hormone:

• Adults, teenagers, and children—At first, 32 milligrams (mg) a day. Some people with very serious conditions caused by too little thyroid hormone may need to take only 16 to 32 mg a day at first. Then, the doctor may want you to increase your dose a little at a time to 65 to 160 mg a day.

For thyroid

• For *oral* dosage form (tablets):

—For replacing thyroid hormone:

• Adults, teenagers, and children—60 milligrams (mg) a day. Some people with very serious conditions caused by too little thyroid hormone may need to take only 15 mg a day at first. Also, some elderly patients may need lower doses at first. Then, your doctor may want to increase your dose a little at a time to 60 to 120 mg a day.

Missed dose—If you miss a dose of this medicine, take it as soon as possible. However, if it is almost time for your next dose, skip the missed dose and go back to your regular dosing schedule. Do not double doses. If you miss 2 or more doses in a row or if you have any questions about this, check with your doctor.

Storage—To store this medicine:

• Keep out of the reach of children.

- Store away from heat and direct light.
- Do not store in the bathroom, near the kitchen sink, or in other damp places. Heat or moisture may cause the medicine to break down.
- Do not keep outdated medicine or medicine no longer needed. Be sure that any discarded medicine is out of the reach of children.

Precautions While Using This Medicine

It is very important that your doctor check your progress at regular visits, to make sure that this medicine is working properly.

If you have certain kinds of heart disease, this medicine may cause chest pain or shortness of breath when you exert yourself. If these occur, do not overdo exercise or physical work. If you have any questions about this, check with your doctor.

Before having any kind of surgery (including dental surgery) or emergency treatment, *tell the medical doctor or dentist in charge that you are taking this medicine.*

Do not take any other medicine unless prescribed by your doctor. Some medicines may increase or decrease the effects of thyroid on your body and cause problems in controlling your condition. Also, thyroid hormones may change the effects of other medicines.

Side Effects of This Medicine

Along with its needed effects, a medicine may cause some unwanted effects. Although not all of these side effects may occur, if they do occur they may need medical attention.

Check with your doctor as soon as possible if any of the

following side effects occur since they may indicate an overdose or an allergic reaction:

Rare

Headache (severe) in children; skin rash or hives

Signs and symptoms of overdose

Chest pain; fast or irregular heartbeat; shortness of breath

For patients taking this medicine for underactive thyroid:

• This medicine usually takes several weeks to have a noticeable effect on your condition. Until it begins to work, you may experience no change in your symptoms. Check with your doctor if the following symptoms continue:

Clumsiness; coldness; constipation; dry, puffy skin; listlessness; muscle aches; sleepiness; tiredness; weakness; weight gain

Other effects may occur if the dose of the medicine is not exactly right. These side effects will go away when the dose is corrected. Check with your doctor if any of the following symptoms occur:

Changes in appetite; changes in menstrual periods; diarrhea; fever; hand tremors; headache; increased sensitivity to heat; irritability; leg cramps; nervousness; sweating; trouble in sleeping; vomiting; weight loss

Other side effects not listed above may also occur in some patients. If you notice any other effects, check with your doctor.

TICLOPIDINE　Systemic

A commonly used brand name in the U.S. and Canada is Ticlid.

Description

Ticlopidine (tye-KLOE-pi-deen) is used to lower the chance of having a stroke. It is given to people who have already had a stroke and to people with certain medical problems that may lead to a stroke. Because ticlopidine can cause serious side effects, especially during the first 3 months of treatment, it is used mostly for people who cannot take aspirin to prevent strokes.

A stroke may occur when a blood vessel in the brain is blocked by a blood clot. Ticlopidine lessens the chance that a harmful blood clot will form, by preventing certain cells in the blood from clumping together. This effect of ticlopidine may also increase the chance of serious bleeding in some people.

This medicine is available in the following dosage forms:

Oral

- Tablets (U.S. and Canada)

Before Using This Medicine

In deciding to use a medicine, the risks of taking the medicine must be weighed against the good it will do. This is a decision you and your doctor will make. For ticlopidine, the following should be considered:

Allergies—Tell your doctor if you have ever had any unusual or allergic reaction to ticlopidine. Also tell your health care professional if you are allergic to any other substances, such as foods, preservatives, or dyes.

Pregnancy—Studies with ticlopidine have not been done in pregnant women. This medicine did not cause birth defects in animal studies. However, it caused other unwanted effects in animal studies when it was given in amounts that were large enough to cause harmful effects in the mother.

Breast-feeding—It is not known whether ticlopidine passes into the breast milk.

Children—There is no specific information comparing use of ticlopidine in children with use in other age groups.

Older adults—This medicine has been tested and has not been shown to cause different side effects or problems in older people than it does in younger adults.

Other medicines—Although certain medicines should not be used together at all, in other cases two different medicines may be used together even if an interaction might occur. In these cases, your doctor may want to change the dose, or other precautions may be necessary. When you are taking ticlopidine, it is especially important that your health care professional know if you are taking any of the following:

- Anticoagulants (blood thinners) or
- Aspirin or
- Heparin (e.g., Hepalean, Liquaemin)—The chance of serious bleeding may be increased

Other medical problems—The presence of other medical problems may affect the use of ticlopidine. Make sure you tell your doctor if you have any other medical problems, especially:

- Blood disease—The chance of serious side effects may be increased
- Blood clotting problems, such as hemophilia, or
- Liver disease (severe) or
- Stomach ulcers—The chance of serious bleeding may be increased
- Kidney disease (severe)—Ticlopidine is removed from the body more slowly when the kidneys are not working properly. This may increase the chance of side effects.

Proper Use of This Medicine

Ticlopidine should be taken with food. This increases the amount of medicine that is absorbed into the body. It may also lessen the chance of stomach upset.

Take this medicine only as directed by your doctor. Ticlopidine will not work properly if you take less of it than directed. Taking more ticlopidine than directed may increase the chance of serious side effects without increasing the helpful effects.

Dosing—*Follow your doctor's orders or the directions on the label.* The following dose was used, and found effective, in studies. However, some people may need a different dose. *If your dose is different, do not change it* unless your doctor tells you to do so:

- For adults—1 tablet (250 mg) two times a day, with food.
- For children—It is not likely that ticlopidine would be used to help prevent strokes in children. If a child needs this medicine, however, the dose would have to be determined by the doctor.

Missed dose—If you miss a dose of this medicine, take it as soon as possible. However, if it is almost time for your next dose, skip the missed dose and go back to your regular dosing schedule. Do not double doses.

Storage—To store this medicine:
- Keep out of the reach of children.
- Store away from heat and direct light.
- Do not store in the bathroom, near the kitchen sink, or in other damp places. Heat or moisture may cause the medicine to break down.
- Do not keep outdated medicine or medicine no longer needed. Be sure that any discarded medicine is out of the reach of children.

Precautions While Using This Medicine

It is very important that blood tests be done every 2 weeks for the first 3 months of treatment with ticlopidine. The tests are needed to find out whether certain side effects are occurring. Finding these side effects early helps to prevent them from becoming serious. Your doctor will arrange for the blood tests to be done. *Be sure that you do not miss any appointments for these tests.* You will probably not need to have your blood tested so often after the first 3 months of treatment, because the side effects are less likely to occur after that time.

Tell all medical doctors, dentists, nurses, and pharmacists you go to that you are taking this medicine. Ticlopidine may increase the risk of serious bleeding during an operation or some kinds of dental work. Therefore, treatment may have to be stopped about 10 days to 2 weeks before the operation or dental work is done.

Ticlopidine may cause serious bleeding, especially after an injury. Sometimes, bleeding inside the body can occur without your knowing about it. Ask your doctor whether there are certain activities you should avoid while taking this medicine (for example, sports that can cause injuries). *Also, check with your doctor immediately if you are injured while being treated with this medicine.*

Check with your doctor immediately if you notice any of the following side effects:

- Bruising or bleeding, especially bleeding that is hard to stop.
- Any sign of infection, such as fever, chills, or sore throat.
- Sores, ulcers, or white spots in the mouth.

After you stop taking ticlopidine, the chance of bleeding may continue for 1 or 2 weeks. During this period of time, continue to follow the same precautions that you followed while you were taking the medicine.

Side Effects of This Medicine

Along with its needed effects, a medicine may cause some unwanted effects. Although not all of these side effects

may occur, if they do occur they may need medical attention.

Check with your doctor immediately if any of the following side effects occur:

> *Less common or rare*
>> Abdominal or stomach pain (severe) or swelling; back pain; blood in eyes; blood in urine; bloody or black, tarry stools; bruising or purple areas on skin; coughing up blood; decreased alertness; dizziness; fever, chills, or sore throat; headache (severe or continuing); joint pain or swelling; nosebleeds; pinpoint red spots on skin; sores, ulcers, or white spots in mouth; paralysis or problems with coordination; stammering or other difficulty in speaking; unusually heavy bleeding or oozing from cuts or wounds; unusually heavy or unexpected menstrual bleeding; vomiting of blood or material that looks like coffee grounds

Also, check with your doctor as soon as possible if any of the following side effects occur:

> *More common*
>> Skin rash

> *Less common or rare*
>> Hives or itching of skin; ringing or buzzing in ears; yellow eyes or skin

Other side effects may occur that usually do not need medical attention. These side effects may go away during treatment as your body adjusts to the medicine. However, check with your doctor if any of the following side effects continue or are bothersome:

> *More common*
>> Abdominal or stomach pain (mild); bloating or gas; diarrhea; nausea

> *Less common*
>> Indigestion; vomiting

Other side effects not listed above may also occur in some patients. If you notice any other effects, check with your doctor.

TORSEMIDE   Systemic†

A commonly used brand name in the U.S. is Demadex.

†Not commercially available in Canada.

Description

Torsemide (TORE-se-mide) belongs to the group of medicines called loop diuretics. Torsemide is given to help reduce the amount of water in the body in certain conditions, such as congestive heart failure, severe liver disease (cirrhosis), or kidney disease. It works by acting on the kidneys to increase the flow of urine.

Torsemide is also used to treat high blood pressure (hypertension). High blood pressure adds to the work load of the heart and arteries. If it continues for a long time, the heart and arteries may not function properly. This can damage the blood vessels of the brain, heart, and kidneys, resulting in a stroke, heart failure, or kidney failure. High blood pressure may also increase the risk of heart attacks. These problems may be less likely to occur if blood pressure is controlled.

Torsemide is available only with your doctor's prescription, in the following dosage forms:

Oral
- Tablets (U.S.)

Parenteral
- Injection (U.S.)

Before Using This Medicine

In deciding to use a medicine, the risks of taking the medicine must be weighed against the good it will do. This is a decision you and your doctor will make. For torsemide, the following should be considered:

Allergies—Tell your doctor if you have ever had any unusual or allergic reaction to bumetanide, ethacrynic acid, furosemide, sulfonamides (sulfa drugs), or thiazide diuretics (water pills). Also, tell your health care professional if you are allergic to any other substances, such as foods, preservatives, or dyes.

Pregnancy—Studies have not been done in pregnant women. In general, diuretics are not useful for normal swelling of feet and hands that occurs during pregnancy. Diuretics should not be taken during pregnancy unless recommended by your doctor.

Breast-feeding—It is not known whether torsemide passes into breast milk. Although most medicines pass into breast milk in small amounts, many of them may be used safely while breast-feeding. Mothers who are taking this medicine and who wish to breast-feed should discuss this with their doctor.

Children—Studies on this medicine have been done only in adult patients, and there is no specific information comparing use of torsemide in children with use in other age groups.

Older adults—Many medicines have not been studied specifically in older people. Therefore, it may not be known whether they work exactly the same way they do in younger adults. Although there is no specific information comparing use of torsemide in the elderly with use in other age groups, this medicine is not expected to cause different side effects or problems in older people than it does in younger adults.

Other medicines—Although certain medicines should not be used together at all, in other cases two different medicines may be used together even if an interaction might occur. In these cases, your doctor may want to change the dose, or other precautions may be necessary. When you are taking torsemide, it is especially important that your health care professional know if you are taking any of the following:

- Acetazolamide (e.g., Diamox) or
- Alcohol or
- Amphotericin B by injection (e.g., Fungizone) or
- Azlocillin (e.g., Azlin) or
- Capreomycin (e.g., Capastat) or
- Carbenicillin by injection (e.g., Geopen) or
- Corticosteroids (cortisone-like medicine) or
- Corticotropin (ACTH) or
- Dichlorphenamide (e.g., Daranide) or
- Diuretics (water pills) or
- Insulin or
- Laxatives (with overdose or chronic misuse) or
- Methazolamide (e.g., Neptazane) or
- Mezlocillin (e.g., Mezlin) or
- Piperacillin (e.g., Pipracil) or
- Salicylates or
- Sodium bicarbonate (e.g., baking soda) or
- Ticarcillin (e.g., Ticar) or
- Ticarcillin and clavulanate (e.g., Timentin) or
- Vitamin B_{12} (e.g., AlphaRedisol, Rubramin-PC) (when used in megaloblastic anemia) or
- Vitamin D—Use of these medicines with torsemide may increase the chance of potassium loss

- Aldesleukin (e.g., Proleukin) or
- Anti-infectives by mouth or by injection (medicine for infection) or
- Carmustine (e.g., BiCNU) or
- Cisplatin (e.g., Platinol) or
- Combination pain medicine containing acetaminophen and

aspirin (e.g., Excedrin) or other salicylates (with large amounts taken regularly) or

- Cyclosporine (e.g., Sandimmune) or
- Deferoxamine (e.g., Desferal) (with long-term use) or
- Gold salts (medicine for arthritis) or
- Inflammation or pain medicine, except narcotics, or
- Methotrexate (e.g., Mexate) or
- Penicillamine (e.g., Cuprimine) or
- Pentamidine (e.g., Pentam 300) or
- Plicamycin (e.g., Mithracin) or
- Streptozocin (e.g., Zanosar) or
- Tiopronin (e.g., Thiola)—Use of these medicines with torsemide may increase the chance of kidney damage
- Anticoagulants (blood thinners)—Torsemide may decrease the effects of these medicines
- Lithium (e.g., Lithane)—Use of lithium with torsemide may increase the chance of kidney damage; also, the chance of side effects of lithium may be increased

Other medical problems—The presence of other medical problems may affect the use of torsemide. Make sure you tell your doctor if you have any other medical problems, especially:

- Diabetes mellitus (sugar diabetes)—Torsemide may increase the amount of sugar in the blood
- Gout or
- Hearing problems—Torsemide may make these conditions worse
- Heart attack (recent)—Use of torsemide after a recent heart attack may make this condition worse
- Kidney disease (severe) or
- Liver disease—Higher blood levels of torsemide may occur, which may increase the chance of side effects

---

Proper Use of This Medicine

This medicine may cause you to have an unusual feeling of tiredness when you begin to take it. You may also notice an increase in the amount of urine or in your frequency of urination. After you have taken the medicine for a while, these effects should lessen.

It is best to plan your dose or doses according to a schedule that will least affect your personal activities and sleep. Ask your health care professional to help you plan the best time to take this medicine.

To help you remember to take your medicine, try to get into the habit of taking it at the same time each day.

For patients taking this medicine for *high blood pressure:*

- In addition to the use of the medicine your doctor has prescribed, treatment for your high blood pressure may include weight control and care in the types of foods you eat, especially foods high in sodium. Your doctor will tell you which of these are most important for you. You should check with your doctor before changing your diet.

- Many patients who have high blood pressure will not notice any signs of the problem. In fact, many may feel normal. It is very important that you *take your medicine exactly as directed* and that you keep your appointments with your doctor even if you feel well.

- Remember that this medicine will not cure your high blood pressure, but it does help control it. Therefore, you must continue to take it as directed if you expect to lower your blood pressure and keep it down. *You may have to take high blood pressure medicine for the rest of your life.* If high blood pressure is not treated, it can cause serious problems, such as heart failure, blood vessel disease, stroke, or kidney disease.

Dosing—The dose of torsemide will be different for different patients. *Follow your doctor's orders or the directions on the label.* The following information includes only the average doses of torsemide. *If your dose is different, do not change it* unless your doctor tells you to do so.

The number of tablets that you take depends on the strength of the medicine. Also, *the length of time you take the medicine depends on the medical problem for which you are taking torsemide.*

- For *oral* dosage form (tablets):
  —For lowering the amount of water in the body:
  - Adults—Dose is usually 5 to 20 milligrams (mg) once a day. However, your doctor may increase your dose as needed.
  - Children—Use and dose must be determined by your doctor.
  —For high blood pressure:
  - Adults—5 to 10 mg once a day.
  - Children—Use and dose must be determined by your doctor.
- For *injection* dosage form:
  —For lowering the amount of water in the body:
  - Adults—Dose is usually 5 to 20 mg injected into a vein once a day. However, your doctor may increase your dose as needed.
  - Children—Use and dose must be determined by your doctor.

Missed dose—If you miss a dose of this medicine, take it as soon as possible. However, if it is almost time for your next dose, skip the missed dose and go back to your regular dosing schedule. Do not double doses.

Storage—To store this medicine:
- Keep out of the reach of children.
- Store away from heat and direct light.
- Do not store in the bathroom, near the kitchen sink, or in other damp places. Heat or moisture may cause the medicine to break down.

- Keep the medicine from freezing. Do not refrigerate.
- Do not keep outdated medicine or medicine no longer needed. Be sure that any discarded medicine is out of the reach of children.

Precautions While Using This Medicine

It is important that your doctor check your progress at regular visits to make sure that this medicine is working properly.

This medicine may cause a loss of potassium from your body:

- To help prevent this, your doctor may want you to:
  —eat or drink foods that have a high potassium content (for example, orange or other citrus fruit juices), or
  —take a potassium supplement, or
  —take another medicine to help prevent the loss of the potassium in the first place.
- It is very important to follow these directions. Also, it is important not to change your diet on your own. This is more important if you are already on a special diet (as for diabetes) or if you are taking a potassium supplement or a medicine to reduce potassium loss. Extra potassium may not be necessary and, in some cases, too much potassium could be harmful.

To prevent the loss of too much water and potassium, tell your doctor if you become sick, especially with severe or continuing nausea and vomiting or diarrhea.

Before having any kind of surgery (including dental surgery) or emergency treatment, make sure the medical doctor or dentist in charge knows that you are taking this medicine.

Dizziness, lightheadedness, or fainting may occur, especially when you get up from a lying or sitting position. This is more likely to occur in the morning. *Getting up slowly may help.* When you get up from lying down, sit on the edge of the bed with your feet dangling for 1 or 2 minutes. Then stand up slowly. If the problem continues or gets worse, check with your doctor.

The dizziness, lightheadedness, or fainting is also more likely to occur if you drink alcohol, stand for long periods of time, or exercise, or if the weather is hot. *While you are taking this medicine, be careful to limit the amount of alcohol you drink. Also, use extra care during exercise or hot weather or if you must stand for long periods of time.*

For *diabetic patients:*

- This medicine may affect blood sugar levels. While you are using this medicine, be especially careful in testing for sugar in your blood or urine.

For patients taking this medicine for *high blood pressure:*

- *Do not take other medicines unless they have been discussed with your doctor.* This especially includes over-the-counter (nonprescription) medicines for appetite control, asthma, colds, cough, hay fever, or sinus problems, since they may tend to increase your blood pressure.

Side Effects of This Medicine

Along with its needed effects, a medicine may cause some unwanted effects. Although not all of these side effects may occur, if they do occur they may need medical attention.

Check with your doctor as soon as possible if any of the following side effects occur:

Less common

> Dryness of mouth; fast or irregular heartbeat; increased thirst; mood or mental changes; muscle pain or cramps; nausea or vomiting; unusual tiredness or weakness

Rare

> Black, tarry stools; dizziness when getting up from a sitting or lying position; ringing or buzzing in the ears or any hearing loss; skin rash

Other side effects may occur that usually do not need medical attention. These side effects may go away during treatment as your body adjusts to the medicine. However, check with your doctor if any of the following side effects continue or are bothersome:

More common

> Constipation; dizziness; headache; stomach upset

TRAZODONE   Systemic

Some commonly used brand names are:

In the U.S.—

Desyrel   Trialodine

Trazon

Generic name product may also be available.

In Canada—

Desyrel

Description

Trazodone (TRAZ-oh-done) belongs to the group of medicines known as antidepressants or "mood elevators." It is used to relieve mental depression and depression that sometimes occurs with anxiety.

Trazodone is available only with your doctor's prescription, in the following dosage form:

Oral

- Tablets (U.S. and Canada)

Before Using This Medicine

In deciding to use a medicine, the risks of taking the medicine must be weighed against the good it will do. This is a decision you and your doctor will make. For trazodone, the following should be considered:

Allergies—Tell your doctor if you have ever had any unusual or allergic reaction to trazodone. Also tell your health care professional if you are allergic to any other substances, such as foods, preservatives, or dyes.

Pregnancy—Studies have not been done in pregnant women. However, studies in animals have shown that trazodone causes birth defects and a decrease in the number of successful pregnancies when given in doses many times larger than human doses.

Breast-feeding—Trazodone passes into breast milk.

Children—Studies on this medicine have been done only in adult patients, and there is no specific information comparing use of trazodone in children with use in other age groups.

Older adults—Drowsiness, dizziness, confusion, vision problems, dryness of mouth, and constipation may be more likely to occur in the elderly, who are usually more sensitive to the effects of trazodone.

Other medicines—Although certain medicines should not be used together at all, in other cases two different medicines may be used together even if an interaction might occur. In these cases, your doctor may want to change the dose, or other precautions may be necessary. When you are taking trazodone, it is especially important that your health care professional know if you are taking any of the following:

• Antihypertensives (high blood pressure medicine)—Taking

these medicines with trazodone may result in low blood pressure (hypotension); the amount of medicine you need to take may change

- Central nervous system (CNS) depressants (medicine that causes drowsiness) or
- Tricyclic antidepressants (medicine for depression)—Taking these medicines with trazodone may add to the CNS depressant effects

Other medical problems—The presence of other medical problems may affect the use of trazodone. Make sure you tell your doctor if you have any other medical problems, especially:

- Alcohol abuse (or history of)—Drinking alcohol with trazodone will increase the central nervous system (CNS) depressant effects
- Heart disease—Trazodone may make the condition worse
- Kidney disease or
- Liver disease—Higher blood levels of trazodone may occur, increasing the chance of side effects

---

Proper Use of This Medicine

To lessen stomach upset and to reduce dizziness and light-headedness, take this medicine with or shortly after a meal or light snack, even for a daily bedtime dose, unless your doctor has told you to take it on an empty stomach.

Take trazodone only as directed by your doctor, to benefit your condition as much as possible.

Sometimes trazodone must be taken for up to 4 weeks before you begin to feel better, although most people notice improvement within 2 weeks.

Dosing—The dose of trazodone will be different for different patients. *Follow your doctor's orders or the directions on the label.* The following information includes only the average doses of trazodone. *If your dose is different, do not change it* unless your doctor tells you to do so:

- Adults—Oral, to start, 50 milligrams per dose taken three times a day, or 75 milligrams per dose taken two times a day. Your doctor may increase your dose if needed.
- Children 6 to 18 years of age—Oral. Your doctor will tell you what dose to take based on your body weight.
- Children up to 6 years of age—Dose must be determined by the doctor.
- Elderly patients—Oral, to start, 25 milligrams per dose taken three times a day. Your doctor may increase your dose if needed.

Missed dose—If you miss a dose of this medicine, take it as soon as possible. However, if it is within 4 hours of your next dose, skip the missed dose and go back to your regular dosing schedule. Do not double doses.

Storage—To store this medicine:

- Keep out of the reach of children.
- Store away from heat and direct light.
- Do not store in the bathroom, near the kitchen sink, or in other damp places. Heat or moisture may cause the medicine to break down.
- Do not keep outdated medicine or medicine no longer needed. Be sure that any discarded medicine is out of the reach of children.

Precautions While Using This Medicine

It is very important that your doctor check your progress at regular visits. This will allow your doctor to check the medicine's effects and to change the dose if needed.

Do not stop taking this medicine without first checking with your doctor. To prevent a possible return of your medical problem, your doctor may want you to reduce gradually the amount of medicine you are using before you stop completely.

Before having any kind of surgery, dental treatment, or emergency treatment, tell the medical doctor or dentist in charge that you are using this medicine. Taking trazodone together with medicines that are used during surgery or dental or emergency treatments may increase the CNS depressant effects.

This medicine will add to the effects of alcohol and other CNS depressants (medicines that slow down the nervous system, possibly causing drowsiness). Some examples of CNS depressants are antihistamines or medicine for hay fever, other allergies, or colds; sedatives, tranquilizers, or sleeping medicine; prescription pain medicine or narcotics; barbiturates; medicine for seizures; muscle relaxants; or anesthetics, including some dental anesthetics. *Check with your doctor before taking any of the above while you are using this medicine.*

This medicine may cause some people to become drowsy or less alert than they are normally. *Make sure you know how you react to this medicine before you drive, use machines, or do anything else that could be dangerous if you are not alert.*

Dizziness, lightheadedness, or fainting may occur, especially when you get up from a lying or sitting position. Getting up slowly may help. If this problem continues or gets worse, check with your doctor.

Trazodone may cause dryness of the mouth. For temporary relief, use sugarless gum or candy, melt bits of ice in your mouth, or use a saliva substitute. However, if your mouth continues to feel dry for more than 2 weeks, check with your medical doctor or dentist. Continuing dryness of the mouth may increase the chance of dental disease, including tooth decay, gum disease, and fungus infections.

Side Effects of This Medicine

Along with its needed effects, a medicine may cause some unwanted effects. Although not all of these side effects may occur, if they do occur they may need medical attention.

Stop taking this medicine and check with your doctor immediately if the following side effect occurs:

Rare

Painful, inappropriate erection of the penis, continuing

Also, check with your doctor as soon as possible if any of the following side effects occur:

Less common

Confusion; muscle tremors

Rare

Fainting; fast or slow heartbeat; skin rash; unusual excitement

Symptoms of overdose

Drowsiness; loss of muscle coordination; nausea and vomiting

Other side effects may occur that usually do not need medical attention. These side effects may go away during treatment as your body adjusts to the medicine. However, check with your doctor if any of the following side effects continue or are bothersome:

More common

Dizziness or lightheadedness; drowsiness; dryness of mouth (usually mild); headache; nausea and vomiting; unpleasant taste

Less common

Blurred vision; constipation; diarrhea; muscle aches or pains; unusual tiredness or weakness

Other side effects not listed above may also occur in some patients. If you notice any other effects, check with your doctor.

ZALCITABINE Systemic

A commonly used brand name in the U.S. and Canada is HIVID.
Another commonly used name is ddC.

Description

Zalcitabine (zal-SITE-a-been) (also known as ddC) is used
in the treatment of the infection caused by the human
immunodeficiency virus (HIV). HIV is the virus that
causes acquired immune deficiency syndrome (AIDS).

Zalcitabine (ddC) will not cure or prevent HIV infection
or AIDS; however, it helps keep HIV from reproducing
and appears to slow down the destruction of the immune
system. This may help delay the development of problems
usually related to AIDS or HIV disease. Zalcitabine will
not keep you from spreading HIV to other people. People
who receive this medicine may continue to have other
problems usually related to AIDS or HIV disease.

Zalcitabine may cause some serious side effects, including
peripheral neuropathy (a problem involving the nerves).
Symptoms of peripheral neuropathy include tingling, burning, numbness, or pain in the hands or feet. Zalcitabine may
also cause pancreatitis (inflammation of the pancreas).
Symptoms of pancreatitis include stomach pain, and nausea
and vomiting. *Check with your doctor if any new health
problems or symptoms occur while you are taking
zalcitabine.*

Zalcitabine is available only with your doctor's prescrip-
tion, in the following dosage form:
  Oral
  • Tablets (U.S. and Canada)

Before Using This Medicine

In deciding to use a medicine, the risks of taking the medicine must be weighed against the good it will do. This is a decision you and your doctor will make. For zalcitabine, the following should be considered:

Allergies—Tell your doctor if you have ever had any unusual or allergic reaction to zalcitabine. Also tell your health care professional if you are allergic to any other substances, such as foods, preservatives, or dyes.

Pregnancy—Zalcitabine has not been studied in pregnant women. However, studies in animals have shown that zalcitabine causes birth defects when given in very high doses. Before taking this medicine, make sure your doctor knows if you are pregnant or if you may become pregnant.

Breast-feeding—It is not known whether zalcitabine passes into the breast milk. However, if your baby does not already have the AIDS virus, there is a chance that you could pass it to your baby by breast-feeding. Talk to your doctor first if you are thinking about breast-feeding your baby.

Children—Zalcitabine can cause serious side effects in any patient. Therefore, it is especially important that you discuss with your child's doctor the good that this medicine may do as well as the risks of using it. Your child must be seen frequently and your child's progress carefully followed by the doctor while the child is taking zalcitabine.

Older adults—Zalcitabine has not been studied specifically in older people. Therefore, it is not known whether it causes different side effects or problems in the elderly than it does in younger adults.

Other medicines—Although certain medicines should not

be used together at all, in other cases two different medicines may be used together even if an interaction might occur. In these cases, your doctor may want to change the dose, or other precautions may be necessary. When you are taking zalcitabine, it is especially important that your health care professional know if you are taking any of the following:

- Alcohol or
- Asparaginase (e.g., Elspar) or
- Azathioprine (e.g., Imuran) or
- Estrogens (female hormones) or
- Furosemide (e.g., Lasix) or
- Methyldopa (e.g., Aldomet) or
- Pentamidine by injection (e.g., Pentam, Pentacarinat) or
- Sulfonamides (e.g., Bactrim, Septra) or
- Sulindac (e.g., Clinoril) or
- Tetracyclines or
- Thiazide diuretics (water pills) (e.g., Diuril, Hydrodiuril) or
- Valproic acid (e.g., Depakote)—Use of these medicines with zalcitabine may increase the chance of pancreatitis (inflammation of the pancreas)
- Aminoglycosides by injection (amikacin [e.g., Amikin], gentamicin [e.g., Garamycin], kanamycin [e.g., Kantrex], neomycin [e.g., Mycifradin], netilmicin [e.g., Netromycin], streptomycin, tobramycin [e.g., Nebcin]) or
- Amphotericin B (e.g., Fungizone) or
- Foscarnet (e.g., Foscavir)—Use of these medicines with zalcitabine may increase the chance of side effects
- Chloramphenicol (e.g., Chloromycetin) or
- Cisplatin (e.g., Platinol) or
- Dapsone (e.g., Avlosulfon) or
- Didanosine (e.g. Videx) or
- Ethambutol (e.g., Myambutol) or
- Ethionamide (e.g., Trecator-SC) or
- Hydralazine (e.g., Apresoline) or
- Isoniazid (e.g., Nydrazid) or
- Lithium (e.g., Eskalith, Lithobid) or
- Metronidazole (e.g., Flagyl) or
- Nitrous oxide or
- Phenytoin (e.g., Dilantin) or

- Stavudine (e.g., d4T) or
- Vincristine (e.g., Oncovin)—Use of these medicines with zalcitabine may increase the chance of peripheral neuropathy (tingling, burning, numbness, or pain in your hands or feet)
- Nitrofurantoin (e.g., Furadantin, Macrodantin)—Use of nitrofurantoin with zalcitabine may increase the chance of side effects, including peripheral neuropathy (tingling, burning, numbness, or pain in your hands or feet) and pancreatitis (inflammation of the pancreas)

Other medical problems—The presence of other medical problems may affect the use of zalcitabine. Make sure you tell your doctor if you have any other medical problems, especially:

- Alcohol abuse or
- Increased blood triglycerides (or a history of) or
- Pancreatitis (or a history of)—Patients with these medical problems may be at increased risk of pancreatitis (inflammation of the pancreas)
- Alcohol abuse, history of, or
- Liver disease—Zalcitabine may make liver disease worse in patients with liver disease or a history of alcohol abuse
- Kidney disease—Patients with kidney disease may have an increased chance of side effects
- Peripheral neuropathy—Zalcitabine may make this condition worse

---

Proper Use of This Medicine

Take this medicine exactly as directed by your doctor. Do not take more of it, do not take it more often, and do not take it for a longer time than your doctor ordered. Also, do not stop taking this medicine without checking with your doctor first.

Keep taking zalcitabine for the full time of treatment, even if you begin to feel better.

This medicine works best when there is a constant amount in the blood. *To help keep the amount constant, do not miss any doses.* If you need help in planning the best times to take your medicine, check with your health care professional.

Only take medicine that your doctor has prescribed specifically for you. Do not share your medicine with others.

Dosing—The dose of zalcitabine will be different for different patients. *Follow your doctor's orders or the directions on the label.* The following information includes only the average doses of zalcitabine. Your dose may be different if you have kidney disease. *If your dose is different, do not change it* unless your doctor tells you to do so:

- For *oral* dosage form (tablets):
- —For treatment of HIV infection:
  - Adults and children 13 years of age and older—0.75 milligrams (mg), together with 200 mg of zidovudine, every eight hours.
  - Children up to 12 years of age—Use and dose are based on body weight and must be determined by your doctor.

Missed dose—If you miss a dose of this medicine, take it as soon as possible. However, if it is almost time for your next dose, skip the missed dose and go back to your regular dosing schedule. Do not double doses.

Storage—To store this medicine:
- Keep out of the reach of children.
- Store away from heat and direct light.
- Do not store in the bathroom, near the kitchen sink, or in other damp places. Heat or moisture may cause the medicine to break down.
- Do not keep outdated medicine or medicine no longer needed. Be sure that any discarded medicine is out of the reach of children.

Precautions While Using This Medicine

It is very important that your doctor check your progress at regular visits.

Do not take any other medicines without checking with your doctor first. To do so may increase the chance of side effects from zalcitabine.

HIV may be acquired from or spread to other people through infected body fluids, including blood, vaginal fluid, or semen. *If you are infected, it is best to avoid any sexual activity involving an exchange of body fluids with other people. If you do have sex, always wear (or have your partner wear) a condom ("rubber").* Only use condoms made of latex, and *use them every time you have vaginal, anal, or oral sex.* The use of a spermicide (such as nonoxynol-9) may also help prevent transmission of HIV if it is not irritating to the vagina, rectum, or mouth. Spermicides have been shown to kill HIV in lab tests. Do not use oil-based jelly, cold cream, baby oil, or shortening as a lubricant—these products can cause the condom to break. Lubricants without oil, such as *K-Y Jelly*, are recommended. Women may wish to carry their own condoms. Birth control pills and diaphragms will help protect against pregnancy, but they will not prevent someone from giving or getting the AIDS virus. *If you inject drugs*, get help to stop. *Do not share needles or equipment with anyone.* In some cities, more than half of the drug users are infected, and sharing even one needle or syringe can spread the virus. If you have any questions about this, check with your health care professional.

Side Effects of This Medicine

Along with its needed effects, a medicine may cause some unwanted effects. Although not all of these side effects

may occur, if they do occur they may need medical attention.

Check with your doctor immediately if any of the following side effects occur:

> *More common*
>> Tingling, burning, numbness, or pain in the hands, arms, feet, or legs

> *Less common*
>> Fever; joint pain; muscle pain; skin rash; ulcers in the mouth and throat

> *Rare*
>> Fever and sore throat; nausea and vomiting; stomach pain (severe)

Other side effects may occur that usually do not need medical attention. These side effects may go away during treatment as your body adjusts to the medicine. However, check with your doctor if any of the following side effects continue or are bothersome:

> *Less common*
>> Diarrhea; headache

Other side effects not listed above may also occur in some patients. If you notice any other effects, check with your doctor.

ZIDOVUDINE Systemic

Some commonly used brand names are:

In the U.S.—
  Retrovir

In Canada—

Apo-Zidovudine	Retrovir
Novo-AZT	

Another commonly used name is AZT.

Description

Zidovudine (zye-DOE-vue-deen) (also known as AZT) is used in the treatment of the infection caused by the human immunodeficiency virus (HIV). HIV is the virus responsible for acquired immune deficiency syndrome (AIDS). Zidovudine is also used to slow the progression of disease in patients infected with HIV who have early symptoms or no symptoms at all.

Zidovudine will not cure or prevent HIV infection or AIDS; however, it helps keep HIV from reproducing and appears to slow down the destruction of the immune system. This may help delay the development of problems usually related to AIDS or HIV disease. Zidovudine will not keep you from spreading HIV to other people. People who receive this medicine may continue to have the problems usually related to AIDS or HIV disease.

Zidovudine may cause some serious side effects, including bone marrow problems. Symptoms of bone marrow problems include fever, chills, or sore throat; pale skin; and unusual tiredness or weakness. These problems may require blood transfusions or temporarily stopping treatment with zidovudine. *Check with your doctor if any new health problems or symptoms occur while you are taking zidovudine.*

Zidovudine is available only with your doctor's prescription, in the following dosage forms:

Oral
- Capsules (U.S. and Canada)
- Syrup (U.S. and Canada)

Parenteral
- Injection (U.S. and Canada)

Before Using This Medicine

In deciding to use a medicine, the risks of taking the medicine must be weighed against the good it will do. This is a decision you and your doctor will make. For zidovudine, the following should be considered:

Allergies—Tell your doctor if you have ever had any unusual or allergic reaction to zidovudine. Also tell your health care professional if you are allergic to any other substances, such as foods, preservatives, or dyes.

Pregnancy—Zidovudine crosses the placenta. Studies in pregnant women have not been completed. However, zidovudine has been shown to decrease the chance of passing HIV to your baby during pregnancy and at birth. Zidovudine has not been shown to cause birth defects in studies in rats and rabbits given this medicine by mouth in doses many times larger than the human dose.

Breast-feeding—It is not known whether zidovudine passes into the breast milk. However, if your baby does not have the AIDS virus, there is a chance that you could pass it to your baby by breast-feeding. Talk to your doctor first if you are thinking about breast-feeding your baby.

Children—Zidovudine can cause serious side effects in any patient. Therefore, it is especially important that you discuss with your child's doctor the good that this medicine may do as well as the risks of using it. Your child must be carefully followed, and frequently seen, by the doctor while he or she is taking zidovudine.

Older adults—Zidovudine has not been studied specifically in older people. Therefore, it is not known whether it causes different side effects or problems in the elderly than it does in younger adults.

Other medicines—Although certain medicines should not

be used together at all, in other cases two different medicines may be used together even if an interaction might occur. In these cases, your doctor may want to change the dose, or other precautions may be necessary. When you are taking zidovudine, it is especially important that your health care professional know if you are taking any of the following:

- Amphotericin B by injection (e.g., Fungizone) or
- Antineoplastics (cancer medicine) or
- Antithyroid agents (medicine for overactive thyroid) or
- Azathioprine (e.g., Imuran) or
- Chloramphenicol (e.g., Chloromycetin) or
- Colchicine or
- Cyclophosphamide (e.g., Cytoxan) or
- Flucytosine (e.g., Ancobon) or
- Ganciclovir (e.g., Cytovene) or
- Interferon (e.g., Intron A, Roferon-A) or
- Mercaptopurine (e.g., Purinethol) or
- Methotrexate (e.g., Mexate) or
- Plicamycin (e.g., Mithracin)—Caution should be used if these medicines and zidovudine are used together; taking zidovudine while you are using or receiving these medicines may make anemia and other blood problems worse
- Clarithromycin (e.g., Biaxin)—Clarithromycin may decrease the amount of zidovudine in the blood
- Probenecid (e.g., Benemid)—Probenecid may increase the amount of zidovudine in the blood, increasing the chance of side effects

Other medical problems—The presence of other medical problems may affect the use of zidovudine. Make sure you tell your doctor if you have any other medical problems, especially:

- Anemia or other blood problems—Zidovudine may make these conditions worse
- Liver disease—Patients with liver disease may have an increase in side effects from zidovudine
- Low amounts of folic acid or vitamin B_{12} in the blood—Zidovudine may worsen anemia caused by a decrease of folic acid or vitamin B_{12}

Proper Use of This Medicine

Patient information sheets about zidovudine are available. Read this information carefully.

Take this medicine exactly as directed by your doctor. Do not take more of it, do not take it more often, and do not take it for a longer time than your doctor ordered. Also, do not stop taking this medicine without checking with your doctor first.

Keep taking zidovudine for the full time of treatment, even if you begin to feel better.

For patients using *zidovudine syrup:*

- Use a specially marked measuring spoon or other device to measure each dose accurately. The average household teaspoon may not hold the right amount of liquid.

This medicine works best when there is a constant amount in the blood. *To help keep the amount constant, do not miss any doses.* If you need help in planning the best times to take your medicine, check with your health care professional.

Dosing—The dose of zidovudine will be different for different patients. *Follow your doctor's orders or the directions on the label.* The following information includes only the average doses of zidovudine. *If your dose is different, do not change it* unless your doctor tells you to do so.

- For the treatment of HIV infection:
  —For *oral* dosage forms (capsules and syrup):
    - Adults and teenagers—100 milligrams (mg) every four hours for a total of 500 or 600 mg a day.
    - Children 3 months to 12 years of age—Dose is

based on body size and must be determined by your doctor.

—For *injection* dosage form:

• Adults and teenagers—Dose is based on body weight and must be determined by your doctor. The usual dose is 1 to 2 mg per kilogram (0.45 to 0.9 mg per pound) of body weight, injected slowly into a vein every four hours around the clock. The injection dosage form is given until you can take zidovudine by mouth.

• Children 3 months to 12 years of age—Dose is based on body size and must be determined by your doctor.

Missed dose—If you do miss a dose of this medicine, take it as soon as possible. However, if it is almost time for your next dose, skip the missed dose and go back to your regular dosing schedule. Do not double doses.

Storage—To store this medicine:

• Keep out of the reach of children.

• Store away from heat and direct light.

• Do not store in the bathroom, near the kitchen sink, or in other damp places. Heat or moisture may cause the medicine to break down.

• Do not keep outdated medicine or medicine no longer needed. Be sure that any discarded medicine is out of the reach of children.

Precautions While Using This Medicine

It is very important that your doctor check your progress at regular visits. This medicine may cause blood problems.

Do not take any other medicines without checking with your doctor first. To do so may increase the chance of side effects from zidovudine.

Zidovudine may cause blood problems. These problems may result in a greater chance of certain infections and slow healing. Therefore, you should be careful when using regular toothbrushes, dental floss, and toothpicks not to damage your gums. Check with your medical doctor or dentist if you have any questions about proper oral hygiene (mouth care) during treatment.

HIV may be acquired from or spread to other people through infected body fluids, including blood, vaginal fluid, or semen. *If you are infected, it is best to avoid any sexual activity involving an exchange of body fluids with other people. If you do have sex, always wear (or have your partner wear) a condom ("rubber").* Only use condoms made of latex, and *use them every time you have vaginal, anal, or oral sex.* The use of a spermicide (such as nonoxynol-9) may also help prevent the spread of HIV if it is not irritating to the vagina, rectum, or mouth. Spermicides have been shown to kill HIV in lab tests. Do not use oil-based jelly, cold cream, baby oil, or shortening as a lubricant—these products can cause the condom to break. Lubricants without oil, such as *K-Y Jelly*, are recommended. Women may wish to carry their own condoms. Birth control pills and diaphragms will help protect against pregnancy, but they will not prevent someone from giving or getting the AIDS virus. *If you inject drugs*, get help to stop. *Do not share needles with anyone.* In some cities, more than half of the drug users are infected, and sharing even one needle can spread the virus. If you have any questions about this, check with your health care professional.

Side Effects of This Medicine

Along with its needed effects, a medicine may cause some unwanted effects. Although not all of these side effects may occur, if they do occur they may need medical attention.

Check with your doctor immediately if any of the following side effects occur:

More common

Fever, chills, or sore throat; pale skin; unusual tiredness or weakness

Note: The above side effects may also occur up to weeks or months after you stop taking this medicine.

Rare

Abdominal discomfort; confusion; convulsions (seizures); general feeling of discomfort; loss of appetite; mood or mental changes; muscle tenderness and weakness; nausea

Other side effects may occur that usually do not need medical attention. These side effects may go away during treatment as your body adjusts to the medicine. However, check with your doctor if any of the following side effects continue or are bothersome:

More common

Headache (severe); muscle soreness; nausea; trouble in sleeping

Less common

Bluish-brown colored bands on nails

Other side effects not listed above may also occur in some patients. If you notice any other effects, check with your doctor.

Additional Information

Once a medicine has been approved for marketing for a certain use, experience may show that it is also useful for other medical problems. Although this use is not included in product labeling, zidovudine is used in certain patients with the following medical condition:

- Human immunodeficiency virus (HIV) infection due to occupational exposure (possible prevention of)

Other than the above information, there is no additional information relating to proper use, precautions, or side effects for this use.

ZOLPIDEM   Systemic†

A commonly used brand name in the U.S. is Ambien.

†Not commercially available in Canada.

Description

Zolpidem (ZOLE-pi-dem) belongs to the group of medicines called central nervous system (CNS) depressants (medicines that slow down the nervous system). Zolpidem is used to treat insomnia (trouble in sleeping). In general, when sleep medicines are used every night for a long time, they may lose their effectiveness. In most cases, sleep medicines should be used only for short periods of time, such as 1 or 2 days, and generally for no longer than 1 or 2 weeks.

This medicine is available only with your doctor's prescription, in the following dosage form:

Oral
   • Tablets (U.S.)

Before Using This Medicine

Sleep medicines may cause a special type of memory loss or "amnesia." When this occurs, a person does not remember what has happened during the several hours between use of the medicine and the time when its effects wear off. This is usually not a problem since most people fall asleep after taking the medicine. In most instances, memory problems can be avoided by taking zolpidem only when you are able to get a full night's sleep (7 to 8 hours) before you need to be active again. Be sure to talk to your doctor if you think you are having memory problems.

In deciding to use a medicine, the risks of taking the medicine must be weighed against the good it will do. This is a decision you and your doctor will make. For zolpidem, the following should be considered:

Allergies—Tell your doctor if you have ever had any unusual or allergic reaction to zolpidem. Also tell your health care professional if you are allergic to any other substances, such as foods, preservatives, or dyes.

Pregnancy—Zolpidem has not been studied in pregnant women. However, studies in pregnant animals have shown that zolpidem slows down the development of the offspring when given to the mother in doses many times the human dose. Before taking this medicine, make sure your doctor knows if you are pregnant or if you may become pregnant.

Breast-feeding—Although zolpidem passes into breast milk, it has not been reported to cause problems in nursing babies.

Children—Studies on this medicine have been done only in adult patients, and there is no specific information comparing use of zolpidem in children with use in other age groups.

Older adults—Confusion and falling are more likely to occur in the elderly, who are usually more sensitive than younger adults to the effects of zolpidem.

Other medicines—Although certain medicines should not be used together at all, in other cases two different medicines may be used together even if an interaction might occur. In these cases, your doctor may want to change the dose, or other precautions may be necessary. When you are taking zolpidem, it is especially important that your health care professional know if you are taking any of the following:

- Other central nervous system (CNS) depressants (medicines that cause drowsiness) or
- Tricyclic antidepressants (amitriptyline [e.g., Elavil], amoxapine [e.g., Asendin], clomipramine [e.g., Anafranil], desipramine [e.g., Pertofrane], doxepin [e.g., Sinequan], imipramine [e.g., Tofranil], nortriptyline [e.g., Aventyl], protriptyline [e.g., Vivactil], trimipramine [e.g., Surmontil])—The CNS depressant effects of either these medicines or zolpidem may be increased, possibly leading to unwanted effects

Other medical problems—The presence of other medical problems may affect the use of zolpidem. Make sure you tell your doctor if you have any other medical problems, especially:

- Alcohol abuse (or history of) or
- Drug abuse or dependence (or history of)—Dependence on zolpidem may develop
- Emphysema, asthma, bronchitis, or other chronic lung disease or
- Mental depression or
- Sleep apnea (temporary stopping of breathing during sleep)—Zolpidem may make these conditions worse
- Kidney disease or
- Liver disease—Higher blood levels of zolpidem may result, increasing the chance of side effects

---

Proper Use of This Medicine

Take this medicine only as directed by your doctor. Do not take more of it, do not take it more often, and do not take it for a longer time than your doctor ordered. If too much is taken, it may become habit-forming (causing mental or physical dependence).

Take zolpidem just before going to bed, when you are ready to go to sleep. This medicine works very quickly to put you to sleep.

Do not take this medicine when your schedule does not permit you to get a full night's sleep (7 to 8 hours). If you must wake up before this, you may continue to feel drowsy and may experience memory problems, because the effects of the medicine have not had time to wear off.

Zolpidem may be taken with or without food or on a full or empty stomach. It may work faster if you take it on an empty stomach. However, if your doctor tells you to take the medicine a certain way, take it exactly as directed.

Dosing—The dose of zolpidem will be different for different patients. *Follow your doctor's orders or the directions on the label.* The following information includes only the average doses of zolpidem. *If your dose is different, do not change it* unless your doctor tells you to do so.

The number of tablets that you take depends on the strength of the medicine.

- For *oral* dosage form (tablets):
  —For the treatment of insomnia (trouble in sleeping):
  - Adults—10 milligrams (mg) at bedtime.
  - Older adults—5 mg at bedtime.
  - Children up to 18 years of age—Use and dose must be determined by the doctor.

Missed dose—If you miss a dose of this medicine, skip the missed dose and go back to your regular dosing schedule. Do not double doses.

Storage—To store this medicine:
- Keep out of the reach of children.
- Store away from heat and direct light.
- Do not store in the bathroom, near the kitchen sink, or in other damp places. Heat or moisture may cause the medicine to break down.

- Do not keep outdated medicine or medicine no longer needed. Be sure that any discarded medicine is out of the reach of children.

Precautions While Using This Medicine

If you think you need to take zolpidem for more than 7 to 10 days, be sure to discuss it with your doctor. Insomnia that lasts longer than this may be a sign of another medical problem.

This medicine will add to the effects of alcohol and other CNS depressants (medicines that slow down the nervous system, possibly causing drowsiness). Some examples of CNS depressants are antihistamines or medicine for hay fever, other allergies, or colds; sedatives, tranquilizers, or sleeping medicine; prescription pain medicine or narcotics; barbiturates; medicine for seizures; muscle relaxants; or anesthetics, including some dental anesthetics. *Check with your doctor before taking any of the above while you are using this medicine.*

This medicine may cause some people, especially older persons, to become drowsy, dizzy, lightheaded, clumsy or unsteady, or less alert than they are normally. Even though zolpidem is taken at bedtime, it may cause some people to feel drowsy or less alert on arising. Also, this medicine may cause double vision or other vision problems. *Make sure you know how you react to zolpidem before you drive, use machines, or do anything else that could be dangerous if you are dizzy, or are not alert or able to see well.*

If you develop any unusual and strange thoughts or behavior while you are taking zolpidem, be sure to discuss it with your doctor. Some changes that have occurred in people taking this medicine are like those seen in people who drink alcohol and then act in a manner that is not normal. Other changes may be more unusual and extreme, such as confusion, hallucinations (seeing, hearing, or feeling things that are not there), and unusual excitement, nervousness, or irritability.

If you will be taking zolpidem for a long time, do not stop taking it without first checking with your doctor. Your doctor may want you to reduce gradually the amount you are taking before stopping completely. Stopping this medicine suddenly may cause withdrawal side effects.

After taking zolpidem for insomnia, you may have difficulty sleeping (rebound insomnia) for the first few nights after you stop taking it.

If you think you or someone else may have taken an overdose of this medicine, get emergency help at once. Taking an overdose of zolpidem or taking alcohol or other CNS depressants with zolpidem may lead to breathing problems and unconsciousness. Some signs of an overdose are severe drowsiness, severe nausea or vomiting, staggering, and troubled breathing.

Side Effects of This Medicine

Along with its needed effects, a medicine may cause some unwanted effects. Although not all of these side effects may occur, if they do occur they may need medical attention.

Check with your doctor as soon as possible if any of the following side effects occur:

Less common

> Clumsiness or unsteadiness; confusion—more common in older adults; mental depression

Rare

> Dizziness, lightheadedness, or fainting; falling—more common in older adults; fast heartbeat; hallucinations (seeing, hearing, or feeling things that are not there);

skin rash; swelling of face; trouble in sleeping; unusual excitement, nervousness, or irritability; wheezing or difficulty in breathing

Symptoms of overdose

Clumsiness or unsteadiness (severe); dizziness (severe); double vision or other vision problems; drowsiness (severe); nausea (severe); troubled breathing; slow heartbeat; vomiting (severe)

Other side effects may occur that usually do not need medical attention. These side effects may go away during treatment as your body adjusts to the medicine. However, check with your doctor if any of the following side effects continue or are bothersome:

Less common

Abdominal or stomach pain; daytime drowsiness; diarrhea; double vision or other vision problems; drugged feelings; dryness of mouth; general feeling of discomfort or illness; headache; memory problems; nausea; nightmares or unusual dreams; vomiting

After you stop using this medicine, your body may need time to adjust. The length of time this takes depends on the amount of medicine you were using and how long you used it. During this time check with your doctor if you notice any of the following side effects:

Abdominal or stomach cramps or discomfort; agitation, nervousness, or feelings of panic; convulsions (seizures); flushing; lightheadedness; muscle cramps; nausea; sweating; tremors; uncontrolled crying; unusual tiredness or weakness; vomiting; worsening of mental or emotional problems

Other side effects not listed above may also occur in some patients. If you notice any other effects, check with your doctor.

Glossary

Abdomen—The body area between the chest and pelvis.

Abortifacient—Medicine that causes abortion.

Abrade—Scrape or rub away the outer cover or layer of a part.

Absorption—Passing into the body; incorporation of substances into or across tissues of the body, for example, digested food into the blood from the small intestine, or poisons through the skin.

Achlorhydria—Absence of acid that normally would be found in the stomach.

Acidifier, urinary—Medicine that makes the urine more acidic.

Acidosis—Too much acidity or loss of alkalinity in the body fluids and tissues.

Acromegaly—Enlargement of the face, hands, and feet because of too much growth hormone.

Acute—Sharp or intense; describes a condition that begins suddenly, has severe symptoms, and usually lasts a short time.

Addison's disease—Disease caused by not enough secretion of corticosteroid hormones by the adrenal glands; causes weakness, salt loss, and low blood pressure.

Adhesion—The union by connective tissue of two parts that are normally separate (such as parts of a joint).

Adjunct—An additional or secondary treatment that is helpful but is not necessary for treatment of a particular condition; not effective for that condition if used alone.

Adjuvant—1. A substance added to or used with another substance to assist its action. 2. Something that assists or enhances the effectiveness of medical treatment.

Adrenal cortex—Outer layer of tissue of the adrenal gland, which produces corticosteroid hormones.

Adrenal glands—Two organs located next to the kidneys. They produce the hormones epinephrine and norepinephrine and corticosteroid hormones, such as cortisol.

Adrenaline—See epinephrine.

Adrenal medulla—Inner part of the adrenal gland, which produces epinephrine and norepinephrine.

Adrenocorticoids—See corticosteroids.

Aerosol—Suspension of very small liquid or solid particles in compressed gas; drugs in aerosol form are dispensed in the form of a mist by releasing the gas.

African sleeping sickness—See Trypanosomiasis, African.

Agent—A force or substance capable of causing a change.

Agoraphobia—Fear of public places or open spaces.

Agranulocytosis—Disorder in which there is a severe decrease in the number of granulocytes normally present in the blood.

AIDS (acquired immunodeficiency syndrome)—Disease caused by human immunodeficiency virus (HIV). The disease results in a breakdown of the body's immune system, which makes a person more likely to get some other infections and some forms of cancer.

Alcohol-abuse deterrent—Medicine used to help alcoholics avoid the use of alcohol.

Alkaline—Having a pH of more than 7. Opposite of acidic.

Alkalizer, urinary—Medicine that makes the urine more alkaline.

Alkalosis—Too much alkalinity or loss of acidity in the body fluids and tissues.

Alopecia—Loss or absence of hair from areas where it normally is present; baldness.

Altitude sickness agent—Medicine used to prevent or lessen some of the effects of high altitude on the body.

Alzheimer's disease—Progressive disorder of thinking and other mental processes, usually beginning in late middle age.

Aminoglycosides—A class of chemically related antibiotics used to treat some serious types of bacterial infections.

Anabolic steroids—Synthetic forms of male hormones.

Analgesic—Medicine that relieves pain without causing unconsciousness.

Anaphylaxis—Sudden, severe allergic reaction.

Androgen—Substance, such as testosterone, that stimulates development of male characteristics.

Anemia—Reduction, to below normal, of hemoglobin in the blood.

Anesthesiologist—A physician who is qualified to give an anesthetic and other medicines to a patient before and during surgery.

Anesthetic—Medicine that causes a loss of feeling or sensation, especially of pain, sometimes through loss of consciousness.

Aneurysm—Abnormal dilatation or saclike swelling of an artery, vein, or the heart.

Angina—Pain, tightness, or feeling of heaviness in the chest, due mostly to lack of oxygen for the heart muscle. The pain may be felt in the left shoulder, jaw, or arm instead of or in addition to the chest. Symptoms often occur during exercise.

Angioedema—Allergic condition marked by continuing swelling and severe itching of areas of the skin.

Anorexia—Loss of appetite for food.

Anoxia—Absence of oxygen. The term is sometimes incorrectly used for hypoxia, which means an abnormally low amount of oxygen in the body.

Antacid—Medicine used to neutralize excess acid in the stomach.

Antagonist—Drug or other substance that blocks or works against the action of another.

Anthelmintic—Medicine used to destroy or expel intestinal worms.

Antiacne agent—Medicine used to treat acne.

Antianemic—Agent that prevents or corrects anemia.

Antianginal—Medicine used to prevent or treat angina attacks.

Antianxiety agent—Medicine used to treat excessive nervousness, tension, or anxiety.

Antiarrhythmic—Medicine used to treat irregular heartbeats.

Antiasthmatic—Medicine used to treat asthma.

Antibacterial—Medicine that kills or stops the growth of bacteria.

Antibiotic—Chemical substance used to treat infections.

Antibody—Special kind of blood protein that helps the body fight infection.

Antibulimic—Medicine used to treat bulimia.

Anticholelithic—Medicine used to dissolve gallstones.

Anticoagulant—Medicine used to prevent formation of blood clots in the blood vessels.

Anticonvulsant—Medicine used to prevent or treat convulsions (seizures).

Antidepressant—Medicine used to treat mental depression.

Antidiabetic agent—Medicine used to control blood sugar levels in patients with diabetes mellitus (sugar diabetes).

Antidiarrheal—Medicine used to treat diarrhea.

Antidiuretic—Medicine used to decrease formation of urine (for example, in patients with diabetes insipidus).

Antidote—Medicine used to prevent or treat harmful effects of another medicine or a poison.

Antidyskinetic—Medicine used to help treat the loss of muscle control caused by certain diseases or by some other medicines.

Antidysmenorrheal—Medicine used to treat menstrual cramps.

Antiemetic—Medicine used to prevent or treat nausea and vomiting.

Antiendometriotic—Medicine used to treat endometriosis.

Antienuretic—Medicine used to help prevent bedwetting.

Antifibrotic—Medicine used to treat fibrosis.

Antiflatulent—Medicine used to help relieve excess gas in the stomach or intestines.

Antifungal—Medicine used to treat infections caused by a fungus.

Antiglaucoma agent—Medicine used to treat glaucoma.

Antigout agent—Medicine used to prevent or relieve gout attacks.

Antihemorrhagic—Medicine used to prevent or help stop serious bleeding.

Antihistamine—Medicine used to prevent or relieve the symptoms of allergies (such as hay fever).

Antihypercalcemic—Medicine used to help lower the amount of calcium in the blood.

Antihyperlipidemic—Medicine used to help lower high levels of lipids in the blood.

Antihyperphosphatemic—Medicine used to help lower the amount of phosphate in the blood.

Antihypertensive—Medicine used to treat high blood pressure.

Antihyperuricemic—Medicine used to prevent or treat gout or other medical problems caused by too much uric acid in the blood.

Antihypocalcemic—Medicine used to increase calcium blood levels in patients with too little calcium.

Antihypoglycemic—Medicine used to increase blood sugar levels in patients with low blood sugar.

Antihypokalemic—Medicine used to increase potassium blood levels in patients with too little potassium.

Anti-infective—Medicine used to treat infection.

Anti-inflammatory—Medicine used to relieve pain, swelling, and other symptoms of inflammation.

Anti-inflammatory, nonsteroidal—An anti-inflammatory medicine that is not a cortisone-like medicine.

Anti-inflammatory, steroidal—A cortisone-like anti-inflammatory medicine.

Antimetabolite—Medicine that interferes with the normal processes within cells, preventing their growth.

Antimuscarinic—Medicine used to block the effects of a certain chemical in the body; often used to reduce smooth muscle spasms, especially abdominal or stomach cramps or spasms.

Antimyasthenic—Medicine used to treat myasthenia gravis.

Antimyotonic—Medicine used to prevent or relieve nighttime leg cramps or muscle spasms.

Antineoplastic—Medicine used to treat cancer.

Antineuralgic—Medicine used to treat neuralgia.

Antiprotozoal—Medicine used to treat infections caused by protozoa.

Antipsoriatic—Medicine used to treat psoriasis.

Antipsychotic—Medicine used to treat certain nervous, mental, and emotional conditions.

Antipyretic—Medicine used to reduce fever.

Antirheumatic—Medicine used to treat arthritis (rheumatism).

Antirosacea—Medicine used to treat rosacea.

Antiseborrheic—Medicine used to treat dandruff and seborrhea.

Antiseptic—Medicine that stops the growth of germs. Used on the surface of the skin to prevent infections in cuts, scrapes, and wounds.

Antispasmodic—Medicine used to reduce smooth muscle spasms (for example, stomach, intestinal, or urinary tract spasms).

Antispastic—Medicine used to treat muscle spasms.

Antithyroid agent—Medicine used to treat an overactive thyroid gland.

Antitremor agent—Medicine used to treat tremors (trembling or shaking).

Antitubercular—Medicine used to treat tuberculosis (TB).

Antitussive—Medicine used to relieve cough.

Antiulcer agent—Medicine used to treat stomach and duodenal ulcers.

Antivertigo agent—Medicine used to prevent dizziness.

Antiviral—Medicine used to treat infections caused by a virus.

Anus—The opening at the end of the digestive tract through which bowel contents are passed.

Anxiety—An emotional state with apprehension, worry, or tension in reaction to real or imagined danger or dread of a situation; accompanied by sweating, increased pulse, trembling, weakness, and fatigue.

Apnea—Temporary absence of breathing.

Apoplexy—See Stroke.

Appendicitis—Inflammation of the appendix.

Appetite stimulant—Medicine used to help increase the desire for food.

Appetite suppressant—Medicine used in weight control programs to help decrease the desire for food.

Arrhythmia—Abnormal heart rhythm.

Arteritis, temporal—Inflammatory disease of arteries, usually of the head; occurs in older people.

Arthralgia—Pain in a joint.

Arthritis, rheumatoid—Chronic disease, especially of the joints, marked by pain and swelling.

Ascites—Accumulation of fluid in the abdominal cavity.

Asthma—Disease marked by inflammation of the bronchial tubes (air passages). During an attack, air passages become constricted, causing wheezing and difficult breathing. Attacks may be brought on by allergens, virus infection, cold air, or exercise.

Atherosclerosis—Common disease of the arteries in which artery walls thicken and harden.

Avoid—To keep away from deliberately.

Bacteremia—Presence of bacteria in the blood.

Bacterium—Tiny, one-celled organism. Different types of bacteria are responsible for a number of diseases and infections.

Bancroft's filariasis—Disease transmitted by mosquitos in which an infection with the filarial worm occurs. Affects the lymph system, producing inflammation.

Beriberi—Disorder caused by too little vitamin B_1 (thiamine), marked by an accumulation of fluid in the body, extreme weight loss, inflammation of nerves, or paralysis.

Bile—Thick fluid produced by the liver and stored in the gallbladder. Bile helps in the digestion of fats.

Bile duct—Tubular passage which carries bile from the liver to the gallbladder, or from the gallbladder to the intestine.

Bilharziasis—See Schistosomiasis.

Biliary—Relating to bile, the bile duct, or the gallbladder.

Bilirubin—The bile pigment that is orange-colored or yellow; an excess in the blood may cause jaundice.

Bipolar disorder—Severe mental illness marked by repeated episodes of depression and mania. Also called *manic-depressive illness.*

Bisexual—One who is sexually attracted to both sexes.

Black fever—See Leishmaniasis, visceral.

Blackwater fever—Condition, marked by dark urine, rarely seen as a complication of malaria.

Bone marrow—Soft material filling the cavities of bones.

Bone marrow depression—Condition in which the production of red blood cells, leukocytes, or platelets by the red bone marrow is decreased.

Bone resorption inhibitor—Medicine used to prevent or treat certain types of bone disorders, such as Paget's disease of the bone; helps prevent bone loss.

Bowel disease, inflammatory, suppressant—Medicine used to treat certain intestinal disorders, such as colitis.

Bradycardia—Slow heart rate, usually less than 60 beats per minute.

Bronchitis—Inflammation of the bronchial tubes (air passages) of the lungs.

Bronchodilator—Medicine used to open up the bronchial tubes (air passages) of the lungs to increase the flow of air through them.

Buccal—Relating to the cheek. A buccal medicine is taken by placing it in the pocket between the cheek and the gum and letting it slowly dissolve.

Bulimia—Disturbance in eating behavior marked by bouts of excessive eating followed by self-induced vomiting and diarrhea, hard exercise, or fasting.

Bursa—Small fluid-filled sac present where body parts move over one another (such as in a joint) to help reduce friction.

Bursitis—Inflammation of a bursa.

Candidiasis of the mouth—Overgrowth of the yeast *Candida* in the mouth marked by white patches on the tongue or inside the mouth. Also called *thrush* or *white mouth*.

Candidiasis of the vagina—Yeast infection of the vagina caused by the yeast *Candida;* associated with itching, burning, and a cheesy or curd-like white discharge.

Cardiac—Relating to the heart.

Cardiac arrhythmia—Irregularity or loss of the normal rhythm of the heartbeat.

Cardiac load–reducing agent—Medicine used to ease the workload of the heart by allowing the blood to flow through the blood vessels more easily.

Cardiotonic—Medicine used to improve the strength and efficiency of the heart.

Caries, dental—Tooth decay, sometimes causing pain, leading to the crumbling of the tooth. Also called *cavities*.

Cataract—An opacity (cloudiness) in the eye lens that impairs vision or causes blindness.

Catheter—Tube inserted into a small opening in the body so that fluids can be put in or taken out.

Caustic—Burning or corrosive agent; irritating and destructive to living tissue.

Cavity—1. Hollow space within the body. 2. Hole in a tooth, caused by dental caries.

Central nervous system—Part of the nervous system that is composed of the brain and spinal cord.

Cerebral palsy—Permanent disorder of motor weakness and loss of coordination due to damage to the brain.

Cervix—Lower end or necklike opening of the uterus to the vagina.

Chemotherapy—Treatment of illness or disease by chemical agents. The term most commonly refers to the use of drugs to treat cancer.

Chickenpox—See Varicella.

Chlamydia—A family of microorganisms that cause a variety of diseases in humans. One form is transmitted by sexual contact.

Cholesterol—Fatlike substance made by the liver but also absorbed from the diet; found only in animal tissues. Too much blood cholesterol is associated with several potential health risks, especially atherosclerosis (hardening of the arteries).

Chromosome—The structure in the cell nucleus that contains the DNA; in humans, there are normally 46.

Chronic—Describes a condition of long duration, which is often of gradual onset and may involve very slow changes. Note that the term ''chronic'' has nothing to do with how serious the condition is.

Cirrhosis—Chronic liver disease marked by destruction of its cells and abnormal tissue growth.

Clitoris—Small, erectile body, being a part of the female external sex organs.

CNS—See Central nervous system.

Cold sores—See Herpes simplex.

Colic—Waves of sudden severe abdominal pain, which are usually separated by relatively pain-free intervals.

Colitis—Inflammation of the colon (bowel).

Colony stimulating factor—Protein that stimulates the production of one or more kinds of cells made in the bone marrow.

Colostomy—Operation in which part of the colon (bowel) is brought through the abdominal wall to create an artificial opening. The contents of the intestine are discharged through the opening, bypassing the rest of the intestines.

Coma—State of unconsciousness from which the patient cannot be aroused.

Coma, hepatic—Disturbances in mental function and the nervous system caused by severe liver disease.

Condom—Thin sheath or cover worn over the penis during sexual intercourse to prevent pregnancy or infection; made of latex (rubber) or animal intestine.

Congestive heart failure—Condition resulting from inability of the heart to pump strongly enough to maintain adequate blood flow; characterized by breathlessness and edema.

Conjunctiva—Delicate mucous membrane covering the front of the eye and the inside of the eyelid.

Conjunctivitis—Inflammation of the conjunctiva.

Constriction—Squeezing together and becoming narrower or smaller, such as constriction of blood vessels or eye pupils.

Contagious disease—Disease that can be transmitted from one person to another.

Contamination—The introduction of germs or unclean material into or on normally sterile substances or objects.

Contraceptive—Medicine or device used to prevent pregnancy.

Contraction—A shortening or tightening, as in the normal function of muscles.

Convulsion—Sudden involuntary contraction or series of jerkings of muscles.

Corticosteroids—Group of cortisone-like hormones that are secreted by the adrenal cortex and are critical to the body. The two major groups of corticosteroids are glucocorticoids, which affect fat and body metabolism, and mineralocorticoids, which regulate salt/water balance. Also called *adrenocorticoids*.

Cortisol—Natural hormone produced by the adrenal cortex, important for carbohydrate, protein, and fat metabolism and for the normal response to stress; synthetic cortisol (hydrocortisone) is used to treat inflammations, allergies, collagen diseases, rheumatic disorders, and adrenal failure.

Cot death—See Sudden infant death syndrome (SIDS).

Cowpox—See Vaccinia.

Creutzfeldt-Jakob disease—Rare disease, probably caused by a slow-acting virus that affects the brain and nervous system.

Crib death—See Sudden infant death syndrome (SIDS).

Crohn's disease—Chronic, inflammatory disease of the digestive tract, usually the lower small intestine.

Croup—Inflammation and blockage of the larynx (voice box) in young children.

Crystalluria—Crystals in the urine.

Cushing's syndrome—Condition in which the adrenal gland produces too much cortisone-like hormone, leading to weight gain, round face, and high blood pressure.

Cycloplegia—Paralysis of certain eye muscles; can be induced by medication for certain eye examinations.

Cycloplegic—Medicine used to induce cycloplegia.

Cyst—Abnormal sac or closed cavity filled with liquid or semisolid matter.

Cystic—Marked by cysts.

Cystic fibrosis—Hereditary disease of children and young adults which predominantly affects the lungs. Exocrine glands do not function normally, and excess mucus is produced.

Cystine—An amino acid found in most proteins; it is produced by the digestion of the protein.

Cystitis, interstitial—Inflammation of the bladder, predominantly in women, with frequent urge to urinate and painful urination.

Cytomegalovirus—One of a group of viruses. One form may be sexually transmitted and can be fatal in patients with weakened immune systems.

Cytoplasm—The contents of a cell outside the nucleus.

Cytotoxic agent—Chemical that kills cells or stops cell division; used to treat cancer.

Decongestant, nasal—Medicine used to help relieve nasal congestion (stuffy nose).

Decongestant, ophthalmic—Medicine used in the eye to relieve redness, burning, itching, or other irritation.

Decubitus—The position taken in lying down.

Decubitus ulcer—Bedsore; damage to the skin and underlying tissues caused by constant pressure.

Dental—Related to the teeth and gums.

Depression, mental—Condition marked by deep sadness; associated with lack of any pleasurable interest in life. Other symptoms include disturbances in sleep, appetite, and concentration, and difficulty in performing day-to-day tasks.

Dermatitis herpetiformis—Skin disease marked by sores and itching.

Dermatitis, seborrheic—Type of eczema found on the scalp and face.

Dermatomyositis—Inflammatory disorder of the skin and underlying tissues, including breakdown of muscle fibers.

Diabetes insipidus—Disorder in which the patient produces large amounts of dilute urine and is constantly thirsty. Also called *water diabetes*.

Diabetes mellitus—Disorder in which the body cannot process sugars to release energy; either the body does not produce enough insulin or the body tissues are unable to use the insulin present. This leads to too much sugar in the blood (hyperglycemia). Also called *sugar diabetes*.

Diagnose—Find out the cause or nature of a disorder by examination and laboratory tests.

Diagnostic procedure—A process carried out to determine the cause or nature of a condition, disease, or disorder.

Dialysis, renal—Artificial technique for removing waste materials or poisons from the blood when the kidneys are not working properly.

Digestant—Agent that will help in digestion.

Diplopia—Awareness of two images of a single object at one time; double vision.

Diuretic—Medicine used to increase the amount of urine produced by helping the kidneys get rid of water and salt. Also called *water pill.*

Diverticulitis—Inflammation of a diverticulum in the intestinal tract.

Diverticulum—Sac or pouch opening from a canal or cavity.

DNA—Deoxyribonucleic acid; the genetic material that controls heredity. DNA is located in the cell nucleus.

Down syndrome—Mental retardation associated with the presence of an extra chromosome 21. Patients with Down syndrome are marked physically by a round head, flat nose, slightly slanted eyes, and short stature. Also called *mongolism.*

Duct—Tube or channel, especially one that serves to carry secretions from a gland.

Dumdum fever—See Leishmaniasis, visceral.

Duodenal ulcer—Open sore in that part of the small intestine closest to the stomach.

Duodenum—First of the three parts of the small intestine.

Dyskinesia—Refers to abnormal, involuntary movement or a defect in voluntary movement.

Dyspnea—Shortness of breath; difficult breathing.

Eczema—Inflammation of the skin, marked by itching and rash.

Edema—Swelling of body tissue due to accumulation of fluids, usually first noticed in the feet or lower legs.

Eighth-cranial-nerve disease—Disease of the eighth cranial nerve, serving the inner ear; results in dizziness, loss of balance, loss of hearing, nausea, or vomiting.

Electrolyte—In medical use, chemicals (ions) in body fluids that are needed for normal functioning of the body. Body electrolytes include bicarbonate, chloride, sodium, potassium, etc.

Embolism—Sudden blocking of a blood vessel by a blood clot or foreign substances carried to the place of obstruction by the blood.

Embryo—In humans, a developing fertilized egg within the uterus (womb) from about two to eight weeks after fertilization.

Emergency—Extremely serious unexpected or sudden happening or situation that calls for immediate action.

Emollient—Substance that soothes and softens an irritated surface, such as the skin.

Emphysema—Lung condition in which destructive changes occur in the air spaces; air is not exchanged normally during the process of breathing in and out.

Encephalitis—Inflammation of the brain.

Encephalopathy—Any degenerative disease of the brain; caused by many different medical conditions.

Endocarditis—Inflammation of the lining of the heart, leading to fever, heart murmurs, and heart failure.

Endocrine gland—A gland that has no duct; releases its secretion directly into the blood.

Endometriosis—Condition in which material similar to the lining of the uterus (womb) appears at other sites within the pelvic cavity, causing pain and bleeding.

Enteric coating—Coating on tablets which allows them to pass through the stomach unchanged before being broken up in the intestine and being absorbed. Used to protect the stomach from the medicine and/or the medicine from the stomach's acid.

Enteritis—Inflammation of the small intestine, usually causing diarrhea.

Enuresis—Urinating while asleep (bedwetting).

Enzyme—Type of protein produced by cells that may bring about or speed up a normal chemical reaction in the body.

Eosinophil—One type of white blood cells readily stained by the dye eosin; important in allergic reactions and parasitic infections.

Eosinophilia—Condition in which the number of eosinophils in the blood is abnormally high.

Epidural space—Area in the spinal column into which medicines (usually for pain) can be administered.

Epilepsy—Any of a group of brain disorders featuring sudden attacks of seizures and other symptoms.

Epinephrine—Hormone secreted by the adrenal medulla. It stimulates the heart, constricts blood vessels, and relaxes some smooth muscles. Also called *adrenaline*.

EPO—See erythropoietin.

Ergot alkaloids—A class of medicines that cause narrowing of blood vessels; used to treat migraine headaches, and to reduce bleeding in childbirth.

Erythropoietin—Hormone secreted by the kidney. It controls the production of red blood cells by the bone marrow; also available as a synthetic drug (EPO).

Esophagus—The part of the digestive tract connecting the pharynx to the stomach.

Estrogen—Principal female sex hormone necessary for the normal sexual development of the female; during the menstrual cycle, its actions help prepare for possible pregnancy. Estrogen is often used to treat discomforts of menopause.

Exocrine gland—Any gland that discharges its secretion through a duct that opens on a surface (not into the blood).

Exophthalmos—Thrusting forward of the eyeballs in their sockets, giving the appearance of the eyes sticking out too far; commonly associated with hyperthyroidism.

Expectorant—Medicine used to help remove mucus or phlegm in the lungs by coughing or spitting it up.

Extrapyramidal symptoms—Movement disorders occurring with certain diseases or with use of certain drugs, including trembling and shaking of hands and fingers, twisting movements of the body, shuffling walk, and stiffness of arms or legs.

Familial Mediterranean fever—Inherited condition involving inflammation of the lining of the chest, abdomen, and joints. Also called *recurrent polyserositis.*

Fasciculation—Small, spontaneous contraction of a few muscle fibers, which is visible through the skin; muscular twitching.

Favism—Inherited condition resulting from sensitivity to broad (fava) beans; marked by fever, vomiting, diarrhea, and acute destruction of red blood cells.

Fertility—Capacity to bring about the start of pregnancy.

Fertilization—Union of an ovum with a sperm.

Fetus—In humans, a developing baby within the uterus (womb) from about the beginning of the third month of pregnancy.

Fibrocystic—Having benign (noncancerous) tumors of connective tissue.

Fibroid tumor—A noncancerous tumor of the uterus formed of fibrous or fully developed connective tissue.

Fibrosis—Condition in which the skin and underlying tissues tighten and become less flexible.

Fistula—Abnormal tubelike passage connecting two internal organs or one that leads from an abscess or internal organ to the body surface.

Flatulence—Excessive amount of air or gas in the stomach or intestine.

Flu—See Influenza.

Flushing—Temporary redness of the face and/or neck.

Fungus—Any of a group of simple organisms, including molds and yeasts.

Fungus infection—Infection caused by a fungus. Some common fungus infections are tinea pedis (athlete's foot), tinea capitis (ringworm of the scalp), tinea cruris (ringworm of the groin or jock itch), and mouth or vaginal candidiasis (yeast infections).

Gait—Manner of walk.

Gamma globulin—The portion of the blood that contains most of the antibodies associated with the body's immunity to infection.

Gastric—Relating to the stomach.

Gastric acid secretion inhibitor—Medicine used to decrease the amount of acid produced by the stomach.

Gastroenteritis—Inflammation of the stomach and intestine.

Gastroesophageal reflux—Backward flow into the esophagus of the contents of the stomach and duodenum. The condition is often characterized by ''heartburn.''

Generic—General in nature; relating to an entire group or class. In relation to medicines, the general name of a drug substance; not owned by one specific group as would be true for a trademark or brand name.

Genital—1. Relating to the organs concerned with reproduction; the sexual organs. 2. Relating to reproduction.

Genital warts—Small growths found on the genitals or around the anus; caused by a virus. The disease may be transmitted by sexual contact.

Gilles de la Tourette syndrome—See Tourette's disorder.

Gingiva—Gums.

Gingival hyperplasia—Overgrowth of the gums.

Gingivitis—Inflammation of the gums.

Glandular fever—See Mononucleosis.

Glaucoma—Condition of abnormally high pressure in the eye; may lead to loss of vision if not treated.

Glomeruli—Clusters of capillaries in the nephrons of the kidney that act as filters of the blood.

Glomerulonephritis—Inflammation of the glomeruli of the kidney not directly caused by infection.

Glucose-6-phosphate dehydrogenase (G6PD) deficiency—Lack of or reduced amounts of an enzyme (glucose-6-phosphate dehydrogenase) that helps the breakdown of certain sugar compounds in the body.

Gluten—Type of protein found primarily in wheat and rye.

Goiter—Enlargement of the thyroid gland that causes the neck to swell. Condition usually results from a lack of iodine or overactivity of the thyroid gland.

Gonadotropin—Any hormone that stimulates the activities of the ovaries or testes.

Gonorrhea—An infectious disease, usually transmitted by sexual contact. It causes infection in the genital organs in both men and women, and may also result in systemic disease.

Gout—Disease in which too much uric acid builds up in the blood and joints, leading to inflammation of the joints.

Granulation—Small, fleshy outgrowths on the healing surface of a wound or ulcer; a normal stage in healing.

Granulocyte—A class of white blood cell.

Granulocytopenia—Abnormal reduction of the number of granulocytes in the blood; agranulocytosis.

Granuloma—A growth or mass of granulation tissue produced in response to chronic infection, inflammation, a foreign body, or unknown causes.

Graves' disease—Disorder that causes thyrotoxicosis, goiter, and exophthalmos. Also called *exophthalmic goiter*.

Groin—The area between the abdomen and thigh.

Guillain-Barré syndrome—Nerve disease marked by sudden numbness and weakness in the limbs that may progress to complete paralysis.

Gynecomastia—Excessive development of the breasts in the male.

Hair follicle—Sheath of tissue surrounding a hair root.

Hansen's disease—See Leprosy.

Hartnup disease—Hereditary disease in which the body has trouble processing certain chemicals, leading to mental retardation, rough skin, and problems with muscle coordination.

Heart attack—See Myocardial infarction.

Hematuria—Presence of blood or red blood cells in the urine.

Hemoglobin—Iron-containing substance found in red blood cells that transports oxygen from the lungs to the tissues of the body.

Hemolytic anemia—Type of anemia resulting from breakdown of red blood cells.

Hemophilia—Hereditary disease in males in which blood clotting is delayed, leading to excessive and uncontrolled bleeding even after minor injuries.

Hemorrhoids—Enlarged veins in the walls of the anus. Also called *piles*.

Hepatic—Relating to the liver.

Hepatitis—Inflammation of the liver.

Hernia, hiatal—Condition in which the stomach passes partly into the chest through the opening for the esophagus in the diaphragm.

Herpes simplex—The virus that causes "cold sores." These are an inflammation of the skin resulting in small, painful blisters. Infection may occur either in or around the mouth or, in the case of genital herpes, on the genitals (sex organs).

Herpes zoster—An infectious disease usually marked by pain and blisters along one nerve, often on the face, chest, stomach, or back. The infection is caused by the virus that also causes chickenpox. Also called *shingles*.

Heterosexual—One who is sexually attracted to persons of the opposite sex.

High blood pressure—See Hypertension.

Hirsutism—Adult male pattern of hair growth in women.

HIV (human immunodeficiency virus)—Virus that causes AIDS.

Hodgkin's disease—Malignant condition marked by swelling of the lymph nodes, with weight loss and fever.

Homosexual—One who is sexually attracted to persons of the same sex.

Hormone—Substance produced in one part of the body (such as a gland), which then passes into the bloodstream and travels to other organs or tissues, where it carries out its effect.

Hot flashes—Sensations of heat of the face, neck, and upper body, often accompanied by sweating and flushing; commonly associated with menopause.

Hydrocortisone—See Cortisol.

Hyperactivity—Abnormally increased activity.

Hypercalcemia—Too much calcium in the blood.

Hypercalciuria—Too much calcium in the urine.

Hypercholesterolemia—Excessive amount of cholesterol in the blood.

Hyperglycemia—Abnormally high blood sugar.

Hyperkalemia—Abnormally high amount of potassium in the blood.

Hyperkeratosis—Overgrowth or thickening of the outer horny layer of the skin.

Hyperlipidemia—General term for an abnormally high level of any or all of the lipids in the blood.

Hyperphosphatemia—Too much phosphate in the blood.

Hypersensitivity—Condition in which the body has an abnormally increased reaction to a foreign substance.

Hypertension—Blood pressure in the arteries (blood vessels) that is higher than normal for the patient's age group. Hypertension may lead to a number of serious health problems. Also called *high blood pressure.*

Hyperthermia—Abnormally high body temperature.

Hyperthyroidism—Excessive secretion of thyroid hormones by the thyroid gland, causing thyrotoxicosis.

Hypocalcemia—Too little calcium in the blood.

Hypoglycemia—Abnormally low blood sugar.

Hypokalemia—Abnormally low amount of potassium in the blood.

Hypotension, orthostatic—Excessive fall in blood pressure that occurs when standing or upon standing up.

Hypothalamus—Area of the brain that controls many body functions, including body temperature, certain metabolic and endocrine processes, and some activities of the nervous system.

Hypothermia—Abnormally low body temperature.

Hypothyroidism—Condition caused by thyroid hormone deficiency, which results in a decrease in metabolism.

Hypoxia—Broad term meaning intake of oxygen or its use by the body is inadequate.

Ileostomy—Operation in which the ileum is brought through the abdominal wall to create an artificial opening. The contents of the intestine are discharged through the opening, bypassing the colon (bowel).

Ileum—Last of the three portions of the small intestine.

Immune deficiency condition—Lack of immune response to protect against infectious disease.

Immune system—Complex network of the body that defends against foreign substances or organisms that may harm the body.

Immunizing agent, active—Agent that causes the body to produce its own antibodies for protection against certain infections.

Immunocompromised—Decreased natural immunity caused by irradiation, certain medicine or diseases, or other conditions.

Immunosuppressant—Medicine that reduces the body's natural immunity.

Impair—To cause to decrease, weaken, or damage, usually because of injury or disease.

Impetigo—Contagious bacterial skin infection common in babies and children in which skin redness develops into blisters that break and form a thick crust.

Implant—1. Special form of medicine, often a small pellet or rod, that is inserted into the body or beneath the skin so that the medicine will be released continuously over a period of time. 2. To insert or graft material or an object into a body site. 3. Material or an object inserted into a body site, such as a lens implant or a breast implant. 4. Action of a fertilized ovum becoming attached or embedded in the uterus.

Impotence—Difficulty or inability of a male to have or maintain an erection of the penis.

Incontinence—Inability to control natural passage of urine or of bowel movements.

Induce—To cause or bring about.

Infertility—Medical condition which results in the difficulty or inability of a woman to become pregnant or of a man to cause pregnancy.

Inflammation—Pain, redness, swelling, and heat in a part of the body, usually in response to injury or illness.

Influenza—Highly contagious respiratory virus infection, marked by coughing, headache, chills, fever, muscle pain, and general weakness. Also called *flu*.

Ingredient—One of the parts or substances that make up a mixture or compound.

Inhalation—1. Act of drawing in the breath or drawing air into the lungs. 2. Medicine that is used when breathed (inhaled) into the lungs. Some inhalations work locally in the lungs, while others produce their effects elsewhere in the body.

Inhibitor—Substance that prevents a process or reaction.

Inner ear—Inner portion of the ear; a liquid filled system of cavities and ducts that make up the organs of hearing and balance.

Insomnia—Inability to sleep or remain asleep.

Insulin—Hormone that increases the efficiency with which the body uses sugar. Injections of insulin are used in the treatment and control of diabetes mellitus (sugar diabetes).

Intra-amniotic—Within the sac that contains the fetus and amniotic fluid.

Intra-arterial—Within an artery.

Intracavernosal—Into the corpus cavernosa (cavities in the penis that, when filled with blood, produce an erection).

Intracavitary—Into a body cavity (for example, the chest cavity or bladder).

Intramuscular—Into a muscle.

Intrauterine device (IUD)—Small plastic or metal device placed in the uterus (womb) to prevent pregnancy.

Intravenous—Into a vein.

Ion—Atom or group of atoms carrying an electric charge.

Irrigation—Washing of a body cavity or wound with a stream of sterile water or a solution of a medicine.

Ischemia—Condition caused by inadequate blood flow to a part of the body; usually caused by constriction or blocking of blood vessels that supply the part of the body affected.

Jaundice—Yellowing of the eyes and skin due to excess bilirubin in the blood.

Jock itch—Ringworm of the groin.

Kala-azar—See Leishmaniasis, visceral.

Kaposi's sarcoma—Malignant tumor of blood vessels; often appears in the skin. One form occurs in immunocompromised patients, for example, transplant recipients and AIDS patients.

Keratolytic—Medicine used to soften hardened areas of the skin, such as warts.

Ketoacidosis—Type of acidosis associated with diabetes.

Lactation—Secretion of breast milk.

Larva—The immature form of life of some insects and other animal groups that hatch from eggs.

Larynx—Organ that serves as a passage for air from the pharynx to the lungs; it contains the vocal cords.

Laxative—Medicine used to encourage bowel movements.

Laxative, bulk-forming—Laxative that acts by absorbing liquid and swelling to form a soft, bulky stool. The bowel is then stimulated normally by the presence of the bulky mass.

Laxative, hyperosmotic—Laxative that acts by drawing water into the bowel from surrounding body tissues. This provides a soft stool mass and increased bowel action.

Laxative, lubricant—Laxative that acts by coating the bowel and the stool mass with a waterproof film. This keeps moisture in the stool. The stool remains soft and its passage is made easier.

Laxative, stimulant—Laxative that acts directly on the intestinal wall. The direct stimulation increases the muscle contractions that move the stool mass along. Also called *contact laxative*.

Laxative, stool softener—Laxative that acts by helping liquids mix into the stool and prevent dry, hard stool masses. The stool remains soft and its passage is made easier. Also called *emollient laxative*.

Legionnaires' disease—Lung infection caused by a certain bacterium.

Leishmaniasis, visceral—Tropical disease, transmitted by sandfly bites, which causes liver and spleen enlargement, anemia, weight loss, and fever. Also called *black fever*, *Dumdum fever*, or *kala-azar*.

Lennox-Gastaut syndrome—Type of childhood epilepsy.

Leprosy—Chronic infectious disease characterized by lesions, especially in the skin and nerves, leading to loss of feeling, paralysis in the hands and feet and deformity. Also called *Hansen's disease*.

Leukemia—Disease of the blood and bone marrow in which too many white blood cells are produced, resulting in anemia, bleeding, and low resistance to infections.

Leukocyte—White blood cell.

Leukoderma—See Vitiligo.

Leukopenia—Abnormal reduction in the total number of leukocytes in the blood.

Lipid—Term applied generally to dietary fat or fatlike substances not soluble in water.

Local effect—Affecting only the area to which something is being applied.

Lugol's solution—Transparent, deep brown liquid containing iodine and potassium iodide.

Lupus—See Lupus erythematosus, systemic.

Lupus erythematosus, systemic—Chronic inflammatory disease most often affecting the skin, joints, and various internal organs. Also called *lupus* or *SLE* (systemic lupus erythematosus).

Lymph—Fluid that bathes the tissues. It is formed in tissue spaces in all parts of the body and circulated by the lymphatic system.

Lymphatic system—Network of vessels that conveys lymph from the spaces between the cells of the body back to the bloodstream.

Lymph node—A small rounded body found at intervals along the lymphatic system. The nodes act as filters for the lymph by keeping bacteria and other foreign particles from entering the bloodstream. They also produce lymphocytes.

Lymphocyte—Any of a number of white blood cells found in the blood, lymph, and lymphatic tissues. They are involved in immunity.

Lymphoma—Malignant tumor of lymph nodes or tissue.

Lyse—To cause breakdown. In cells, damage or rupture of the membrane results in destruction of the cell.

Macrobiotic—Vegetarian diet consisting mostly of whole grains.

Malaria—Tropical blood infection caused by a protozoa; symptoms include chills, fever, sweats, headaches, and anemia. Malaria is spread to humans by the bite of an infected mosquito.

Malignant—Describing a condition that becomes continually worse if untreated; also used to mean cancerous.

Malnutrition—Condition caused by unbalanced or insufficient diet.

Mammogram—X-ray picture of the breast.

Mania—Mental state in which fast talking and excited feelings or actions are out of control.

Mast cells—Cells in the connective tissue that store histamine; they release substances that bring about inflammation and produce signs of allergic reactions.

Mastocytosis—Accumulation of too many mast cells in tissues.

Mediate—To bring about or accomplish indirectly.

Megavitamin therapy—Taking very large doses of vitamins to prevent or treat certain medical problems.

Melanoma—Highly malignant cancer tumor, usually occurring on the skin.

Menière's disease—Disease affecting the inner ear that is characterized by ringing in the ears, hearing loss, and dizziness.

Meningitis—Inflammation of the tissues that surround the brain and spinal cord.

Menopause—The time in a woman's life when the ovaries no longer produce an egg cell at regular times and menstruation stops.

Methemoglobin—Substance formed when hemoglobin has been oxidized; in this form, hemoglobin cannot act as an oxygen carrier.

Methemoglobinemia—Presence of methemoglobin in the blood.

Middle ear—Chamber of the ear lying behind the eardrum and containing the structures that conduct sound.

Migraine—Throbbing headache, usually affecting one side of the head; often accompanied by nausea, vomiting, and sensitivity to light.

Miotic—Medicine used in the eye that causes the pupil to constrict (become smaller).

Mongolism—See Down syndrome.

Mono—See Mononucleosis.

Monoclonal—Derived from a single cell; related to production of drugs by genetic engineering, such as monoclonal antibodies.

Mononucleosis—Infectious viral disease occurring mostly in adolescents and young adults, marked by fever, sore throat, swelling of the lymph nodes in the neck and armpits, and severe fatigue. Also called *mono* or *glandular fever*.

Motility—Ability to move without outside aid, force, or cause.

Motor—Relating to structures that bring about movement, such as nerves and muscles.

Mucolytic—Medicine that breaks down or dissolves mucus.

Mucosal—Relating to the mucous membrane.

Mucous membrane—Moist layer of tissue surrounding or lining many body structures and cavities, including the mouth, lips, inside of nose, anus, and vagina.

Mucus—Thick fluid produced by the mucous membranes and glands.

Multiple sclerosis (MS)—Chronic, inflammatory nerve disease marked by weakness, unsteadiness, shakiness, and speech and vision problems.

Myasthenia gravis—Chronic disease marked by abnormal weakness, and sometimes paralysis, of certain muscles.

Mydriatic—Medicine used in the eye that causes the pupil to dilate (become larger).

Myelogram—X-ray picture of the spinal cord.

Myeloma, multiple—Cancerous bone marrow disease.

Myocardial infarction—Interruption of blood supply to the heart, leading to sudden, severe chest pain, and damage to the heart muscle. Also called *heart attack*.

Myocardial reinfarction prophylactic—Medicine used to help prevent additional heart attacks in patients who have already had one attack.

Myotonia congenita—Hereditary muscle disorder marked by difficulty in relaxing a muscle or releasing a grip after any strong effort.

Narcolepsy—Extreme tendency to fall asleep suddenly.

Nasal—Relating to the nose.

Nasogastric (NG) tube—Tube that is inserted through the nose, down the throat, and into the stomach. It may be used to remove fluid or gas from the stomach or to administer medicine, food, fluid, or nutrients to the patient.

Nebulizer—Instrument that administers liquid in the form of a fine spray.

Necrosis—Death of tissue, cells, or a part of a structure or organ, surrounded by healthy parts.

Neoplasm—New and abnormal growth of tissue in or on a part of the body, in which the multiplication of cells is uncontrolled and progressive. Also called *tumor*.

Nephron—Unit of the kidney that acts as a filter of the blood in forming urine.

Neuralgia—Severe stabbing or throbbing pain along the course of one or more nerves.

Neuralgia, trigeminal—Severe burning or stabbing pain along certain nerves in the face. Also called *tic douloureux*.

Neuritis, optic—Disease of the nerves in the eye.

Neuritis, peripheral—Inflammation of terminal nerves or the nerve endings, usually associated with pain, muscle wasting, and loss of reflexes.

Neutropenia—Abnormally small number of neutrophils in the blood.

Neutrophil—The most common type of granulocyte; important in the body's protection against infection.

Nodule—Small, rounded mass, lump, or swelling.

Nonsuppurative—Not discharging pus.

NSAID (nonsteroidal anti-inflammatory drug)—See Anti-inflammatory, nonsteroidal.

Nucleus—The part of the cell that contains the chromosomes.

Nystagmus—Rapid, rhythmic, involuntary movements of the eyeball; may be from side to side, up and down, or around.

Obesity—Excess accumulation of fat in the body along with an increase in body weight that exceeds the healthy range for the body's frame.

Obstetrics—Field of medicine concerned with the care of women during pregnancy and childbirth.

Obstruction—Something that blocks or closes up a passage or structure.

Occlusive dressing—Dressing (such as plastic kitchen wrap) that completely cuts off air to the skin.

Occult—Concealed, hidden, or of unknown cause; cannot be seen by the human eye; detectable only by microscope or chemical testing, as for occult blood in the stools or feces.

Ophthalmic—Relating to the eye.

Opioid—1. Any synthetic narcotic with opium-like actions; not derived from opium. 2. Natural chemicals that produce opium-like effects by acting at the same cell sites where opium exerts action.

Oral—Relating to the mouth.

Orchitis—Inflammation of the testis.

Osteitis deformans—See Paget's disease.

Osteomalacia—Softening of the bones due to lack of vitamin D.

Osteoporosis—Loss of calcium from bone tissue, resulting in bones that are brittle and easily fractured.

OTC (over the counter)—Refers to medicine or devices available without a prescription.

Otic—Relating to the ear.

Otitis media—Inflammation of the middle ear.

Ototoxicity—Having a harmful effect on the organs or nerves of the ear concerned with hearing and balance.

Ovary—Female sex organ that produces egg cells and sex hormones. The two ovaries are in the lower abdomen, one on each side.

Overactive thyroid—See hyperthyroidism.

Ovulation—Process by which an ovum is released from the ovary. In human menstruating females, this usually occurs once a month.

Ovum—Mature female sex or reproductive cell, or egg cell. It is capable of developing into a new organism if fertilized.

Paget's disease—Chronic bone disease, marked by thickening of the bones and severe pain. Also called *osteitis deformans*.

Pancreatitis—Inflammation of the pancreas.

Pancytopenia—Reduction in the number of red cells, all types of white cells, and platelets in the blood.

Paralysis agitans—See Parkinson's disease.

Parathyroid glands—Four small bodies situated beside the thyroid gland; secrete parathyroid hormone that regulates calcium and phosphorus metabolism.

Parenteral—Any method of administering medicine when the medicine cannot be given by mouth; most often refers to injecting a medicine into the body using a needle and syringe.

Parkinsonism—See Parkinson's disease.

Parkinson's disease—Brain disease marked by tremor (shaking), stiffness, and difficulty in moving. Also called *Parkinsonism, paralysis agitans,* or *shaking palsy.*

Patent ductus arteriosus (PDA)—Condition in babies in which an important blood vessel adjacent to the heart fails to close as it should, resulting in faulty circulation and serious health problems.

Pediculicide—Medicine that kills lice.

Pediculosis—Infestation of the body, pubis, or scalp with lice.

Pellagra—Disease caused by too little niacin, which results in scaly skin, diarrhea, and mental depression.

Pemphigus—Skin disease marked by successive outbreaks of blisters.

Peptic ulcer—Open sore in esophagus, stomach, or duodenum.

Peritoneum—Membrane sac lining the abdominal wall and covering the liver, stomach, spleen, gallbladder, and intestines.

Peritonitis—Inflammation of the peritoneum.

Peyronie's disease—Dense, fiber-like growth in the penis, which can be felt as an irregular hard lump, and which usually causes bending and pain when the penis is erect.

Pharynx—Space just behind the mouth that serves as a passageway for food from the mouth to the esophagus and for air from the nose and mouth to the larynx.

Phenol—Substance used as a preservative for some injectable medicines.

Pheochromocytoma—Tumor of the adrenal medulla.

Phlebitis—Inflammation of a vein.

Phlegm—Thick mucus produced in the respiratory passages.

Piles—See Hemorrhoids.

Pituitary gland—Pea-sized body located at the base of the skull. It produces a number of hormones that are essential to normal body growth and functioning.

Placebo—Medicine that, unknown to the patient, has no active medicinal substance; its use may relieve or improve a condition because the patient believes it will. Also called *sugar pill.*

Plaque, dental—Mixture of saliva, bacteria, and carbohydrates that forms on the teeth, leading to caries (cavities) and gum disease.

Platelet—Small, disk-shaped body found in the blood that plays an important role in blood clotting.

Platelet aggregation inhibitor—Medicine used to help prevent the platelets in the blood from clumping together. This effect reduces the chance of heart attack or stroke in certain patients.

Pleura—Membrane covering the lungs and lining the chest cavity.

Pneumococcal—Relating to certain bacteria that cause pneumonia.

Pneumocystis carinii—Organism that causes pneumocystis carinii pneumonia.

Pneumocystis carinii pneumonia—A pulmonary disease of infants and weakened persons, including those with

AIDS or those receiving drugs that weaken the immune system.

Polymorphous light eruption—A skin problem in certain people, which results from exposure to sunlight.

Polymyalgia rheumatica—A rheumatic disease, most common in elderly patients, which causes aching and stiffness in the shoulders and hips.

Polyp—Tumor or mass of tissue attached with a stalk or broad base; found in cavities such as the nose, uterus, or rectum.

Porphyria—A group of uncommon, usually inherited diseases of defective porphyrin metabolism.

Porphyrin—One of a number of pigments occurring in living organisms throughout nature; porphyrins are constituents of bile pigment, hemoglobin, and certain enzymes.

Prevent—To stop or to keep from happening.

Priapism—Prolonged abnormal, painful erection of the penis.

Proctitis—Inflammation of the rectum.

Progesterone—Natural steroid hormone responsible for preparing the uterus for pregnancy. If fertilization occurs, progesterone's actions carry on or maintain the pregnancy.

Progestin—A natural or synthetic hormone that has progesterone-like actions.

Prolactin—Hormone secreted by the pituitary gland that stimulates and maintains milk flow in women following childbirth.

Prolactinoma—A pituitary tumor; results in secretion of excess prolactin.

Prophylactic—1. Agent or medicine used to prevent the occurrence of a specific condition. 2. Condom.

Prostate—Gland surrounding the neck of the male urethra just below the base of the bladder. It secretes a fluid that constitutes a major portion of the semen.

Prosthesis—Any artificial substitute for a missing body part.

Protozoa—Tiny, one-celled animals; some cause diseases in humans.

Psoralen—Chemical found in plants and used in certain perfumes and medicines. Exposure to a psoralen and then to sunlight may increase the risk of severe burning.

Psoriasis—Chronic skin disease marked by itchy, scaly, red patches.

Psychosis—Severe mental illness marked by loss of contact with reality, often involving delusions, hallucinations, and disordered thinking.

Purpura—Condition marked by bleeding into the skin; skin rash or spots are first red, darken to purple, then fade to brownish-yellow.

PUVA—Treatment for psoriasis by use of a psoralen, such as methoxsalen or trioxsalen, and long-wave ultraviolet light.

Rachischisis—See Spina bifida.

Radiopaque agent—Substance that makes it easier to see an area of the body with x-rays. Radiopaque agents are used to help diagnose a variety of medical problems.

Radiopharmaceutical—Radioactive agent used to diagnose certain medical problems or treat certain diseases.

Raynaud's syndrome—Condition marked by paleness, numbness, and discomfort in the fingers when they are exposed to cold.

Rectal—Relating to the rectum.

Renal—Relating to the kidneys.

Reye's syndrome—Serious disease affecting the liver and brain that sometimes occurs after a virus infection, such as influenza or chickenpox. It occurs most often in young children and teenagers. The first sign of Reye's syndrome is usually severe, prolonged vomiting.

Rheumatic heart disease—Heart disease marked by scarring and chronic inflammation of the heart and its valves, occurring after rheumatic fever.

Rhinitis—Inflammation of the mucous membrane inside the nose.

Rickets—Bone disease usually caused by too little vitamin D, resulting in soft and malformed bones.

Ringworm—See Tinea.

Risk—The possibility of injury or of suffering harm.

River blindness—Tropical disease produced by infection with worms of the Onchocerca type. The condition usually causes severe itching and may cause blindness. Also called *Roble's disease, blinding filarial disease,* and *craw-craw.*

Rosacea—Skin disease of the face, usually in middle-aged and older persons. Also called *adult acne.*

Sarcoidosis—Chronic disorder in which the lymph nodes in many parts of the body are enlarged, and small fleshy swellings develop in the lungs, liver, and spleen.

Scabicide—Medicine used to treat scabies (itch mite) infection.

Scabies—Contagious dermatitis caused by a mite burrowing into the skin; characterized by tiny skin eruptions and severe itching.

Schistosomiasis—Tropical infection in which worms enter the skin from infested water and settle in the bladder or intestines, causing inflammation and scarring. Also called *bilharziasis.*

Schizophrenia—Severe mental disorder in which thinking, mood, and behavior are disturbed.

Scintigram—Image obtained by detecting radiation emitted from a radiopharmaceutical introduced into the body.

Scleroderma—Chronic disease first characterized by hardening, thickening, and shrinking of the skin; later, certain organs also are affected.

Scotoma—Area of decreased vision or total loss of vision in a part of the visual field; blind spot.

Scrotum—Sac that holds the testes (male sex glands).

Scurvy—Disease caused by a deficiency of vitamin C (ascorbic acid), marked by bleeding gums, bleeding beneath the skin, and body weakness.

Sebaceous gland—Skin gland that secretes sebum.

Seborrhea—Skin condition caused by the excess release of sebum from the sebaceous glands, accompanied by dandruff and oily skin.

Sebum—Fatty secretion produced by sebaceous (oil) glands of the skin.

Secretion—1. Process in which a gland in the body or on the surface of the body releases a substance for use. 2. The substance released by the gland.

Sedative-hypnotic—Medicine used to treat excessive nervousness, restlessness, or insomnia.

Sedation—A profoundly relaxed or calmed state.

Seizure—A sudden attack or convulsion, as in epilepsy or other disorders.

Semen—Fluid released from the penis at sexual climax. It is made up of sperm suspended in secretions from the reproductive tract.

Severe—Of a great degree, such as very serious pain or distress.

Shaking palsy—See Parkinson's disease.

Shingles—See Herpes zoster.

Shock—Severe disruption of cellular metabolism associated with reduced blood volume and blood pressure too low to supply adequate blood to the tissues.

Shunt—Surgical tube used to transfer blood or other fluid from one part of the body to another.

SIADH (secretion of inappropriate antidiuretic hormone) syndrome—Disease in which the body retains (keeps) more fluid than normal.

Sickle cell anemia—Hereditary disorder that predominantly affects blacks; caused by abnormal hemoglobin.

The name comes from the sickle-shaped red blood cells found in the blood of patients.

Sinusitis—Inflammation of a sinus.

Sjögren's syndrome—Condition usually occurring in older women, marked by dry eyes, dry mouth, and rheumatoid arthritis.

Skeletal muscle relaxant—Medicine used to relax certain muscles and help relieve the pain and discomfort caused by strains, sprains, or other injury to the muscles.

SLE—See Lupus erythematosus, systemic.

Soluble—Able to be dissolved in a fluid.

Spasticity—Increase in normal muscular tone, causing stiff, awkward movements.

Spastic paralysis—Paralysis marked by muscle rigidity or spasticity in the part of the body that is paralyzed.

Sperm—Mature male reproductive or sex cell.

Spermicide—Substance that kills sperm.

Spina bifida—Birth defect in which the infant's spinal cord is partially exposed through a hole in the backbone. Also called *rachischisis*.

Stenosis—Abnormal narrowing of a passage or duct of the body.

Sterility—1. Inability to produce offspring. 2. The state of being free of living microorganisms.

Stimulant, respiratory—Medicine used to stimulate breathing.

Stomatitis—Inflammation of the mucous membrane of the mouth.

Streptokinase—Enzyme that dissolves blood clots.

Stroke—Very serious event which occurs when an artery to the brain becomes clogged by a blood clot or bursts and causes hemorrhage. Stroke can affect speech, memory behavior, and other life patterns, and may result in paralysis. Also called *apoplexy*.

Stye—Infection of one or more sebaceous glands of the eyelid, marked by swelling.

Subcutaneous—Under the skin.

Sublingual—Under the tongue. A sublingual medicine is taken by placing it under the tongue and letting it slowly dissolve.

Sudden infant death syndrome (SIDS)—Death of an infant, usually while asleep, from an unknown cause. Also called *crib death* or *cot death.*

Sugar diabetes—See Diabetes mellitus.

Sugar pill—See Placebo.

Sulfite—Type of preservative; causes allergic reactions, such as asthma, in sensitive patients.

Sunscreen—Substance, usually a cream or lotion, that blocks ultraviolet light and helps prevent sunburn when applied to the skin.

Suppository—Mass of medicated material shaped for insertion into the rectum, vagina, or urethra. Suppository is solid at room temperature but melts at body temperature.

Suppressant—Medicine that stops an action or condition.

Suspension—A form of medicine in which the drug is mixed with a liquid but is not dissolved in it. When left standing, particles settle at the bottom of the liquid and the top portion turns clear. When shaken it is ready for use.

Syncope—Sudden loss of consciousness due to inadequate blood flow to the brain; fainting.

Syphilis—An infectious disease, usually transmitted by sexual contact. The three stages of the disease may be separated by months or years.

Syringe—Device used to inject liquids into the body, remove material from a part of the body, or wash out a body cavity.

Systemic—Term used for general effects throughout the body; applies to most medicines when taken by mouth or given by injection.

Tachycardia—Abnormal rapid beating of the heart, usually at a rate over 100 beats per minute in adults.

Temporomandibular joint (TMJ)—Hinge that connects the lower jaw to the skull.

Tendinitis—Inflammation of a tendon.

Teratogenic—Causing abnormal development in an embryo or fetus resulting in birth defects.

Testosterone—Principal male sex hormone.

Tetany—Condition marked by spasm and twitching of the muscles, particularly those of the hands, feet, and face; caused by a decrease in the calcium ion concentration in the blood.

Therapeutic—Relating to the treatment of a specific condition.

Thimerosal—Chemical used as a preservative in some medicines, and as an antiseptic and disinfectant.

Thrombolytic agent—Substance that dissolves blood clots.

Thrombophlebitis—Inflammation of a vein accompanied by the formation of a blood clot.

Thrombus—Blood clot that obstructs a blood vessel or a cavity of the heart.

Thrush—See Candidiasis of the mouth.

Thyroid gland—Gland in the lower front of the neck. It releases thyroid hormones, which control body metabolism.

Thyrotoxicosis—Condition resulting from excessive amounts of thyroid hormones in the blood, causing increased metabolism, fast heartbeat, tremors, nervousness, and increased sweating.

Tic—Repeated involuntary movement or spasm of a muscle.

Tic douloureux—See Neuralgia, trigeminal.

Tinea—Fungus infection of the surface of the skin, particularly the scalp, feet, and nails. Also called *ringworm*.

Tone—The slight, continuous tension present in resting muscles.

Topical—Term used for local effects when applied directly to the skin.

Tourette's disorder—Condition usually marked with motor tics (jerking movements) and vocal tics (grunts, sniffs). Also called *Gilles de la Tourette syndrome.*

Toxemia—Blood poisoning caused by bacterial production of toxins.

Toxemia of pregnancy—Condition occurring in pregnant women marked by hypertension, edema, excess protein in the urine, convulsions, and possibly coma.

Toxic—Poisonous; related to or caused by a toxin or poison.

Toxin—A substance produced by an animal or plant that is poisonous to another organism.

Toxoplasmosis—Disease caused by a blood protozoan, usually transmitted to humans from cats or by eating raw meat; generally the symptoms are mild and self-limited.

Tracheostomy—A surgical opening through the throat into the trachea (windpipe) to bypass an obstruction to breathing.

Tranquilizer—Medicine that produces a calming effect. It is used to relieve mental anxiety and tension.

Transdermal—A means of administering medicine into the body by use of skin patches or disks, or ointment; medicine contained in the patch or disk or the ointment is absorbed through the skin.

Trichomoniasis—Infection of the vagina resulting in inflammation of genital tissues and discharge. It can be passed on to males.

Triglyceride—A molecular form in which fats are present in food and the body; triglycerides are stored in the body as fat.

Trypanosome fever—See Trypanosomiasis, African.

Trypanosomiasis, African—Tropical disease, transmitted by tsetse fly bites, which causes fever, headache, and chills, followed by enlarged lymph nodes and anemia. Months or even years later, the disease affects the central nervous system, causing drowsiness and lethargy, coma, and death. Also called *African sleeping sickness.*

Tuberculosis (TB)—Infectious disease which may affect any organ but most commonly the lungs; symptoms include fever, night sweats, weight loss, and spitting up blood.

Tumor—Abnormal growth or enlargement in or on a part of the body.

Tyramine—Chemical present in many foods and beverages. Its structure and action in the body are similar to epinephrine.

Ulcer—Open sore or break in the skin or mucous membrane; often fails to heal and is accompanied by inflammation.

Ulcerative colitis—Chronic, recurrent inflammation and ulceration of the colon.

Ulceration—1. Formation or development of an ulcer. 2. Condition of an area marked with ulcers loosely associated with one another.

Underactive thyroid—See Hypothyroidism.

Ureter—Tube through which urine passes from the kidney to the bladder.

Urethra—Tube through which urine passes from the bladder to the outside of the body.

Urticaria—Hives; an eruption of itching wheals on the skin.

Vaccine—Medicine given by mouth or by injection to produce immunity to a certain infection.

Vaccinia—The skin and sometimes body reactions associated with smallpox vaccine. Also called *cowpox.*

Vaginal—Relating to the vagina.

Varicella—Very infectious virus disease marked by fever and itchy rash that develops into blisters and then scabs. Also called *chickenpox*.

Vascular—Relating to the blood vessels.

Vasodilator—Medicine that dilates the blood vessels, permitting increased blood flow.

Ventricular fibrillation—Life-threatening condition of fine, quivering, irregular movements of many individual muscle fibers of the ventricular muscle; replaces the normal heartbeat and interrupts pumping function.

Ventricle—A small cavity, such as one of the two lower chambers of the heart or one of the several cavities of the brain.

Vertigo—Sensation of whirling motion or dizziness, either of oneself or of one's surroundings.

Veterinary—Relating to animals and their diseases and treatment.

Virus—Any of a group of simple microbes too small to be seen by a light microscope. They can grow and reproduce only in living cells. Many cause diseases in humans, including the common cold.

Vitiligo—Condition in which some areas of skin lose pigment and turn white. Also called *leukoderma*.

von Willebrand's disease—Hereditary blood disease in which blood clotting is delayed, leading to excessive and uncontrolled bleeding even after minor injuries.

Water diabetes—See Diabetes insipidus.

Water pill—See Diuretic.

Wheal—Temporary, small, raised area of the skin, usually accompanied by itching or burning; welt.

Wheezing—A whistling sound made when there is difficulty in breathing.

White mouth—See Candidiasis of the mouth.

Wilson's disease—Inborn defect in the body's ability to process copper. Too much copper may lead to jaundice, cirrhosis, mental retardation, or symptoms like those of Parkinson's disease.

Zollinger-Ellison syndrome—Disorder in which the stomach produces too much acid, leading to ulcers.

USP Division of Information Development Advisory Panels*

Members who serve as Chairs are listed first.

The information presented in this text represents an ongoing review of the drugs contained herein and represents a consensus of various viewpoints expressed. The individuals listed below have served on the USP Advisory Panels and have contributed to the development of the USP DI database. Such listing does not imply that these individuals have reviewed all of the material in this text or that they individually agree with all statements contained herein.

Anesthesiology
Paul F. White, Ph.D., M.D., *Chair*, Dallas, TX; David R. Bevan, M.B., FFARCS, MRCP, Vancouver, British Columbia; Eugene Y. Cheng, M.D., Milwaukee, WI; Charles J. Cotá, M.D., Chicago, IL; Robert Feinstein, M.D., St. Louis, MO; Peter S.A. Glass, M.D., Durham, NC; Michael B. Howie, M.D., Columbus, OH; Beverly A. Krause, C.R.N.A., M.S., St. Louis, MO; Carl Lynch, III, M.D., Ph.D., Charlottesville, VA; Carl Rosow, M.D., Ph.D., Boston, MA; Peter S. Sebel, M.B., Ph.D., Atlanta, GA; Walter L. Way, M.D., Greenbrae, CA; Matthew B. Weinger, M.D., San Diego, CA; Richard Weiskopf, M.D., San Francisco, CA; David H. Wong, Pharm.D., M.D., Long Beach, CA

---

*as of July 31, 1995

Cardiovascular and Renal Drugs

Burton E. Sobel, M.D., *Chair*, St. Louis, MO; William P. Baker, M.D., Ph.D., Bethesda, MD; Nils U. Bang, M.D., Indianapolis, IN; Emmanuel L. Bravo, M.D., Cleveland, OH; Mary Jo Burgess, M.D., Salt Lake City, UT; James H. Chesebro, M.D., Boston, MA; Peter Corr, Ph.D., St. Louis, MO; Dwain L. Eckberg, M.D., Richmond, VA; Ruth Eshleman, Ph.D., W. Kingston, RI; William H. Frishman, M.D., Bronx, NY; Edward D. Frohlich, M.D., New Orleans, LA; Martha Hill, Ph.D., R.N., Baltimore, MD; Norman M. Kaplan, M.D., Dallas, TX; Michael Lesch, M.D., Detroit, MI; Manuel Martinez-Maldonado, M.D., Decatur, GA; Patrick A. McKee, M.D., Oklahoma City, OK; Dan M. Roden, M.D., Nashville, TN; Michael R. Rosen, M.D., New York, NY; Jane Schultz, R.N., B.S.N., Rochester, MN; Robert L. Talbert, Pharm.D., San Antonio, TX; Raymond L. Woosley, M.D., Ph.D., Washington, DC

Clinical Immunology/Allergy/Rheumatology

Albert L. Sheffer, M.D., *Chair*, Boston, MA; John A. Anderson, M.D., Detroit, MI; Emil Bardana, Jr., M.D., Portland, OR; John Baum, M.D., Rochester, NY; Debra Danoff, M.D., Montreal, Quebec; Daniel G. de Jesus, M.D., Ph.D., Vanier, Ontario; Elliott F. Ellis, M.D., Jacksonville, FL; Patricia A. Fraser, M.D., Boston, MA; Frederick E. Hargreave, M.D., Hamilton, Ontario; Evelyn V. Hess, M.D., Cincinnati, OH; Jean M. Jackson, M.D., Boston, MA; Stephen R. Kaplan, M.D., Buffalo, NY; Sandra M. Koehler, Milwaukee, WI; Richard A. Moscicki, M.D., Newton, MA; Shirley Murphy, M.D., Albuquerque, NM; Gary S. Rachelefsky, M.D., Los Angeles, CA; Robert E. Reisman, M.D., Buffalo, NY; Robert L. Rubin, Ph.D., La Jolla, CA; Daniel J. Stechschulte, M.D., Kansas City, KS; Virginia S. Taggert, Bethesda, MD; Joseph A. Tami, Pharm.D., San Antonio, TX; John H. Toogood, M.D., London, Ontario; Martin D. Valentine, M.D., Baltimore, MD; Michael Weinblatt, M.D., Boston, MA; Dennis Michael Williams, Pharm.D., Chapel Hill, NC; Stewart Wong, Ph.D., Annandale, VA

Clinical Toxicology/Substance Abuse

Theodore G. Tong, Pharm.D., *Chair*, Tucson, AZ; John Ambre, M.D., Ph.D., Chicago, IL; Usoa E. Busto, Pharm.D., Toronto, Ontario; Darryl Inaba, Pharm.D., San Francisco, CA; Edward P. Krenzelok, Pharm.D., Pittsburgh, PA; Michael Montagne, Ph.D., Boston, MA; Sven A. Normann, Pharm.D., Tampa, FL; Gary M. Oderda, Pharm.D., Salt Lake City, UT; Paul

Pentel, M.D., Minneapolis, MN; Rose Ann Soloway, R.N., Washington, DC; Daniel A. Spyker, M.D., Ph.D., Rockville, MD; Anthony R. Temple, M.D., Ft. Washington, PA; Anthony Tommasello, Pharm.D., Baltimore, MD; Joseph C. Veltri, Pharm.D., Salt Lake City, UT; William A. Watson, Pharm.D., Kansas City, MO

Consumer Interest/Health Education

Gordon D. Schiff, M.D., *Chair*, Chicago, IL; Michael J. Ackerman, Ph.D., Bethesda, MD; Barbara Aranda-Naranjo, R.N., San Antonio, TX; Frank J. Ascione, Pharm.D., Ph.D., Ann Arbor, MI; Judith I. Brown, Silver Spring, MD; Jose Camacho, Austin, TX; Margaret A. Charters, Ph.D., Syracuse, NY; Jennifer Cross, San Francisco, CA; William G. Harless, Ph.D., Bethesda, MD; Louis H. Kompare, Lake Buena Vista, FL; Margo Kroshus, R.N., B.S.N., Rochester, MN; Marilyn Lister, Wakefield, Quebec; Margaret Lueders, Seattle, WA; Frederick S. Mayer, R.Ph., M.P.H., Sausalito, CA; Nancy Milio, Ph.D., Chapel Hill, NC; Irving Rubin, Port Washington, NY; T. Donald Rucker, Ph.D., River Forest, IL; Stephen B. Soumerai, Sc.D., Boston, MA; Carol A. Vetter, Rockville, MD

Critical Care Medicine

Catherine M. MacLeod, M.D., *Chair*, Chicago, IL; William Banner, Jr., M.D., Salt Lake City, UT; Philip S. Barie, M.D., New York, NY; Thomas P. Bleck, M.D., Charlottesville, VA; Roger C. Bone, M.D., Toledo, OH; Susan S. Fish, Pharm.D., Boston, MA; Edgar R. Gonzalez, Pharm.D., Richmond, VA; Robert Gottesman, Rockville, MD; John W. Hoyt, M.D., Pittsburgh, PA; Sheldon A. Magder, M.D., Montreal, Quebec; Joseph E. Parrillo, M.D., Chicago, IL; Sharon Peters, M.D., St. John's, Newfoundland; Domenic A. Sica, M.D., Richmond, VA; Martin G. Tweeddale, M.B., Ph.D., Vancouver, British Columbia

Dentistry

Sebastian G. Ciancio, D.D.S., *Chair*, Buffalo, NY; Donald F. Adams, D.D.S., Portland, OR; Karen A. Baker, M.S. Pharm., Iowa City, IA; Stephen A. Cooper, D.M.D., Ph.D., Philadelphia, PA; Frederick A. Curro, D.M.D., Ph.D., Jersey City, NJ; Paul J. Desjardins, D.M.D., Ph.D., Newark, NJ; Tommy W. Gage, D.D.S., Ph.D., Dallas, TX; Stephen F. Goodman, D.D.S., New York, NY; Daniel A. Haas, D.D.S., Ph.D., Toronto, Ontario; Richard E. Hall, D.D.S., Ph.D., Buffalo, NY; Lireka P. Joseph, Dr.P.H., Rockville, MD; Janice Lieberman, Fort Lee, NJ; Laurie Lisowski, Lewiston, NY; Clarence L. Trummel, D.D.S., Ph.D., Farmington, CT; Joel M. Weaver, II, D.D.S., Ph.D., Columbus, OH; Clifford W. Whall, Jr., Ph.D., Chicago, IL; Raymond P. White, Jr., D.D.S., Ph.D., Chapel Hill, NC; Ray C. Williams, D.M.D., Boston, MA

Dermatology

Robert S. Stern, M.D., *Chair*, Boston, MA; Beatrice B. Abrams, Ph.D., Somerville, NJ; Richard D. Baughman, M.D., Hanover, NH; Michael Bigby, M.D., Boston, MA; Janice T. Chussil, R.N., M.S.N., Portland, OR; Stuart Maddin, M.D., Vancouver, British Columbia; Milton Orkin, M.D., Robbinsdale, MN; Neil H. Shear, M.D., Toronto, Ontario; Edgar Benton Smith, M.D., Galveston, TX; Dennis P. West, M.S. Pharm., Lincolnshire, IL; Gail M. Zimmerman, Portland, OR

Diagnostic Agents—Nonradioactive

Robert L. Siegle, M.D., *Chair*, San Antonio, TX; Kaizer Aziz, Ph.D., Rockville, MD; Robert C. Brasch, M.D., San Francisco, CA; Nicholas Harry Malakis, M.D., Bethesda, MD; Robert F. Mattrey, M.D., San Diego, CA; James A. Nelson, M.D., Seattle, WA; Jovitas Skucas, M.D., Rochester, NY; Gerald L. Wolf, Ph.D., M.D., Charlestown, MA

Drug Information Science

James A. Visconti, Ph.D., *Chair*, Columbus, OH; Marie A. Abate, Pharm.D., Morgantown, WV; Ann B. Amerson, Pharm.D., Lexington, KY; Philip O. Anderson, Pharm.D., San Diego, CA; Danial E. Baker, Pharm.D., Spokane, WA; C. David Butler, Pharm.D., M.B.A., Naperville, IL; Linda L. Hart, Pharm.D., Saddle River, NJ; Edward J. Huth, M.D., Philadelphia, PA; John M. Kessler, Pharm.D., Chapel Hill, NC; R. David Lauper, Pharm.D., Emeryville, CA; Domingo R. Martinez, Pharm.D., Birmingham, AL; William F. McGhan, Pharm.D., Ph.D., Philadelphia, PA; John K. Murdoch, B.Sc.Phm., Toronto, Ontario; Kurt A. Proctor, Ph.D., Alexandria, VA; Arnauld F. Scafidi, M.D., M.P.H., Rockville, MD; John A. Scarlett, M.D., Austin, TX; Gary H. Smith, Pharm.D., Tucson, AZ; Dennis F. Thompson, Pharm.D., Oklahoma City, OK; William G. Troutman, Pharm.D., Albuquerque, NM; Lee A. Wanke, M.S., Houston, TX

Drug Utilization Review

Judith K. Jones, M.D., Ph.D., *Chair*, Arlington, VA; John F. Beary, III, M.D., Washington, DC; James L. Blackburn, Pharm.D., Saskatoon, Saskatchewan; Richard S. Blum, M.D., East Hills, NY; Amy Cooper-Outlaw, Pharm.D., Stone Mountain, GA; Joseph W. Cranston, Jr., Ph.D., Chicago, IL; W. Gary Erwin, Pharm.D., Philadelphia, PA; Jere E. Goyan, Ph.D., Saddle River, NJ; Duane M. Kirking, Ph.D., Ann Arbor, MI; Karen E. Koch, Pharm.D., Tupelo, MS; Aida A. LeRoy, Pharm.D., Arlington, VA; Jerome Levine, M.D., Baltimore, MD; Richard W. Lindsay, M.D., Charlottesville, VA; M. Laurie Mashford, M.D., Melbourne, Victoria, Australia; Deborah M. Nadzam, R.N., Ph.D., Oakbrook Terrace, IL; William Z. Potter, M.D., Ph.D., Bethesda, MD; Louise R. Rodriquez, M.S., Washington, DC; Stephen P. Spielberg, M.D., Ph.D., West Point, PA; Suzan M. Streichenwein, M.D., Houston, TX; Brian L. Strom, M.D., Philadelphia, PA; Michael Weintraub, M.D., Rockville, MD; Antonio Carlos Zanini, M.D., Ph.D., São Paulo, Brazil

Endocrinology

Maria I. New, M.D., *Chair*, New York, NY; Ronald D. Brown, M.D., Oklahoma City, OK; R. Keith Campbell, Pharm.D., Pullman, WA; David S. Cooper, M.D., Baltimore, MD; Betty J. Dong, Pharm.D., San Francisco, CA; Andrea Dunaif, M.D., New York, NY; Anke A. Ehrhardt, Ph.D., New York, NY; Nadir R. Farid, M.D., Durham, N.C.; John G. Haddad, Jr., M.D., Philadelphia, PA; Michael M. Kaplan, M.D., Southfield, MI; Harold E. Lebovitz, M.D., Brooklyn, NY; Marvin E. Levin, M.D., Chesterfield, MO; Marvin M. Lipman, M.D., Scarsdale, NY; Barbara J. Maschak-Carey, R.N., M.S.N., Philadelphia, PA; James C. Melby, M.D., Boston, MA; Walter J. Meyer, III, M.D., Galveston, TX; Rita Nemchik, R.N., M.S., C.D.E., Florence, NJ; Daniel A. Notterman, M.D., New York, NY; Ron Gershon Rosenfeld, M.D., Stanford, CA; Paul Saenger, M.D., Bronx, NY; Leonard Wartofsky, M.D., Washington, DC

Family Practice

Robert M. Guthrie, M.D., *Chair*, Columbus, OH; Jack A. Brose, D.O., Athens, OH; Jannet M. Carmichael, Pharm.D., Reno, NV; Jacqueline A. Chadwick, M.D., Scottsdale, AZ; Mark E. Clasen, M.D., Ph.D., Dayton, OH; Lloyd P. Haskell, M.D.,

West Borough, MA; Luis A. Izquierdo-Mora, M.D., Rio Piedras, PR; Edward L. Langston, M.D., Houston, TX; Stephen T. O'Brien, M.D., Enfield, CT; Charles D. Ponte, Pharm.D., Morgantown, WV; Jack M. Rosenberg, Pharm.D., Ph.D., Brooklyn, NY; John F. Sangster, M.D., London, Ontario; Theodore L. Yarboro, Sr., M.D., M.P.H., Sharon, PA

Gastroenterology

Gordon L. Klein, M.D., *Chair*, Galveston, TX; Karl E. Anderson, M.D., Galveston, TX; William Balistreri, M.D., Cincinnati, OH; Paul Bass, Ph.D., Madison, WI; Rosemary R. Berardi, Pharm.D., Ann Arbor, MI; Raymond F. Burk, M.D., Nashville, TN; Thomas Q. Garvey, III, M.D., Potomac, MD; Donald J. Glotzer, M.D., Boston, MA; Flavio Habal, M.D., Toronto, Ontario; Paul E. Hyman, M.D., Torrance, CA; Bernard Mehl, D.P.S., New York, NY; William J. Snape, Jr., M.D., Torrance, CA; Ronald D. Soltis, M.D., Minneapolis, MN; C. Noel Williams, M.D., Halifax, Nova Scotia; Hyman J. Zimmerman, M.D., Bethesda, MD

Geriatrics

Robert E. Vestal, M.D., *Chair*, Boise, ID; Darrell R. Abernethy, M.D., Washington, DC; William B. Abrams, M.D., West Point, PA; Jerry Avorn, M.D., Boston, MA; Robert A. Blouin, Pharm.D., Lexington, KY; S. George Carruthers, M.D., Halifax, Nova Scotia; Lynn E. Chaitovitz, Rockville, MD; Terry Fulmer, R.N., Ph.D., New York, NY; Philip P. Gerbino, Pharm.D., Philadelphia, PA; Pearl S. German, Sc.D., Baltimore, MD; David J. Greenblatt, M.D., Boston, MA; Martin D. Higbee, Pharm.D., Tucson, AZ; Brian B. Hoffman, M.D., Palo Alto, CA; J. Edward Jackson, M.D., San Diego, CA; Joseph V. Levy, Ph.D., San Francisco, CA; Paul A. Mitenko, M.D., FRCPC, Nanaimo, British Columbia; John E. Morley, M.B., B.Ch., St. Louis, MO; Jay Roberts, Ph.D., Philadelphia, PA; Louis J. Rubenstein, R.Ph., Alexandria, VA; Janice B. Schwartz, M.D., San Francisco, CA; Alexander M.M. Shepherd, M.D., San Antonio, TX; William Simonson, Pharm.D., Portland, OR; Daniel S. Sitar, Ph.D., Winnipeg, Manitoba; Mary K. Walker, R.N., Ph.D., Lexington, KY; Alastair J. J. Wood, M.D., Nashville, TN

Hematologic and Neoplastic Disease

John W. Yarbro, M.D., Ph.D., *Chair*, Springfield, IL; Joseph S. Bailes, M.D., McAllen, TX; Laurence H. Baker, D.O., Ann Arbor, MI; Barbara D. Blumberg-Carnes, Albuquerque, NM;

Helene G. Brown, B.S., Los Angeles, CA; Nora L. Burnham, Pharm.D., Princeton, NJ; William J. Dana, Pharm.D., Houston, TX; Connie Henke-Yarbro, R.N., B.S.N., Springfield, IL; William H. Hryniuk, M.D., San Diego, CA; B. J. Kennedy, M.D., Minneapolis, MN; Barnett Kramer, M.D., Rockville, MD; Michael J. Mastrangelo, M.D., Philadelphia, PA; David S. Rosenthal, M.D., Cambridge, MA; Richard L. Schilsky, M.D., Chicago, IL; Rowena N. Schwartz, Pharm.D., Pittsburgh, PA; Roy L. Silverstein, M.D., New York, NY; Samuel G. Taylor, IV, M.D., Chicago, IL; Raymond B. Weiss, M.D., Washington, DC

Infectious Disease Therapy

Donald Kaye, M.D., *Chair*, Philadelphia, PA; Robert Austrian, M.D., Philadelphia, PA; C. Glenn Cobbs, M.D., Birmingham, AL; Joseph W. Cranston, Jr., Ph.D., Chicago, IL; John J. Dennehy, M.D., Danville, PA; Courtney V. Fletcher, Pharm.D., Minneapolis, MN; Earl H. Freimer, M.D., Toledo, OH; Marc LeBel, Pharm.D., Quebec, Quebec; John D. Nelson, M.D., Dallas, TX; Lindsay E. Nicolle, M.D., Winnipeg, Manitoba; Alvin Novick, M.D., New Haven, CT; Charles G. Prober, M.D., Stanford, CA; Douglas D. Richman, M.D., San Diego, CA; Spotswood L. Spruance, M.D., Salt Lake City, UT; Roy T. Steigbigel, M.D., Stony Brook, NY; Paul F. Wehrle, M.D., San Clemente, CA

International Health

Rosalyn C. King, Pharm.D., M.P.H., *Chair*, Silver Spring, MD; Walter M. Batts, Rockville, MD; Eugenie Brown, Pharm.D., Kingston, Jamaica; Alan Cheung, Pharm.D., M.P.H., Washington, DC; Mary Couper, M.D., Geneva, Switzerland; Gabriel Daniel, Washington, DC; S. Albert Edwards, Pharm.D., Lincolnshire, IL; Enrique Fefer, Ph.D., Washington, DC; Peter H. M. Fontilus, Curaçao, Netherlands Antilles; Gan Ee Kiang, Penang, Malaysia; Marcellus Grace, Ph.D., New Orleans, LA; George B. Griffenhagen, Washington, DC; Margareta Helling-Borda, Geneva, Switzerland; Thomas Langston, Silver Spring, MD; Thomas Lapnet-Moustapha, Yaounde, Cameroon; David Lee, B.A., M.D., Arlington, VA; Aissatov Lo, Ka-Olack, Senegal; Stuart M. MacLeod, M.D., Hamilton, Ontario; Russell E. Morgan, Jr., Dr.P.H., Chevy Chase, MD; David Ofori-Adjei, M.D., Accra, Ghana; S. Ofosu-Amaah, M.D., New York, NY; James Rankin, Arlington, VA; Olikoye Ransome-

Kuti, M.D., Lagos, Nigeria; Budiono Santoso, M.D., Ph.D., Yogyakarta, Indonesia; Carmen Selva, Ph.D., Madrid, Spain; Valentin Vinogradov, Moscow, Russia; Fela Viso-Gurovich, Mexico City, Mexico; William B. Walsh, M.D., Chevy Chase, MD; Lawrence C. Weaver, Ph.D., Minneapolis, MN; Albert I. Wertheimer, Ph.D., Glen Allen, VA

Neurology
Stanley van den Noort, M.D., *Chair*, Irvine, CA; William T. Beaver, M.D., Washington, DC; Elizabeth U. Blalock, M.D., Anaheim, CA; James C. Cloyd, Pharm.D., Minneapolis, MN; David M. Dawson, M.D., West Roxbury, MA; Kevin Farrell, M.D., Vancouver, British Columbia; Kathleen M. Foley, M.D., New York, NY; Anthony E. Lang, M.D., Toronto, Ontario; Ira T. Lott, M.D., Orange, CA; James R. Nelson, M.D., La Jolla, CA; J. Kiffin Penry, M.D., Winston-Salem, NC; Neil H. Raskin, M.D., San Francisco, CA; Alfred J. Spiro, M.D., Bronx, NY; M. DiAnn Turek, R.N., Holt, MI

Nursing Practice
Rosemary C. Polomano, R.N., M.S.N., *Chair*, Philadelpia, PA; Mecca S. Cranley, R.N., Ph.D., Buffalo, NY; Jan M. Ellerhorst-Ryan, R.N., M.S.N., Cincinnati, OH; Linda Felver, Ph.D., R.N., Portland, OR; Hector Hugo Gonzalez, R.N., Ph.D., San Antonio, TX; Mary Harper, R.N., Ph.D., Rockville, MD; Ada K. Jacox, R.N., Ph.D., Baltimore, MD; Patricia Kummeth, R.N., M.S., Rochester, MN; Ida M. Martinson, R.N., Ph.D., San Francisco, CA; Carol P. Patton, R.N., Ph.D., J.D., Detroit, MI; Ginette A. Pepper, R.N., Ph.D., Englewood, CO; Geraldine A. Peterson, R.N., M.A., Potomac, MD; Linda C. Pugh, R.N., Ph.D., York, PA; Sharon S. Rising, R.N., C.N.M., Cheshire, CT; Marjorie Ann Spiro, R.N., B.S., C.S.N., Scarsdale, NY

Nutrition and Electrolytes
Robert D. Lindeman, M.D., *Chair*, Albuquerque, NM; Hans Fisher, Ph.D., New Brunswick, NJ; Walter H. Glinsmann, M.D., Washington, DC; Helen Andrews Guthrie, M.S., Ph.D., State College, PA; Steven B. Heymsfield, M.D., New York, NY; K. N. Jeejeebhoy, M.D., Toronto, Ontario; Leslie M. Klevay, M.D., Grand Forks, ND; Linda S. Knox, M.S.N., Philadelphia, PA; Bonnie Liebman, M.S., Washington, DC; Sudesh K. Mahajan, M.D., Grosse Point Woods, MI; Craig

J. McClain, M.D., Lexington, KY; Jay M. Mirtallo, M.S., Columbus, OH; Sohrab Mobarhan, M.D., Maywood, IL; Robert M. Russell, M.D., Boston, MA; Harold H. Sandstead, M.D., Galveston, TX; William J. Stone, M.D., Nashville, TN; Carlos A. Vaamonde, M.D., Miami, FL; Stanley Wallach, M.D., New York, NY

Obstetrics and Gynecology

Douglas D. Glover, M.D., *Chair*, Morgantown, WV; Rudi Ansbacher, M.D., Ann Arbor, MI; Florence Comite, M.D., New Haven, CT; James W. Daly, M.D., Columbia, MO; Marilynn C. Frederiksen, M.D., Chicago, IL; Charles B. Hammond, M.D., Durham, NC; Barbara A. Hayes, M.A., New Rochelle, NY; Art Jacknowitz, Pharm.D., Morgantown, WV; William J. Ledger, M.D., New York, NY; Andre-Marie Leroux, M.D., Ottawa, Ontario; William A. Nahhas, M.D., Dayton, OH; Warren N. Otterson, M.D., Shreveport, LA; Samuel A. Pasquale, M.D., New Brunswick, NJ; Johanna Perlmutter, M.D., Boston, MA; Robert W. Rebar, M.D., Cincinnati, OH; Richard H. Reindollar, M.D., Boston, MA; G. Millard Simmons, M.D., Morgantown, WV; J. Benjamin Younger, M.D., Birmingham, AL

Ophthalmology

Herbert E. Kaufman, M.D., *Chair*, New Orleans, LA; Steven R. Abel, Pharm.D., Indianapolis, IN; Jules Baum, M.D., Boston, MA; Lee R. Duffner, M.D., Miami, FL; David L. Epstein, M.D., Durham, NC; Allan J. Flach, Pharm.D., M.D., Corte Madera, CA; Vincent H. L. Lee, Ph.D., Los Angeles, CA; Steven M. Podos, M.D., New York, NY; Kirk R. Wilhelmus, M.D., Houston, TX; Thom J. Zimmerman, M.D., Ph.D., Louisville, KY

Otorhinolaryngology

Leonard P. Rybak, M.D., Ph.D., *Chair*, Springfield, IL; Robert E. Brummett, Ph.D., Portland, OR; Robert A. Dobie, M.D., San Antonio, TX; Linda J. Gardiner, M.D., Fort Myers, FL; David Hilding, M.D., Price, UT; David B. Hom, M.D., Minneapolis, MN; Helen F. Krause, M.D., Pittsburgh, PA; Richard L. Mabry, M.D., Dallas, TX; Lawrence J. Marentette, M.D., Ann Arbor, MI; Robert A. Mickel, M.D., Ph.D., San Francisco, CA; Randal A. Otto, M.D., San Antonio, TX;

Richard W. Waguespack, M.D., Birmingham, AL; William R. Wilson, M.D., Washington, DC

Parasitic Disease

Jay S. Keystone, M.D., *Chair*, Toronto, Ontario; Michele Barry, M.D., New Haven, CT; Frank J. Bia, M.D., M.P.H., Guilford, CT; David Botero, M.D., Medellin, Colombia; David O. Freedman, M.D., Birmingham, AL; Elaine C. Jong, M.D., Seattle, WA; Dennis D. Juranek, M.D., Atlanta, GA; Donald J. Krogstad, M.D., New Orleans, LA; Douglas W. MacPherson, M.D., Hamilton, Ontario; Edward K. Markell, M.D., Berkeley, CA; Theodore Nash, M.D., Bethesda, MD; Murray Wittner, M.D., Bronx, NY

Patient Counseling (Ad Hoc)

Frank J. Ascione, Pharm.D., Ph.D., *Chair*, Ann Arbor, MI; John E. Arradondo, M.D., Houston, TX; Candace Barnett, Atlanta, GA; Karin Bolte, Washington, DC; Allan H. Bruckheim, M.D., Harrison, NY; Mark Clasen, M.D., Ph.D., Dayton, OH; Amy Cooper-Outlaw, Pharm.D., Stone Mountain, GA; Frederick A. Curro, D.M.D., Ph.D., Jersey City, NJ; Robin DiMatteo, Ph.D., Riverside, CA; Diane B. Ginsburg, Austin, TX; Denise Grimes, R.N., Jackson, MI; Richard Herrier, Tucson, AZ; Barry Kass, R.Ph., Boston, MA; Thomas Kellenberger, Pharm.D., Montvale, NJ; Alice Kimball, Darnestown, MD; Pat Kramer, Bismarck, ND; Patti Kummeth, R.N., Rochester, MN; Ken Leibowitz, Philadelphia, PA; Colleen Lum Lung, R.N., Denver, CO; Louise Matte, Quebec, Canada; Scotti Milley, Richmond, VA; Constance Pavlides, R.N., D.N.Sc., Rockville, MD; Lisa Tedesco, Ph.D., Ann Arbor, MI

Pediatric Anesthesiology (Ad Hoc)

Charles J. Coté, M.D., *Chair*, Chicago, IL; J. Michael Badgwell, M.D., Lubbock, TX; Barbara Brandon, M.D., Pittsburgh, PA; Ryan Cook, M.D., Pittsburgh, PA; John J. Downes, M.D., Philadelphia, PA; Dennis Fisher, M.D., San Francisco, CA; John E. Forestner, M.D., Fort Worth, TX; Helen W. Karl, M.D., Seattle, WA; Harry G. G. Kingston, M.B., Portland, OR; Anne Marie Lynn, M.D., Seattle, WA; Mark Shriner, M.D., Philadelphia, PA; Victoria Simpson, M.D., Ph.D., Denver, CO; Meb Watcha, M.D., St. Louis, MO

Pediatrics

Philip D. Walson, M.D., *Chair*, Columbus, OH; Susan Alpert, Ph.D., M.D., Rockville, MD; Jacob V. Aranda, M.D., Ph.D.,

Montreal, Quebec; Cheston M. Berlin, Jr., M.D., Hershey, PA; Nancy Jo Braden, M.D., Phoenix, AZ; Patricia J. Bush, Ph.D., Washington, DC; Marion J. Finkel, M.D., Morris Township, NJ; George S. Goldstein, M.D., Briarcliff Manor, NY; Ralph E. Kauffman, M.D., Detroit, MI; Gideon Koren, M.D., Toronto, Ontario; Joan M. Korth-Bradley, Pharm.D., Ph.D., Philadelphia, PA; Richard Leff, Pharm.D., Kansas City, KS; Carolyn Lund, R.N., M.S., San Francisco, CA; Wayne Snodgrass, M.D., Galveston, TX; Celia A. Viets, M.D., Ottawa, Canada; John T. Wilson, M.D., Shreveport, LA; Sumner J. Yaffe, M.D., Bethesda, MD; Karin E. Zenk, Pharm.D., Irvine, CA

Pharmacy Practice

Thomas P. Reinders, Pharm.D., *Chair*, Richmond, VA; Olya Duzey, M.S., Big Rapids, MI; Yves Gariepy, B.Sc.Pharm., Quebec, Quebec; Ned Heltzer, M.S., New Castle, DE; Lester S. Hosto, B.S., Little Rock, AR; Martin J. Jinks, Pharm.D., Pullman, WA; Frederick Klein, B.S., Montvale, NJ; Calvin H. Knowlton, Ph.D., Lumberton, NJ; Patricia A. Kramer, B.S., Bismarck, ND; Dennis McCallum, Pharm.D., Minneapolis, MN; Shirley P. McKee, B.S., Houston, TX; William A. McLean, Pharm.D., Ottawa, Ontario; Gladys Montañez, B.S., Santurce, PR; Donald L. Moore, B.S., Kokomo, IN; John E. Ogden, M.S., Washington, DC; Henry A. Palmer, Ph.D., Storrs, CT; Lorie G. Rice, B.A., M.P.H., San Francisco, CA; Mike R. Sather, M.S., Albuquerque, NM; Albert Sebok, B.S., Hudson, OH; William E. Smith, Pharm.D., Ph.D., Boston, MA; Susan East Torrico, B.S., Orlando, FL; J. Richard Wuest, Pharm.D., Cincinnati, OH; Glenn Y. Yokoyama, Pharm.D., Pasadena, CA

Psychiatric Disease

Burton J. Goldstein, M.D., *Chair*, Williams Island, FL; Magda Campbell, M.D., New York, NY; Alex A. Cardoni, M.S. Pharm., Hartford, CT; James L. Claghorn, M.D., Houston, TX; N. Michael Davis, M.S., Miami, FL; Larry Ereshefsky, Pharm.D., San Antonio, TX; W. Edwin Fann, M.D., Houston, TX; Alan J. Gelenberg, M.D., Tucson, AZ; Tracy R. Gordy, M.D., Austin, TX; Paul Grof, M.D., Ottawa, Ontario; Russell T. Joffe, M.D., Toronto, Ontario; Harriet P. Lefley, Ph.D., Miami, FL; Nathan Rawls, Pharm.D., Memphis, TN; Ruth Robinson, Saskatoon, Saskatchewan; Matthew V. Rudorfer,

M.D., Rockville, MD; Karen A. Theesen, Pharm.D., Omaha, NE

Pulmonary Disease

Harold S. Nelson, M.D., *Chair*, Denver, CO; Richard C. Ahrens, M.D., Iowa City, IA; Eugene R. Bleecker, M.D., Baltimore, MD; William W. Busse, M.D., Madison, WI; Christopher Fanta, M.D., Boston, MA; Mary K. Garcia, R.N., Sugarland, TX; Nicholas Gross, M.D., Hines, IL; Leslie Hendeles, Pharm.D., Gainesville, FL; Elliot Israel, M.D., Boston, MA; Susan Janson-Bjerklie, R.N., Ph.D., San Francisco, CA; John W. Jenne, M.D., Hines, IL; H. William Kelly, Pharm.D., Albuquerque, NM; James P. Kemp, M.D., San Diego, CA; Henry Levison, M.D., Toronto, Ontario; Gail Shapiro, M.D., Seattle, WA; Stanley J. Szefler, M.D., Denver, CO

Radiopharmaceuticals

Carol S. Marcus, Ph.D., M.D., *Chair*, Torrance, CA; Capt. William H. Briner, B.S., Durham, NC; Ronald J. Callahan, Ph.D., Boston, MA; Janet F. Eary, M.D., Seattle, WA; Joanna S. Fowler, Ph.D., Upton, NY; David L. Gilday, M.D., Toronto, Ontario; David A. Goodwin, M.D., Palo Alto, CA; David L. Laven, N.Ph., C.R.Ph., FASCP, Bay Pines, FL; Andrea H. McGuire, M.D., Des Moines, IA; Peter Paras, Ph.D., Rockville, MD; Barry A. Siegel, M.D., St. Louis, MO; Edward B. Silberstein, M.D., Cincinnati, OH; Dennis P. Swanson, M.S., Pittsburgh, PA; Mathew L. Thakur, Ph.D., Philadelphia, PA; Henry N. Wellman, M.D., Indianapolis, IN

Surgical Drugs and Devices

Lary A. Robinson, M.D., *Chair*, Tampa, FL; Gregory Alexander, M.D., Rockville, MD; Norman D. Anderson, M.D., Baltimore, MD; Alan R. Dimick, M.D., Birmingham, AL; Jack Hirsh, M.D., Hamilton, Ontario; Manucher J. Javid, M.D., Madison, WI; Henry J. Mann, Pharm.D., Bloomington, MN; Kurt M. W. Niemann, M.D., Birmingham, AL; Robert P. Rapp, Pharm.D., Lexington, KY; Ronald Rubin, M.D., West Newton, MA

Urology

John A. Belis, M.D., *Chair*, Hershey, PA; Culley C. Carson, M.D., Chapel Hill, NC; Richard A. Cohen, M.D., Red Bank, NJ; B. J. Reid Czarapata, R.N., North Potomac, MD; Jean B. de Kernion, M.D., Los Angeles, CA; Warren Heston, Ph.D.,

New York, NY; Mark V. Jarowenko, M.D., Hershey, PA; Mary Lee, Pharm.D., Chicago, IL; Marguerite C. Lippert, M.D., Charlottesville, VA; Penelope A. Longhurst, Ph.D., Philadelphia, PA; Tom F. Lue, M.D., San Francisco, CA; Michael G. Mawhinney, Ph.D., Morgantown, WV; Martin G. McLoughlin, M.D., Vancouver, British Columbia; Randall G. Rowland, M.D., Ph.D., Indianapolis, IN; J. Patrick Spirnak, M.D., Cleveland, OH; William F. Tarry, M.D., Morgantown, WV; Keith N. Van Arsdalen, M.D., Philadelphia, PA

Veterinary Medicine

Lloyd E. Davis, D.V.M., Ph.D., *Chair*, Urbana, IL; Arthur L. Aronson, D.V.M., Ph.D., Raleigh, NC; Gordon W. Brumbaugh, D.V.M., Ph.D., College Station, TX; Peter Conlon, D.V.M., Ph.D., Guelph, Ontario; Gordon L. Coppoc, D.V.M., Ph.D., West Lafayette, IN; Sidney A. Ewing, D.V.M., Ph.D., Stillwater, OK; Stuart D. Forney, M.S., Fort Collins, CO; William G. Huber, D.V.M., Ph.D., Sun City West, AZ; Vernon Corey Langston, D.V.M., Ph.D., Mississippi State, MS; Mark G. Papich, D.V.M., Raleigh, NC; John W. Paul, D.V.M., Somerville, NJ; Thomas E. Powers, D.V.M., Ph.D., Columbus, OH; Charles R. Short, D.V.M., Ph.D., Baton Rouge, LA; Richard H. Teske, D.V.M., Ph.D., Rockville, MD; Jeffrey R. Wilcke, D.V.M., M.S., Blacksburg, VA

Index

Brand names appear in italics. Generic or family names appear in standard typeface.

Accupril, 32
Acebutolol, 226
Acetaminophen & Codeine, 833
Acetaminophen, Codeine, & Caffeine, 833
Acetohexamide, 108
Acetophenazine, 1006
Achromycin, 1187
Achromycin V, 1187
Acrivastine, 145
Acrivastine & Pseudoephedrine, 169
Actagen, 166
Actagen-C Cough, 453
Actifed, 166
Actifed with Codeine Cough, 453
Actifed Head Cold & Allergy Medicine, 166
Acyclovir, Systemic, 3
Adalat CC, 318
Adatuss D.C. Expectorant, 453

Adrenalin Chloride, 244
Adrenalin Chloride Solution, 265
Advil, 906
Advil Caplets, 906
Advil, Children's, 906
Airet, 244
Alamine, 166
Alamine Expectorant, 453
Alamine-C Liquid, 453
Albert Glyburide, 108
Albuterol, 245, 265
Aldomet, 792
Alersule, 166
Aleve, 906
Alka-Seltzer Plus Cold & Cough, 453
Alka-Seltzer Plus Night-Time Cold, 453
Allent, 166
Aller-Chlor, 143
Allercon, 166
Allerdryl, 144
Allerest, 166
Allerest, Children's, 166

Allerest Maximum Strength, 166
Allerest 12 Hour, 166
Allerest 12 Hour Caplets, 166
Allerfrim, 166
Allerfrin, 166
Allerfrin with Codeine, 453
Allergy Cold, 166
Allergy Formula Sinutap, 166
Allergy Relief Medicine, 166
AllerMax Caplets, 143
Aller-med, 143
Allerphed, 166
All-Nite Cold Formula, 453
Allopurinol, Systemic, 10
Alprazolam, 203
Altace, 32
Alupent, 244, 265
Amantadine, Systemic, 17
Amaril D, 166
Amaril D Spantab, 166
Ambay Cough, 453
Ambenyl Cough, 453
Ambenyl-D Decongestant Cough Formula, 453
Ambien, 1244
Ambophen Expectorant, 453
Amen, 1084
Amgenal Cough, 453
Ami-Drix, 166
Amiloride, 550
Aminophylline, 285

Ami-Tex LA, 453
Amitriptyline, 91
Amlodipine, Systemic, 26
Amoxapine, 91
Amoxicillin, 970
Amoxicillin & Clavulanate, 992
Amoxil, 969
Ampicillin, 970
Ampicillin & Sulbactam, 992
Anafranil, 90
Ana-Guard, 265
Anamine, 166
Anamine HD, 453
Anamine T.D., 166
Anaplex, 166
Anaplex HD, 453
Anaplex S.R., 166
Anaprox, 906
Anaprox DS, 906
Anatuss, 453
Anatuss with Codeine, 453
Anatuss DM, 453
Anatuss LA, 453
Anergan 25, 183
Anergan 50, 183
Angiotensin-Converting Enzyme (ACE) Inhibitors, Systemic, 32
Anisindione, 57
Anisotropine, 45
Ansaid, 906
Anticholinergics/ Antispasmodics, Systemic, 44
Anticoagulants, Systemic, 57

Anticonvulsants, Hydantoin, Systemic, 66
Antidepressants, Monoamine Oxidase (MAO) Inhibitor, Systemic, 79
Antidepressants, Tricyclic, Systemic, 90
Antidiabetics, Oral, Systemic, 108
Antidyskinetics, Systemic, 122
Antifungals, Azole, Systemic, 132
Antihistamines, Phenothiazine-Derivative, Systemic, 183
Antihistamines, Systemic, 143
Antihistamines & Decongestants, Systemic, 166
Antinaus 50, 183
Anti-Tuss DM Expectorant, 453
Anxanil, 143
Apo-Allopurinol, 10
Apo-Amitriptyline, 91
Apo-Carbamazepine, 333
Apo-Chlorpropamide, 108
Apo-Dimenhydrinate, 144
Apo-Glyburide, 108
Apo-Guanethidine, 658
Apo-Haloperidol, 665
Apo-Hydroxyzine, 144
Apo-Imipramine, 91
Apo-Methyldopa, 792
Apo-Metoclop, 799

Apo-Metronidazole, 806
Apo-Nitrofurantoin, 900
Apo-Quinidine, 1097
Apo-Sulfatrim, 1137
Apo-Sulfatrim DS, 1137
Apo-Tolbutamide, 108
Apo-Trimip, 91
Apo-Zidovudine, 1236
Apresoline, 711
Aprodine with Codeine, 453
Aprodrine, 166
Aquest, 594
A.R.M. Maximum Strength Caplets, 166
Arm-a-Med Isoetharine, 244
Arm-a-Med Metaproterenol, 244
Asacol, 786
Asendin, 90
Aspirin, Caffeine, & Dihydrocodeine, 844
Aspirin & Codeine, 844
Aspirin, Codeine, & Caffeine, 844
Aspirin, Codeine, & Caffeine, Buffered, 844
Astemizole, 145
AsthmaHaler Mist, 244
AsthmaNefrin, 245
Atarax, 143
Atenolol, 226
Atrohist Pediatric, 166
Atrohist Sprinkle, 166
Atropine, 45
Atrovent, 734
Augmentin, 992

Aventyl, 90
Avirax, 3
Axid, 692
Aygestin, 1084
Azatadine, 145
Azatadine & Pseudoe-
  phedrine, 169
Azithromycin, Systemic,
  197
Azmacort, 406
Azulfidine, 1147
Azulfidine EN-Tabs, 1147

Bacampicillin, 970
Bactrim, 1137
Bactrim DS, 1137
Banex, 453
Banex-LA, 453
Banex Liquid, 453
Banophen, 143
Banophen Caplets, 143
Bayaminic Expectorant,
  453
Bayaminicol, 453
Baycodan, 453
Baycomine, 453
Baycomine Pediatric, 453
BayCotussend Liquid, 453
Baydec DM Drops, 453
*Bayer Select Chest Cold
  Caplets*, 453
*Bayer Select Flu Relief
  Caplets*, 453
*Bayer Select Head &
  Chest Cold Caplets*,
  453
*Bayer Select Ibuprofen
  Caplets*, 906

*Bayer Select Night Time
  Cold Caplets*, 453
Bayhistine DH, 453
Bayhistine Expectorant,
  453
Baytussin AC, 453
Baytussin DM, 453
Beclomethasone, 407, 425
Beconase AQ, 425
Beldin, 143
Belix, 143
Belladonna, 45
Bena-D 10, 143
Bena-D 50, 143
Benadryl, 143
Benadryl Decongestant,
  166
Benadryl Kapseals, 143
Benadryl 25, 143
Benahist 10, 143
Benahist 50, 143
Ben-Allergin-50, 143
Benazepril, 32
Bendroflumethiazide, 561
Benemid, 1066
Benoject-10, 143
Benoject-50, 143
Benuryl, 1066
Benylin Cough, 143
Benylin Decongestant,
  166
*Benylin Expectorant
  Cough Formula*, 453
Benzodiazepines, Sys-
  temic, 202
Benzthiazide, 561
Benztropine, 122
Bepridil, 319

Beta-Adrenergic Blocking Agents, Systemic, 225
Betamethasone, 435
Betaxolol, 226
Biaxin, 373
Bifenabid, 1073
Biperiden, 122
Biphetane DC Cough, 453
Bisoprolol, 226
Bitolterol, 245
Brethaire, 245
Brethine, 265
Brevicon, 612
Brexin, 453
Brexin L.A., 166
Bricanyl, 265
Brofed, 166
Bromaline, 166
Bromanate, 166
Bromanate DC Cough, 453
Bromanyl, 453
Bromarest DX Cough, 453
Bromatane DX Cough, 453
Bromatap, 166
Bromatapp, 166
Bromazepam, 203
Bromfed, 166
Bromfed-DM, 453
Bromfed-PD, 166
Bromodiphenhydramine, 145
Bromophen T.D., 166
Bromotuss with Codeine, 453
Bromphen, 143, 166

Bromphen DC with Codeine Cough, 453
Bromphen DX Cough, 453
Brompheniramine, 145
Brompheniramine & Phenyleprine, 169
Brompheniramine, Phenylephrine, & Phenylpropanolamine, 169
Brompheniramine & Phenylpropanolamine, 169
Brompheniramine, Phenyltoloxamine, & Phenylephrine, 169
Brompheniramine & Pseudoephedrine, 169
Brompheril, 166
Bronchodilators, Adrenergic, Inhalation, 244
Bronchodilators, Adrenergic, Oral/Injection, 265
Bronchodilators, Xanthine-Derivative, Systemic, 284
Broncholate, 453
Bronitin Mist, 245
Bronkaid Mist, 245
Bronkephrine, 265
Bronkometer, 245
Bronkosol, 245
Bronkotuss Expectorant, 453
Brontane DX Cough, 453
Budesonide, 407, 425
Buffered Insulin Human, 718

Bumetanide, 539
Bumex, 539
Buprenorphine, 820
Bupropion, Systemic, 294
BuSpar, 299
Buspirone, Systemic, 299
Butalbital & Aspirin, 305
Butalbital, Aspirin, & Caffeine, 305
Butalbital & Aspirin, Systemic, 304
Butorphanol, 820
Bydramine Cough, 143

Cafergot, 675
Cafertine, 675
Cafetrate, 675
Calan SR, 318
Calcidrine, 453
Calcium Channel
   Blocking Agents, Systemic, 318
Calm X, 143
Capoten, 32
Captopril, 32
Carbamazepine, Systemic, 333
Carbenicillin, 970
Carbidopa & Levodopa, 753
Carbinoxamine, 145
Carbinoxamine & Pseudoephedrine, 169
*Carbinoxamine
   Compound,* 453
*Carbinoxamine
   Compound-Drops,* 453
Carbiset, 166

Carbiset-TR, 166
Carbodec, 166
Carbodec DM Drops, 453
Carbodec TR, 166
Carbolith, 762
Cardec DM, 453
Cardec DM Drops, 453
Cardec DM Pediatric, 453
Cardec-S, 166
Cardioquin, 1097
Cardizem CD, 318
Cardura, 576
Carisoprodol, 1124
Carteolol, 226
Cataflam, 906
Catapres, 385
Catapres-TTS, 385
Ceclor, 344
Cefaclor, 345
Cefadroxil, 345
Cefamandole, 345
Cefazolin, 345
Cefixime, 345
Cefmetazole, 345
Cefonicid, 345
Cefoperazone, 345
Cefotaxime, 345
Cefotetan, 345
Cefoxitin, 345
Cefpodoxime, 345
Cefprozil, 345
Ceftazidime, 345
Ceftin, 345
Ceftizoxime, 346
Ceftriaxone, 346
Cefuroxime, 346
Cefzil, 345
Cenafed Plus, 166

Cephalexin, 346

Cephalosporins, Systemic, 344

Cephalothin, 346

Cephapirin, 346

Cephradine, 346

Cerose-DM, 453

Cetirizine, 145

Charitin, 143

Cheracol, 453

Cheracol D Cough, 453

Cheracol Plus, 453

Cheracol Sinus, 166

Children's Dramamine, 143

Children's Formula Cough, 454

Children's Tylenol Cold Multi Symptom Plus Cough, 454

Children's Vicks NyQuil Cold/Cough Relief, 454

Chlo-Amine, 143

Chlorafed, 166

Chlorafed H.S. Timecelles, 166

Chlorafed Timecelles, 166

Chlorate, 143

Chlordiazepoxide, 203

Chlordrine S.R., 166

Chlorgest-HD, 454

Chlor-Niramine, 143

Chlor-100, 143

Chlorothiazide, 561

Chlorotrianisene, 595

Chlorphed, 143

Chlorphedrine SR, 166

Chlorphenesin, 1124

Chlorpheniramine, 145

Chlorpheniramine, Phenindamine, & Phenylpropanolamine, 169

Chlorpheniramine & Phenylephrine, 169

Chlorpheniramine, Phenylephrine, & Phenylpropanolamine, 169

Chlorpheniramine & Phenylpropanolamine, 169

Chlorpheniramine, Phenyltoloxamine, & Phenylephrine, 169

Chlorpheniramine, Phenyltoloxamine, Phenylephrine, & Phenylpropanolamine, 169

Chlorpheniramine & Pseudoephedrine, 169

Chlorpheniramine, Pyrilamine, & Phenylephrine, 169

Chlorpheniramine, Pyrilamine, Phenylephrine, & Phenylpropanolamine, 169

Chlor-Pro, 143

Chlor-Pro 10, 143

Chlorpromazine, 1006

Chlorpropamide, 108

Chlor-Rest, 166

Chlorspan-12, 143

Chlortab-4, 143

Chlortab-8, 143
Chlorthalidone, 561
Chlor-Trimeton, 143
Chlor-Trimeton Allergy, 143
Chlor-Trimeton 4 Hour Relief, 166
Chlor-Trimeton Repetabs, 143
Chlor-Trimeton 12 Hour Relief, 166
Chlor-Tripolon, 144
Chlorzoxazone, 1124
Chodehist DH, 454
Cholestyramine, Oral, 362
Chomhist LA, 166
Cibalith-S, 762
Cimetidine, 692
Cin-Quin, 1097
Cipro, 635
Ciprofloxacin, 635
Cisapride, Systemic, 368
Citra Forte, 454
Clarithromycin, Systemic, 373
Claritin, 144
Clemastine, 145
Clemastine & Phenylpro-panolamine, 169
Cleocin, 378
Cleocin Pediatric, 378
Clidinium, 45
Clinagen LA 40, 594
Clindamycin, Systemic, 378
Clinoril, 906
Clomipramine, 91
Clonazepam, 203

Clonidine, Systemic, 385
Clopra, 799
Clorazepate, 203
Cloxacillin, 970
Clozapine, Systemic, 394
Clozaril, 394
Co-Apap, 454
Codamine, 454
Codamine Pediatric, 454
Codan, 454
Codegest Expectorant, 454
Codeine, 820
Codiclear DH, 454
Codimal-A, 143
Codimal DH, 454
Codimal DM, 454
Codimal Expectorant, 454
Codimal-L.A., 166
Codimal PH, 454
Codistan No.1, 454
Cognex, 1174
Colestid, 400
Colestipol, Oral, 400
Colfed-A, 166
Coltab Children's, 166
Comhist, 166
Compazine, 1005
Compoz, 143
Comtrex Cough Formula, 454
Comtrex Daytime Caplets, 454
Comtrex Daytime Maxi-mum Strength Cold, Cough, & Flu Relief, 454
Comtrex Daytime Maxi-

mum Strength Cold & Flu Relief, 454

Comtrex Hot Flu Relief, 454

Comtrex Maximum Strength Liqui-Gels, 454

Comtrex Multi-Symptom Cold Reliever, 454

Comtrex Multi-Symptom Non-Drowsy Caplets, 454

Comtrex Nighttime, 454

Comtrex Nighttime Maximum Strength Cold, Cough, & Flu Relief, 454

Comtrex Nighttime Maximum Strength Cold & Flu Relief, 454

Concentrin, 454

Condrin-LA, 166

Conex, 454

Conex with Codeine Liquid, 454

Conex D.A., 166

Congess JR, 454

Congess SR, 454

Congestac Caplets, 454

Conjec-B, 143

Contac Cough & Chest Cold, 454

Contac Cough & Sore Throat, 454

Contac Day Caplets, 454

Contac Jr. Children's Cold Medicine, 454

Contac Maximum

Strength 12-Hour Caplets, 166

Contac Night Caplets, 454

Contac Severe Cold & Flu Formula Caplets, 454

Contac Severe Cold Formula, 454

Contac Severe Cold Formula Night Strength, 454

Contac 12-Hour, 166

Contac 12 Hour Allergy, 143

Contuss, 454

Cophene-B, 143

Cophene No.2, 166

Cophene-S, 454

Cophene-X, 454

Cophene-XP, 454

Co-Pyronil 2, 166

Corticosteroids, Inhalation, 406

Corticosteroids, Nasal, 425

Corticosteroids/ Corticotropin, Glucocorticoid Effects, Systemic, 433

Corticotropin, 435

Cortisone, 435

Cotrim, 1137

Cotrim DS, 1137

Co-Tuss V, 454

Cotylbutazone, 906

CoTylenol Cold Medication, 454

Cough/Cold Combinations, Systemic, 453

Coumadin, 57
Cramp End, 906
Cromolyn, Inhalation, 495
C-Tussin Expectorant, 454
Curretab, 1084
Cyclobenzaprine, Systemic, 509
Cyclothiazide, 561
Cycoflex, 509
Cycrin, 1084
Cyproheptadine, 145
Cytotec, 815

Dalacin C, 378
Dalacin C Palmitate, 378
Dalacin C Phosphate, 378
Dallergy-D, 166
Dallergy Jr., 166
Darvocet-N 100, 832
Darvon, 819
Darvon with A.S.A., 844
Darvon Compound, 844
Darvon Compound-65, 844
Darvon-N, 819
Darvon-N with A.S.A., 844
Daypro, 906
DayQuil Multi-Symptom Cold/Flu LiquiCaps, 454
DayQuil Non-Drowsy Cold/Flu, 454
DayQuil Sinus Pressure & Congestion Relief Caplets, 454
Declomycin, 1187
Decohistine DH, 454

Deconamine, 167
Deconamine SR, 167
Decongestabs, 167
Deconsal Pediatric, 454
Deconsal Sprinkle, 454
Deconsal II, 454
Dehist, 143, 167
Deladiol-40, 594
Delestrogen, 594
Deltasone, 434
Demadex, 1216
Demazin, 167
Demazin Repetabs, 167
Demeclocycline, 1187
Demerol, 819
Demerol-APAP, 832
Demulen 1/35, 612
Demulen 1/50, 612
depGynogen, 594
Depo-Estradiol, 594
Depogen, 594
Depo-Provera, 1084
Deproist Expectorant with Codeine, 454
Desipramine, 91
Desogen, 612
Desogestrel & Ethinyl Estradiol, 613
Despec, 454
Desyrel, 1224
De-Tuss, 454
Detussin Expectorant, 454
Detussin Liquid, 454
Dexafed Cough, 454
Dexamethasone, 407, 425, 435
Dexaphen SA, 167

Dexbrompheniramine & Pseudoephedrine, 169

Dexchlor, 143

Dexchlorpheniramine, 145

Dexophed, 167

Dey-Lute Isoetharine S/F, 245

Dey-Lute Metaproterenol, 245

D.H.E. 45, 675

DiaBeta, 108

Diabetic Tussin DM, 454

Diabinese, 108

Diamine T.D., 143

Diazepam, 203

Diclofenac, 908

Dicloxacillin, 970

Dicumarol, 57

Dicyclomine, 45

Didanosine, Systemic, 516

Diethylstilbestrol, 595

Diflucan, 132

Diflunisal, 908

Digitalis Medicines, Systemic, 525

Digitoxin, 525

Digoxin, 525

Dihistine, 167

Dihistine DH, 454

Dihistine Expectorant, 454

Dihydrocodeine, Acetaminophen, & Caffeine, 833

Dihydroergotamine, 676

Dilacor-XR, 318

Dilantin, 66

Dilaudid Cough, 454

Diltiazem, 319

Dimacol Caplets, 454

Dimaphen, 167

Dimaphen S.A., 167

Dimenhydrinate, 145

Dimetabs, 143

Dimetane, 143

Dimetane-DC Cough, 455

Dimetane Decongestant, 167

Dimetane Decongestant Caplets, 167

Dimetane-DX Cough, 455

Dimetane Extentabs, 143

Dimetapp, 167

Dimetapp Allergy, 143

Dimetapp Allergy Liqui-Gels, 143

Dimetapp Cold & Allergy, 167

Dimetapp DM, 455

Dimetapp DM Cold & Cough, 455

Dimetapp Extentabs, 167

Dimetapp 4-Hour Liquigels Maximum Strength, 167

Dinate, 143

Dioval 40, 594

Dioval XX, 594

Dipentum, 943

Diphen Cough, 143

Diphenacen-50, 143

Diphenadryl, 143

Diphenhist, 143

Diphenhist Captabs, 143

Diphenhydramine, 145

Diphenhydramine & Pseu-
    doephedrine, 170
Diphenylpyraline, 145
Disobrom, 167
Disophrol, 167
Disophrol Chronotabs,
    167
Disopyramide, Systemic,
    532
Diuretics, Loop, Sys-
    temic, 539
Diuretics, Potassium-Spar-
    ing, Systemic, 550
Diuretics, Thiazide, Sys-
    temic, 561
Dixarit, 385
Dolgesic, 906
Dolobid, 906
Dommanate, 143
Donatussin, 455
Donatussin DC, 455
Donatussin Drops, 455
Dondril, 455
Dopamet, 792
*Dorcol Children's Cold
    Formula,* 167
Dorcol Children's Cough,
    455
Dormarex 2, 143
Dormin, 143
Doryx, 1187
Doxazosin, Systemic, 576
Doxepin, 91
Doxy, 1187
Doxy-Caps, 1187
Doxycycline, 1187
Doxylamine, 145
Dramamine, 143

Dramamine Chewable,
    143
Dramamine Liquid, 143
Dramanate, 143
Dramocen, 143
Dramoject, 143
Dristan Allergy, 167
Dristan Cold & Flu, 455
*Dristan Juice Mix-in
    Cold, Flu, & Cough,*
    455
Drixoral, 167
Drixoral Cold & Allergy,
    167
Drize, 167
Dura-Estrin, 594
Duragen-20, 594
Duragen-40, 594
Dura-Gest, 455
Duralex, 167
Duralith, 762
Duraquin, 1097
Dura-Tap PD, 167
Duratuss, 455
Duratuss HD, 455
Dura-Vent, 455
Dura-Vent/A, 167
Duricef, 345
Dymelor, 108
Dymenate, 143
DynaCirc, 318
Dyphylline, 285

E-Cypionate, 594
Ed A-Hist, 167
ED-TLC, 455
ED Tuss HC, 455
E.E.S., 582

Effective Strength Cough Formula, 455
Effective Strength Cough Formula with Decongestant, 455
Efficol Cough Whip (Cough Suppressant/ Decongestant), 455
Efficol Cough Whip (Cough Suppressant/ Decongestant & Antihistamine), 455
Efficol Cough Whip (Cough Suppressant/ Expectorant), 455
Elavil, 90
Emex, 799
Enalapril, 32
Enalaprilat, 32
Endafed, 167
Endagen-HD, 455
Endal, 455
Endal Expectorant, 455
Endal-HD, 455
Endal-HD Plus, 455
Endep, 90
Enomine, 455
Enovil, 90
Enoxacin, 635
E.N.T., 167
Entex, 455
Entex LA, 455
Entex Liquid, 455
Entex PSE, 455
Entuss-D, 455
Entuss Expectorant, 455
Entuss Pediatric Expectorant, 455

Ephedrine, 265
Epinephrine, 245, 265
EpiPen Auto-Injector, 265
EpiPen Jr. Auto-Injector, 265
Epitol, 333
Ercaf, 675
Ergo-Caff, 675
Ergomar, 675
Ergostat, 675
Ergotamine, 676
Ergotamine & Caffeine, 676
Ergotamine, Caffeine, & Belladonna Alkaloids, 676
Ergotamine, Caffeine, Belladonna Alkaloids, & Pentobarbital, 676
Ergotamine, Caffeine, & Cyclizine, 676
Ergotamine, Caffeine, & Dimenhydrinate, 676
Ergotamine, Caffeine, & Diphenhydramine, 676
Ery-Tab, 582
Erythrityl Tetranitrate, 881
Erythromycin Base, 583
Erythromycin Estolate, 583
Erythromycin Ethylsuccinate, 583
Erythromycin Gluceptate, 583
Erythromycin Lactobionate, 583

Erythromycin Stearate, 583

Erythromycins, Systemic, 582

Eskalith, 762

Eskalith CR, 762

Estazolam, 203

Estinyl, 594

Estrace, 594

Estraderm, 594

Estradiol, 595

Estragyn 5, 594

Estragyn LA 5, 594

Estra-L 40, 594

Estratab, 594

Estro-A, 594

Estro-Cyp, 594

Estrofem, 594

Estrogens, Conjugated, 595

Estrogens, Esterified, 595

Estrogens, Systemic, 594

Estrogens & Progestins—Oral Contraceptives, Systemic, 612

Estroject-LA, 594

Estro-L.A., 594

Estrone, 595

Estrone '5', 594

Estropipate, 595

Estro-Span, 594

Estrovis, 594

Ethacrynic Acid, 539

Ethinyl Estradiol, 595

Ethopropazine, 122

Ethotoin, 66

Ethylnorepinephrine, 265

Ethynodiol Diacetate & Ethinyl Estradiol, 613

Etodolac, 908

Eudal-SR, 455

Euglucon, 108

E-Vista, 143

Excedrin IB, 906

Excedrin IB Caplets, 906

Exgest LA, 455

Extended Insulin Zinc, 718

Extended Insulin Zinc, Human, 718

Extra Action Cough, 455

Famciclovir, Systemic, 627

Famotidine, 692

Famvir, 627

Father John's Medicine Plus, 455

Fedahist, 167

Fedahist Decongestant, 167

Fedahist Gyrocaps, 167

Fedahist Timecaps, 167

Feldene, 906

Felodipine, 319

Fendol, 455

Fenoprofen, 908

Fenoterol, 245, 265

Finasteride, Systemic, 630

Flagyl, 806

Flagyl I.V., 806

Flagyl I.V. RTU, 806

Flexeril, 509

Floctafenine, 908

Floxin, 635

Flucloxacillin, 970
Fluconazole, 132
Flumadine, 1104
Flunarizine, 319
Flunisolide, 407, 425
Fluoroquinolones, Systemic, 635
Fluoxetine, Systemic, 643
Fluphenazine, 1006
Flurazepam, 203
Flurbiprofen, 908
Fluvastatin, 704
Fosinopril, 32
Furadantin, 900
Furalan, 900
Furatoin, 900
Furosemide, 539
Fynex, 143

Gabapentin, Systemic, 649
Genac, 167
Genahist, 143
Gen-Allerate, 143
Genamin, 167
Genatap, 167
Genatuss DM, 455
GenCept 0.5/35, 612
GenCept 1/35, 612
GenCept 10/11, 612
Gencold, 167
Gen-D-phen, 143
Gen-Glybe, 108
Genite, 455
Genora 0.5/35, 612
Genora 1/35, 612
Genora 1/50, 612
Genpril, 906

Genpril Caplets, 906
Gesterol 50, 1084
Glipizide, 109
Glucotrol, 108
Glyburide, 109
Glycofed, 455
Glycopyrrolate, 45
Glycotuss-DM, 455
Glydeine Cough, 455
Glynase PresTab, 108
Gotamine, 675
GP-500, 455
Granisetron, Systemic, 655
Gravol, 144
Gravol L/A, 144
Guaifed, 455
Guaifed-PD, 455
GuaiMAX-D, 455
Guaipax, 455
Guaitab, 455
Guanethidine, Systemic, 658
GuiaCough CF, 455
GuiaCough PE, 455
Guiamid D.M. Liquid, 455
Guiatuss A.C., 455
Guiatuss CF, 455
Guiatuss DAC, 455
Guiatuss-DM, 455
Guiatuss PE, 455
Guiatussin with Codeine Liquid, 455
Guiatussin DAC, 455
Guiatussin with Dextromethorphan, 455
Gynogen L.A. 20, 594
Gynogen L.A. 40, 594

Habitrol, 866
Halazepam, 203
Haldol, 665
Haldol Decanoate, 665
Haldol LA, 665
Haloperidol, Systemic, 665
Halotussin-DM Expectorant, 455
Haltran, 906
Hayfebrol, 167
Headache Medicines, Ergot Derivative—Containing, Systemic, 675
Hismanal, 143
Histafed C, 455
Histaject Modified, 143
Histalet, 167
Histalet Forte, 167
Histalet X, 455
Histamic, 167
Histamine H$_2$-Receptor Antagonists, Systemic, 692
Histantil, 183
Histatab Plus, 167
Histatan, 167
Histatuss Pediatric, 455
Hista-Vadrin, 167
Histine DM, 455
Histor-D, 167
Histussin HC, 455
HIVID, 1230
HMG-CoA Reductase Inhibitors, Systemic, 704
Homatropine, 45
Humibid DM, 455

Humibid DM Sprinkle, 455
Humulin 50/50, 717
Humulin 70/30, 717
Humulin L, 717
Humulin N, 717
Humulin R, 717
Humulin U Ultralente, 717
Hycodan, 455
Hycomine, 455
Hycomine Compound, 455
Hycomine Pediatric, 455
Hycotuss Expectorant, 455
Hydralazine, Systemic, 711
Hydramine, 143
Hydramine Cough, 143
Hydramyn, 143
Hydrate, 143
Hydril, 143
Hydrochlorothiazide, 562
Hydrocodone, 820
Hydrocodone & Acetaminophen, 833
Hydrocodone & Aspirin, 844
Hydrocodone, Aspirin, & Caffeine, 844
Hydrocortisone, 435
Hydroflumethiazide, 562
Hydromet, 455
Hydromine, 455
Hydromine Pediatric, 456
Hydromorphone, 820
Hydropane, 456
Hydrophen, 456

Hydroxyprogesterone, 1085
Hydroxyzine, 145
Hy/Gestrone, 1085
Hylutin, 1085
Hyoscyamine, 45
Hyrexin-50, 143
Hytrin, 1180
Hyzine-50, 143

Ibifon 600 Caplets, 906
Ibren, 906
Ibu, 906
Ibu-4, 907
Ibu-6, 907
Ibu-8, 907
Ibu-200, 906
Ibuprin, 907
Ibuprofen, 908
Ibuprohm, 907
Ibuprohm Caplets, 907
Ibu-Tab, 907
Imipramine, 91
Imitrex, 1167
Impril, 91
Improved Sino-Tuss, 456
Indocin, 907
Indocin SR, 907
Indomethacin, 908
Insomnal, 144
Insulin, 717
Insulin, Systemic, 717
Insulin Human, 717
Insulin Zinc, 718
Insulin Zinc, Human, 718
Intal, 495
Iophen-C Liquid, 456
Iophen DM, 456

Ipratropium, Inhalation, 734
Ipsatol Cough Formula for Children, 456
Ismelin, 658
Isoclor, 167
Isoclor Timesules, 167
Isoetharine, 245
Isophane Insulin, 718
Isophane Insulin, Human, 718
Isophane Insulin, Human & Insulin Human, 718
Isophane Insulin & Insulin, 718
Isopropamide, 45
Isoproterenol, 245, 265
Isosorbide Dinitrate, 881
Isradipine, 319
Isuprel, 245, 265
Isuprel Glossets, 265
Isuprel Mistometer, 245
Itraconazole, 132

Jenest, 612

K-Dur, 1043
Kestrone-5, 594
Ketazolam, 203
Ketoconazole, 132
Ketoprofen, 908
Ketorolac, Systemic, 745
Kiddy Koff, 456
KIE, 456
Klerist-D, 167
Klonopin, 202

Klor-Con 10, 1043
Kolephrin/DM Caplets, 456
Kolephrin GG/DM, 456
Kolephrin NN Liquid, 456
Kophane, 456
Kophane Cough & Cold Formula, 456
Kronofed-A Jr. Kronocaps, 167
Kronofed-A Kronocaps, 167
Kwelcof Liquid, 456
Kytril, 655

Labetalol, 226
Lanatuss Expectorant, 456
Lanoxin, 525
Lasix, 539
Lente Iletin I, 717
Lente Iletin II, 717
Lente Insulin, 717
Lente L, 717
Leponex, 394
Lesterol, 1073
Levate, 91
Levlen, 612
Levodopa, 753
Levodopa, Systemic, 753
Levonorgestrel & Ethinyl Estradiol, 613
Levorphanol, 820
Levothyroxine, 1202
Liothyronine, 1202
Liotrix, 1202
Lisinopril, 32
Lithane, 762
Lithium, Systemic, 762

Lithizine, 762
Lithobid, 762
Lithonate, 762
Lithotabs, 762
Lodine, 907
Lodrane LD, 167
Loestrin 1/20, 612
Loestrin 1.5/30, 612
Lomefloxacin, 635
Lo/Ovral, 612
Lopressor, 225
Lopurin, 10
Loratadine, 145
Loratadine & Pseudoephedrine, 170
Lorazepam, 203
Lorcet Plus, 832
Lorelco, 1073
Losec, 947
Lotensin, 32
Lovastatin, 704
Loxapac, 770
Loxapine, Systemic, 770
Loxitane, 770
Loxitane C, 770
Loxitane IM, 770
Ludiomil, 779
Lurselle, 1073

Macrobid, 900
Macrodantin, 900
Mapap Cold Formula, 456
Maprotiline, Systemic, 779
Marcof Expectorant, 456
Marmine, 143
Marplan, 79

Maxair, 245
Maxeran, 799
Meclofenamate, 908
Meclomen, 907
Meda Syrup Forte, 456
Medi-Flu, 456
Medi-Flu Caplets, 456
Medihaler-Epi, 245
Medihaler-Iso, 245
Medipren, 907
Medipren Caplets, 907
*Mediquell Decongestant
    Formula,* 456
Medroxyprogesterone,
    1085
Mefenamic Acid, 908
Megace, 1085
Megestrol, 1085
Menaval-20, 594
Menest, 594
Mepenzolate, 45
Meperidine, 820
Meperidine & Acetamino-
    phen, 833
Mephenytoin, 66
Mesalamine, Oral, 786
Mesasal, 786
Mesoridazine, 1006
Metaprel, 245, 265
Metaproterenol, 245, 265
Metaxalone, 1124
Methadone, 820
Methantheline, 45
Methdilazine, 183
Methicillin, 970
Methocarbamol, 1124
Methotrimeprazine, 1006
Methscopolamine, 45

Methyclothiazide, 562
Methyldopa, Systemic,
    792
Methylprednisolone, 435
Metoclopramide,
    Systemic, 799
Metolazone, 562
Metoprolol, 226
Metric 21, 806
Metro I.V., 806
Metronidazole, Systemic,
    806
Mevacor, 704
Mezlocillin, 970
Miconazole, 132
Mirco-K 10, 1043
Micronase, 108
microNefrin, 245
Micronor, 1085
Midahist DH, 456
Midol IB, 907
Migergot, 675
Minipress, 1059
Minocin, 1187
Minocycline, 1187
Misoprostol, Systemic,
    815
Mobenol, 108
ModiCon, 612
Monistat i.v., 132
Monodox, 1187
Morphine, 820
Motrin, 907
Motrin, Children's, 907
Motrin-IB, 907
Motrin-IB Caplets, 907
Multipax, 144
Mycotussin, 456

Myhistine DH, 456
Myhistine Expectorant, 456
Myhydromine, 456
Myhydromine Pediatric, 456
Myidil, 144
Myminic Expectorant, 456
Myminicol, 456
Myphetane DC Cough, 456
Myphetane DX Cough, 456
Myphetapp, 167
Mytussin AC, 456
Mytussin DAC, 456
Mytussin DM, 456

Nabumetone, 908
Nadolol, 226
Nafcillin, 970
Nalbuphine, 820
Naldecon, 167
Naldecon-CX Adult Liquid, 456
Naldecon-DX Adult Liquid, 456
Naldecon-DX Children's Syrup, 456
Naldecon-DX Pediatric Drops, 456
Naldecon-EX, 456
Naldecon-EX Pediatric Drops, 456
Naldecon Pediatric Drops, 167
Naldecon Pediatric Syrup, 167

Naldecon Senior DX, 456
Naldelate, 167
Naldelate DX Adult, 456
Naldelate Pediatric Syrup, 167
Nalfon, 907
Nalfon 200, 907
Nalgest, 167
Nalgest Pediatric, 167
Napril, 167
Naprosyn, 907
Naproxen, 908
Narcotic Analgesics & Acetaminophen, Systemic, 832
Narcotic Analgesics & Aspirin, Systemic, 844
Narcotic Analgesics—For Pain Relief, Systemic, 819
Nardil, 79
Nasacort, 425
Nasahist, 167
Nasahist B, 144
Nasatab LA, 456
Nauseatol, 144
ND Clear T.D., 167
ND-Stat Revised, 144
Nedocromil, Inhalation, 858
N.E.E. 1/35, 612
N.E.E. 1/50, 612
Nelova 0.5/35E, 612
Nelova 1/35E, 612
Nelova 1/50M, 612
Nelova 10/11, 612
Nelulen 1/35E, 612
Nelulen 1/50E, 612

Nephron, 245
Nervine Nighttime Sleep-Aid, 144
Neurontin, 649
New-Decongest Pediatric Syrup, 167
New-Decongestant Pediatric, 167
Nicardipine, 319
Nicoderm, 866
Nicorette, 866
Nicorette DS, 866
Nicotine, Systemic, 866
Nicotrol, 866
Nico-Vert, 144
Nidryl, 144
Nifedipine, 319
Nimodipine, 319
Nisaval, 144
Nitrates—Lingual Aerosol, Systemic, 875
Nitrates—Sublingual, Chewable or Buccal, Systemic, 881
Nitrates—Topical, Systemic, 892
Nitrazepam, 203
Nitro-Dur, 892
Nitrofuracot, 900
Nitrofurantoin, Systemic, 900
Nitroglycerin, 881
Nitroglycerin Ointment, 893
Nitroglycerin Transdermal Patches, 893
Nitrolingual, 875
Nitrostat, 881

Nizatidine, 693
Nizoral, 132
Nolahist, 144
Nolamine, 167
Nolex LA, 456
Nonsteroidal Anti-Inflammatory Drugs, Systemic, 906
Noradryl, 144
Noraminic, 167
Noratuss II Liquid, 456
Nordette, 612
Nordryl Cough, 144
Norethin 1/35E, 612
Norethin 1/50M, 612
Norethindrone, 1085
Norethindrone Acetate & Ethinyl Estradiol, 613
Norethindrone & Ethinyl Estradiol, 613
Norethindrone & Mestranol, 613
Norfloxacin, 635
Norfranil, 90
Norgesic, 952
Norgesic Forte, 952
Norgestimate & Ethinyl Estradiol, 613
Norgestrel, 1085
Norgestrel & Ethinyl Estradiol, 613
Norinyl 1+35, 612
Norinyl 1+50, 612
Norlutate, 1085
Norlutin, 1085
Normatane, 167
Normatane DC, 456
Norpace, 532

Norpace CR, 532
Norphadrine, 952
Norphadrine Forte, 952
Norpramin, 90
Nor-QD, 1085
Nortriptyline, 91
Nortussin with Codeine, 456
Norvasc, 26
Novafed A, 167
Novagest Expectorant with Codeine, 456
Novahistine, 167
Novahistine DH Liquid, 456
Novahistine DMX Liquid, 456
Novahistine Expectorant, 456
Nova-Terfendadine, 144
Novo-AZT, 1236
Novo-Butamide, 108
Novocarbamaz, 333
Novo-Dimenate, 144
Novo-Doxepin, 91
Novo-Glyburide, 108
Novo-Hydroxyzin, 144
Novo-Hylazin, 711
Novolin 70/30, 717
Novolin L, 717
Novolin N, 717
Novolin R, 717
Novomedopa, 792
Novonidazol, 806
Novo-Peridol, 665
Novo-Pheniram, 144
Novopramine, 91
Novo-Propamide, 108

Novoquinidin, 1097
Novotrimel, 1137
Novotrimel DS, 1137
Novo-Tripramine, 91
Novotriptyn, 91
NPH Iletin I, 717
NPH Iletin II, 717
NPH Insulin, 717
NPH-N, 717
N3 Gesic, 953
N3 Gesic Forte, 953
Nucochem, 456
Nucochem Pediatric Expectorant, 456
Nucofed, 456
Nucofed Expectorant, 456
Nucofed Pediatric Expectorant, 456
Nucohem Expectorant, 456
Nu-Cotrimox, 1137
Nu-Cotrimox DS, 1137
Nucotuss Expectorant, 456
Nucotuss Pediatric Expectorant, 456
Nuprin, 907
Nuprin Caplets, 907
Nytcold Medicine, 456
Nytime Cold Medicine Liquid, 456
Nytol with DPH, 144
Nytol Maximum Strength, 144

Octamide, 799
Octamide PFS, 799
Ofloxacin, 635

Ogen .625, 594
Ogen 1.25, 594
Ogen 2.5, 594
Olsalazine, Oral, 943
Omeprazole, Systemic, 947
Omnicol, 456
Opium Injection, 820
Optimine, 144
Oraminic Spancaps, 167
Oraminic II, 144
Ordrine AT, 456
Orinase, 108
Ornade Spansules, 167
Ornex Severe Cold No Drowsiness Caplets, 456
Orphenadrine & Aspirin, Systemic, 952
Orphenagesic, 953
Orphenagesic Forte, 953
Ortho-Cept, 612
Ortho-Cyclen, 612
Ortho-Est, 594
Ortho-Novum 1/35, 612
Ortho-Novum 1/50, 612
Ortho-Novum 10/11, 612
Ortho-Novum 7/7/7, 612
Ortho Tri-Cyclen, 612
Orthoxicol Cough, 456
Orudis, 907
Oruvail, 907
Ovcon-35, 612
Ovcon-50, 612
Ovral, 612
Ovrette, 1085
Oxacillin, 971
Oxaprozin, 908

Oxazepam, 203
Oxprenolol, 226
Oxtriphylline, 285
Oxycodone, 820
Oxycodone & Acetaminophen, 833
Oxycodone & Aspirin, 845
Oxymorphone, 820
Oxyphencyclimine, 45
Oxytetracycline, 1187

Pamelor, 90
Pamprin-IB, 907
Panectyl, 183
Panesclerina, 1073
Panmycin, 1187
Para-Hist HD, 456
Par-Drix, 167
Parhist SR, 167
Parnate, 79
Paroxetine, Systemic, 963
Partapp, 167
Partapp TD, 167
Partuss LA, 456
Paxil, 963
PBZ, 144
PBZ-SR, 144
PediaCare Allergy Formula, 144
PediaCare Children's Cough-Cold, 456
PediaCare Cold Formula, 167
PediaCare Cough-Cold, 456

PediaCare Night Rest Cough-Cold Liquid, 456
Pediacof Cough, 456
Pedituss Cough, 456
Pelamine, 144
Penbutolol, 226
Penicillin G, 971
Penicillin V, 971
Penicillins, Systemic, 969
Penicillins & Beta-Lactamase Inhibitors, Systemic, 992
Pentasa, 786
Pentazine, 183
Pentazine VC with Codeine, 456
Pentazocine, 821
Pentazocine & Acetaminophen, 833
Pentazocine & Aspirin, 845
Pentoxifylline, Systemic, 1001
Pepcid, 692
Pepcid I.V., 692
Percocet, 832
Periactin, 144
Pericyazine, 1006
Peridol, 665
Perphenazine, 1006
Pertofrane, 91
Pertussin All Night CS, 456
Pertussin All Night PM, 456
Pfeiffer's Allergy, 144
Phanadex, 456

Phanatuss, 457
Phenameth DM, 457
Phenameth VC with Codeine, 457
Phenazine 25, 183
Phenazine 50, 183
Phencen-50, 183
Phendry, 144
Phendry Children's Allergy Medicine, 144
Phenelzine, 79
Phenergan, 183
Phenergan with Codeine, 457
Phenergan with Dextromethorphan, 457
Phenergan Fortis, 183
Phenergan Plain, 183
Phenergan VC, 167
Phenergan VC with Codeine, 457
Phenerzine, 183
Phenetron, 144
Phenetron Lanacaps, 144
Phenhist DH with Codeine, 457
Phenhist Expectorant, 457
Phenindamine, 145
Pheniramine & Phenylephrine, 170
Pheniramine, Phenyltoloxamine, Pyrilamine, & Phenylpropanolamine, 170
Pheniramine, Pyrilamine, & Phenylpropanolamine, 170
Phenoject-50, 183

Phenothiazines, Systemic, 1005
Phenylbutazone, 908
Phenylfenesin L.A., 457
Phenytoin, 66
Pherazine with Codeine, 457
Pherazine DM, 457
Pherazine VC, 168
Pherazine VC with Co-deine, 457
Pilocarpine, Systemic, 1037
Pindolol, 226
Piperacillin, 971
Piperacillin & Tazobac-tam, 992
Pipotiazine, 1007
Pirbuterol, 245
Pirenzepine, 45
Piroxicam, 908
Pivampicillin, 971
Pivmecillinam, 971
PMS-Dimenhydrinate, 144
PMS Haloperidol, 665
PMS Sulfasalazine, 1147
PMS Sulfasalazine E.C., 1147
Pneumotussin HC, 457
Poladex T.D., 144
Polaramine, 144
Polaramine Expectorant, 457
Polaramine Repetabs, 144
Poly-Histine-CS, 457
Poly-Histine-D, 168
Poly-Histine-D Ped, 168
Poly-Histine-DM, 457

Polythiazide, 562
Ponstel, 907
Potassium Acetate, 1044
Potassium Bicarbonate, 1044
Potassium Bicarbonate & Potassium Chloride, 1044
Potassium Bicarbonate & Potassium Citrate, 1044
Potassium Chloride, 1044
Potassium Chloride, Pot-assium Bicarbonate, & Potassium Citrate, 1044
Potassium Gluconate, 1044
Potassium Gluconate & Potassium Chloride, 1044
Potassium Gluconate & Potassium Citrate, 1044
Potassium Supplements, Systemic, 1043
Pravachol, 704
Pravastatin, 704
Prazepam, 203
Prazosin, Systemic, 1059
Prednisolone, 435
Prednisone, 435
Prehist, 168
Premarin, 594
Premarin Intravenous, 594
Prilosec, 947
Primatene Mist, 245

Primatene Mist Suspension, 245
Primatuss Cough Mixture 4, 457
Primatuss Cough Mixture 4D, 457
Prinivil, 32
Pro-50, 183
Probalan, 1066
Probenecid, Systemic, 1066
Probucol, Systemic, 1073
Procainamide, Systemic, 1078
Procan SR, 1078
Procardia XL, 318
Procaterol, 245
Prochlorperazine, 1007
Procyclidine, 122
Pro-Depo, 1085
Prodrox, 1085
Progesterone, 1085
Progestins, Systemic, 1084
Promacot, 183
Promazine, 1007
Pro-Med 50, 183
Promet, 183
Prometa, 265
Prometh with Dextromethorphan, 457
Prometh VC with Codeine, 457
Prometh VC Plain, 168 183
Promethazine DM, 457
Promethazine & Phenylephrine, 170

Promethazine VC, 168
Promethazine VC with Codeine, 457
Promethist with Codeine, 457
Promine, 1078
Prominic Expectorant, 457
Prominicol Cough, 457
Promist HD Liquid, 457
Prompt Insulin Zinc, 718
Pronestyl, 1078
Pronestyl-SR, 1078
Propacet 100, 832
Propantheline, 45
Propoxyphene, 821
Propoxyphene & Acetaminophen, 833
Propoxyphene & Aspirin, 845
Propoxyphene, Aspirin, & Caffeine, 845
Propranolol, 226
Propulsid, 368
Prorex-25, 183
Prorex-50, 183
Proscar, 630
Pro-Span, 1085
ProStep, 866
Protamine Zinc Insulin, 718
Prothazine, 183
Prothazine Plain, 183
Protostat, 806
Protriptyline, 91
Proventil, 245, 265
Proventil Repetabs, 265
Provera, 1085

Prozac, 643
Pseudo-Car DM, 457
Pseudo-Chlor, 168
Pseudodine C Cough, 457
Pseudo-gest Plus, 168
Purinol, 10
P-V-Tussin, 457
Pyribenzamine, 144
Pyrilamine, 145

Quadra-Hist, 168
Quadra-Hist Pediatric, 168
Quazepam, 203
Quelidrine Cough, 457
Questran, 362
Questran Light, 362
Quiess, 144
Quinaglute Dura-tabs, 1097
Quinalan, 1097
Quinapril, 32
Quinate, 1097
Quinestrol, 595
Quinethazone, 562
Quinidex Extentabs, 1097
Quinidine, Systemic, 1097
Quinora, 1097

Racepinephrine, 245
Ramipril, 32
Ranitidine, 693
Reactine, 144
Reclomide, 799
Reglan, 799
Regular Iletin I, 717
Regular Iletin II, 717

Regular (Concentrated) Iletin II, U-500, 717
Regular Insulin, 717
Relafen, 907
Remcol-C, 457
Rentamine Pediatric, 457
Resaid S.R., 168
Rescaps-D S.R., 457
Rescon, 168
Rescon-DM, 457
Rescon-ED, 168
Rescon-GG, 457
Rescon Jr., 168
Respaire-60 SR, 457
Respaire-120 SR, 457
Retrovir, 1236
Rhinatate, 168
Rhinolar-EX, 168
Rhinolar-EX 12, 168
Rhinosyn, 168
Rhinosyn-DM, 457
Rhinosyn-DMX Expectorant, 457
Rhinosyn-PD, 168
Rhinosyn-X, 457
Rhotrimine, 91
Rimantadine, Systemic, 1104
Rinade B.I.D., 168
Robafen AC Cough, 457
Robafen CF, 457
Robafen DAC, 457
Robafen DM, 457
Robitet, 1187
Robitussin A-C, 457
Robitussin-CF, 457
Robitussin Cold & Cough Liqui-Gels, 457

Robitussin-DAC, 457

Robitussin-DM, 457

Robitussin Maximum Strength Cough & Cold, 457

Robitussin Night Relief, 457

Robitussin Night Relief Colds Formula Liquid, 457

Robitussin-PE, 457

Robitussin Pediatric Cough & Cold, 457

Robitussin Severe Congestion Liqui-Gels, 457

Rolatuss Expectorant, 457

Rolatuss with Hydrocodone, 457

Rolatuss Plain, 168

Rondamine-DM Drops, 457

Rondec, 168

Rondec-DM, 457

Rondec-DM Drops, 457

Rondec Drops, 168

Rondec-TR, 168

Roubac, 1137

Roxicet, 832

R-Tannamine, 168

R-Tannamine Pediatric, 168

R-Tannate, 168

R-Tannate Pediatric, 168

Rufen, 907

Ru-Tuss, 168

Ru-Tuss DE, 457

Ru-Tuss Expectorant, 457

Ru-Tuss with Hydrocodone Liquid, 457

Ru-Tuss II, 168

Rymed, 457

Rymed Liquid, 457

Rymed-TR Caplets, 457

Ryna, 168

Ryna-C Liquid, 457

Ryna-CX Liquid, 457

Rynatan, 168

Rynatan Pediatric, 168

Rynatan-S Pediatric, 168

Rynatuss, 457

Rynatuss Pediatric, 457

Rythmodan, 532

Rythmodan-LA, 532

Safe Tussin, 457

Salagen, 1037

Salazopyrin, 1147

Salazopyrin EN-Tabs, 1147

Saleto-CF, 457

Salmeterol, Inhalation, 1108

Salofalk, 786

S.A.S. Enteric-500, 1147

S.A.S.-500, 1147

Scopolamine, 45

Scot-Tussin DM, 457

Seldane, 144

Seldane Caplets, 144

Seldane-D, 168

Semprex-D, 168

Septra, 1137

Septra DS, 1137

Serevent, 1108

Sertraline, Systemic, 1119

Shogan, 183
Siladryl, 144
Silexin Cough, 457
Silphen Cough Syrup, 144
Simvastatin, 704
Sinequan, 90
Sinucon Pediatric Drops, 168
Sinufed Timecelles, 457
Sinupan, 457
SINUvent, 457
Skeletal Muscle Relaxants, Systemic, 1124
Sleep-Eze 3, 144
Slo-bid, 284
Snaplets-D, 168
Snaplets-DM, 457
Snaplets-EX, 457
Snaplets-Multi, 457
Sominex Formula 2, 144
Sotalol, 226
Spironolactone, 550
Sporanox, 132
SRC Expectorant, 457
S-T Forte, 458
S-T Forte 2, 458
Stamoist E, 457
Stamoist LA, 458
Statuss Green, 458
Stavudine, Systemic, 1131
Stilphostrol, 594
S-2, 245
Sudafed Cold & Cough Liquid Caps, 458
Sudafed Cough, 458
Sudafed Plus, 168
Sudafed Severe Cold Formula Caplets, 458

Sulfacytine, 1157
Sulfadiazine, 1157
Sulfamethizole, 1157
Sulfamethoprim, 1137
Sulfamethoprim DS, 1137
Sulfamethoxazole, 1157
Sulfamethoxazole & Trimethoprim, Systemic, 1137
Sulfaprim, 1137
Sulfaprim DS, 1137
Sulfasalazine, Systemic, 1147
Sulfatrim, 1137
Sulfatrim DS, 1137
Sulfisoxazole, 1157
Sulfonamides, Systemic, 1157
Sulfoxaprim, 1137
Sulfoxaprim DS, 1137
Sulindac, 908
Sumatriptan, Systemic, 1167
Sumycin, 1187
Superlipid, 1073
Suprax, 345
Surmontil, 91
Sus-Phrine, 265
Symadine, 17
Symmetrel, 17
Synthroid, 1202
Syracol Liquid, 458

Tacaryl, 183
TACE, 594
Tacrine, Systemic, 1174
Tagamet, 692
Tamine S.R., 168

Tanoral, 168
Tavist, 144
Tavist-D, 168
Tavist-1, 144
T-Dry, 168
T-Dry Junior, 168
Tega-Vert, 144
Tegretol, 333
Tegretol Chewtabs, 333
Tegretol CR, 333
Telachlor, 144
Teldrin, 144
Temaril, 183
Temazepam, 203
Temazin Cold, 168
Tenormin, 225
Tenoxicam, 908
Terazosin, Systemic, 1180
Terbutaline, 245, 265
Terfenadine, 145
Terfenadine & Pseudoe-
    phedrine, 170
Terramycin, 1187
Tetracycline, 1187
Tetracyclines, Systemic,
    1187
Tetracyn, 1187
Theo-Dur, 284
Theophylline, 285
*TheraFlu/Flu, Cold &
    Cough Medicine,* 458
*TheraFlu Maximum
    Strength Non-Drowsy
    Formula Flu, Cold &
    Cough Medicine,* 458
*TheraFlu Nighttime Maxi-
    mum Strength,* 458
Thiopropazate, 1007

Thioproperazine, 1007
Thioridazine, 1007
Threamine DM, 458
Threamine Expectorant,
    458
Thyroglobulin, 1202
Thyroid, 1202
Thyroid Hormones, Sys-
    temic, 1202
Tiaprofenic Acid, 908
Ticarcillin, 971
Ticarcillin & Clavulanate,
    992
Ticlid, 1210
Ticlopidine, Systemic,
    1210
Tija, 1187
Tilade, 858
Timolol, 226
Tipramine, 91
T-Koff, 458
Tofranil, 91
Tofranil-PM, 91
Tolamide, 108
Tolazamide, 109
Tolbutamide, 109
Tolectin 200, 907
Tolectin 400, 907
Tolectin 600, 907
Tolinase, 108
Tolmetin, 908
Tol-Tab, 108
Tolu-Sed Cough, 458
Tolu-Sed DM, 458
Toradol, 745
Toradol IM, 745
Toradol Oral, 745
Tornalate, 245

Torsemide, Systemic, 1216

Touro A & H, 168

Touro LA Caplets, 458

Traminic Cold, 168

Tranylcypromine, 79

Travamine, 144

Traveltabs, 144

Trazodone, Systemic, 1224

Trazon, 1224

Trendar, 907

Trental, 1001

Triacin C Cough, 458

Triadapin, 91

Triafed, 168

Triafed with Codeine, 458

Trialodine, 1224

Triamcinolone, 407, 425, 435

Triaminic Allergy, 168

Triaminic Chewables, 168

Triaminic-DM Cough Formula, 458

Triaminic Expectorant, 458

Triaminic Expectorant with Codeine, 458

Triaminic Expectorant DH, 458

Triaminic Nite Light, 458

Triaminic Oral Infant Drops, 168

Triaminic Sore Throat Formula, 458

Triaminic TR, 168

Triaminic-12, 168

Triaminicol Multi-Symptom Relief, 458

Triaminicol Multi-Symptom Relief Colds with Coughs, 458

Triamterene, 550

Triazolam, 203

Triazole, 1137

Triazole DS, 1137

Trichlormethiazide, 562

Tricodene Cough & Cold, 458

Tricodene Forte, 458

Tricodene NN, 458

Tricodene Pediatric, 458

Tricodene Sugar Free, 458

Tridihexethyl, 45

Trifed, 168

Trifed-C Cough, 458

Trifluoperazine, 1007

Triflupromazine, 1007

Trihexyphenidyl, 122

Trikacide, 806

Trikates, 1044

Tri-Levlen, 612

Trimeprazine, 183

Trimeth-Sulfa, 1137

Triminol Cough, 458

Trimipramine, 91

Trimox, 970

Trinalin Repetabs, 168

Trind, 168

Tri-Nefrin Extra Strength, 168

Trinex, 458

Tri-Norinyl, 612

Triofed, 168

Triotann, 168
Triotann Pediatric, 168
Tripalgen Cold, 168
Tripelennamine, 145
Triphasil, 612
Tri-Phen-Chlor, 168
Tri-Phen-Chlor Pediatric, 168
Tri-Phen-Chlor T.R., 168
Triphenyl, 168
Triphenyl Expectorant, 458
Triphenyl T.D., 168
Triposed, 168
Triprolidine, 145
Triprolidine & Pseudoephedrine, 170
Triptil, 91
Triptone Caplets, 144
Trisulfam, 1137
Tritann, 168
Tritann Pediatric, 168
Tri-Tannate, 168
Tri-Tannate Pediatric, 168
Tri-Tannate Plus Pediatric, 458
Trymegen, 144
Tusquelin, 458
Tuss-Ade, 458
Tussafed, 458
Tussafed Drops, 458
Tussafin Expectorant, 458
Tuss Allergine Modified T.D., 458
Tussanil DH, 458
Tussanil Plain, 168
Tussar DM, 458

Tussar SF, 458
Tussar-2, 458
Tuss-DM, 458
Tussex Cough, 458
Tussgen, 458
Tuss-Genade Modified, 458
Tussigon, 458
Tussionex, 458
Tussi-Organidin DM Liquid, 458
Tussi-Organidin Liquid, 458
Tussirex with Codeine Liquid, 458
Tuss-LA, 458
Tusso-DM, 458
Tussogest, 458
Tusstat, 144
12-Hour Cold, 167
Twilite Caplets, 144
2/G-DM Cough, 455
Ty-Cold Cold Formula, 458
Tylenol with Codeine, 832
Tylenol with Codeine No.1, 832
Tylenol with Codeine No.2, 832
Tylenol with Codeine No.3, 832
Tylenol with Codeine No.4, 832
Tylenol Cold & Flu, 458
Tylenol Cold & Flu No Drowsiness Powder, 458

Tylenol Cold Medication, 458

Tylenol Cold Medication Non-Drowsy, 458

Tylenol Cold Night Time, 458

Tylenol Cough with Decongestant Maximum Strength, 458

Tylenol Maximum Strength Cough, 458

Tylenol Maximum Strength Flu Gelcaps, 458

Tyrodone, 458

ULR-LA, 458

ULTRAbrom PD, 168

Ultralente U, 717

Uni-Bent Cough, 144

Uni-Decon, 168

Unisom Nighttime Sleep Aid, 144

Unisom SleepGels Maximum Strength, 144

Uni-tussin DM, 458

Unproco, 458

Uroplus DS, 1137

Uroplus SS, 1137

Utex-S.R., 458

Valergen-10, 594

Valergen-20, 594

Valergen-40, 594

Valium, 202

Vancenase AQ, 425

Vanceril, 406

Vanex Expectorant, 459

Vanex Forte Caplets, 168

Vanex-HD, 459

Vanex-LA, 459

Vaponefrin, 245

Vasotec, 32

V-Dec-M, 459

Veetids, 970

Velosulin Human, 717

Veltane, 144

Veltap, 168

Ventolin, 245, 265

Ventolin Nebules, 245

Ventolin Rotacaps, 245

Verapamil, 319

Verelan, 318

Versacaps, 459

Vertab, 144

V-Gan-25, 183

V-Gan-50, 183

Vibramycin, 1187

Vibra-Tabs, 1187

Vicks Children's NyQuil Allergy/Head Cold, 168

Vicks DayQuil 4 Hour Allergy Relief, 168

Vicks DayQuil 12 Hour Allergy Relief, 168

Vicks 44 Cough & Cold Relief LiquiCaps, 459

Vicks 44D Dry Hacking Cough & Head Congestion, 459

Vicks 44M Cough, Cold & Flu Relief, 459

Vicks 44M Cough, Cold & Flu Relief LiquiCaps, 459

Vicks NyQuil Multi-Symptom Cold/Flu Relief, 459

Vicks NyQuil Multi-Symptom LiquiCaps, 459

Vicks Pediatric Formula 44D Cough & Decongestant, 459

Vicks Pediatric Formula 44E, 459

Vicks Pediatric Formula 44M Multi-Symptom Cough & Cold, 459

Vicodin Tuss, 459

Videx, 516

Viro-Med, 459

Vistaject-25, 144

Vistaject-50, 144

Vistaril, 144

Vistazine 50, 144

Vivactil, 91

Volmax, 265

Voltaren, 907

Warfarin, 57

Wehdryl-10, 144

Wehdryl-50, 144

Wehgen, 594

Wellbutrin, 294

Wigraine, 675

Xanax, 202

Zalcitabine, Systemic, 1230

Zantac, 692

Zephrex, 459

Zephrex-LA, 459

Zerit, 1131

Zestril, 32

Zidovudine, Systemic, 1236

Zithromax, 197

Zocor, 704

Zoloft, 1119

Zolpidem, Systemic, 1244

Zovirax, 3

Zyloprim, 10